TREATMENT OF BIPOLAR ILLNESS

A Casebook for Clinicians and Patients

TREATMENT OF BIPOLAR ILLNESS

A Casebook for Clinicians and Patients

Robert M. Post, M.D.

Gabriele S. Leverich, LCSW, BCD

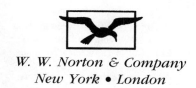

W. W. Norton & Company
New York • London

For information about permission to reproduce selections from this book, write to Permissions,
W. W. Norton & Company, Inc., 500 Fifth Avenue, New York, NY 10110

For information about special discounts for bulk purchases, please contact W. W. Norton Special Sales
at specialsales@wwnorton.com or 800-233-4830.

Manufacturing by Courier Westford
Book design by Bytheway Publishing Services
Production Manager: Leeann Graham

Library of Congress Cataloging-in-Publication Data
Post, Robert M.
Treatment of bipolar illness : a casebook for clinicians and patients / Robert M. Post and
Gabriele S. Leverich. — 1st ed.
    p. ; cm.
    "A Norton professional book."
    Includes bibliographical references and index.
ISBN-13: 978-0-393-70537-9 (hardcover)   1. Manic-depressive illness—Chemotherapy.
2. Psychotropic drugs.   I. Leverich, Gabriele S.   II. Title.
[DNLM: 1. Bipolar Disorder—drug therapy—Case Reports. 2. Psychotropic Drugs—
therapeutic use—Case Reports. WM 207 P857t 2008]

RC516.T73 2008
616.89′5061—dc22   2007016332

ISBN 13: 978-0-393-70537-9

W. W. Norton & Company, Inc., 500 Fifth Avenue, New York, N.Y. 10110
www.wwnorton.com
W. W. Norton & Company Ltd., Castle House, 75/76 Wells St., London W1T 3QT

1 2 3 4 5 6 7 8 9 0

To my wife Susan, daughter Laura, and son David who have been a continuing source of joy and inspiration for me.
—RMP

To my son Peter and my daughter Alexandra, who never cease to bring love, curiosity, and inspiration into my life, and to Yolande whose own work and dedication made everything meaningful and imperative.
—GSL

Contents

PART III. PHARMACOLOGY AND NEUROBIOLOGY OF BIPOLAR ILLNESS

PART IV. RESPONSE TO MOOD STABILIZERS

LITHIUM

CARBAMAZEPINE

VALPROIC ACID

Acknowledgments

The idea for this book largely grew out of our experience with patients who had difficult to treat (refractory) bipolar illness who volunteered to come to an inpatient Clinical Research Unit of the Biological Psychiatry Branch of the National Institute of Mental Health (NIMH) at the National Institutes of Health Clinical Center in Bethesda, Maryland, for study and treatment. By virtue of their prior failure to respond to multiple psychopharmacological interventions in the community, these treatment-refractory patients were referred to us for study and exposure to novel and nontraditional treatment approaches. After patients finished participation in formal double-blind protocols approved by the NIMH Institutional Review Board, they were offered a period of treatment optimization so that they could be discharged in the most stabilized phase of illness possible. This period of treatment optimization allowed us to make use of the patients' detailed past history of any response (illustrated in the retrospective life chart), clinical and biological information gleaned from their inpatient stay and response to protocols, and the collective wisdom of a staff of extraordinary clinical investigators (noted below).

We have thus seen a large group of patients with difficult to manage forms of bipolar illness. In particular, we have a wealth of experience with this subgroup of patients who were not responsive to the traditional treatment of lithium carbonate, as well as many of the other now widely used modalities. While some may argue that this patient population is thus atypical and nonrepresentative, a very large literature and clinical experience now indicate that the phenomenon of lithium resistance in particular and illness resistance in general is also very widespread in the bipolar population at large. These views were reinforced by our observations of less than ideal responses to traditional psychopharmacological regimens in a large series of outpatients studied by our collaborative group.

Thus, of the 1–3% of the population in most countries with a diagnosis of bipolar disorder, there is a very substantial group who have major difficulties with the management of their illness. It is to that group of patients, as well as their families, that this book is dedicated, with the hope that this series of case examples and case studies will help patients and physicians arrive more rapidly at the best treatment outcomes that can be achieved for a given patient.

In this regard, we are greatly indebted to the inpatients and outpatients who not only volunteered for participation in the clinical research studies and donated their time and their bodies (in the form of blood tests, spinal fluid, positron emission tomography studies of brain activity, and the like) but also allowed us to use their life charts as illustrations in each chapter in the hope that doing so would provide important information and assistance to others with similar problems. Each gave and signed informed consent for participation in each research protocol and for use of their data. All of their data have been included in previous NIMH publications emanating from the intramural program. In addition, we obtained another written consent more recently (about 2004 to 2006) to insure that patients were still willing to share their essentially unaltered life chart, but with all personal identifiers removed in this publication. Renewed consent was always given, and in the very few instances where this was unavailable, we moderately changed the graphic and the details of their case, so that their identity would be further obscured.

We are similarly appreciative of the patients who volunteered from 1995 to 2002 to participate so intensively in the Stanley Foundation Bipolar Network, now renamed the Bipolar Collaborative Network. The generous contributions of Theodore and Vada Stanley of the Stanley Medical Research Institute were also invaluable in allowing us the privilege to study and treat outpatients longitudinally as well as in depth. Our coinvestigators in the BCN now include: Lori Altshuler and Mark Frye at UCLA; Trisha Suppes in Dallas; Susan McElroy and Paul Keck Jr. in Cincinatti; the authors in Bethesda; Willem Nolen and Ralph Kupka in Utrecht, Netherlands; and Heinze Grunze in Munich, Germany. Each of these individuals have contributed friendship, knowledge of the illness and its treatment, and unending energy and commitment to excellence in patient care and scholarship in facilitating the work of this book.

The support of the Dalio Family Foundation in this and related publications from the BCN is also deeply appreciated. We thank the nursing staff for intensive observation, rating, and care of patients through what have been, at times, most difficult phases of illness management. In addition, a host of clinical associate physicians in the former Biological Psychiatry Branch have made a major impact on this project and, in many cases, contributed the essential ideas for the novel observations made in the case management.

In this regard, we would particularly like to recognize the contributions of a series of unit administrators who have made profound and lasting contributions to the clinical investigation, patient care, and therapeutics of patients with refractory unipolar and bipolar illness. Among other physicians, these ward chiefs include Drs. John Carman, Fred Stoddard, Robert Gerner, David Jimerson, James Ballenger, Charles Kellner, Thomas Uhde, Peter P. Roy-Byrne, Edward Silberman, Terence A. Ketter, Mark Frye, and Andrew Speer.

Each of these doctors made major sacrifices to their own career pursuits in an attempt to foster excellence of clinical care and research on the unit, and made major impacts on the outcome of patients' lives, and on the gleaning of new information about the mechanisms underlying manic-depressive illness and its therapeutics. In addition, a large number of clinical research associates have made equally important contributions to this project and to many of the case studies presented. These include Drs. Victor Reus, Alex C. Rey, Neal R. Cutler, David R. Rubinow, Frank W. Putnam, Wade S. Berretini, Russell T. Joffe, Lori L. Altshuler, Keith G. Kramlinger, Peter Hauser, Peggy Jo Pazzaglia, Ann Callahan, Lauren Marangell, Mark S. George, Kirk Denicoff, Timothy Kimbrell, Beth Osuch, and Gabriella Obrocea.

A series of research assistants have also made substantial contributions to the systematization and collection of life chart data, including Kathleen Squillace, Melissa Spearing, Amy Thiebault, Nancy Palmer, Tina Goldstein, Melissa Brotman, Karen Autio, Emily Fergus, Maria Martinez, Kendra Scouten, and Maria Martin. Chris Gavin and Harriet Brightman made invaluable editorial and manuscript production contributions.

Introduction

THE COMMON PROBLEM OF INITIAL OR ACQUIRED TREATMENT RESISTANCE IN BIPOLAR DISORDER

When attempting to distill some of the practice and principles of the psychopharmacotherapeutics of bipolar illness, the authors faced a number of daunting tasks. Clinical trials assessing the efficacy of psychopharmacological agents for the treatment of bipolar illness have lagged far behind those conducted in the unipolar depressive disorders or in the other major psychotic disorder, schizophrenia. Clinical trials comparing the efficacy and effectiveness of one agent to another have been even more sparse.

Thus, the treatment guidelines for bipolar illness have been established largely on the basis of an uncontrolled literature and expert opinion (Keck et al., 2004). In many instances, the guidelines are sufficient for initial suggestions about psychopharmacological approaches, but data are virtually absent for guiding second- and third-line options, and beyond, for those with treatment-refractory bipolar illness.

This is particularly problematic because treatment resistance in bipolar illness has been grossly underestimated. While response rates to lithium carbonate, for example, have been routinely cited at 70–80% based on results of earlier randomized controlled trials (RCTs), lithium's real-world clinical effectiveness is more in the range of 25–30%. A number of reasons account for this apparent discrepancy. RCTs, by their very nature, usually eliminate patients with the most difficult-to-treat illnesses, including those with a current suicidal risk; additional psychiatric, substance abuse, and medical comorbidities; rapid cycling and other subtypes poorly responsive to treatment; and, of course, those with psychotic presentations that often make the informed consent process unacceptably difficult. Therefore, RCTs tend to study patients with less severe and unrepresentative presentations of bipolar illness. In addition, clinical trials are often a short several weeks' duration, and success is often measured on the basis of criteria such as 50% improvement in severity of manic or depressive symptoms. With these criteria for response, patients can accurately be called responders but continue to have substantial residual symptoms.

In contrast, in clinical practice, one is striving for the achievement and maintenance of a remission wherein the illness continues to have a minimal impact on the patient's social, educational, and occupational roles and other daily activities. For a variety of reasons, including the enormous cost constraints, most of the anticonvulsants and atypical psychotics used in the treatment of bipolar illness have been first studied in acute mania and for only 3 to 4 weeks. What happens after this period of time is a mystery. Do the few patients who achieve the equivalent of clinical remission in this brief time frame maintain it? Do those with substantial partial improvement continue to follow this trajectory to remission or do they "stall out"? What adjunctive treatments are required to achieve full stabilization for the much improved or minimally improved patient? All of these critical clinical questions remain relatively unaddressed in the literature.

Even the studies that do begin to address long-term prevention typically follow the patient for relatively short periods of time (e.g., 6 months to 1 year). Data from a number of long-term follow-up clinics such as that of Maj, Pirozzi, Magliano, and Bartoli (1998) indicate that even patients with an initial excellent lithium response, that is, complete remission for at least 2 years, upon longer term follow-up may begin to show breakthrough episodes. In some patients, this can progress to a complete loss of responsiveness in a pattern suggestive of a process of tolerance development. In others, effectiveness is lost secondary to noncompliance, which may be in the range of 50% of patients in usual treatment, but much lower during carefully monitored studies. Thus, short-term perspectives may yield a highly skewed view of real longer term clinical outcomes.

Another factor leading to the underestimation of treatment resistance is the fact that what was considered lithium monotherapy often includes the use of many other agents, including adjunctive antidepressants, minor tranquilizers, and major tranquilizers for manic and psychotic breakthroughs. Therefore, when lithium is called effective, it may in reality already represent quite complex combination therapy.

However, even when such monotherapy is examined over the long term, substantially less than 50% of the patients are considered responders in most clinical series (Gitlin, Swendsen, Heller, & Hammen, 1995). In the outpatient studies of Denicoff, Smith-Jackson, Disney, et al. (1997) in our group, patients were randomized to a year of treatment with lithium or carbamazepine and crossed over to the other agent in a double-blind fashion in the second year. As in clinical practice, adjunctive treatment with antidepressants, neuroleptics, and benzodiazepines was allowed as necessary. Despite these additions, fewer than one third of the outpatients were considered responders to either a year of carbamazepine or lithium monotherapy. The responder, moreover, consisted of only a very small group with Clinical Global Impressions (CGI) scale scores of *very much improved* (i.e., an A grade, or a virtual remission) and a much larger group of those who were *much improved* (i.e., substantial and clinically relevant improvement, but some residual symptomatology remains; a grade B). Approximately 50% of the individuals responded during a third year in the clinic on a combination of lithium and carbamazepine, but even with a year of the addition of valproate (plus or minus lithium) where necessary, or another year on all three mood stabilizers in combination, some 37% of the initial group of outpatients remained without any single year of the five achieving *much* to *very much improved* ratings on the CGI (Denicoff, Smith-Jackson, Bryan, et al., 1997; Denicoff, Smith-Jackson, Disney, et al., 1997). These data are highly consistent with others in the literature, and indicate the very substantial need for clarification of further therapeutic approaches that may be more successful in helping patients achieve better mood stabilization (Gitlin et al., 1995; Goldberg, Harrow, & Leon, 1996; Post, Speer, & Leverich, 2003).

This book thus focuses on the longitudinal course of manic-depressive illness and some of the nuances of clinical decision making in its long-term treatment. This, in itself, sets it apart from most other books in the field, which tend to concentrate primarily on the therapeutic approaches to acute episodes of mania or depression based only on a controlled clinical trials literature.

ORGANIZATION OF THE BOOK

This longitudinal perspective is all the more necessary since acute periods of wellness and remission may be part of the natural course of illness rather than response to treatment, and the long-term prevention of episode recurrence is the only reliable and effective way of assessing the true impact of psychopharmacological regimens for any patient. Given the increasing recognition of the difficulties and complexities of approaching this issue of long-term remission, we decided to organize this book in a somewhat unusual format, with almost all chapters focused on an individual's course of illness and response to treatment.

Chapter Formats

1. Mood chart: Using the NIMH Life Chart Methodology (NIMH-LCM) to delineate both course of illness and response to treatment, almost every chapter shows a graphic depiction of a given patient's illness, which illustrates a particularly important theme in the approach to therapeutics.

2. Case description: Each case study is also presented in a written summary form in order to highlight the salient points embedded in the patient's illness and treatment response.

3. Background literature: For those interested in more details, a background section briefly reviews the scientific literature pertinent to a given point of therapeutics. A selected set of references are cited in this section, and can be found in the combined bibliography at the end of the series of chapters.

4. Principles of the case: The chief principles derived from each chapter are listed, possible treatment options other than the ones employed are outlined, and the strength of the evidence supporting these suggestions and conclusions is indicated.

The evidence is rated as follows:

+++ = Robustly studied and usually verified in controlled trials
++ = Substantial evidence primarily from open, uncontrolled studies in the literature
+ = Some support based on published case series
± = Highly preliminary and speculative

This rating of the range of supporting evidence may be of particular importance to the reader, since, by nature of the current state of the art, a substantial part of the clinical therapeutics of the long-term course of bipolar illness is based on clinical inference, expert consensus, and only on a very scant controlled-trials database. Accordingly, while some principles of illness course and treatment are well documented (++ and +++), many others are listed in a highly preliminary form in order to highlight controversies and the potential problems involved in the choice of one set of agents over another, and to suggest theoretically or conceptually based possibilities requiring further systematic study.

   5. Summary statement: Finally, one or two sentences give a take-home message or bottom line on the main point illustrated in the chapter for those who wish to see the most concise descriptor in order to decide whether they should further explore the specifics of the chapter.

   A life chart is chosen as the focus of each chapter for its ability to summarize and present extensive longitudinal data in a concise and clear fashion. Given the inherent variability of bipolar illness and its potential for an almost infinite series of differences in patterns of presentation and clinical response, it seemed that the life chart approach to case presentations suits the aphorism that a picture is worth a thousand words. Moreover, we have found that the life chart itself becomes a useful clinical tool and may help trigger earlier and different therapeutic interventions by uncovering illness patterns and by displaying early trends in a patient's course and response to treatment that are not otherwise easily evident from even very extensive written hospital and outpatient records. Instructions for how to complete a retrospective and prospective life chart for adults or children are given in Appendix 3.

Audience: Physicians, Clinicians, Patients, and Family Members

Since this book is intended for a dual audience—both treating physicians and clinicians, and sophisticated patients—each might maximally benefit from such focused life chart case presentations and discussions. Additionally, the life chart format appeared particularly user-friendly for this book in view of the increasing recognition of the benefit that patients derive from generating retrospective and prospective graphic depictions of their illness and its response to treatment.

   Utilizing the life chart method either on their own or in collaboration with their treating physician or therapist, patients will be able to take a more active role in discussing, evaluating, and helping choose therapeutic options. Thus, we thought that people would be able to read selected chapters that were especially pertinent to their own illness or that of their friends or family members and absorb the salient points and principles. Physicians and other treating clinicians would similarly be able to focus on and read about a given set of problems and their possible solutions as summarized. In addition, both physicians and patients would also have available an introduction to the relevant literature.

   In this fashion, each chapter can be viewed as a stand-alone treatment exploration or discovery story with the graphic illustration of a given patient and problem, a case history, pertinent literature review, a series of possible therapeutic maneuvers, and an overall moral or important message embedded in the story. We do, however, recommend that the book generally be read in sequence, since it is organized around general thematic presentations that progress in a fairly systematic fashion from simple and well-founded treatment principles to extremely complex and tenuous ones. Initially, possible adversities in the course of illness are illustrated, followed by an orienting psychopharmacological overview, chapters on traditional treatments, and then treatments of increasing atypicality.

Sequence of Contents

Thus, the first chapters (1–8) emphasize the historical, descriptive, and phenomenological aspects of the longitudinal course of bipolar illness and some of the principles and implications for treatment that they illustrate. Chapters 9 and 10 briefly overview the general psychopharmacology of bipolar illness and some of its recently emerging neurobiology, respectively. These two chapters thus pave the way for the series of chapters that emphasize potential therapeutic interventions with lithium and the related mood-stabilizing anticonvulsants valproate and carbamazepine, and now lamotrigine as well. The ongoing controversies regarding the appropriate role and sequencing of the use of the traditional unimodal antidepressants in the treatment of bipolar depression, as well as similar issues related to the addition of antipsychotics for manic episodes, are then addressed in a series of chapters on augmentation strategies. Furthermore, with new classes of drugs and somatic treatments just becoming available for the therapeutics of bipolar illness, there is an attempt to highlight many of these emerging approaches, even if their efficacy has only been suggested in a preliminary form.

While not the primary focus of this book, we conclude with several chapters relating to the psychopharmacology of childhood-onset bipolar disorders, which are increasingly being recognized, but for which there are many fewer controlled studies than for the adult-onset forms.

Paradoxically, the epilogue on getting well and staying well may be a good place to start reading this book for the patient or family member who wants to do all the right things from the start. For many, the illness can be kept in excellent check with a concerted and active approach and respectful attitude toward its grave potential for suffering and harm. For those who have already had many problems and recurrences, we hope that many chapters will be pertinent and helpful to the successful management of their illness, and that the epilogue will aid in the continuation and maintenance of their improvement.

Finally, a series of appendices may provide the interested reader with more details about a particular rating form, question, or topic. The generic (chemical) name for a drug is used throughout the book, but the marketed (brand) name is easily obtained in Appendix 1 in two alphabetized lists and in a list of drugs by their class or mechanism of action.

Implications for Future Studies

Additionally, it is hoped that the book will represent a suitable and coherent set of teaching case examples, that it will clarify themes important for long-term therapeutics and highlight many of the topics that delineate future clinical research needs for the academician and investigator interested in the study of bipolar illness. One will see that virtually every chapter deserves a series of derivative studies that, if conducted, would allow more precise answers about the relative risk-to-benefit ratio of a given therapeutic approach. However, given the current relative absence of controlled trials to address most therapeutic dilemmas (not only in the acute therapeutics of bipolar depression but also in approaches to the long-term course of illness in particular), we, as treating clinicians, are often forced to opt for potential therapeutic approaches based only on a minimum of systematic data. The small scope of systematic clinical trials literature that is available to inform clinicians and patients at most of the critical choice points in bipolar illness, that is, the surfeit of suggestions with only weak (+ to ±) support, may actually help illustrate the magnitude of the existing problem. It is hoped that recognition of these knowledge gaps might eventually help accelerate the funding of a series of more systematic approaches to the therapeutics of this markedly understudied field.

Thus, the book is intended to be very much a work in progress, with the potential for many additional chapters as new therapeutic approaches to the illness become available. Hopefully, in future editions we will be able to rapidly revise the rank order and strength of therapeutic suggestions as new information becomes available. While we lament the relative lack of systematic study of bipolar illness over the past several decades, the book simultaneously emphasizes and presents an optimistic view of current clinical therapeutics of the bipolar disorders; adjuncts for symptom breakthrough; drugs targeted for the many comorbidities of bipolar illness; and use of multiple drugs in combination.

Part I

INTRODUCTION

1

Emil Kraepelin and the History of the Development of the Detailed Mood Chart

The majority of this book is written using psychiatric case reports, graphically displayed using the life chart method developed at the National Institute of Mental Health (NIMH). Therefore, we thought it might be useful to provide a brief historical outline of the development and rationale for a detailed, descriptive, longitudinal approach to the mapping of bipolar episodes.

It was Hippocrates, a physician in the 4th and 5th centuries (460–375 B.C.), who provided the first classification of mental disorders with a description of melancholia and mania. He built on the premise of Alcmaeon of Crotona and other pre-Hippocratic Greek physicians who thought that alterations in mental states were based on disturbed interactions of body fluids (such as bile) with the brain. Based on his supposition that the brain was the organ of mental functions that included mental disturbances and other disorders, Hippocrates wrote, "The people ought to know that the brain is the sole provider of pleasures and joys, laughter and jests, sadness and worry as well as dysphoria and crying" (as quoted by Angst & Marneros, 2001).

Aretaeus, a famous Greek physician in the first century A.D., provided a detailed description of the attributes of mania and melancholia but saw the two states as a single disease, with mania being a worsening of melancholia (Marneros & Brieger, 2002). It was Jean-Pierre Fal-

ret, a 19th-century French psychiatrist, who, based on his longitudinal observations of the psychopathology of manic and melancholic episodes, in 1851 introduced the concept of *la folie circulaire* (circular insanity) because "patients afflicted with this illness live out their lives in a perpetual circle of depression and manic excitement interrupted by a period of lucidity, which is typically brief but occasionally long lasting" (Sedler, 1983). However, he perceived the sequence of these "three specific states occurring in a determinate, predictable, unalterable order" and further stated "it will suffice to describe one of these cycles in order to give an exact idea of all the others, since they resemble one another in any given patient" (Sedler, 1983).

Karl Kahlbaum in Germany took up Falret's concept of circular insanity as *Cyklisches Irresein* (1882) and made a further differentiation between mental illnesses that were remitting and did not end in progressive deterioration in the intervening period between illness episodes, compared to those that often did (i.e., the schizophrenia-like illnesses; Kahlbaum, 1863). Based on his observations, he grouped circular insanity, although not curable, into the remitting category.

Emil Kraepelin (1856–1926), a German psychiatrist, built on Kahlbaum's work and in 1921 not only differentiated manic-depressive illness (*manic-depressive insanity* or *Das manisch-*

3

depressive Irresein) from schizophrenia, but also crystallized the critical observations on the longitudinal unfolding of the illness, which even today provide a most comprehensive topography of manic-depressive illness.

Kraepelin agreed with Kahlbaum's differentiation of long-term outcome between the remitting disorders and those that can lead to progressive deterioration: "The universal experience is striking, that the attacks of manic-depressive insanity . . . never lead to profound dementia, not even when they continue throughout life almost without interruption" (1921, p. 3). He included all morbid mood states (including depression only, i.e., what we now call unipolar depression) in the domain of manic-depressive illness, but it was primarily his observations about the course and variability of manic-depressive illness (now called bipolar disorder) that furthered the understanding of this illness presentation as a separate entity.

Kraepelin depicted the illness course of each individual patient (*Lebenslauf*) in a diagrammatic form, charting the occurrences of mania, depression, and well intervals on a monthly basis in order "to give a more exact view of the varieties of course in manic-depressive insanity" (1921, p. 139). We include an example of a Kraepelinian life chart or diagram of a patient's course of illness based on longitudinal observations (Figure 1.1). He noted the age of the patient on the left side of the diagram and the months of the year across the top row, with shades of blue indicating the severity of the depressions and, correspondingly, shades of red signifying the severity levels of mania. Additionally, he further distinguished characteristics of different presentations of mania or depression by adding crosshatching in the opposite color to differentiate angry, explosive mania, manic stupor, or mixed states (the simultaneous experience of manic and depressive symptoms with blue crosshatching for mixed mania) and, on the opposite pole, agitated or irritable depression (red crosshatching for irritable depression).

In some of Kraepelin's life charts we can also recognize the depiction of switches between mania and depression within a month, which we now categorize as *ultrarapid* cycling

(episodes lasting a week or less) and *ultradian* cycling (mood switches within a single day). Kraepelin included 18 examples of these life charts in his book on manic-depressive illness but stated, "If we give no more examples, that is not because those already given represent adequately the multiplicity of the courses taken by manic-depressive insanity; it is absolutely inexhaustible. The cases reported only show that there can be no talk of even an approximate regularity in the course, as has formerly been frequently assumed on the ground of certain isolated observations" (1921, p. 149). His colleague Otto Rehm, who collaborated with Kraepelin in constructing the charts (Rehm, 1919), provided us with more life charts in his monograph *Manic-Melancholic Insanity* (*Das Manisch-Melancholische Irresein*), each of which depicts further aspects of the variability of the illness.

Although Kraepelin felt that one could certainly observe in the individual attacks of a patient a certain "photographic similarity" (1921, p. 136) of behavior, the frequency and duration of the episodes, however, were "extremely varied" (p. 139). Based on his longitudinal observations, Kraepelin disagreed with Falret's view of the illness as having a "determinate, predictable, unalterable order" and stated, "I am convinced that that kind of effort at classification must of necessity wreck on the irregularity of the disease. The kind and duration of the attacks and the intervals by no means remain the same in the individual case but may frequently change, so that the case must be reckoned always to new forms" (p.139).

When considering causes for the emergence of bipolar disorder in a given individual, Kraepelin (1921, p. 165) observed a hereditary factor in some patients, especially in children from bilineal families (in which both parents have the illness). He furthermore felt that "the real, the deeper cause in the malady is to be sought in a permanent morbid state which must also continue to exist in the intervals between episodes" (p. 117), thus presuming an underlying continuous biological vulnerability factor even when the illness is quiescent.

When looking at external causes for the occurrence of an episode, Kraepelin felt that they

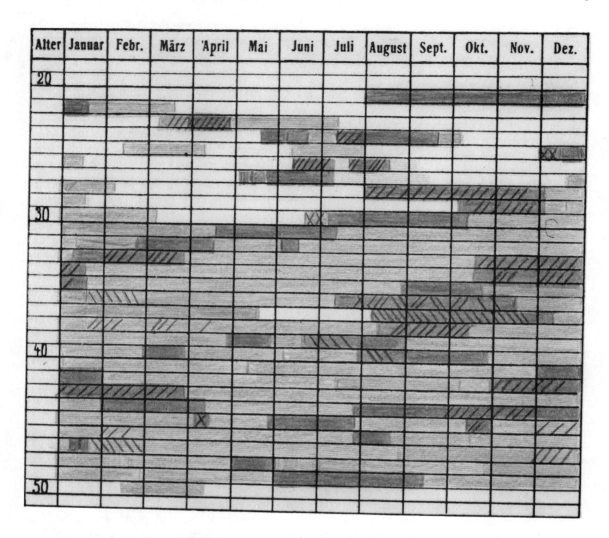

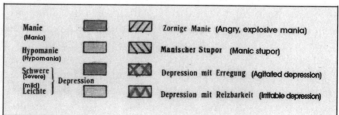

Figure 1.1 Depiction of a patient's progression from intermittent episodes to continuous cycling as recorded by Emil Kraepelin. This patient started with intermittent episodes, which became essentially continuous after age 30.

played a "very subordinate" role compared to the "innate predisposition" (1921, p. 177). However, he delineated some of the types of external events or stressors to which one can ascribe a contributory role in the emergence of an episode, such as "bodily illnesses," or the death of a spouse, near relative, or other important losses. He felt that one could regard all these factors as "possibly sparks for the discharge of the individual attacks" (p. 180). Yet the real cause for the illness "must be sought in *permanent internal changes*," especially since despite the removal of the "discharging cause" the episode follows its independent progression.

Additionally, based on his detailed longitudinal observations, he not only elucidated the variability and essential unpredictability of the illness evolution but also expounded general principles of illness evolution; over time, (a) the well intervals between initial episodes tend to become shorter, and (b) episodes become progressively more independent of precipitating factors ("quite without external occasion," p. 181). Although he acknowledged the fact that in some patients a regular, almost rhythmic pattern of episode and well interval occurrence could be observed, he also described a waxing and waning in cycle frequency for the individual patient, so that the long-term illness patterns could not be predicted with certainty.

The value and necessity of long-term recording of all pertinent factors in a patient's medical and psychiatric history were reemphasized by Adolf Meyer, an American psychiatrist, who held Kraepelin and his work in high regard. In *The Collected Papers of Adolf Meyer* (1951), we find a chapter excerpted from "Contributions to Medical and Biological Research" (1919) titled, "The Life Chart and the Obligation of Specifying Positive Data in Psychopathological Diagnosis," in which he emphasized the physician's responsibility to be aware of all factors pertaining to a patient's presenting problems that can only be fully understood in the context of a longitudinal perspective.

To gain such a comprehensive overview, however, the physician would have to examine what are often quite substantial charts and records, and "it is the length of the records and their apparent lack of pointedness that make many physicians shun the task" (Meyer, 1951). Thus, Meyer presents a charting system, which he calls Life Chart, and expands Kraepelin's diagrams by allowing for the charting of a psychosocial history in the form of life events (starting with the patient's date of birth), the occurrence of medical illnesses, and the emergence of psychiatric symptoms. At the end of his chapter, which includes examples of his life chart method, he states that "this brief note may illustrate the objective practical procedure of modern psychopathological studies, and how simply, controllably, and suggestively the facts can be brought into a record."

Kraepelin's contributions to our current understanding of manic-depressive illness and its variable and recurrent nature, as well as his supposition of the biological underpinnings, even during periods of illness quiescence, assume even greater significance in this era of psychopharmacology and other somatic treatments. Kahlbaum (1882), in the prepsychopharmacological era, stated at the end of his paper "On Circular Insanity" that it was of "utmost importance" for the general practitioner to be provided with some diagnostic clarity and anchor points based on longitudinal observations by the psychiatric specialist, so that the practicing physician could arrive at a more certain earlier diagnostic decision as to course, prognosis, and treatment of the presenting mental illness.

Clearly, in this era of the availability of a wide armamentarium of psychotropic medications, it is of further great importance that the treating physician or psychiatrist be keenly aware of the retrospective and prospective longitudinal data on the effectiveness of a given drug or regimen for a patient, so that the best treatment choices are offered and made at each juncture in the illness. Acute responses alone may not inform us sufficiently about the effectiveness of a given drug and what other treatments may be necessary in order to achieve and sustain a full remission.

The work of Baastrup and Schou (1967) is a poignant example of the need for longitudinal observations. With the recognition of the therapeutic efficacy of lithium by Cade (1977), long-term observations were required to establish its potential usefulness not only acutely but also as a prophylactic agent in the treatment of manic-depressive illness. Baastrup and Schou in Denmark recruited patients in 1960 for a study of the long-term effects of lithium on the course of affective illness. They published the results of the study in 1967, based on 6 years of observation, and on an additional 3-year extension in 1973, in the form of "diagrammatic case histories" (Baastrup & Schou, 1967; Schou, 1973).

Their method very much resembles Kraepelin's longitudinal approach, with the modification of recording illness episodes following a timeline that allowed for the coding of medications, in this case lithium, above the episodes. A reproduction of the "diagrammatic case histories" can be found in Schou's (1973) article, in which pre- and postlithium longitudinal case histories for each patient in the study effectively demonstrate lithium's prophylactic effect for the great majority of patients, the relapses in some patients who discontinued lithium, and then, generally, re-responsiveness once lithium was reinstituted.

We chose to adopt Kraepelin's basic format, his life events, and Baastrup and Schou's drug coding in the development of our life chart method (LCM) and added a number of other components (Leverich & Post 1996, 1998; Post, Roy-Byrne, & Uhde, 1988; Squillace, Post, Savard, & Erwin-Gorman, 1984). We made provisions for rating mania and depression at three levels of retrospective severity (on a monthly basis) and at four levels of severity prospectively (on a daily basis). We added an hours of sleep measure and space to track comorbid symptoms as well as provisions for documenting medications used and psychosocial stressors experienced (Figure 1.2). In the latest personal calendar version, medication side effects can also be recorded on a daily basis. Nearly identical formats of our life chart are available for a patient to complete self-ratings (which we highly recommend) and for clinicians' ratings (Appendix 3).

The occurrence of early onset bipolar disorder in childhood and adolescence, already illustrated in some of Kraepelin's life charts, is now increasingly recognized and accepted. The impact on the young patients' lives and on their families often is enormous. Diagnostic issues,

however, still abound as to what illness criteria need to be met so that a bipolar disorder would be considered to be present in a child or adolescent (Chapters 67 and 68).

To circumvent some of the diagnostic controversies and ambiguities, which often inhibit starting appropriate treatment, we have also developed a children's life chart to help parents track their children's symptoms and behaviors, as described in Chapters 67 and 68 and illustrated in Appendix 3. Rather than defining illness phases as mania or depression, we categorized mood symptoms and behaviors as activated or inhibited/withdrawn, and at what level of severity they occurred based on the associated functional impairment at home, in school, or with their friends (Leverich & Post, 1998). In this fashion, an accurate portrayal of the illness and its severity, frequency, and variability can be mapped free of arbitrary diagnostic presumptions. Thus, a clearer view of the presenting symptomatology and its variation can be achieved, and treatment interventions can be instituted and assessed accordingly.

We have noted the many advantages to completing a life chart (Table 1.1), and we also hope that the use of a life chart in almost every chapter in the book further emphasizes the utility of such an approach. We echo Adolf Meyer's sentiments about unwieldy and unfocused stacks of patient records. We firmly believe, along with Kraepelin, Meyer, and Schou, that a carefully completed life chart may be one of the most important tools in the search for optimal treatments for this too often difficult to treat illness.

The life chart can reveal different patterns of illness progression that have very different treatment implications. For example, with the use of the life chart method, we were able to uncover two different types of loss of responsiveness to lithium in a subgroup of patients that were initially highly responsive. One was lithium discontinuation-related refractoriness resulting from stopping lithium (as described in Chapter 12). Another was gradual loss of efficacy while remaining on the drug via the development of tolerance (as discussed in Chapter 11 and Chapters 19, 24, 27, and 38 for other drugs).

Others have begun to record similar observations (Kukopulos, Reginaldi, Giradi, & Tondo,

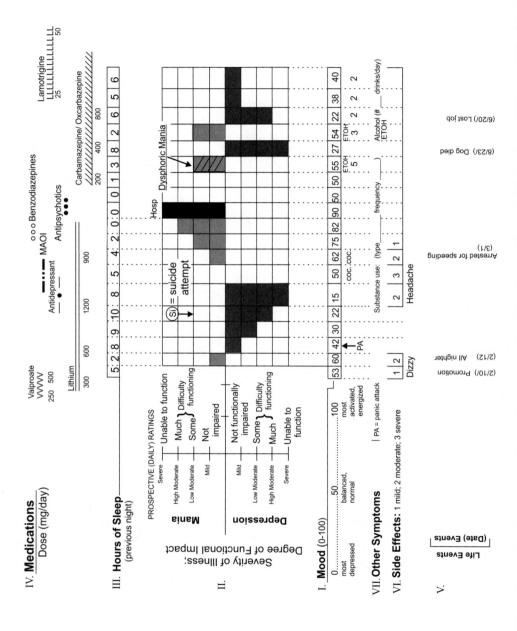

Figure 1.2 Schema for graphing the course of affective illness: prospective daily ratings of (I) mood, (II) functioning, (III) sleep, (IV) medications (top); (V) life events, (VI) side effects, and (VII) other symptoms (bottom). Kraepelin's method of mapping of the topography of bipolar episodes led us to the development of the more detailed National Institute of Mental Health Life Chart Method for graphing the course of affective illness. We expanded the schema to include a retrospective version rated at three levels of manic and depressive severity (on a monthly basis). The more detailed prospective version is rated daily at four levels of severity depending on the degree of functional impact of the affective symptoms. We added additional components in order to record medications and doses, other symptoms (e.g., psychosis, dysphoric mania, panic attacks, anxiety, alcohol consumption, etc.), side effects, and life events. A patient self-version is also available and includes ratings of mood on a 0–100 scale, number of switches per day, and hours of sleep (see Appendix 2).

8

Table 1.1 *The Benefits of Systematically Charting the Course of Bipolar Illness*

Document Prior Course (Retrospective LCM)	Patient as Active Partner	Applicability for Clinical Research (Prospective LCM)
Assess partial treatment responses	Directs future clinical trials based on prior responses (sequential trials and rational polypharmacy)	Illness variables quantitated based on:
Maintains continuity between retrospective and prospective assessments	Provides educational opportunity	Daily prospective ratings
Elucidates:	Focuses on targeted psychotherapy	Mapping of severity, duration, and patterning of affective disturbances
Psychosocial precipitants	Increases compliance	Episode number
Seasonal variation	Enables development of an early warning system	Detailed evaluation of drug responsiveness possible
Tolerance patterns	Helps medicalize illness	Validity:
Manic switches or cycle acceleration (TCA, MAOI, SSRI)	Is a portable history if care provider changes	Clinician version well-validated
Ultrarapid and ultradian cycling	Facilitates consultations among physicians if needed	Utility:
Medication discontinuation-induced relapses	Self-rated prospective version provides easy graphic representation of response in multiple domains (i.e., mood, functional impairment, sleep, and side effects	Used in many academic and industry studies
	Daily monitoring of mood (like blood sugar in diabetes) helps patient actively participate in care	Systematic longitudinal assessments comparable across patients and sites
Daily Prospective Ratings:	Helps in titration of drug doses (using response vs. side effects)	Automated computer-based analysis available
Essential for detailed evaluation of course of illness and response to treatment	Assists in establishing contribution of new agents in complex combination therapy	
	Helps treat to remission	

1975; Maj, Pirozzi, & Kemali, 1989) of both tolerance and lithium discontinuation-induced refractoriness. For example, Maj et al. (1989), in their report of the results of the long-term outcome of lithium prophylaxis, found that of the 49 excellent responders (who had experienced complete remissions for 2 or more years), 14 eventually relapsed over the next 5 years (despite demonstrated medication compliance). These examples reveal the dangers of breakthrough episodes that require alternative psychopharmacological or somatic interventions in order to maintain remission. The dangers inherent in stopping effective treatment are also crystallized by the LCMs in Chapter 12.

The need for longitudinal outcome measures, in addition to cross-sectional ratings, has increasingly been recognized by the pharmaceutical industry as well. Now many studies have begun to utilize the LCM format in studies of prophylactic efficacy. With the appreciation that as many as 40% to 50% of patients in some academic settings experience rapid or faster cycling, even frequent cross-sectional or intermittent ratings will miss significant illness fluctuations. Typical cross-sectional rating scales for depression cover only 1 week, or, for mania with the Young Mania Rating Scale (Young, Biggs, & Ziegler, 1978), 48 hours. Thus, the actual long-term efficacy of an agent for a given individual may be misinterpreted, based on the usual intermittent ratings. For example, the significantly better long-term antimanic effects of lithium compared with carbamazepine were not seen with the typical once-a-month measures for 1 year on each drug, but were clearly revealed by ratings on the prospective LCM (Denicoff, Smith-Jackson, Disney, et al., 1997).

Thus, tools based on Kraepelin's longitudinal approach to bipolar disorder, such as the life chart and similar methods, can offer the patient, clinician, and researcher a productive way to systematically and comprehensively evaluate the course of bipolar illness and treatment responses to existing and novel agents for the most effective management of this illness.

Part II

PHENOMENOLOGY OF
ILLNESS COURSE

2

Acceleration in Cycle Frequency

CASE HISTORY

The classic pattern of cycle acceleration observed and described earlier by Kraepelin in untreated patients is illustrated in the life chart of this patient (Figure 2.1). Between some of the initial episodes, the patient was well for months to several years. Early in 1981, while being treated with antidepressants and lithium in combination, the patient began to cycle more rapidly and regularly in a relatively continuous fashion without any well intervals. This pattern continued for the next 2 years with approximately the same frequency and intensity when a new phase of dramatic cycle acceleration emerged after a more prolonged depression. This occurred despite many different treatment attempts with antidepressants—lithium, electroconvulsive therapy, and other similar treatments.

Illness Progression to a Phase of Ultra-UltraRapid (Ultradian) Cycling

Episodes then became more arrhythmic (in 1984) and finally progressed to ultrarapid and ultra-ultrarapid (ultradian) cycling in a chaotic pattern (in 1985). Embedded in this process are several phenomena that can be characteristic of the course of bipolar illness: (1) cycle acceleration (shorter well intervals between successive episodes); (2) progression to continuous cycling (in 1982); and (3) emergence of ultradian cycling (i.e., distinct and dramatic mood oscillations

within a single day; 1995). Figure 2.1 (bottom) also illustrates: (4) good response of ultradian cycling to combination therapy (carbamazepine and lithium; 1986–1989); (5) reemergence of episode or development of treatment resistance (1988–1990) to previously effective combination therapy; (6) response to lithium plus an antidepressant (1991–1993), and (7) a reresponse to a second trial of carbamazepine (1994–1995).

This patient was one of the first who convinced us that ultra-ultrarapid cycling (i.e., multiple switches within a 24-hour period, also called ultradian cycling; see enlargement of pattern in Figure 2.2) could occur in patients who had otherwise exhibited a pattern and course of classic manic-depressive illness. Heretofore, most in the field had surmised that patients who showed these rapid, dramatic oscillations in mood and behavior had personality rather than primary affective disorders, and that patients with classic manic-depressive illness could not cycle faster than once every 48 hours. Multiple case reports by Bunney and Hartmann and others had reported this striking pattern of 48-hour cycling (i.e., one day up, the next day down). However, Kramlinger and Post (1996), and George, Jones, Post, Mikalauskas, and Leverich (1992), based on this and other patients' self-reports and objective observations by nurses with detailed ratings every 2 hours, indicated that mood oscillations could reach another level and jump to very high frequency with essentially random fluctuations in a pattern consistent with the mathematics of chaos.

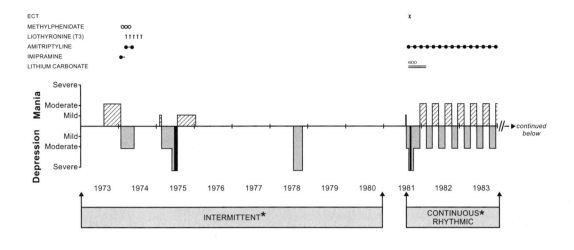

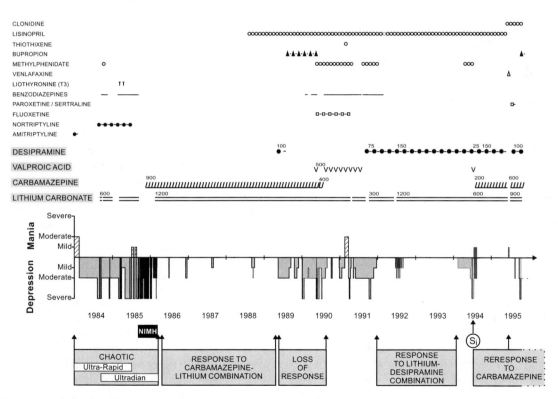

Figure 2.1 Phases in illness evolution and treatment response in a bipolar female. This patient's course of illness demonstrates a process of phase transitions from a pattern of illness characterized by isolated, intermittent episode occurrence with a progression to a continuous, rhythmic phase (top line) and ultimately to ultrarapid and ultradian cycling (bottom, left).

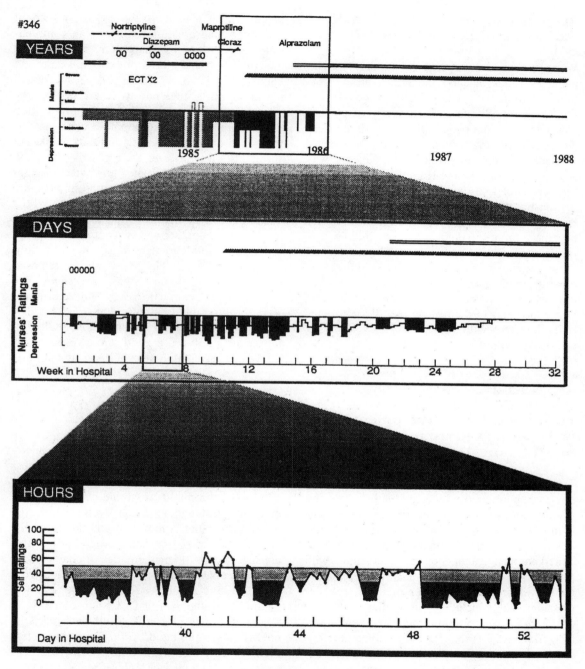

Figure 2.2 Zooming in on similar patterns of affective fluctuations apparent in monthly, daily, and hourly ratings. Ultradian fluctuations in mood observed in the patient's 2-hour ratings are illustrated (bottom row) as sequentially enlarged from the daily nursing ratings (middle) and the monthly life chart ratings (top). These fluctuations within a day are evident during a period of what would otherwise look like slower, more intermittent cycling based on daily nursing ratings (middle row). They still reflect a pattern of ultrarapid cycling between immobilizing depression (shaded) and milder depression or essential euthymia (unshaded). This chaotic pattern responded well to a combination of carbamazepine and lithium (hospital week 28) when neither drug alone, or in combination with other agents, had proven effective.

Response to the Combination of Carbamazepine and Lithium

When carbamazepine was substituted for the patient's blind placebo medicines at the National Institutes of Mental Health, some attenuation in the amplitude and frequency of cycling was achieved. The patient, however, did not get well until lithium, which had been previously ineffective despite addition of other agents, was added to carbamazepine (Figure 2.1, 1986). On this combination therapy, the patient slowly demonstrated a deceleration in the frequency and amplitude of her depressive cycles, until she became euthymic (Figure 2.2, see middle row for detailed view). She was able to be discharged on this regimen of carbamazepine-lithium combination therapy and did exceedingly well over the next 3 or 4 years, suffering only brief and minor episodes of depression that did not materially interfere with her ability to work as an operating room nurse.

Renewed Cycle Acceleration Despite Continuation of Treatment: The Development of Treatment Resistance (or Tolerance)

These minor episodic breakthrough depressions, however, continued with a gradually increasing severity and rapidity of recurrence despite ongoing treatment with carbamazepine and lithium. Finally, episodes of moderate severity required adjunctive antidepressant intervention with a variety of agents that were, however, not effective in preventing further breakthrough depressions. These included nortriptyline (Pamelor), desipramine (Norpramin), bupropion (Wellbutrin), fluoxetine (Prozac), and minor tranquilizers of the benzodiazepines: oxazepam (Serax) and clorazepate (Tranxene). Enalapril (Vasotec) had earlier been added for control of the patient's high blood pressure. Two hospitalizations were required for severe depression with suicidal ideation.

This episode pattern conforms to a pattern of tolerance development that can occur in a small percentage of patients to the positive effects of carbamazepine or lithium alone or in combination (as discussed in Chapters 12 and 19). The patient was transferred from carbamazepine to valproate in 1990, which helped get her out of the unremitting moderate to severe depression. This switch was predicated on the proposition that carbamazepine and valproate work via different mechanisms of action and thus would not show cross-tolerance to their effects on mood. This response to valproate, however, was not sustained for a significant period of time (Figure 2.1), and after a breakthrough depression with a switch into a moderate mania and subsequent depression, valproate was discontinued. The addition of an antidepressant (desipramine) to lithium eventually brought 18 months of renewed good functioning, but significant depressive breakthroughs started to recur with a progression to ultrarapid and ultradian cycling. The reinstitution of carbamazepine along with lithium again produced a good initial response, as it had in 1985, with a year of good functioning.

BACKGROUND LITERATURE

Particularly striking in the issues of cycle acceleration are the distinct phases or shifts in illness patterning from intermittent episodes in the beginning to continuous rhythmic cycling, and finally ultrafast and ultradian cycling. Potential reasons for such illness progression are discussed in Chapter 10. Such a progression is also consistent with the mathematics of chaos theory (George et al., 1992; Gottschalk, Bauer, & Whybrow, 1995; Kramlinger & Post, 1996).

Similar to the data of Di Costanzo and Schifano (1991) and Denicoff, Smith-Jackson, Disney, et al. (1997), rapid-cycling patients are less likely to respond to lithium or carbamazepine treatment alone (about 25% response rates) but are more likely to respond to the combination of both drugs (about 50% response rates). This patient's course of illness is a clear demonstration of intermittent episodes again reemerging through treatment with eventual progression to a complete loss of efficacy.

We believe that this process of loss of efficacy occurs not on the basis of lowered blood levels of carbamazepine or lithium, but because the illness is finding a way to circumvent existing effects of the drugs. In the face of tolerance development, a switch to a new drug with a different mechanism of action, or having a period of time off the original drug, can lead to a renewed response to the drug. The caveat should be reemphasized that this period of time off a drug should be reserved as a highly experimental option to be used only when an initially good response to that drug had occurred but was gradually lost with the development of tolerance. In contrast, a period of time off drug in a patient who is continuing to respond to that drug may have extremely adverse consequences, including severe relapses and even the possibility of the development of unresponsiveness or refractoriness to that drug in the future (Post, Leverich, Altshuler, & Mikalauskas, 1992; Post, Leverich, Pazzaglia, Mikalauskas, & Denicoff, 1993; see Chapter 13).

When this patient was transferred from carbamazepine to valproate, she failed to show a sustained response. This could be because either: (1) she would have been a valproate nonresponder in any event; or (2) there was some degree of cross-tolerance between carbamazepine and valproate in this patient's affective illness, just as there is for some types of seizures (Weiss, Clark, Rosen, Smith, & Post, 1995).

When carbamazepine treatment was reinitiated in 1994 (as augmentation of lithium and desipramine), the patient showed a renewed response to the drug.

PRINCIPLES OF THE CASE — STRENGTH OF EVIDENCE

1. Many patients show an overall pattern of cycle acceleration in their course of illness; this can be halted by effective treatment. +++

2. Tricyclic antidepressants may have been involved in this patient's conversion from intermittent to continuous cycling, yet this did not recur in 1992 with lithium plus desipramine. ±

3. Some patients with classic bipolar illness may show mood cycling within a single day, that is, what is called ultra-ultrarapid (or ultradian) cycling in a highly irregular or chaotic pattern. ++

4. Patients with ultradian cycling may be more resistant to routine pharmacotherapies. +

5. Ultra-ultrarapid (ultradian) cycling patterns may occur in bipolar illness in the absence of a personality disorder; such patients often show an excellent response to more complex combination therapy. +

6. Response to the combination of lithium and carbamazepine occurs in about 50% of rapid-cycling patients (even when there is inadequate response to either agent alone). +++

7. Tolerance can develop to the long-term prophylactic response to several types of medications in a small subgroup of patients. ++

8. At times, the discontinuation of medicine in the face of tolerance development may lead to the renewal of clinical responsiveness to that medication. ±

9. Note: Discontinuation of effective medications should be resisted in the face of sustained clinical improvement, since it is likely to result in relapse or, rarely, treatment nonresponsiveness (see Chapter 13). +++

10. In the face of an initial good response to medication and subsequent loss of response via tolerance, several different options may be tried in careful sequence using each patient as a systematic clinical trial in order to find an optimum therapeutic regimen.

These principles can be based on:

a. Increasing the dose of drug;   ±+

b. Augmenting the treatment with a new agent;   ±

c. Switching to a drug with a different mechanism of action that does not show cross tolerance; or   ±

d. Retreatment with the drug after a period of time off.   ±

TAKE-HOME MESSAGE

Even though episode recurrence can speed up over time, extended periods of complete remission can be achieved. Careful charting of illness course and treatment response will help in finding and maintaining the best therapeutic regimens for each individual patient.

3

Increasing Depressive Episode Frequency and Severity, and Baseline Dysfunction Between Episodes

CASE HISTORY

This patient is a 38-year-old computer programmer whose illness history showed intermittent depressive episodes of mild to moderate severity (1967–1969), progressing to episodes associated with complete dysfunction occurring on an intermittent basis. Following his episodes in 1982, his illness was transformed, in that he began to fail to return to his baseline euthymic mood state and continued to have twice-yearly (winter and spring) severe episodes emerging from a more chronic or dysthymic baseline level of depression (i.e., double depressions; Figure 3.1).

In the several years prior to his NIMH admission, the patient had increasing numbers of severe depressed episodes per year punctuated by the new phenomenon of brief periods of hypomania. This persisted until 1988 with the emergence of additional periods of depression, with a distinctly less seasonal pattern and a more severe level of baseline depression. Finally, prior to the NIMH hospitalization in 1989 and continuing at the NIMH off medications, these periods of depression were punctuated by distinct periods of hypomania with increased energy, rambunctiousness, euphoric mood, and bizarre be-

havior, including moving rapidly up and down the corridor of the unit, flapping his elbows as if they were wings, and quacking like a duck. These episodes had discrete onsets and offsets and, at times, lasted less than 24 hours (Figure 3.2). During these phases, the patient would change rapidly from having marked psychomotor retardation and being almost mute to moving rapidly about the ward. These periods of mood elevation were of variable duration, lasting as little as 30 minutes to 1 hour, averaging about 3 or 4 hours, sometimes occurring for 12 to 24 hours. They were terminated with a rapid onset of full-blown incapacitating depression.

Thus, this overall pattern of increasing cycle frequency, severity of baseline depression, and emergence of hypomanias occurred during various attempts to treat the depression with traditional antidepressants, monoamine oxidase inhibitors (MAOIs), selective serotonin reuptake inhibitors (SSRIs), and mood stabilizers such as lithium. These drugs were largely without effect, and their potential influence on the hypomanic inductions remains undetermined, because they also could have occurred as part of the natural course of illness (as previously described by Kraepelin and others prior to the advent of antidepressants).

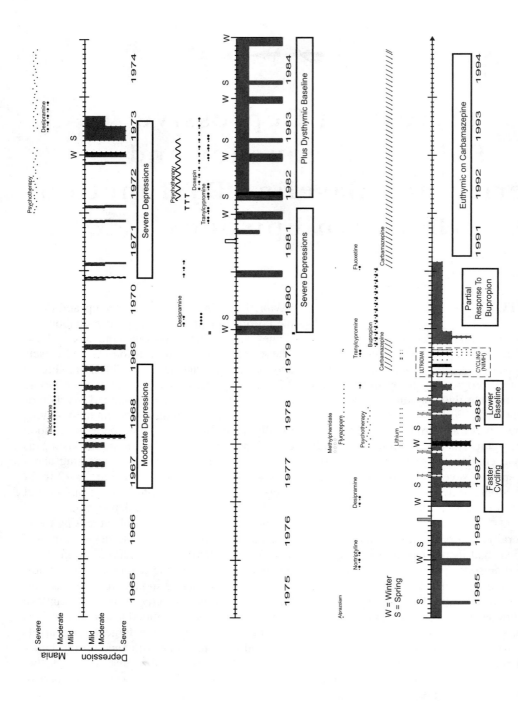

Figure 3.1 The onset of recurrent episodic depressions, generally widely spaced at the beginning of the illness, with cycle acceleration and increasing severity of baseline mood dysfunction, progressing from wellness (euthymia) to mild depression (dysthymia), and then to greater levels of depression in between more severe episodes. This progression occurred despite a variety of antidepressant manipulations and culminated in the eventual emergence of episodic bursts of distinct hypomania (i.e., bipolar II depressions).

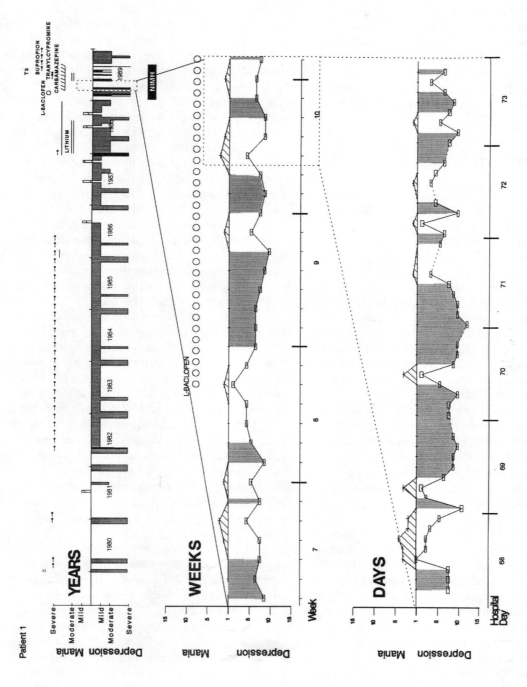

Figure 3.2 Successive telescopic representations of this patient's course of illness with the traditional life chart ratings on the top, nurses' daily ratings in the middle, and the patient's self-ratings performed on an every 2 (Q2) hourly basis on the bottom line, to illustrate the ultra-ultrarapid cycling aspect of this patient's course in terms of distinct mood changes occurring faster than once every 24 hours (i.e., ultradian cycling; bottom row) and the self-similarity of illness patterns at different gross to fine grained levels of temporal resolution and analysis.

At the NIMH, the patient showed a good antidepressant response when carbamazepine (Tegretol) was blindly substituted for placebo. Responsiveness was not complete, so bupropion (Wellbutrin) was added to the carbamazepine, with additional clinical improvement sufficient to allow the patient to be discharged in only a mildly dysthymic state, as further described in Chapter 39.

BACKGROUND LITERATURE

This patient's illness progression shows a classic pattern described originally by Kraepelin and documented in many articles since that time. It is also highly representative of a course of presumptive unipolar depression that Dr. Paul Grof has followed in many patients, showing that with illness maturation and age of the patient, episodes of depression tend to occur with greater frequency over time in patients not undergoing prophylactic treatment (Grof, Angst, & Haines, 1974). In this instance, the patient also eventually received treatment that was either inadequate or may have actually exacerbated the course of illness.

The period of more chronic low-level baseline depression dysthymia from which more severe episodes emerged is typical of the pattern labeled double depression (Keller & Shapiro, 1982). A seasonal pattern of winter onsets of the depression is often typical of seasonal affective disorder, but unusual for this patient was the second depression occurring on a yearly basis independent of apparent daylight entrainment by the winter season. However, as is the case in some patients with seasonal affective disorder, the timing of these episodes eventually broke away from this semiregular pattern and began to emerge independently of any season (Bauer, 1992). The hypomanias emerged during treatment with an antidepressant initially and then proceeded to occur spontaneously as well.

This case illustrates the fallibility of the current *DSM-IV* diagnostic system (American Psychiatric Association, 1994) because hypomanias emerging during antidepressant treatment are not formally considered bipolar II illness but are considered substance induced. However, this patient would later meet criteria for bipolar II, as the manias were then observed during a period without treatment with medications (as also repeatedly observed by Akiskal et al., 1995). At the NIMH, the patient would have met criteria only for bipolar not otherwise specified (BP-NOS), since none of the distinct periods of hypomania lasted 4 days or longer as required for a bipolar II diagnosis.

The potential diagnostic importance of such a bipolar II or a BP-NOS diagnosis is readily revealed by the patient's life chart. It was not until treatment with another mood stabilizer (carbamazepine), with a different mechanism of action than lithium carbonate, that the patient's illness began to show amelioration from its steady, progressive deterioration, despite treatment with a variety of antidepressant modalities with or without lithium carbonate.

Extremely frequent mood shifts may occur in otherwise classical bipolar patients (see Chapters 2 and 53), and although these patients often need more complex regimens or combination therapies to induce remission, the pattern of ultrarapid or ultra-ultrarapid (ultradian) cycling does not preclude an eventual positive outcome as in this patient (Kramlinger & Post, 1996). Many more patients with classic bipolar illness are now experiencing these extreme ultradian cycle frequencies, including 18% in one study of outpatients (Kupka et al., 2005; Nolen et al., 2004; Post, Denicoff, et al., 2003). These rapid mood shifts can occur in the absence of major personality disorders.

However, the syndrome of borderline personality disorder can often present with similar ultrarapid variability and lability in mood. Patients with borderline personality disorder can be distinguished from patients with uncomplicated bipolar illness, in that they usually do not have substantial periods of wellness, with good work, social, and interpersonal functioning between episodes (as did the patient illustrated here). However, bipolar illness often co-occurs with a variety of psychiatric disorders, and many patients with bipolar illness have traumatic early experiences that can further predispose them to post-traumatic stress disorder (PTSD) and the development of personality disorders.

PRINCIPLES OF THE CASE	STRENGTH OF EVIDENCE
1. Mild episodes may signal more severe episodes if untreated or inadequately treated.	++
2. Isolated, intermittent episodes may lead to more frequent episodes with a rhythmic or dysrhythmic pattern of occurrence.	+++
3. Some patients may acquire a pattern of double depression in which they do not return to their baseline euthymic state in between affective episodes.	+
4. When antidepressants in conjunction with lithium are not successful in treating patients with recurrent mood disorders, other mood stabilizers (such as carbamazepine, valproate, or lamotrigine) may be necessary.	++
5. Hypomanic episodes may emerge, even after many depressions and many years without such an occurrence. However, the likelihood of a manic episode after three successive major depressive episodes is small, estimated to be about 17% by Angst.	++
6. Patients may move from a regular pattern of depressive occurrences to a more unpredictable or chaotic pattern associated with ultrarapid and ultra-ultra-rapid (ultradian) cycling, as observed in Figure 3.2.	++

TAKE-HOME MESSAGE

This life chart indicates that even after a decade of progressively more frequent depression, patients can regain a euthymic state with appropriate pharmacotherapy. Do not give up hope, even after many years of depressive cycling refractory to many typical medication approaches. A wealth of new treatment options is available, and in the face of inadequate response to conventional approaches, one should be encouraged to explore others, as outlined in many chapters throughout this book.

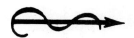

Increasing Episode Duration
and Shorter Well Intervals

CASE HISTORY

Patient 1

This 30-year-old patient experienced a variety of severe early childhood traumas prior to the onset of her recurrent major depressive illness. It was not until approximately 10 depressive episodes had occurred that a first hypomanic period emerged at 10 years of age. At approximately age 14, these hypomanic periods became more extended and the patient essentially cycled continuously between moderately severe depression and severe hypomania. In the third decade of life depressions continued to increase in both severity and duration, resulting in three hospitalizations for depression and two for mania.

Patient 2

This patient showed a highly similar but condensed version of the pattern seen in Figure 4.1. It is noteworthy that this apparently bipolar II patient, with hypomanias and mild to severe depression in 1992 and 1993, was first treated with psychotherapy and an antidepressant without a mood stabilizer as depression increased in severity (see also parallel treatment with fluoxetine in 1993 and 1994 in Patient 1).

Patient 2 had a prolonged severe depression in 1994 during treatment with venlafaxine, was hospitalized twice in 1995, and then experi-

enced a full-blown mania in the fall of 1995. Three manic hospitalizations ensued, with the manic hospitalization in 1999 occurring while not on antidepressants, confirming her transition from a bipolar II to a bipolar I subtype.

BACKGROUND LITERATURE

The patients in Figures 4.1 and 4.2 are examples of individuals who appear to have a unipolar recurrent depressive pattern, but then convert (without intervening antidepressant treatment) to a clear pattern of cycling, with hypomanias between depressions of mild to moderate severity. In the later phases of illness, the depressions continued to increase in both severity and duration and became essentially incapacitating. Angst showed that after three recurrent major depressions, a small proportion of patients still go on to experience a bipolar course of illness, as illustrated by these patients. His newer data (Angst, Sellaro, Stassen, & Gamma, 2005) showed that there is continued vulnerability to convert to bipolar illness over the entire course of recurrent unipolar illness.

These patients are also a disturbing example of the very long delays in diagnosis and treatment often seen in bipolar illness. They were not treated for many years of their illness, and then with antidepressants without mood stabilizers. In Patient 1, this represents an approximately 20-year delay before treatment was initi-

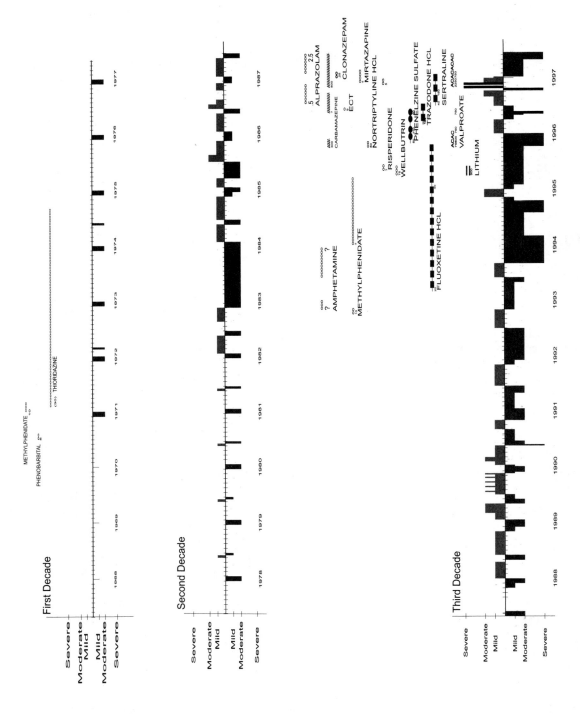

Figure 4.1 This patient experienced multiple depressions of moderate severity in years 4 through 11 of her life (top row). In her second decade, these recurrent depressions became punctuated by hypomanic periods prior to depression onset (middle row, left side), and then a pattern of continuous cycling between more prolonged hypomanias and depressions of varying duration but generally increased severity (middle row, right side). In the third decade of life, the depressions became more severe and prolonged, with a similar trend for increased severity of the intervening hypomanic to manic episodes (bottom row). Regrettably, the patient remained essentially untreated until the last 5 years of her illness, when antidepressants and other agents were instituted, but these did not have a positive effect and other approaches would be needed.

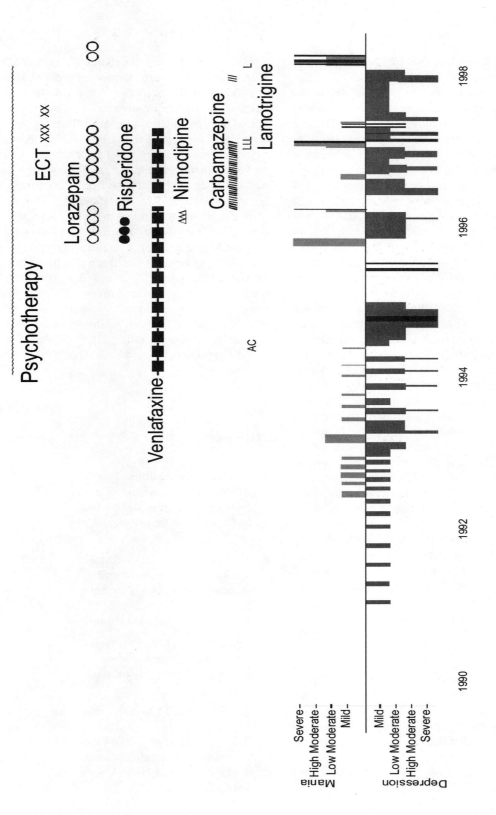

Figure 4.2 Increasing duration and severity of depressions and manias in a patient with delayed onset of appropriate treatment. This patient showed a similar, but much faster, time frame of worsening of both duration and severity of manic and depressive episodes than the previous patient in Figure 4.1.

ated for clearly evident, and increasingly severe, bipolar II continuous cycling illness.

This disturbing delay in onset of treatment parallels that observed in our larger outpatient experience in the Stanley Foundation Bipolar Network, wherein there was an average delay of 10 years between first symptoms associated with dysfunction and first treatment. We also found that the delays of onset of illness to first treatment for depression or mania were longer as a function of younger ages of onset. Our outpatients with onsets of their bipolar illness in childhood (before age 13), had averages delays to first treatment of more than 15 years (Leverich et al. 2007). Patient 1's long period of untreated, recurrent bipolar illness may have contributed to her relative treatment resistance when mood stabilizer treatment was initiated only in the later part of the 1990s. Similar to data reported by Hirschfeld, Calabrese, and colleagues (2003), a large number of patients with bipolar illness in the community remain undiagnosed, and those who do have a bipolar diagnosis are often treated inappropriately, that is, with antidepressants without mood stabilizers, as occurred with these two patients for several years. As discussed in Chapter 9, one can only surmise that if there had been earlier appropriate psychopharmacological intervention, much of these patients' illness and dysfunction could have been avoided.

With the exception of several years of early treatment with thioridazine, Patient 1's first 25 years illustrate the general view, emphasized by Kraepelin, that untreated illness may progress, in this instance not so much with more frequent episodes, but with more severe ones of greater duration, and then to continuous cycling without a well interval.

These two patients thus, unfortunately, become examples of what can happen if the illness is ignored or left poorly treated, as opposed to the dramatic clinical improvement that we illustrate in so many of the following chapters with a variety of psychopharmacological manipulations.

A recent analysis of more than 500 outpatients with bipolar illness rated prospectively on a daily basis for 1 year (Kupka et al., 2005) found that average time depressed remained relatively constant whether or not there were one to eight separate depressive episodes in the year, whereas time manic increased linearly as a function of number of manic episodes. This suggests that on the average, as the number of depressive episodes increases, they generally become shorter, such that time depressed remains, on average, about 30% of the year.

In the follow-up studies in recurrent unipolar depression of Keller and Boland (1998) and Thase (2001), with each additional depressive episode there was a 10% chance that the depression would become chronic and treatment refractory. Perhaps these patients illustrate the point that many recurrences of depression can render a bipolar patient relatively difficult to treat as well (Kupka et al., 2005; Nolen et al., 2004; Post, Denicoff, et al., 2003).

PRINCIPLES OF THE CASE	STRENGTH OF EVIDENCE
1. In some patients, illness progression may be evident in increasing duration of depressive and manic episodes (Patients 1 and 2).	±
2. An acceleration of episode frequency (shorter well interval) accompanied by either increasing (or decreasing) duration of depressions is more common.	++
3. Increasing severity of episode is also not uncommon in untreated or inadequately treated individuals.	++
4. The patients in Figures 4.1 and 4.2 illustrate too long a delay in diagnosis and treatment of bipolar illness, which unfortunately is all too common in the United States.	+++

5. Initiating treatment with antidepressants without the cover of a mood stabilizer is not recommended, because in both patients it appeared to eventually exacerbate rather than ameliorate the course of illness. +++

6. Whether earlier appropriate intervention could have spared these individuals the experience of many years of depressions and manias of increasing severity remains unknown but is a clinical approach worth considering in every individual in the hope that it might. ±

TAKE-HOME MESSAGE

In many individuals, recurrent depressions and then hypomanias can show a pattern of increasing severity and duration if left untreated or inadequately treated. However, as outlined in subsequent chapters in this volume, systematic psychopharmacological intervention and exploration can almost always result in illness improvement or remission.

5

An Unusual Case of
Traumatic Stress Acutely
Precipitating Both PTSD
and Bipolar Illness

CASE HISTORY

This patient was a healthy young woman in her early 20s who prided herself on social consciousness, physical fitness, and close and trusting relationships. She was an avid athlete and her life's dream was to play professional soccer. She had no history of psychiatric illness and was happily and gainfully employed as a bank auditor. While jogging one evening, she observed a house on fire and reflexively took up the role of Good Samaritan, knocking on the front door of a nearby house to alert them to the fire.

Unaccountably, a Rottweiler dog was released from the household and set upon her in a ferocious attack. She attempted to fend off the attack, but the dog bit her several times in the buttocks and calf and ripped tendons in her knee, resulting in a long-term limp. A bewildering series of events continued to unfold including emergency room visits, lack of support by police and firemen, a return to the scene to attempt to rationalize what had happened, progressive anxiety, agitation, and total insomnia, and a sense of unreality and uninterpretability of the incident.

The patient sought medical help in an emergency room, and later, because of her prolonged continuous insomnia, saw a psychiatrist. She was given an atypical antipsychotic and the benzodiazepine lorazepam, but these did not stop an evolving, then full-blown, manic psychosis. This psychosis finally resolved after some weeks and was followed by a severe depression with anxiety, apathy, irritability, inability to concentrate, sleep disturbance, loss of interest in usual activities, inability to relate to friends as usual, and inability to perform even routine tasks at work. She began regularly cycling from depression to hypomania and back to depression without a well interval.

She also experienced all of the classic signs and symptoms of PTSD, including marked sleep disturbance, nightmares replaying aspects of the attack, daytime flashbacks, hyperstartle and hyperirritability to noise, and feelings of progressive numbing and unreality.

The medications initially prescribed included lithium and antidepressants (with or without adjunctive treatment with carbamazepine or valproate) and were only partially effective in ameliorating her cyclic mood disorder and PTSD symptoms to any marked degree. She was able to return to work, but depressive phases and PTSD symptoms limited the complexity of projects she could now manage.

BACKGROUND LITERATURE

Differential Precipitants of PTSD and Affective Illness

Although the onset of manic-depressive illness is often associated with psychosocial stressors in the initial episodes, it is relatively uncommon in our experience for the illness to be precipitated by such an acute physical or life-threatening stressor. Rather, these are typical etiological factors in the initiation of PTSD. That the two syndromes of bipolar illness and PTSD occurred concomitantly in this patient suggests that at least in some instances, some overlapping psychobiological and neurochemical events can be involved (Figure 5.1). In the literature on precipitation of depression, it is more commonly believed that stressors are related to marital, family, and self-esteem issues as well as those around personal loss, the threat thereof, and threats to one's finances or employment. The first mania occurring at a funeral of an immediate family member is not rare, particularly if it is a death of a mother or sibling by suicide.

In the case described, it may be construed that many losses and potential losses occurred in the context of the vicious dog attack, in that the patient lost her sense of invulnerability as a world-class athlete and faced the potential threats of loss of her job and of a secure and self-assured personal identity. The added potential etiological contribution of the five successive days of complete sleep loss to the precipitation of the full-blown manic episode also cannot be dismissed.

As noted in other chapters (6, 7, and 10), Dr. Emil Kraepelin (1921) observed that stress was often associated with the first episodes of bipolar illness, but that successive episodes might occur more autonomously. Kraepelin recognized both a genetic and environmental or experiential component of the vulnerability to bipolar illness. Subsequent work has supported his initial observations as documented in meta-analyses (Post, 1992, 1996) and the more recent elegant studies of Kendler, Thornton, and Gardner (2000, 2001) in unipolar depression. We have

had the opportunity of assessing the potential effects of psychosocial stressors in a cohort of bipolar patients as well.

Impact of Childhood Traumas on Course of Bipolar Illness in Adults

Leverich, McElroy, et al. (2002) found that compared with those patients with bipolar illness who did not report early traumatic events of physical or sexual abuse, those who did have these experiences in childhood had an earlier age of onset of bipolar illness and a more severe retrospective and prospective course of illness as adults. Compared with those without abuse, those with such early traumatic histories also experienced more time depressed, more Axis I and II comorbidities, and more medical comorbidities (Axis III). Those with histories of physical abuse (Figures 5.2 and 5.3) had an increased severity of manic episodes, and those with sexual abuse had an increased incidence of medically serious suicide attempts (Leverich, McElroy, et al., 2002; Leverich et al., 2003).

These early traumatic life experiences appeared to interact with a positive family history of affective disorders. Those patients with neither risk factor had the latest age of onset of bipolar illness (at an average age of 22 to 24 years), whereas those with both risk factors had the earliest age of onset (10 to 12 years). Those patients with either a positive family history of affective illness or early environmental stressors had intermediate ages of illness onset.

Interestingly, those patients who had these stressful childhood life experiences more often reported stressful life events also at the onset of their bipolar illness than those without such a history, consistent with the stress sensitization model discussed in Chapter 10. These data could be interpreted in several ways, however. Patients with these early stressful life experiences could be putting themselves in position for the experience of more negative life events, or these events may have sensitized the individuals to the neuropsychobiological impact of subsequent stressors that become able to precip-

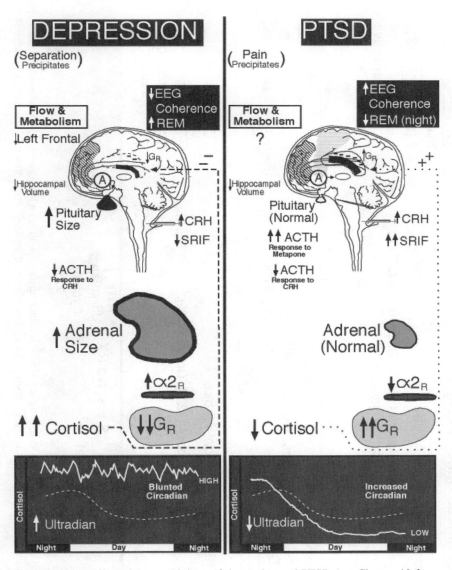

Figure 5.1 Overlapping and differential neurobiology of depression and PTSD (see Chapter 10 for more details).

itate future episodes of the illness (Post and Post, 2004: Post and Leverich, 2006).

In addition, those with these early traumatic histories continued to have an accumulation of more negative life events over the course of their illness, as revealed by the events occurring prior to the most recent episode (at an average age of about 40 at study entry). The incidence of serious suicide attempts was also associated with these negative life events, such as loss of confidants and significant others and loss of health care insurance and access to medical care (Figure 5.3).

As in the case of studies of neonatal stressors in the laboratory, adults with bipolar illness with a history of childhood adversity have lower BDNF levels compared to those without this history (Kauer Sant'Anna et al., 2007). This may

Average Course of Illness Schematized in:

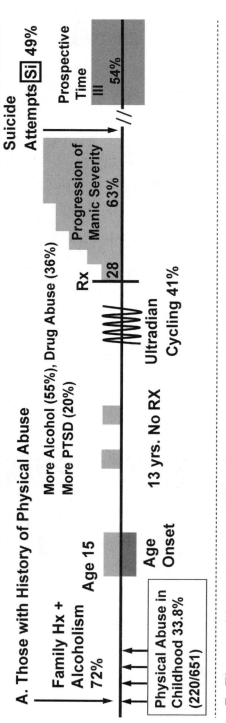

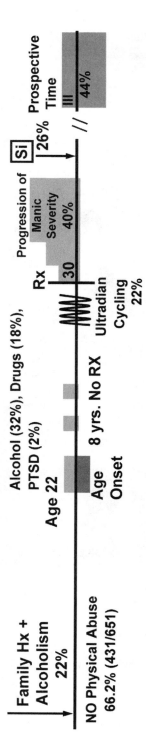

Figure 5.2 A variety of factors associated with a more adverse course of bipolar illness in adult outpatients with A.) a history of severe psychosocial traumas (physical abuse) in childhood or adolescence compared with B.) those without such a history. All findings illustrated are significantly different from history-negative individuals (Leverich, McElroy, et al., 2002).

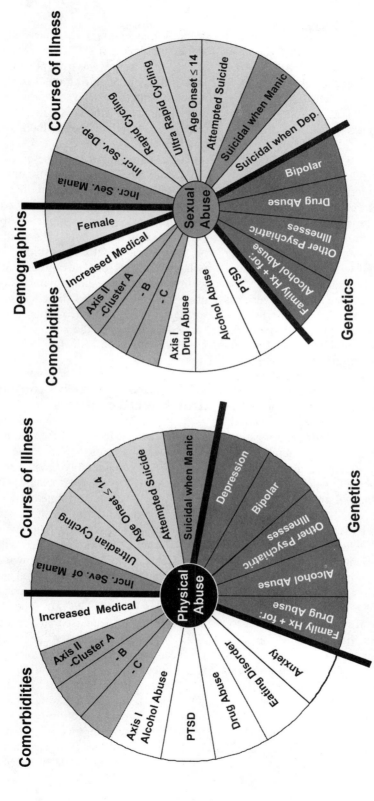

Figure 5.3 Multiple domains and correlates of early physical and sexual abuse (Leverich, McElroy, et al., 2002). Each spoke of the wheel represents a variable that is significantly different from the course and history of bipolar patients without these life stressors.

reflect changes in the brain, and combine with genetic vulnerability mediated by BDNF variants and adult stressors (which also lower BDNF) to increase risk of illness onset (see chapter 10).

Other Comorbidities and Their Prevention

Thus, it would appear that environmental and genetic vulnerabilities interact not only at illness onset, but also over its evolution, with the occurrence of negative life events in some individuals affecting the unfolding of the illness in an ongoing and complex manner. These early traumas were also associated with an increased development of personality disorders and increased likelihood of substance abuse (Leverich, McElroy, et al., 2002). As indicated in Chapter 63, substance abuse can have an additional negative impact on gene expression, as well as on the ability to maintain relationships with significant others and access appropriate health care.

It therefore appears most important to prevent, with adequate treatment, such a negative downward spiral, particularly when it is based on the convergence of both familial (genetic) and experiential (environmental) vulnerabilities. A preventive focus on substance abuse would also appear to be indicated. Adolescents with bipolar illness are at ninefold greater risk of acquiring alcohol or substance abuse than those without bipolar disorder (Wilens et al., 2004). Psychopharmacological-educational programs and support for the patient and family may be of crucial importance, not only in avoiding a second major psychiatric diagnosis with its own set of disabilities (i.e., either alcohol or substance abuse), but also in helping the patient to maintain and strengthen his or her social and medical support systems.

Breslau et al. (2000) commented on the potential relationships between PTSD and affective illness. In their epidemiological findings, they indicated that the occurrence of PTSD placed patients at high risk for subsequent major depression, similar to that observed in other anxiety disorders. Interestingly, the diagnosis of primary major affective illness also led to a higher incidence of PTSD, presumably by two routes. One route was the potential increased vulnerability to acquiring the disorder following a psychosocial stressor, but the second route was apparently through an increased exposure rate to potentially PTSD-inducing stimuli as a function of the affective illness.

The eventual impact of the co-occurrence of PTSD and bipolar illness on treatment outcome has not been systematically studied, but it is our impression that, like other comorbid diagnoses, each additional illness complicates the treatment perspective of the other. This would appear to be even clearer with comorbid PTSD and bipolar illness, as one envisions that the PTSD symptomatology could remain residually, even after the primary mood disorder is successfully treated, or vice versa. However, see Chapter 66 for a description of the successful treatment of both syndromes.

Differential Neurobiology of PTSD and Affective Illness

As schematized in Figure 5.1, the neurobiology of the two syndromes (PTSD and affective illness) differs considerably (Post, 1996). Whereas depression is typically associated with increases in the adrenal stress hormone cortisol, a blunted cortisol circadian rhythm, and resistance of cortisol to suppression by the synthetic steroid dexamethasone, PTSD is associated with the opposite effects, that is, an overall lower excretion of cortisol and an enhanced diurnal variation and increased sensitivity to suppression by dexamethasone (Yehuda, 2000). The neuropeptide somatostatin is decreased in the cerebrospinal fluid (CSF) of patients with primary affective disorder, but is increased in those with PTSD. Lymphocyte and platelet glucocorticoid receptors are downregulated in affective disorder but unregulated in PTSD, perhaps accounting for inhibiting cortisol secretion by way of negative feedback from receptors in the hippocampus. Both syndromes, however, appear to be associated with increased levels of the hypothalamic peptide corticotropin-releasing factor (CRF) in CSF. CRF has been linked to both anxiety and depression and there are attempts to develop CRF antagonists as potential antidepressants.

Whereas depression is typically associated with left frontal cortical hypometabolism, several studies have recently indicated that PTSD is associated with frontotemporal hypermetabolism (especially on the right), either at baseline or in the context of recalling memories of the traumatic event (Osuch, McCann, et al., 2001; Rauch et al., 1996; Semple et al., 1993; Shin et al., 1997). Thus, despite the convergences and co-occurrence of PTSD and primary affective illness, it appears that many of the biochemical and physiological concomitants of the two illnesses can differ considerably.

It is of particular interest that in women with major depression, a smaller hippocampal volume was found exclusively in those patients with a history of childhood trauma, and not with patients with depression only (Vythilingam et al., 2002). Smaller hippocampal volumes are seen in most studies of PTSD (Kitayama et al., 2005), but it is not certain whether it is a predisposing factor or a consequence. In the case noted in this chapter, one would not predict a smaller hippocampus, because there was no history of childhood trauma. Whether smaller hippocampal size would be associated with a history of childhood trauma in bipolar patients remains to be systematically explored.

PRINCIPLES OF THE CASE	STRENGTH OF EVIDENCE
1. Psychosocial stresses are often associated with the onset of bipolar illness.	++
2. In some instances, horrific threats to body integrity and the self, typically associated with PTSD, can also be associated with the onset of bipolar illness.	±
3. Bipolar illness and PTSD may coexist and make treatment approaches more complicated and difficult, because the optimal treatment for PTSD has not yet been well defined either as a single or comorbid syndrome.	+
4. One treatment strategy is to proceed with the drugs most useful in bipolar illness and then treat the PTSD symptomatically as necessary. However, one may look for drugs with a two-for-one efficacy profile (see 5–8 below, and Chapter 66).	±
5. Preliminary literature suggests that carbamazepine and valproate both have a role to play in the sleep disturbance and paroxysmal expression of memory intrusions and flashbacks.	+
6. One small controlled study report also suggests that lamotrigine may be helpful but will not likely improve the sleep disorder, and other agents may be needed for this purpose (as in 5 and 7).	±
7. Unpublished vignettes also suggest that gabapentin may be helpful for sleep and anxiety in some patients with PTSD.	±
8. Topiramate has been reported to be particularly effective in PTSD in a substantial case series.	+

9. Many of the newer mood-stabilizing anticonvulsant drugs may have assets over the high-potency benzodiazepines in the treatment of PTSD and comorbid anxiety syndromes in the context of bipolar disorder, because the

mood-stabilizing anticonvulsants lack the tolerance and addiction liability of the benzodiazepines.   +

10. Serotonin-selective antidepressants help some patients with PTSD and are approved for this indication in PTSD uncomplicated by bipolar disorder.   ++

11. Yohimbine and lactate both appear capable of precipitating panic attacks and flashbacks in patients with panic disorder and PTSD, which implicates alpha-2 noradrenergic receptors in the illness and potential ionic dysregulations, respectively.   +

12. Conversely, the noradrenergic alpha 1 receptor antagonist (prasosin, used in the treatment of high blood pressure) is helpful in the treatment of trauma nightmares of PTSD (Raskind et al. 2007).   +++

13. Formal controlled clinical trials indicate the effectiveness of immediate and extended social support and psychotherapeutic intervention following severe traumas.   +++

14. EMDR (eye movement desensitization therapy) appears to be more helpful for adult compared to childhood onset PTSD.   ++

15. Disappointingly, in our adult outpatients with bipolar disorder, those with a history of traumatic events in childhood have a significantly longer delay between the onset of first bipolar affective symptoms (associated with dysfunction) and first treatment, that is, about 12 years on average compared with about 8 years in those without these early adversities.   +

16. Early environmental adversity is a risk factor for early onset of bipolar illness that interacts with a positive family for bipolar illness in first degree relatives. When both are present, one should be particularly alert to early symptoms, and recommend treatment as indicated.   +++

17. In the case of severe losses and traumas in childhood, support by the other parent, a family member, or other adult can increase the child's resilience and mitigate many of the negative effects.   +

TAKE-HOME MESSAGE

Psychological and, more rarely, physical traumas can be involved in the triggering of bipolar illness. Immediate medical intervention and psychotherapeutic and family support may abort the occurrence of PTSD following a traumatic life event and may help prevent an adverse course of affective illness and the dual risk of development of comorbid substance abuse.

6

$$\sim\!\!\sim\!\!\rightarrow$$

The Role of Psychosocial Stressors
as Triggers for Episode Recurrence

CASE HISTORY

The role of stressful life events as precipitants of a first or subsequent episode is well recognized in the longitudinal course of unipolar and bipolar illness (Chapters 5 and 7). The literature is rich with studies exploring the possible pathogenic role of certain events and the interaction of psychosocial and biological factors in the evolution and progression of the illness. The life chart presented here illustrates the principle that stresses can be involved not only at the onset of illness (either depression or mania) but can also apparently be influential in the precipitation of episodes that break through otherwise effective treatment.

This patient was admitted to NIMH in 1984 after a 20-year history of bipolar disorder. Hospitalized at age 19 for a manic episode, with four more hospitalizations and a suicide attempt, she was started on lithium in 1973 (not illustrated). After several years of good functioning, symptoms of anxiety and dysphoria emerged, necessitating additional medications. After treatment with a tricyclic antidepressant (Chapter 38), the patient became manic, requiring another hospitalization in 1979, as illustrated in Figure 6.1. A pattern of continuous rapid cycling (shown in dotted lines, indicating that the timing and duration of these episodes is only approximate) eventually led to a hospitalization in 1983. Admitted to NIMH in 1984, the

patient responded to carbamazepine (Tegretol), and the response was further confirmed when she relapsed during blinded drug discontinuation and responded to the reinstitution of the combination of lithium and carbamazepine. She did well upon discharge and enjoyed being at home with her husband and small child, resuming all her activities. However, a series of stressors occurred that appeared to destabilize her illness.

The first move to another state, due to her husband's job change, (1) in Figure 6.1, was accomplished without difficulty and the patient continued to function well on her lithium-carbamazepine combination therapy. She also grieved for the death of a close relative, but did not become depressed. She settled into her new environment and described herself as having a good support system.

The possibility of another move in September 1985 because of a second potential job change for her husband was subjectively experienced as stressful, but it did not affect the patient's mood and ability to function.

When a new job assignment became official in January 1986, with all the necessities of selling and buying a house, the patient began to feel the anticipation of renewed loss of home and friends more acutely, and by early March was experiencing a mood swing into a dysphoric hypomania. Although she restabilized on steady medications, she became significantly depressed

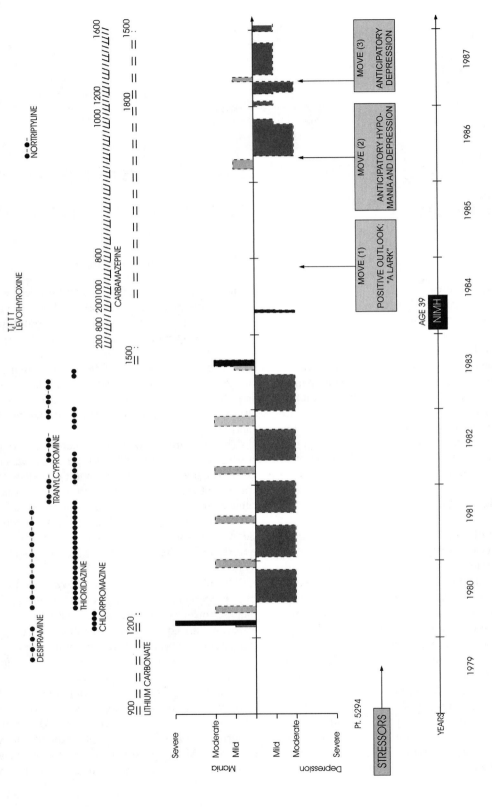

Figure 6.1 This patient responded well to lithium plus carbamazepine, but began to have breakthrough episodes with the stress of three successive moves of her household in 1984–1987.

40

once the second move (2) was accomplished. She felt suicidal, "psychologically battered," grieved the loss of her friends, missed her social support system, and struggled to help her child adjust to a new environment. An increase in both carbamazepine and lithium brought a good response within a week, and she remained stable and active for the remainder of the year.

In January 1987, however, she again became depressed when she heard of the likelihood of another job change and a third move (3) to another city. She responded to an increase in carbamazepine, but became depressed again in March when it became certain that she would have to move again and lose her familiar environment and friends. Both lithium and carbamazepine were increased again with a good response. A possible mild euphoria occurred once the move was accomplished. However, she continued to experience her repeated losses quite intensely, stating that "things are always taken away from me." By early June, she became depressed again after the move and remained depressed for several months, feeling more lonely and "vulnerable" to changes in her environment, more apprehensive about future responses to stressful life events, and expressing great concern over the reactivation of her illness.

BACKGROUND LITERATURE

Both Freud (1957/1917) and Kraepelin (1921) drew attention to a possible pathogenic role of certain events or experiences at the onset of the illness, producing melancholia or manic excitement. The life chart presented here highlights that repeated stressors can be involved not only in the precipitation or evolution of the illness in its early phase but also apparently in the reactivation of the illness in a well-stabilized patient. We know from a meta-analysis of the pertinent literature (Post, 1992) that about 60% of first episodes of recurrent unipolar or bipolar illness are precipitated by stress, but stressor occurrence is typically a less critical or necessary factor for the onset of episodes later in the illness. However, when stressors do occur, some pa-

tients remain highly susceptible to their effects, as suggested here.

A set of the neurobiological mechanisms potentially involved in this phenomenon is postulated and discussed in detail in Chapter 10. Briefly, stresses in childhood may be capable of leaving long-lasting biochemical changes or memory-like residues that can serve as vulnerability factors in the precipitation of affective episodes as an adult (Post, Weiss, & Leverich, 1994; Post et al., 1996). These long-lasting effects likely occur because stressors can influence what genes in the body get expressed. Stressors furthermore can turn on, or off, the expression of growth factors (neurotrophins) that are first involved in synaptic and structural modifications in brain pathways during embryonic development, and later in adulthood are necessary for long-term memory formation. Neurotrophins may also play a role in determining what cells survive or die by programmed cell death (apoptosis). Infants are born with about twice the number of neurons they need, and these are pruned back by programmed cell death (i.e., cell suicide or apoptosis) in latency and adolescence.

What are the clinical implications of these types of mechanisms mediating the long-lasting consequences of early stressors? This is not fully known, but it is important to emphasize that not all stress-induced changes in gene expression are pathological. Data from Meaney et al. (1988) and Plotsky and Meaney (1993) indicate that mild stressors early in life may even protect against neuronal loss and memory decline in adulthood. However, we now know that initial psychosocial stresses early in life may leave one more vulnerable to later stressor-precipitated depression (Caspi et al., 2003). The experience of parental loss early in childhood, for example, can predispose individuals to depression in adulthood, unless moderated by the caring presence of the other parent or another caretaker (Bifulco, Brown, & Harris, 1987; Breier et al., 1988). If deprivation of selected sensory systems can change the gross anatomy of the part of the brain mediating that sensation, as shown in animal studies, one could also expect that similar processes could be occurring in central nervous system structures that are important for the modulation of emotion, interpersonal communication, and social affiliation, when deprivation is severe enough (e.g., as in Romanian orphanages), or when discrete traumas occur. In animals, early reversal of the critical adversities may ameliorate the brain changes. Early intervention to ameliorate the effects of loss and deprivation may similarly be important in preventing developmental and long-range consequences in humans.

A second perspective has been presented by Dr. Mark Smith, who found that antidepressant drugs, in addition to their many effects on neurotransmitters, induced changes in the neurotrophic factors. Whereas repeated stress decreased brain-derived neurotrophic factor (BDNF) and increased neurotrophin-3 in the hippocampus (Smith, Makino, Kvetnansky, & Post, 1995b), Smith, Makino, Altemus, et al. (1995) found that chronic administration of tricyclic antidepressants that block norepinephrine uptake, as well as electroconvulsive therapy, affects neurotrophic factor expression in a manner exactly opposite to that induced by acute and chronic stressors. These findings, replicated by Nibuya et al. (1995), that chronic pretreatment with antidepressants blocks some of the effects of stress in decreasing BDNF in the hippocampus and other important areas of the brain, raise the possibility that antidepressants could have multiple levels of beneficial effect when used in long-term prophylaxis of recurrent unipolar depression. Not only will they prevent future episodes of unipolar depression, but they could lessen the neurochemical impact of stressors (and episodes by their prevention), and thereby reduce vulnerability to future recurrences.

Although all these propositions are hypothetical and remain to be directly tested, the fact that long-term prophylaxis markedly diminishes the rate of relapse in recurring unipolar depression has been unequivocally demonstrated with continuation of multiple antidepressants versus their discontinuation with placebo. Davis, Wang, and Janicak (1993) found that the likelihood of such positive results being due to chance are infinitesimally small ($p < 10^{-34}$). Thus, the hope would also be that early, sustained prophylactic treatment with lithium, carbamazepine, and valproate (which also increase BDNF) would not only prevent future episodes of bipolar illness, but would also help decrease vulnerability by increasing BDNF and other neuroprotective factors (Manji, Moore, & Chen, 2000) and prevent stress- and episode-induced lowering of BDNF.

It may be important to recognize one's own vulnerability to certain types of stressors (such as loss, separation, etc.) and use targeted "stress-immunization" psychotherapy and social support to decrease the perception and neurobiological impact of such stressors. The patient in Figure 6.1 benefited from additional doses of medication but may have needed some targeted psychotherapeutic work as well in attempting to completely abort the breakthrough depressions.

The need for opportunities to learn to cope with and manage stressful events points to the crucial role of social support and psychotherapeutic intervention to help acquire and instill a sense of mastery and adaptation to life events to lessen their negative impact and potential for pathological changes (Post and Post 2004; Post and Leverich, 2006; Miklowitz et al., 2007). We know this from the learned helplessness paradigm, in which the animals that receive a mild shock stress but do not have control over shutting it off acquire more profound and depressive-like behaviors and biochemical consequences than animals who receive the identical physical shock but are given the opportunity of coping with it actively by initiating its termination (with a nose poke or lever press; Glazer & Weiss, 1976; Maier & Jackson, 1977). In depressed patients several different types of systematic psychotherapeutic interventions were each more effective than treatment as usual in helping to achieve and maintain remission (Miklowitz et al., 2007). Interestingly in contrast, the antidepressants (either bupropion or paroxetine) were no more effective than placebo when used adjunctively to mood stabilizers in the treatment of bipolar depression (Sachs et al., 2007).

PRINCIPLES OF THE CASE	STRENGTH OF EVIDENCE
1. Mood stabilizers in combination can be effective in preventing recurrent depression and continuous cycling when antidepressants and MAOIs are not.	+
2. In addition to a role in the initial triggering of the illness, stressors can be involved in the precipitation of episodes breaking through otherwise effective treatment.	++
3. Vulnerability to repeated stressors (matching events) may be decreased through targeted psychotherapeutic intervention and social support.	+
4. Antidepressants without adequate mood stabilization can cause manic switches and continuous cycling (as seen 1980 and 1983).	+
5. Antidepressants may help lessen the negative impact of stressful life events, including preventing the lowering of neurotrophic factors (such as BDNF) in unipolar depression, but there roles in bipolar depression remains controversial.	++
6. Although lithium and valproate also increase BDNF and Bcl-2, they have not yet been shown to prevent stress-induced depletions in hippocampal BDNF, as have the antidepressants. Lithium has been shown to increase cortical grey matter volume in patients with bipolar disorder.	++
7. The atypical antipsychotics quetiapine and ziprasidone have been shown to block the effects of stress on BDNF.	++

TAKE-HOME MESSAGE

A reactivation of the underlying illness in the face of significant stressors for an individual can occur in a well-stabilized patient and highlights the importance of increased pharmacological and social support at times of heightened individual vulnerability.

7

Anniversary Reactions

CASE HISTORY

This 39-year-old woman, when admitted to the NIMH in the mid-1970s, presented with a course of bipolar illness that initially appeared to be closely linked to endocrine and stressful psychosocial events in her life. As illustrated in the life chart, she experienced a minor depression at the onset of menarche and a postpartum depression after the birth of her first child (Figure 7.1). Manic and depressive episodes in 1969 were apparently related to her husband's absence and the death of her sister-in-law.

The convergence of multiple events, including the patient's wedding anniversary, the anniversary of a friend's death, emergence of depression in another friend, and the loss of her pet cat (coupled with an inability to save its kittens), led for the first time to a full-blown major depression and subsequent switch into mania. When severely depressed again, the patient made a suicide attempt, was hospitalized, and began treatment with the tricyclic antidepressant amitriptyline (Elavil) and neuroleptics, without a notable effect on her continued manic and depressive oscillations. She was admitted to the NIMH in 1973, where antidepressant discontinuation was associated with a slight slowing of her manic-depressive cycling compared with her cycling observed on amitriptyline, but both manic and depressive phases remained largely incapacitating.

Relatively specific psychosocial stresses appeared to be associated with most of her rapid-cycling phase changes, which was generally un-

characteristic of the majority of our inpatients. On Day 3 of her hospitalization, her first depression on the unit occurred with a mood switch during her second psychotherapy hour with her physician, and a manic switch occurred in association with major marital issues on Thanksgiving Day during her first pass home. A second depression coincided with her second pass home and renewed conflict with her husband. Her second mania occurred when she walked out of an argumentative couples meeting. Her third depression occurred on Valentine's Day when she did not receive a card from her husband, and her third mania appeared on her own birthday. Her fourth depression again emerged during a stressful psychotherapy hour, and her fourth mania occurred on Easter Sunday.

As elucidated in a more detailed record of this patient's illness (Stoddard, Post, & Bunney, 1977), it appeared that passes home, issues with her husband, holidays, and important psychosocial events may have been associated with some of the patient's mood switches in the latter half of her hospitalization, despite treatment with lithium carbonate. Even upon discharge, minor episodes continued to occur in apparent close temporal relationship to birthdays and holidays (as in Chapter 6), and other life events including denial of bank loans and the birth of her first grandchild (Figure 7.1). These occurred despite an otherwise excellent response to long-term lithium treatment, which markedly decreased the rapidity and amplitude of her cyclic mood disorder (see also Chapter 11).

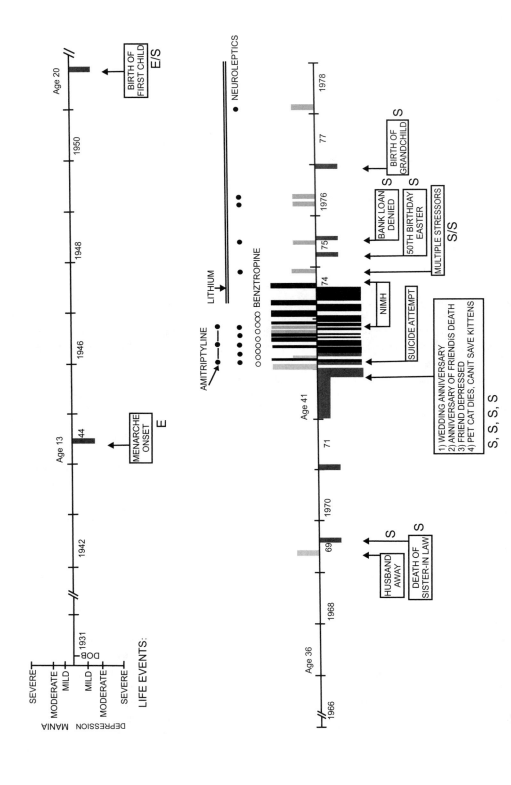

Figure 7.1 This patient's life chart illustrates the endocrine-related (E) and psychosocial stress (S) concomitants to most of her first minor and major affective episodes, with a subsequent more rapid cycling course. However, the timing of episodes continued to appear to be linked to important psychosocial precipitants in the patient's environment. An excellent response to lithium was eventually observed, even in this very rapid-cycling manic-depressive patient, but stressors continued to likely be related to minor breakthrough episodes.

46

BACKGROUND LITERATURE

Freud (1957/1917) as well as Kraepelin (1921) emphasized the role of both perceived and real losses interacting with constitutional factors in the precipitation of episodes:

> In melancholia, the occasions which give rise to the illness extend for the most part beyond the clear case of a loss by death, and include all those situations of being slighted, neglected, or disappointed which can impart opposed feelings of love and hate into the relationship or reinforce an already existing ambivalence. This conflict, due to ambivalence, which sometimes arises more from real experience, sometimes more from constitutional factors, must not be overlooked among the preconditions of melancholia. (Freud, 1957/ 1917, p. 251)

Cohen, Hammen, Henry, and Daley (2004) made similar arguments for manic precipitation by psychosocial stresses, and there is a wealth of literature concerning the more technical aspects of "funeral mania," in which an otherwise grief-precipitating situation of the loss of a loved one can result in a full-blown manic episode instead (Kubacki, 1986; Ranga, Krishnan, Swartz, Larson, & Santoliquido, 1984; Rickarby, 1977). Kessing, Agerbo, and Mortensen (2004) observed that the death of one's mother or a sibling by suicide was uniquely associated with hospitalization for mania.

Potential neurobiological explanations of this transformation from depression to mania are available from more recent biological literature, which describes how either the original or conditioned opposing mechanisms could be precipitated by the appearance of psychosocial stresses or their cued (conditioned) components (Post, Rubinow, & Ballenger, 1984). Although we have emphasized that psychosocial triggers of major episodes are more likely to be present prior to the onset of initial episodes (Post, 1992), the current case suggests that, in many patients, psychosocial stresses continue to be potential precipitating factors in subsequent episodes as well (Chapter 6; Hammen & Gitlin, 1997; Post and Post 2004; Post and Leverich 2006).

This explanation is convergent with a literature that is substantial in this regard, and even includes the early observations that many of the patients who relapsed during lithium discontinuation in the initial studies of Baastrup, Schou, and colleagues (Ahlfors et al., 1981; Baastrup, Hollnagel, Sorensen, & Schou, 1976; Baastrup, Poulsen, Schou, Thomsen, & Amdisen, 1970; Baastrup & Schou, 1967) did so with the added provocation of a variety of precipitating factors. The occurrence of more minor episodes during lithium prophylaxis in this patient and in the patient discussed in Chapter 5 suggest that psychosocial precipitants can also be involved in relapses during otherwise stable maintenance medications. This viewpoint further supports the importance of psychotherapy in addition to medication management, in the treatment of bipolar patients (Miklowitz et al., 2007).

Recent preclinical studies of the biochemical consequences of stress indicate that merely placing an animal back in an environment in which it received a stressor or a cocaine injection is sufficient (by conditioning) to reproduce many of the neurochemical effects of that stressor or the increases in dopamine overflow normally associated with cocaine. Moreover, data from Pert (1998) in our laboratory demonstrate that these kinds of biochemical alterations are sufficient to induce immediate early genes and nuclear transcription factors that then can affect which genes are subsequently turned on and off for longer-term neuronal regulation.

These kinds of data thus provide a bridge to considering how otherwise psychological events, or even their cued or conditioned correlates such as anniversary reactions and related stressors or symbols, could begin to impact some of the same neurochemical systems that are dysregulated by the illness itself and eventually become sufficient to trigger episodes, even in the relative absence of major life events.

To the extent that, for some patients, there remains this very close correlation between selective psychosocial vulnerabilities and the recurrence of new episodes (in either the unmedicated or medicated state), there is clearly a role for added psychotherapeutic and augmenting pharmacotherapeutic approaches during such times of potentially increased vulnerability. Moreover, to the degree that the unique individual sensitivities to specific types of stressful life events can be clarified, one could conceptualize the importance of targeted psychotherapeutic maneuvers to lessen the impact of such future stressors.

This would appear to be of considerable consequence as well, based on preclinical laboratory experimentation. As noted previously, animals that are given some degree of control over the termination of stressful experiences compared to their yoked controls, do not experience major neurochemical changes and depressive-like inhibition of motor and cognitive behaviors (Seligman & Beagley, 1975; Seligman & Maier, 1967).

Thus, if psychotherapy can help increase a patient's confidence of being able to cope with expected stressors more effectively, it may help decrease the perceived magnitude of the stressor and its associated changes in gene expression, thus potentially limiting its impact as a reprecipitator of episodes of illness. The data on coping are also highlighted by the study of Coplan et al. wherein primate mothers and their offspring were exposed to three different kinds of environmental manipulations involving the availability of food. In one instance, food was plentiful and readily obtainable; in the second, it was extremely scarce and the mother had to expend considerable effort to prevent the family from starving; in the third, availability of food was entirely unpredictable.

Corticotropin-releasing factor (CRF) in the cerebrospinal fluid of the preadolescent offspring of the mother was elevated only when the conditions for the mother were unpredictable. In the highly stressful condition of scarce food availability that was predictable and in which the mother apparently developed appropriate coping strategies, there were no increases in CRF in the offspring.

	STRENGTH OF EVIDENCE
PRINCIPLES OF THE CASE	
1. Endocrine-related events may be associated with initial precipitation of affective episodes that can then begin to occur in the absence of these triggers.	+++
2. Postpartum depression often heralds the onset of bipolar illness.	++
3. Life events and losses, as well as anniversary reactions, may precipitate episodes during medication-free intervals or even during treatment with otherwise apparently adequate medications.	+++
4. Lithium may be highly effective in preventing both manic and depressive episodes in some rapid-cycling patients as emphasized here and by Tondo, Hennen, and Baldessarini (2003), despite the lower incidence of response in rapid-cycling compared with non-rapid-cycling patients.	++
5. New data suggest that lithium can increase neurotrophic factors BDNF and Bcl-2 and decrease cell death factors such as BAX and p53 (Chen & Chuang, 1999; Chen et al., 1999). Valproate and carbamazepine also increase BDNF.	++
6. During times of anticipated or unanticipated increased stress, both psychopharmacological and psychosocial interventions may have an important added role.	++
7. If coping strategies can be developed to lessen the impact of anticipated stressors, it would be particularly important for those with actual or conditioned stress or sensitivity.	+
8. As-needed use of benzodiazepines or other sleep-assisting medications during periods of acute grief reaction may be helpful in lessening associated sleep loss and decreasing liability of the induction of mania	

through a sleep-loss mechanism. +

9. Adjunctive use of a mood stabilizer or increased dose of an ongoing regimen may also be considered at these times of increased vulnerability. ++

10. Increased psychosocial support by family members and significant others at times of anticipated high stress could also be built into the treatment regimen when the patient is in the well state. +

TAKE-HOME MESSAGE

Internal endocrine and external life events may both be associated with the precipitation of affective episodes and provide a paradigm for considering how both physiological and psychological occurrences can affect neurobiological systems potentially involved in the triggering of affective episodes. Lithium and other drugs affecting neurotrophic factors may play a key role in the amelioration of such triggered and automatic affective vulnerabilities in many individuals.

8

The Development of Two Different Types of Treatment Resistance: Tolerance Versus Treatment Discontinuation and Loss of Efficacy Following Relapse

BACKGROUND LITERATURE

The life chart figures illustrating tolerance to the long-term effects of lithium, carbamazepine, and valproate appear in Chapters 12, 19, and 24, respectively. The discussions of lithium discontinuation refractoriness and associated life charts are in Chapters 11 and 12. This chapter is a general introduction (without a specific life chart) to the theme of the involvement of differential mechanisms when losing a response to a previously effective drug, because this may have differential therapeutic implications as well. This discussion may also be a useful prelude to the general presentation of the psychopharmacology and neurobiology of bipolar illness in the next two chapters.

Tolerance

Tolerance is a form of treatment resistance that slowly develops over time after an initial successful response to a given agent. It is most cogently demonstrated during long-term treatment of a recurrent illness when there is substantial and sustained clinical improvement; that is, a remission is achieved that is many times longer than the longest previous well interval. This would suggest that initial clinical responsiveness to a given agent has been demonstrated. However, with a further extension of chronic treatment, episodes of affective illness may begin to progressively emerge with increasing frequency, severity, or duration, such that the drug is clearly no longer effective.

In this example, we are not referring to the development of tolerance as commonly used in describing drug addiction, where one is able to tolerate increasingly large doses of opiates, for example, but rather the progressive emergence of breakthrough affective episodes during long-term prophylactic treatment (with the same doses that were originally clinically effective). This type of treatment resistance does not appear to be related to altered blood levels of the drug but to emergence of episodes despite ongoing treatment with the same dose achieving the same blood levels. Thus, we call this type of tolerance *pharmacodynamic* (related to drug actions and efficacy) rather than *pharmacokinetic* (related to drug levels in blood and brain).

The development of tolerance is a well-recognized phenomenon in a variety of neuropsychiatric syndromes, perhaps best illustrated in the paroxysmal pain syndrome of trigeminal neuralgia. In this illness, patients experience recurrent episodes of brief but intolerable shooting facial pain along the distribution of the facial (or trigeminal) nerve. The syndrome almost invariably responds dramatically to treatment with an anticonvulsant such as carbamazepine or oxcarbazepine. However, with long-term administration of carbamazepine, a substantial percentage of patients begin to reexperience the paroxysms of shooting facial pain despite maintenance of doses similar to those previously effective and, in some instances, in spite of increases in dose and blood levels in an attempt to regain responsivity (Pazzaglia & Post, 1992).

Similar phenomena appear to occur with the treatment of panic attacks in some patients (Wesner & Noyes, 1988) and in the long-term prevention of manic and depressive episodes. Tolerance has been observed during long-term treatment with lithium (Post, Leverich, Pazzaglia, Mikalauskas, & Denicoff, 1993; Koukopoulos et al., 1995), carbamazepine (Post, Leverich, Rosoff, & Altshuler, 1990), and valproate (Post, Ketter, Denicoff, Leverich, & Mikalauskas, 1993). It has also been reported in a subgroup of patients with unipolar depression who lost response to antidepressants (Cohen & Baldessarini, 1985) and monoamine oxidase inhibitors (Mann, 1983) after a considerable period of therapeutic efficacy. In some instances, this progression of episode reemergence breaking through long-term pharmacotherapy mirrors the initial progression of episodes in the medication-free condition in which, as noted in Chapters 2, 3, and 4, there is an overall tendency for increasing frequency, severity, or duration of episodes over time.

Potential neurobiological mechanisms related to the development of tolerance and possible pharmacological approaches to its occurrence are discussed in the specific case presentations and chapters to follow as noted above. A general principle in approaching tolerance is to attempt to circumvent it by using another effective agent that acts via a new biochemical mechanism, such that there is not cross-tolerance

from the first to the second drug. In the face of loss of efficacy of a drug by a tolerance process, a period of time off the previously effective medication may also be a useful consideration in eventually reestablishing efficacy to that same drug (Pazzaglia & Post, 1992).

Treatment Discontinuation and Related Refractoriness

An entirely different illness pattern and process appears to be occurring in instances of lithium discontinuation-induced refractoriness, as discussed in Chapter 13. This phenomenon differs from tolerance in that patients do not begin to experience relapses until they have tapered or discontinued treatment altogether with the effective agent. Once an episode has reemerged in the subsequent medication-free condition, a small percentage (perhaps 10–15%) of patients who were initially highly responsive to lithium fail to have as good a response as they originally had, despite reinstitution of the drug at similar or higher doses and blood levels (Maj, Pirozzi, & Magliano, 1995; Post, Leverich, et al., 1992, 1993). In these instances, we believe that the recurrence of the episode in a medication-free period leads to increased aggressiveness of the illness and more complex neuropathological processes that may be sufficient to overwhelm the mechanisms of action of the drug that were originally effective in preventing episodes.

We highlight the distinction between these two patterns of treatment resistance because their mechanisms and treatment approaches appear to be radically different, and therefore the patterns need to be distinguished. In the case of tolerance development, illness gradually reemerges despite maintenance of the previously effective treatment. In this instance, a period off the medication may, in fact, be helpful. In the instances of treatment refractoriness induced by discontinuation of lithium, the discontinuation of treatment is, in fact, the apparent cause of the refractoriness, since it leads not only to episode reemergence in a high proportion of patients, but also in a small number of patients to the failure of lithium to again be as effective as previously, once it is restarted. In some studies, this lesser effectiveness is revealed by the need for higher concomitant doses of antipsychotic medication than were previously necessary. In other isolated cases, this can manifest as a complete failure to rerespond to lithium at maximally tolerated doses, and even with the addition of other adjunctive treatments regaining responsiveness may be difficult.

Some of the ways of dealing with these two different types of unfortunate occurrence are listed in the next section. Both tolerance and lithium discontinuation-related loss of previous good response obviously need to be differentiated from another common type of treatment resistance, that is, the failure to respond to a given treatment from the outset.

PRINCIPLES OF THE CASE
STRENGTH OF EVIDENCE

1. Even after the institution of a fully successful drug treatment or combination drug regimen, a pattern of progressive episode breakthroughs may occasionally occur, leading to a loss of treatment responsiveness via tolerance. +

2. This loss of responsiveness can occur with all the major mood stabilizers, but perhaps to a lesser degree with valproate compared with carbamazepine or lamotrigine, although this has not been directly assessed. ±

3. Tolerance can also occur with the most established treatments such as electroconvulsive therapy and possibly with experimental approaches such as repetitive transcranial magnetic stimulation of the brain. +

4. When tolerance occurs to maximally tolerated doses of a drug, the general approach has been to add or switch to alternative drugs with novel mechanisms of action (i.e., ones that will not possess cross-tolerance). +

5. An alternative to this approach, but essentially an untested possibility, is a period of time off the medication that has lost efficacy (via tolerance) followed by reinstitution of the previously effective regimen at a later time. ±

6. Ways of avoiding tolerance development from the outset have not been adequately studied or delineated. However, several possibilities have been considered based on preclinical data or anecdotal observations in individual patients, including the following:

   a. Using highly effective regimens from the outset, that is, ones that produce remission of symptoms. ++

   b. Instituting treatment earlier rather than later in the course of the illness, before multiple neural systems may become involved. +

   c. Using moderate doses of drugs rather than those that are marginally or minimally effective, and that subsequently require dose escalation in order to maintain response. ±

   d. Preventing other factors that can increase pathological "illness drive," such as avoiding alcohol and drugs of abuse that may provide neurobiological perturbations that add to those of the primary affective disorder. ++

   e. Using combination therapy or complex combination therapy, as it is thought that employing drugs with multiple mechanisms of therapeutic action may result in a reduced likelihood of illness reemergence and loss of treatment response. ±

   f. Possibly using thyroid augmentation (see Chapter 62). +

   g. Not lowering the dose of an effective treatment unnecessarily (i.e., when side effects are not a problem), as this maneuver may render one more vulnerable to breakthrough episodes. ++

h. Not withdrawing or discontinuing one component of an effective treatment combination regimen. This consideration adds to evaluation of the risk-to-benefit ratio of attempting to simplify an effective complex combination regimen merely on aesthetic or philosophical grounds rather than when it is really needed to reduce the side-effects burden. +

7. Principles of avoiding lithium discontinuation-induced refractoriness:

a. Be aware of the extensive range of potential dangers of discontinuing lithium when it has been a sustained effective treatment:

   i. 50% of patients will relapse in the first 5 months off lithium. ++

   ii. Even a slow taper may not reduce the risk of relapse. +

   iii. Some may lose jobs, disrupt marriages, or require hospitalization. ++

   iv. Reresponse may take a substantial period of time or require more medicines than were originally needed. ++

   v. Suicide risk increases dramatically in those off compared with those on lithium treatment. +++

   vi. A small subgroup (about 10–15%) may not reacquire the same degree of response to lithium that they had previously experienced. +

   vii. Stopping lithium could result in progression of the neurobiological alterations associated with the illness. There is increasing evidence that lithium protects the brain; for example, lithium increases the production of neurons and their growth factors; increases the production of glia and their growth factors; helps keep nerve cells alive by decreasing programmed cell death; decreases the size of a stroke and the amount of neurological deficit; and increases brain gray matter (nerve cell bodies) in patients with bipolar disorder. Removing this protection could thus renew, increase, or accelerate unwanted changes in the brain that make reresponse more difficult. +

b. Be conservative. Do not stop an effective treatment, even if one is feeling all better. ++

c. Reconceptualize the illness as a long-term, potentially progressive brain disorder similar to multiple sclerosis or epilepsy that must be rigorously treated to avoid relapses. ++

d. When sustained remissions do occur in the course of treatment, treasure having no disability and no episodes, and do not risk any of the grave consequences listed in 7a. ++

TAKE-HOME MESSAGE

When remission is achieved and sustained, be conservative and stay the course without further unnecessary medication alterations. Conversely, in the face of illness reemergence through previously adequate treatment, be more radical and continue to alter the pharmacotherapeutic regimen until a good effect is achieved.

Part III

PHARMACOLOGY AND NEUROBIOLOGY OF BIPOLAR ILLNESS

9

Fundamentals of Psychopharmacology Pertinent to Treatment of the Bipolar Disorders

Although any detailed approach to psychopharmacology is beyond the scope of this book, it would appear useful for the well-informed lay reader and bipolar patient to have some background introduction to the neurobiology of bipolar illness (Chapter 10) and the potential mechanisms of action of different drugs used to treat it.

ANATOMY AND PHYSIOLOGY

The major mechanism for communication between nerve cells and the brain is the electrical firing of one cell, which releases a packet of neurochemical substances (transmitters) into the area between cells (the synapse). There they bind and activate the receptors of the next cell (Figure 9.1), which, in turn, then fires electrically. When a nerve cell fires, the balance of ions outside and inside the cell changes dramatically. With firing (or depolarization), sodium and calcium ions rush inside the cell, while potassium and chloride ions move to the outside of the cell more slowly to repolarize it. The major drugs used in the treatment of the mood disorders are thought to act directly on either the transmitters that convey messages between cells or on ion balances within the nerve cells.

Three chemical biogenic amine messenger systems, in particular, have been implicated in depression and mania (Figure 9.2). These include the catecholamines norepinephrine (NE) and dopamine (DA), and the indoleamine serotonin (5-HT). Cells that contain these chemicals are strategically located for their widespread effects on brain functioning. The cell bodies containing these amines are located in the brain stem or midbrain, and their long axonal processes reach to virtually every area of the forebrain and cerebral cortex.

Although relatively few cells contain NE (about 10,000 in the compact area called the locus coeruleus located in the middle of the brain stem), their diffuse ramifications are capable of altering mood, anxiety, and arousal in widespread areas of the brain. Similarly, serotonin neurons are located largely in the slightly higher midline structure in the brain stem called the raphe nucleus.

The dopamine cell bodies are located in the midbrain area, called the substantia nigra because of the black pigment contained in these dopamine cell bodies. The dopamine cells in the nigra that project to the striatum that are involved in Parkinson's disease are located in the more lateral or A9 area, whereas the dopamine neurons that project to the frontal cortex (in-

57

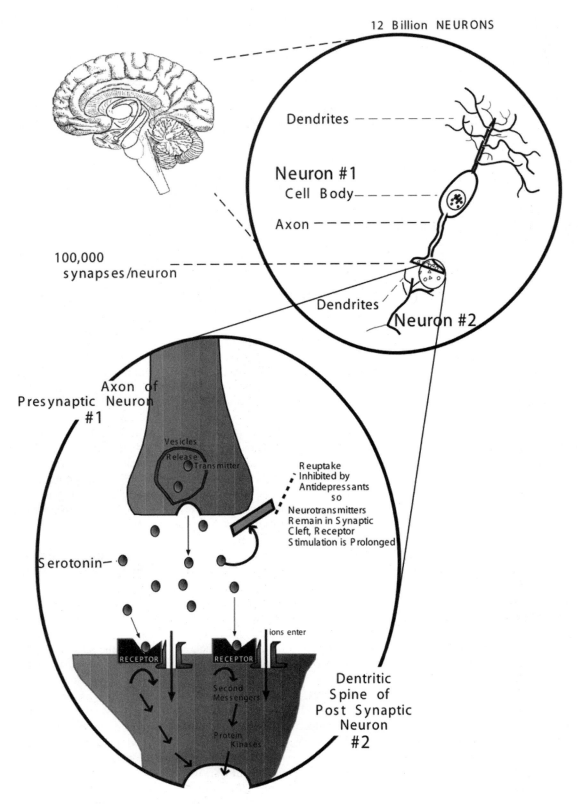

Figure 9.1 An inside look at neurochemistry. The brain (top, left) is made up of 12 billion neurons (top circle), and communication between neurons occurs with synaptic release of chemicals such as serotonin, which act as receptors on the next neuron and then are taken back up presynaptically, by the serotonin transporter, to inactivate the process of chemical transmission.

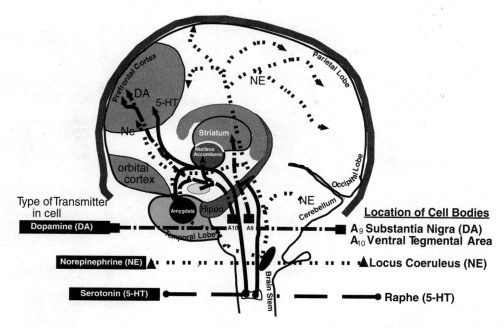

Figure 9.2 Amine systems implicated in mood. Different cell groups contain different neurotransmitters. Dopamine neurons in the substantia nigra are lost in parkinsonism.

volved in stress management, memory, and planning), the amygdala (conditioning and emotion), and nucleus accumbens (activating and reward areas of the brain) are located more medially in area A10, also called the ventral tegmental area (VTA). Possible relationships of these brain areas and their upstream target areas to some of the signs and symptoms of depression are schematized in Figure 9.3.

CATEGORIES OF TREATMENT FOR BIPOLAR ILLNESS AND THEIR ACTIONS

Antidepressants

The major treatment for bipolar illness can be roughly categorized into three groups (Figure 9.4). Unimodal antidepressants have been studied and approved for unipolar depression, but their use in bipolar disorder remains highly controversial. Not only may they not be very effective in bipolar depression (Sachs et at., 2007), but they may cause an overswing into a hypo-

mania or mania (Post et al., 2006; Leverich et al., 2006). Similarly, the older typical antipsychotics as unimodal antimanics treat mania but may exacerbate depression. Some of the newer or atypical antipsychotics, however, also improve depression. The mood stabilizers (lithium, carbamazepine, valproate, and to some extent lamotrigine) help in both phases of the illness. Each class is discussed in detail below. Some general biochemical effects of each drug thought to be important in their action are simplified in Figure 9.5, along with a general coding of the level of evidence for their efficacy in mania (symbols on left) and depression (symbols on right).

Effects of Serotonin in Depression: Serotonin-Active Treatments Considerable data now indicate a prominent role for serotonin in depression. Many of the antidepressants act on serotonin systems and if serotonin function is interfered with, the antidepressant effects of these substances are temporarily lost. How do the antidepressants exert effects on the serotonin system? When packets of serotonin are released

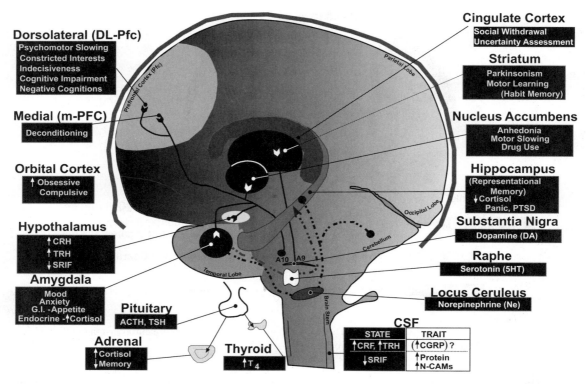

Figure 9.3 Possible regional neurobiology of depressive symptoms. CRH, corticotropin-releasing hormone; TRH, thyrotropin-releasing hormone; SRIF, somatostatin; G.I., gastrointestinal; ACTH, adrenocorticotropin hormone; TSH, thyroid stimulating hormone; CGRP, calcitonin gene-related peptide; N-CAMs, neural cell adhesion molecule.

with electrical impulses, they remain in the space between the neurons, that is, the synapse, and periodically attach in a specific fashion to receptors on the next neuron in a key-in-lock fashion (Figure 9.1). The effect of serotonin at its receptors is terminated by active reuptake of serotonin back into the nerve terminal (Figure 9.6). Most antidepressants block this process of serotonin reuptake or inactivation. This makes more serotonin available at the synapse for a longer time, which leads to more stimulation of the serotonin receptors on the next nerve cell. There are 17 different types of serotonin receptors, and the serotonin-related antidepressants nonspecifically enhance serotonin tone at all of them by increasing synaptic serotonin levels.

The older tricyclic antidepressants (TCAs) tended to be relatively weak blockers of serotonin reuptake and not at all specific or selective. They had a variety of other actions, some of which were associated with substantial side effects. The newer generation of selective serotonin reuptake inhibitors (SSRIs) are both more potent and more selective for serotonin. They tend to be associated with fewer side effects compared with the older antidepressants of the TCA class, which often are associated with constipation, dry mouth, blurry vision (because of their effects of blocking acetylcholine), sedation, and low blood pressure (because of their effects of blocking adrenergic systems and histamine). The older TCAs were also more toxic in overdose than many of the newer agents. The secondary amine antidepressants desmethylimipramine (DMI; Norpramine) and nortriptyline (Pamelor) have fewer side effects than their older tertiary amine structural relatives—imipramine (Tofranil) and amitriptyline (Elavil), respectively, which have three methyl groups instead of two.

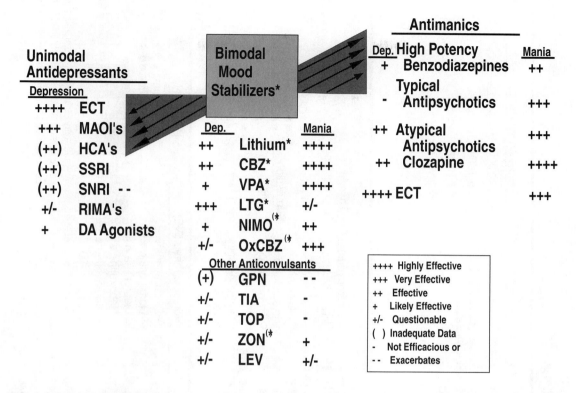

Figure 9.4 Categories of treatments used in manic-depressive illness. Unimodal antidepressants highly effective in unipolar depression may not be as effective in bipolar depression and may exacerbate mania. ECT, electroconvulsive therapy; MAOIs, monoamine oxidase inhibitors; HCAs, heterocyclic antidepessants; SSRI, selective serotonin reuptake inhibitors; SNRI, serotonin and norepinephrine reuptake inhibitors; RIMAs, reversible inhibitors of monoamine oxidase type A; TCA, tricyclic antidepressants; DA, dopamine; CBZ, carbamazepine; VPA, valproate; LTG, lamotrigine; GPN, gabapentin; TOP, topiramate; NIMO, nimodipine; OxCBZ, oxcarbazepine; *, likely mood stabilizers.

At the same time, the SSRIs as a class—which include fluoxetine (Prozac), sertraline (Zoloft), paroxetine (Paxil), fluvoxamine (Luvox), citalopram (Celexa), and escitalopram (Lexapro)—are also effective in panic anxiety disorders and obsessive-compulsive disorder. Nefazodone (Serzone) blocks serotonin reuptake in a potent fashion (like the SSRIs), and inhibits or blocks serotonin type-2 receptors as well. This latter effect is shared by trazodone (Desyrel) and is thought to account for the ability of nefazodone to increase slow wave (or deep) sleep in both normal volunteers and in patients with affective disorders. Conversely, the SSRIs may produce insomnia as a side effect, along with headache and stomach upset.

Carbamazepine increases serotonin levels in the hippocampus by mechanisms that are not clearly delineated. However, carbamazepine also decreases levels of somatostatin in spinal fluid and increases substance P levels in striatum. These findings are of interest because serotonin coexists with the peptides thyrotropin-releasing hormone (TRH) and substance P in the raphe neurons, and these neurons project diffusely to structures thought to be involved in the modulation of mood and behavior, including impulsivity, aggression, and suicide. TRH may be an endogenous antidepressant substance, as administering it often alleviates depression.

Thus, increasing serotonergic tone is generally thought to be involved in the mechanism of action of the antidepressants as well as drugs active in anxiety disorders, aggression, and im-

Drug Efficacy

In ●● Mania ●● In Depression

Antimanics (AMs)

Benzodiazepines
↑Cl⁻ influx
potentiate GABA
●Clonazepam ○
●Lorazepam ○
Indirect
○Levetiracetam ○

Typical Antipsychotics
$Block\ D_2\ Receptors$
●● Trifluperazine –
●● Haloperidol –
●● Molindone –

●● Atypical Antipsychotics (AA) to ○ to ●●
Block mesolimbic dopamine D_1, D_2, D_4 and 5-HT$_2$ receptors
Clozapine, Risperidone, Olanzapine, Quetiapine, Ziprasidone
Partial Agonist at D_1, D_2, D_3 & 5HT$_{1A}$-R
Aripiprazole

Atypicals Antipsychotics?
●● Clozapine ○
●● Risperidone ○
●● Olanzapine ●
●● Quetiapine ●●
●● Ziprasidone ○
●● Aripiprazole ●

Mood Stabilizers*, Anticonvulsants(AC), Others

↓2nd Messengers, G Proteins, ↓calcium influx
●●Lithium ●*
●●Carbamazepine ●*
●●Oxcarbazepine○
●●Valproate ●*

↑brain GABA
●●(Valproate) ●*
––(Gabapentin) ○
–(Tiagabine) ○
–(Topiramate) ○

↓Glutamate release (via ↓Na⁺)
●●Carbamazepine ●*
●●Lamotrigine ●●*
–(Topiramate)○
–Zonisamide○
↓Glutamate (AMPA-R)
–(Topiramate) ○

(Dihydropyridine) ↓L-type Ca⁺⁺ Channels
● Nimodipine●
○ Isradipine○
○ Amlodipine○
(Phenylalkylamine)
●Verapamil –

Thyroid: Augmentation
○T$_3$ ○
Supression
High Dose
○T$_4$ ○

Antidepressants (ADs)

Dopamine (DA)
– Bupropion ●●
– Pramipexole ●

Serotonin (5-HT)
– Fluoxetine ●●
– Sertraline ●●
– Paroxetine ●●
– Fluvoxamine ●●
– Citalopram ●●

5-HT Plus
– Nefazodone ●●
– Mirtazapine ●●

Norepinephrine (NE)
– Desipramine ●●
– Nortriptyline ●●
– Maprotiline ●
– Reboxetine ●
– Atomoxetine ●

5-HT and Ne
– Clomipramine ●●
–– Venlafaxine ●●
– Duloxetine ●●

Figure 9.5 Mechanistic classes of medications used in bipolar illness. Symbols on left refer to the level of evidence for antimanic efficacy and on the right for antidepressant effects. Dark circles indicate definite to likely effectiveness; open circles and minus symbol indicate possible to not effective. Cl, chloride; GABA, gamma-aminobutyric acid. Antidepressant effectiveness is based on studies in unipolar depression and these drugs are not recommended in monotherapy for bipolar depression and even as adjuncts to mood stabilizers may not be very efficacious in bipolar illness.

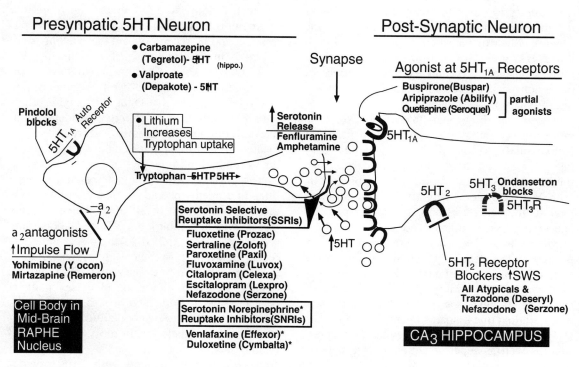

Figure 9.6 Mechanisms of antidepressant action. 5-HT, serotonin.

pulse dyscontrol disorders, and possibly in the prevention of suicide. How the serotonergic system gets reset by the serotonin-active drugs, and how this relates to the neuropeptide changes, remains to be delineated. Peptide cotransmitters such as TRH typically exert their effects over much longer periods than those of the classical neurotransmitters, and the reset of these peptide systems potentially occurring within the serotonin neurons could be important to their longer-term antidepressant effects.

The antianxiety drug buspirone directly activates 5-HT$_{1A}$ receptors, which could explain its effects in generalized anxiety disorders and in treatment of mild depression. Trazodone, like nefazodone, also has the ability to block 5-HT$_2$ receptors, perhaps accounting for its widespread use as a sleep-augmenting strategy in addition to its traditional role as an antidepressant. Trazodone is also an antidepressant that can be used at night with monoamine oxidase inhibitors (MAOIs) if these are associated with sleep disruption, as they very often are.

It is interesting that all of the atypical antipsychotics block 5-HT$_2$ receptors (in addition to their primary effect in blocking dopamine receptors), and it is thought that 5-HT$_2$ receptor blockade could account for their better antidepressant properties than the older antipsychotics, which did not possess this effect. Thus, as noted below, the antipsychotic clozapine could exert its putative mood-stabilizing effects through its unique profile of not only blocking D$_2$ and other dopamine receptors (thought to be related to its antimanic and antipsychotic effects), but also through its ability to block alpha 2, 5-HT$_2$, and many other receptors.

Norepinephrine in Depression Some antidepressants appear to work through selective blockade of NE reuptake in the terminal regions (such as the hippocampus and cortex) of the axon extensions of the cells in the locus coeruleus. These drugs, including the older DMI, nortriptyline, and maprotiline (Ludiomil), and the newer atomoxetine (Strattera) are relatively selective in their ability to block the reuptake of NE, making this substance increasingly available at the synapse. Most of the older TCAs affected both the 5-HT and NE neurotransmitter systems rather nonselectively and exerted a variety of other nonspecific effects including sedation and high toxicity in overdoses.

The newer drugs venlafaxine (Effexor) and duloxetine (Cymbalta) are potent and more selective inhibitors of both 5-HT and NE reuptake, that is, serotonin-norepinephrine reuptake inhibitors. Perhaps because of its potency on both of these systems, venlafaxine is reported to have antidepressant effects in a larger percentage of depressed patients and in some patients refractory to SSRIs. Like the older TCA chlorpromazine (Anafranil), which affects both 5-HT and NE reuptake, venlafaxine is also helpful in the treatment of a variety of pain syndromes because of its dual transmitter effects. A new drug—duloxetine—shares venlafaxine's dual (5-HT and NE) action, conveying antidepressant, as well as superior antipain effects (compared to the SSRIs).

Mirtazapine (Remeron) indirectly increases neuronal firing, the release of both 5-HT and NE (by blocking presynaptic inhibitory NE alpha 2 receptors).

Dopamine The antidepressant effects of drugs working on dopamine systems are much less well developed (Figure 9.7). An older drug, nomifensine, selectively blocked dopamine reuptake, but was removed from the market because of problematic side effects. Bupropion (Wellbutrin) does not appear to be a very potent blocker of dopamine reuptake, but it does increase synaptic levels of dopamine in areas of the brain thought to be involved with mood, motivation, reward, and drug self-administration (i.e., the nucleus accumbens or ventral striatum).

The dorsal striatum or caudate nucleus is more related to motor activity and is affected in Parkinson's disease (motor slowing and tremor). A blockade of the dopamine receptor in the caudate causes the side effects, such as Parkinsonism and tardive dyskinesia of the older major tranquilizers (neuroleptics or typical antipsy-

chotics). Pramipexole (Mirapex) and ropinirole hydrochloride (Requip) directly stimulate dopamine D_2 and D_3 receptors, and these agonists are effective in the treatment of Parkinson's disease. Pramipexole now appears to have good antidepressant effects as well. Bromocriptine (Parlodel) is a selective D_2 agonist, and if pramipexole proves a more effective antidepressant, it would implicate D_3 agonism. D_3 receptors are located in perilimbic areas that are implicated in mood regulation.

The psychomotor stimulants cocaine, pemoline, and methylphenidate (Ritalin and Dexadrine) block uptake of all three amine systems (5-HT, NE, dopamine), but effects on dopamine are most closely linked to their activating effects (Figure 9.7). In the case of amphetamines, because of their robust and acute effects on the dopamine system, they cause increases in attention, energy, activity, and arousal in the short term, but tend not to be good antidepressants for long-term administration in most patients. Psychomotor stimulants are used as augmentation strategies in some patients with refractory depression and are also used in some elderly patients who do not tolerate the side effects of some of the other antidepressant compounds. They and the related stimulant pemoline are widely used in the treatment of attention-deficit/hyperactivity disorder (ADHD) in children. Bupropion also has positive effects in ADHD. The newer FDA-approved drug atomoxetine has a selective effect on NE and is one of the drugs used for ADHD not acting on dopamine.

Another nonstimulant drug effective in ADHD and approved for the treatment of narcolepsy is modafinil (Provigil). Its mechanism of action is not well described, but it appears highly promising as an adjunctive treatment in bipolar patients with residual symptoms of depression, fatigue, and poor concentration (Frye et al., 2007). It appears to convey sustained antidepressant augmentation effects without inducing switches into mania.

MAOIs In contrast to the traditional TCAs and heterocyclics (bupropion has one ring and maprotiline has four rings), as well as the newer antidepressants that are inhibitors of NE or 5-

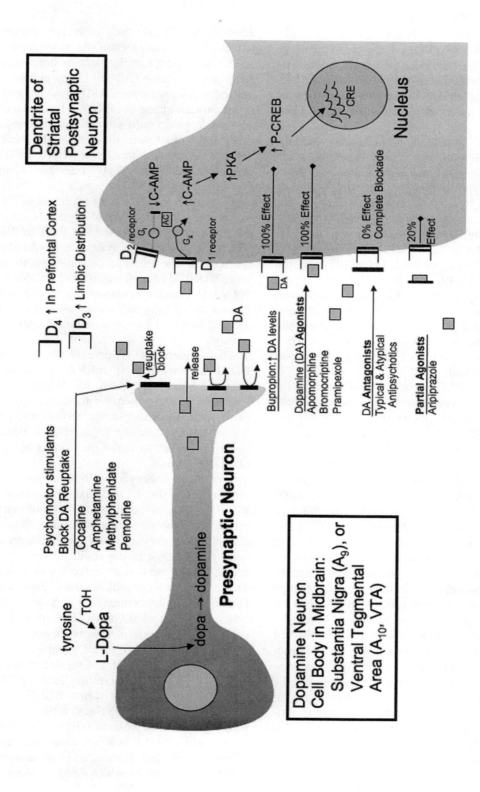

Figure 9.7 Drug actions at the dopamine synapse. DA, dopamine; TOH, tyrosine hydroxylase; C-AMP, cyclic-adenosine monophosphate; PKA, protein kinase A; P-CREB, phosphorylated cyclic AMP response element binding protein; CRE, cyclic-AMP response element (on DNA).

HT reuptake, the MAOIs appear to act by inhibiting the breakdown of these amines in the nerve terminal by an enzyme called monoamine oxidase. Thus, with the use of an MAOI, more biogenic amines remain in the presynaptic nerve terminal for potential release with each electrical impulse.

With the traditional nonselective MAOIs, which inhibit both the A and B forms of the enzyme, there was a risk of high blood pressure, that is, a hypertensive crisis caused by foods that contain tyramine, a potent releaser of NE. With tyramine, large amounts of NE (that cannot be rapidly broken down because of the inhibition of MAO) are released, causing the extreme high blood pressure. If one is taking the traditional MAOIs, one should carry a 10 mg pill of nifedipine (Procardia, a calcium channel blocker), which will inhibit a high blood pressure reaction and the associated headache while the patient is on the way to the doctor's office or emergency room to have his or her blood pressure checked.

There are MAOIs that are also selective for the A-type enzyme that is thought to mediate the antidepressant effects of the drug but are much less likely to cause hypertensive crises. The A-selective drugs include clorgyline and brofaramine (which are not available), and moclobemide (Manerix), which is approved in Canada and is available from most Canadian pharmacies. Moclobemide is a reversible inhibitor of monoamine oxidase type A (RIMA). With this drug, diet is of less importance and the chances for a high blood pressure reaction following ingestion of substances containing high concentrations of tyramine is virtually absent, although most investigators think moclobemide is less effective than the older nonselective MAOIs.

Selegiline is a new type A selective MAOI antidepressant that comes in a skin patch formulation. It has not been studied in bipolar depression, and some feel relatively high doses of the drug, where it is no longer A selective, are required for good antidepressant efficacy in unipolar depression.

Effects of Antidepressants on Brain-Derived Neurotrophic Factor As a group, antidepressants have the ability, via their aminergic effects, to affect intracellular mechanisms resulting in the induction of new proteins such as brain-derived neurotrophic factor (BDNF). They enhance the second messenger cyclic AMP (cAMP) and activate protein kinase A (PKA), which attaches a phosphate group onto a variety of proteins and enzymes in order to facilitate or inhibit their actions. One protein that is activated by PKA phosphorylation is cAMP response element binding protein (CREB), which binds to DNA and is needed to activate the synthesis of a variety of new proteins. Antidepressants increase the amount of phosphorylated CREB (pCREB), which is necessary to stimulate the DNA to begin transcribing the message (via mRNA) to make more BDNF (Figure 9.8, left side). BDNF is involved in cellular communication as a neurotransmitter and in cell survival as a growth factor, and is necessary for long-term learning and memory.

The antidepressants increase the amount of BDNF message (BDNF mRNA) in the hippocampus. Messenger RNA for BDNF is then translated at the protein synthesizing apparatus of the cell (the endoplasmic reticulum), where amino acids are strung together in a beadlike fashion in order to make the correct sequence of BDNF protein.

Smith and colleagues (1995) in our laboratory were the first to find that stress decreased BDNF mRNA in the hippocampus and that this effect was opposite to that of antidepressants. If animals were stressed while they were on antidepressants, some of the ability of stress to decrease BDNF and other effects was blocked. These findings were replicated and extended by Duman (2002) and colleagues at Yale, with the observation that most known antidepressants increased this cascade of effects, beginning with increased NE or 5-HT in the synapse; receptor activation; activation of the second messenger cAMP, PKA, the transcription factor pCREB; and finally the synthesis of new BDNF. Duman et al. proposed that BDNF was a final common pathway for antidepressant effects (Figure 9.8). Interestingly, BDNF is active in animal models of depression, and represents an attractive potential mechanism by which antidepressants (in-

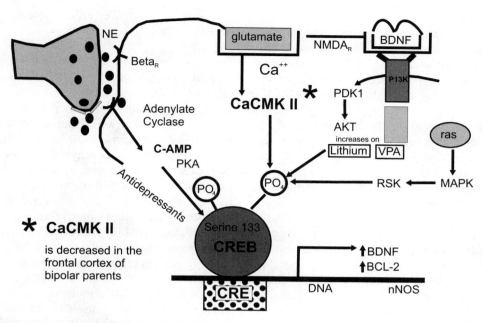

Figure 9.8 Pathways to phosphorylation of CREB and activation of cell survival factors. NE, norepinephrine; Beta$_R$, beta receptors; C-AMP, cyclic adenosine monophosphate; PKA, protein kinase A; Ca, calcium; CaCMKII, calcium calmodulin kinase II; NMDA$_R$, *N*-methyl-D-aspartate receptor; BDNF, brain-derived neurotrophic factor; CREB, c-AMP response element binding protein; RSK, ribosomal kinase; MAPK, mitogen-activated protein kinase; VPA, valproate; PDK, pyruvate dehydrogenase kinase; nNOS, neuronal nitric oxide synthase; CRE, cyclic AMP response element; AKT, also known as protein kinase B; PO$_4$, phosphorylated.

cluding ECT) with initially diverse mechanisms of action may exert a common effect.

Mood Stabilizers: Lithium, Carbamazepine, Valproate, and Lamotrigine

Effects on Cell Excitability The first three mood stabilizers (lithium, carbamazepine, and valproate) are so named not only because of their ability to treat mania acutely, but also because they prevent the recurrence of both manic and depressive episodes in bipolar patients during long-term (prophylactic) administration (Figure 9.4). These agents include the classic drug for bipolar illness, lithium carbonate (Eskalith, Lithane, and Cibalith), and the more recently used mood-stabilizing anticonvulsants carbamazepine (Tegretol, Carbatrol, and Equetro) and valproate (Depakene and the coated enteric form,

divalproex sodium or Depakote). The recently approved drug lamotrigine (Lamictal) is not an effective acute antimanic drug but prevents the recurrence of depressive, mixed, and manic episodes.

These four drugs have diverse effects on both neurotransmitter and receptor systems, as well as affecting a variety of intracellular signaling systems (second messengers), which in turn link membrane receptor effects to other intracellular processes (Figure 9.5) associated with neuronal firing and the long-term regulation of cell excitability by effects on gene expression. Which of these effects is crucial to the mood-stabilizing properties of lithium, carbamazepine, valproate, and lamotrigine is not known, but all four drugs do share some common effects. These shared effects include the ability to enhance serotonin function indirectly, decrease turnover of gamma-aminobutyric acid (GABA, the major inhibitory neurotransmitter in the brain), increase GABA$_B$

receptors in the hippocampus with chronic administration, decrease dopamine and arachidonic acid turnover, block the inositol transporter, and inhibit calcium influx through the glutamate N-methyl-D-aspartate (NMDA) receptor and exert other effects on intracellular calcium.

These drugs also affect G proteins, which magnify or inhibit receptor signals and produce other cellular functions. G proteins have been candidates for the mood-stabilizing effects of these compounds because they have the ability to dampen a number of overactivated systems that have been postulated to occur in both mania and depression. Because mania and depression are both thought to be associated with excessive activation of excitatory or inhibitory systems normally associated with mood swings in either direction, the ability to dampen these excessive activations could be important to the action of mood-stabilizing drugs.

It is of considerable interest that all four major mood stabilizers have some ability to dampen overexcited systems at multiple levels of neuronal activation, including transmitter release, receptor activation, second messengers, protein kinases, transcription factors, DNA activation, and the production of new proteins.

The second messenger systems include: (a) activation of adenylate cyclases that are coupled to receptors by G proteins (either stimulatory, G_s; or inhibitory, G_i); (b) intracellular signaling mechanisms related to phosphoinositol turnover (where receptors activate phospholipase C [PLC] to cause the breakdown of PIP_2 to diacylglycerol) and inositol 1,4,5-triphosphate (IP_3, which releases intracellular calcium); and (c) a variety of other intercellular calcium (Ca^{++}) signaling mechanisms.

Second messengers are not only involved in the acute messages related to firing of cells and neurotransmitter and peptide release, but also initiate a cascade of intracellular events that affect what genes get expressed in the nucleus (Figure 9.8). Thus, there is a mechanism for the longer-lasting impact of acute events on cellular responsivity necessary for memory, and mechanisms that can convey the long-term adaptations necessary for the full effect of some drug treatments.

Delay in Onset of Action This route, from the receptors on the outside of the cell to the nucleus of the cell, to affect gene expression is likely of importance in relation to the delayed onset of the full action of antidepressants and some mood stabilizers. Most of the antidepressant treatments require days to weeks before they exert their therapeutic effects, and weeks to a month or more before their therapeutic effects are maximized. It is thought that this delay in onset of antidepressant effects is related to the time required for systems to be reregulated by the reprogramming of cellular DNA for new levels of gene expression in transmitter, peptide, and growth factor (such as BDNF) systems thought to be important in depression.

Depressed mood by itself is not unalterable in a brief period of time. It is simply that the current antidepressant manipulations require a moderate amount of time (usually several weeks) to achieve their full effects. Rapid onset of antidepressant effects (literally overnight) can be achieved in about one half of severely depressed patients, paradoxically by one night of complete sleep deprivation or partial deprivation of sleep in the last part of the night (see Chapter 59). In other instances, patients can also respond rapidly to pharmacological probes such as stimulants or the neuropeptide TRH (see Chapters 61 and 62). The effects of these acute manipulations tend not to last long, however. The effects of one night's sleep deprivation are usually reversed by going back to sleep the next night (unless this recovery relapse is blocked by lithium or other sleep phase manipulations), and the rapid-onset antidepressant effects of the psychomotor stimulants are often not sustainable during more chronic administration. Several groups have reported very rapid onset of antidepressant effect with a drug ketamine that affects the main excitatory neurotransmitter in brain glutamate. In this instance, effects last some 3 to 5 days.

Neurotrophic and Neuroprotective Effects In addition to the variety of effects of lithium on neurotransmitters, receptors, and second messenger systems, effects on gene expression (the activation of DNA and synthesis of new proteins) have recently been elucidated. These effects may be of clinical importance because they appear relevant to the effects of lithium in a variety of cells, in animal models, and in man. Lithium increases nerve cell survival in tissue cultures by increasing cell survival factors such as Bcl-2 and BDNF (Figure 9.8, right side), and by decreasing cell death factors such as Bax and p53, which are proteins involved in the active process of preprogrammed cell death (apoptosis). Lithium exerts these and related effects at therapeutically relevant concentrations, and lithium is able to decrease the amount of brain damage caused by a stroke (from ligation of the middle cerebral artery in rodents). As shown by Chuang and colleagues (2002) in our laboratory, lithium is also able to decrease the amount of brain damage caused in the animal model of Huntington's chorea, wherein a toxin is placed in the striatum.

These data suggest that lithium may exert neuroprotective effects (Figure 9.9). Whether these effects are relevant to the mechanism of action of lithium in the affective disorders remains to be delineated. However, data of Manji, Moore, & Chen (2000) suggest that four weeks of treatment with lithium increases a magnetic resonance spectroscopy measure of neuronal integrity in the brain (i.e., *N*-acetylaspartate) and increases the amount of gray matter measured on magnetic resonance imaging. Since a number of studies have linked decreased numbers of neurons or glia to the pathophysiology of bipolar illness (see Chapter 10), it is of considerable interest that one of the mainstays of treatment appears to exert neurotrophic and glial protective effects. Interestingly, valproate shares lithium's ability to increase BDNF and Bcl-2 (Figures 9.8 and 9.9), but other mechanisms remain to be explored.

The new molecular insights about the possible neurotrophic effects (BDNF gene expression) of the antidepressants, and of neurotrophic and potentially neuroprotective effects of lithium carbonate, should begin to be incorporated into our clinical perspectives. Although many patients are worried about possible long-term adverse effects of these agents on the brain, the new evidence suggests that they may have protective or ameliorative effects against stressos and other brain insults (Figure 9.9).

Repeated stressors are able to decrease BDNF in the hippocampus, and this can be at least partially prevented by antidepressants. This effect could theoretically be linked to the long-term preventive effects of the antidepressants in the recurrence of depressive relapses. To the extent that stressors are often involved in the precipitation of depressive episodes, blunting some of the biochemical effects of stress could help prevent the triggering of depressive episodes as well as moderating the potential adverse effects of stress on neuronal function and survival.

It has recently been discovered that the generation of new neurons (neurogenesis) takes place even in the adult brain. Stress decreases neurogenesis, whereas the antidepressants and lithium increase its rate. This neurogenesis takes place predominantly in the walls of the ventricular system, containing cerebrospinal fluid lining the insides of deep brain structures such as the hippocampus. New neurons that are born in this (subependymal) layer actually migrate into the hippocampus, become new neurons (dentate granule cells) or glia cells, and begin to form new synapses in some instances. Based on the (not so radical) assumption that having more surviving neurons is a good thing, it is intriguing that the antidepressants and lithium not only facilitate the generation of new neurons in the hippocampus (neurogenesis) but also increase survival of existing cells (via effects on neurotrophic factors).

New data indicate that lithium can increase the birth and development of glial cells as well. Glial cells are 10 times more prevalent in the brain than neurons (about 10 billion neurons and 100 billion glia) and are necessary for normal neural function at the synapse, and for the production of myelin necessary for adequate nerve conduction.

Even though these new molecular mechanisms have not been directly linked to the thera-

	Stress	Gluco-corticoids	Lithium	VPA	ADs
Transcription factor CREB	↓	↓	↑		↑
Neurotrophic factor BDNF	↓	↓	↑	↑	↑
Neuroprotective factor BCL-2 (Anti-Apoptotic)			↑↑	↑	
Neurite sprouting (*in vitro*)		↓	↑		
Neurogenesis (*in vivo*)	↓	↓	↑	↑	↑
Neuronal viability NAA by MRS (in human)			↑	−	
Increased gray matter (in human)		↓	↑ ctx.		↑ hippo. vol.

Figure 9.9 Opposite effects of stress and psychotropic drugs on gene expression, neuroprotection, and brain structure. BDNF, brain-derived neurotrophic factor; CREB, c-AMP response element binding protein; NAA, N-acetyl-aspartate; MRS, magnetic resonance spectroscopy; VPA, valproate; ADs, antidepressants; ctx, cortex; hippo, hippocampus.

peutic effects of the antidepressants or lithium, this information may be of additional assistance to patients who are deciding on the relative assets and liabilities of long-term antidepressant prophylaxis for unipolar depression, or lithium, carbamazepine, and valproate prophylaxis for bipolar illness. In other words, these agents may actually be beneficial rather than harmful to some types of brain function. Since willingness to take pharmacotherapy for long-term prevention of bipolar illness is a key element of good response and positive long-term outcome, helping to dispel concerns that these agents only have toxic side effects may be one valuable component of patients' ability to actively commit to long-term treatment strategies. Lamorigine, which has not yet been studied for its effects on BDNF, would still theoretically have important neuroprotective effects by preventing episodes of depression, and to a lesser extent mania, which themselves are associated with decrements in BDNF in serum.

Calcium Channel Blockers and Actions of Mood Stabilizers on Calcium Influx Other possible mood stabilizers include the calcium channel blockers, particularly those working at the L-type calcium channel. This efficacy of calcium channel blockers in bipolar disorder may be related to calcium influx into the neuron when it is depolarized. These drugs are of considerable interest, because increased intracellular calcium is reported in depressed patients in more than a dozen studies, as assessed by the amount of intracellular Ca^{++} in platelet and lymphocyte blood elements (which may model what happens in nerve cells).

Different types of L-type calcium channel blockers work at different places in the calcium channel. The phenylalkylamine drug verapamil (Calan) binds at the outside of the channel, whereas the dihydropyridines apparently block the channels deeper inside and have differential effects on a variety of biochemical systems, including the ability to block cocaine-induced hyperactivity and its associated dopamine over-flow in dopamine-rich parts of the brain. The dihydropyridines include nimodipine (Nimotop), isradapine (DynaCirc), and amlodipine (Norvasc).

These differential effects at the same calcium channel are potentially clinically relevant, as verapamil has been reported to be effective in some controlled studies of acute manic patients, but is not widely used for this purpose and does not appear to have significant antidepressant properties. In contrast, in preliminary studies, the dihydropyridines have been shown to be effective in some affectively ill patients with recurrent brief depression, treatment-refractory depression, rapid cycling, and, in some instances, in patients with extreme ultradian cycling (see Chapters 32 and 33).

The relative efficacy of these differentially acting calcium channel blockers among the different subtypes and the actions of other classes of mood stabilizers on calcium remain to be more clearly delineated in larger numbers of patients. For example, valproate, zonisamide, and ethosuximide block T-type (T for transient) calcium channels, which is thought to relate to their efficacy in petit mal or absence seizures. Lithium has a variety of complex effects on calcium via actions on cyclases, G proteins, and PI turnover.

Carbamazepine blocks calcium influx through a receptor for the excitatory amino acid glutamate, specifically at the NMDA subtype of glutamate receptor. This action is also shared by valproate, lithium, and lamotrigine. Carbamazepine also blocks excitatory amino acid release, as does lamotrigine, and thus indirectly affects calcium via the NMDA receptor. These latter two putative mood-stabilizing anticonvulsants (carbamazepine and lamotrigine) also block sodium channels, effects shared with phenytoin, topiramate, and valproate.

Increasing (GABA) inhibition or blocking (glutamate) overexcitation Thus, we can roughly divide the world of the anticonvulsants into two general categories (Figure 9.10)—those that decrease effects of the excitatory neurotransmitter glutamine (left side) and those that enhance the main inhibitory neurotransmitter in the brain (GABA, right side). Increasing brain GABA is not sufficient to exert antimanic effects, because three of the four drugs that increase brain GABA levels are not primary antimanic agents, that is, gabapentin, tiagabine, and topiramate.

Carbamazepine's effects on sodium channels are use-dependent. That is, the action is greater the more the cell is overactivated with increased firing and greater amounts of depolarization. This type of use-dependent action is of considerable interest in the potential treatment of the epilepsies, paroxysmal pain syndromes, and paroxysmal disorders of affect regulation, because it could explain the ability of these drugs to inhibit overactive systems while leaving normal degrees of function intact. This use-dependent property also appears to be the case with carbamazepine's action at the NMDA receptor, and with lithium's action on phosphoinositol turnover, also making these key candidate systems for therapeutic effects in the absence of major effects on normal systems. More potent blockers of the NMDA receptor can have rapid onset of antidepressant effects that last about 5 days (Zarate et al., 2006; Preskorn et al., 2007).

Typical and Atypical Antipsychotics

Older Typical Antipsychotics (Neuroleptics) Neuroleptics refer to a category of drugs that block dopamine receptors (Figure 9.7) and are therefore major tranquilizers or antipsychotic agents. In the past, the antipsychotics were usually associated with some degree of parkinsonian (extrapyramidal) side effects because of this blockade of the dopamine system (Figure 9.11). In the non-drug-induced form of parkinsonism, there is a dropout of dopamine cells in the midbrain (substantia nigra A9) area that travel up to the caudate nucleus of the striatum. The hypofunction of these neurons is partially replaced by treatment with levodopa (which increases the synthesis of dopamine in the remaining neurons), or by direct-acting dopamine agonists

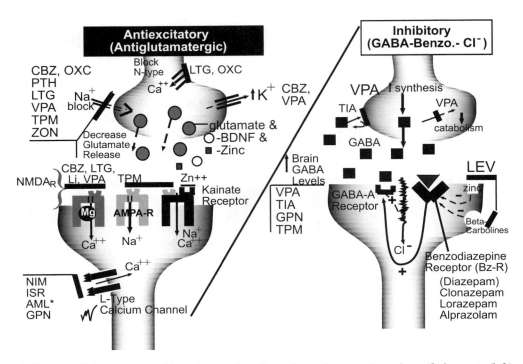

Figure 9.10 Dual mechanisms of anticonvulsant action. Some drugs decrease the actions of glutamate (left), while others increase inhibition by enhancing chloride (Cl⁻) influx at the GABA-benzodiazepine receptor chloride iontophore (right). CBZ, carbamazepine; VPA, valproate; LTG, lamotrigine; GPN, gabapentin; TPM, topiramate; NIM, nimodipine; OXC, oxcarbazepine; ZON, zonisamide; LEV, levetiracetam; PTH, phenytoin; Na, sodium; BDNF, brain-derived neurotrophic factor; Li, lithium; Zn, zinc; AMPA, 2-amino-3-(3-hydroxy-5-methyl-4-isoxazolyl)propionic acid; Ca, calcium; ISR, isradipine; AML, amlodipine; TIA, tiagabine; GABA, gamma-aminobutyric acid.

such as bromocriptine or pramipexole (which imitate the effects of dopamine).

In the case of drug-induced parkinsonism, there is not a loss of dopamine neurons, but rather an inhibition or blockade of dopamine throughput or function, because the dopamine receptors in the striatum are blocked by the neuroleptics (Figure 9.7). These drug-induced parkinsonian side effects are very much like those in the neuronal dropout syndrome that occurs naturally and includes tremor, masked faces (face is inscrutable), slow or festinating gait, loss of muscle flexibility (cog wheel rigidity), and slowness in initiating motor movements. In both syndromes, the effects are partially ameliorated by anticholinergic drugs including benztropine (Cogentin), procyclidine (Kemadrin), and biperiden (Akineton). These anticholinergic drugs change the dopamine-acetylcholine balance in the striatum and provide considerable relief from these side effects.

In addition, the drugs, particularly the older high-potency antipsychotics, in some instances can induce acute dystonic (rigid muscle) side effects and include the more frightening effects of opisthotonos (eyes rolling up in the back of the head, arching of the back, and awkward cramping of the tongue and other muscle groups in the body). These effects are rapidly relieved by IV or oral Benedryl. Among the classic antipsychotics, these reactions are least likely to happen with drugs such as thioridazine (Mellaril), which have some anticholinergic properties built into the drug itself, and are more likely to occur with high-potency drugs such as haloperidol and fluphenazine. The original antipsychotics were the phenothiazines, such as chlorpromazine (Thorazine) and thioridazine, which were

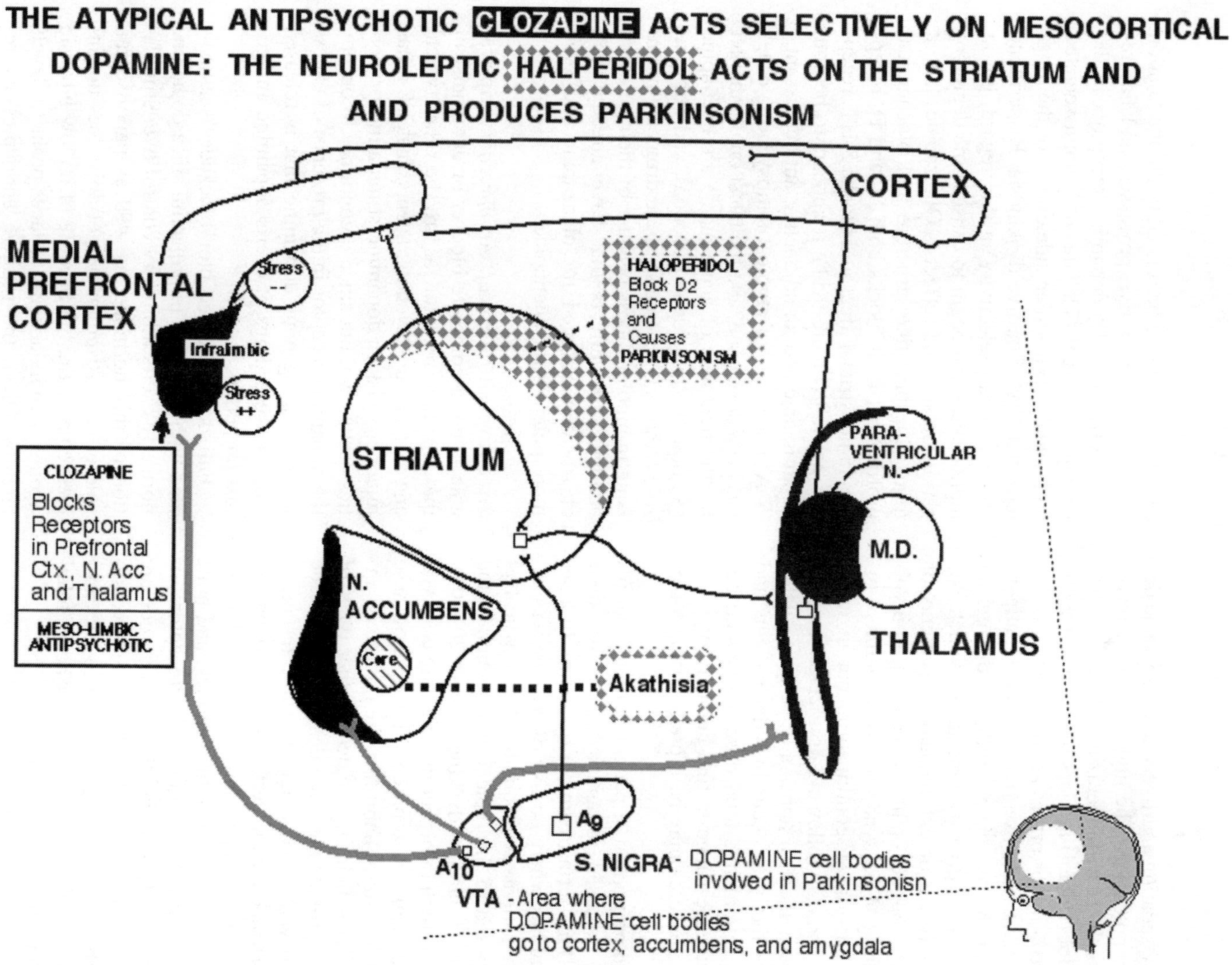

THE ATYPICAL ANTIPSYCHOTIC CLOZAPINE ACTS SELECTIVELY ON MESOCORTICAL DOPAMINE: THE NEUROLEPTIC HALPERIDOL ACTS ON THE STRIATUM AND PRODUCES PARKINSONISM

Figure 9.11 The atypical antipsychotic clozapine acts selectively on mesocortical dopamine and causes few extrapyramidal side effects. The typical antipsychotic (or neuroleptic) haloperidol acts on the striatum and produces parkinsonism and following long-term administration—tardive dyskinesia. N. accumbens, nucleus accumbens; VTA, ventral tegmental area; M.D., Medial dorsal nucleus of the thalamus; S. nigra, substantia nigra.

also fairly sedating and likely to cause some degree of hypotension. The high-potency antipsychotics such as trifluoperazine (Stelazine) and haloperidol (Haldol) are less likely to cause untoward sedation or orthostatic hypotension.

After long-term use, the classical antipsychotics can be associated with the disfiguring syndrome of tardive dyskinesia, in which adventitious (extra or extraneous) movements of the mouth, tongue, or limbs occur on an involuntary basis. This syndrome is sometimes reversible on drug discontinuation, but in many instances persists following drug cessation, and can be permanent. It appears to be dose related and more likely to occur in older patients and females. Cumulative total dose is relevant, but some evidence suggests that numbers of intermittent exposures may be a predisposing factor as well.

A high proportion of patients with bipolar illness are exposed to antipsychotics for their acute or long-term treatment of mania. In a series of studies where tardive dyskinesia was assessed in patients with bipolar illness who had been exposed to the typical antipsychotics, the incidence of tardive dyskinesia was 20–40%, which is as high or higher than the rate observed in patients with schizophrenia. Because of these potential long-term liabilities, the traditional antipsychotics should be avoided if other types of drugs can provide the same degree of antimanic and antipsychotic coverage. In some instances, use of the mood stabilizers lithium, carbamazepine, valproate, and lamotrigine can reduce or eliminate the need for antipsychotics, and none of these drugs block dopamine receptors or cause tardive dyskinesia. If antipsychotics are needed, the atypical antipsychotics are recommended because of their lower liability for causing tardive dyskinesia, and for their better tolerability and antidepressant effects.

Newer Atypical Antipsychotics Recent drug developments have provided alternative antipsychotic treatments that have lower liability for tardive dyskinesia, and yet are potent antipsychotics, and in some cases probable mood stabilizers. Clozapine (Clozaril) blocks dopamine D_2 and D_4 receptors in mesolimbic and mesocorti-

cal areas thought to be related to the modulation of mood and cognitive processes, and has reduced effects on D_2 dopamine receptors in the striatum (Figure 9.11). Thus, it is not associated with acute parkinsonian side effects or the long-term liability of tardive dyskinesia. Risperidone also has some selectivity in this regard, but at higher doses can begin to cause some degree of parkinsonian side effects. Olanzapine has a more clozapine-like structure and biochemical profile; that is, it blocks both D_2 and D_4 receptors in nonstriatal areas and blocks 5-HT_2 receptors as well (Figure 9.11); it appears to be both an antimanic and an adjunctive antidepressant.

A new series of atypical antipsychotic drugs has been developed, and the latest on the market for the treatment of acute mania are quetiapine (Seroquel), ziprasidone (Geodon), and aripiprazole (Abilify). As a class, these drugs are promising in bipolar illness because of their potential antidepressant effects that have already been clearly demonstrated for olanzapine and even more potently for quetiapine.

The "Atypical" Atypical: Aripiprazole Aripiprazole is not a complete blocker or antagonist of the dopamine receptor, as are the other typical and atypical antipsychotic agents. Instead, it has minor agonist or dopamine-stimulating properties on its own, but since it continues to occupy the dopamine receptor in the presence of excess local or endogenous dopamine that is released from nerve endings, it exerts dopamine antagonist properties as well.

Full dopamine receptor blockade is associated with increases in prolactin, since dopamine normally exerts inhibitory control over stimulation of this hormone, as well as parkinsonian side effects. Aripiprazole not only does not increase prolactin, but because of its low intrinsic agonist activity actually reduces prolactin levels slightly. Given the positive antidepressant reports of the D_2 and D_3 dopamine agonist pramipexole (used in the treatment of Parkinson's disease) for bipolar depression, one is hopeful that an agent such as aripiprazole would have not only antimanic but also antidepressant properties.

In this regard, it is of interest that aripiprazole is a partial agonist, not only for D_2 receptors, but also for D_3 receptors and 5-HT_{1A} receptors (Figure 9.6). As 5-HT_{1A} receptors are thought to be involved in the antidepressant effects of compounds such as buspirone, this aspect of aripiprazole's mechanism could also be of the-

oretical utility in the depressive phase of bipolar illness. In addition, aripiprazole is, like nefazodone, an antagonist of 5-HT_2 receptors, whose blockade has been associated with increases in deep sleep (slow wave sleep).

10

Causes and Mechanisms
of Bipolar Illness Onset
and Progression

INTRODUCTION

Although the precise causes and mechanisms involved in the onset and progression of bipolar illness have not been conclusively identified, much evidence is accumulating about the general types of processes involved. We know that bipolar illness runs strongly in families, with genetics playing a role in the vulnerability to illness onset in approximately 50% of adult patients with bipolar illness. It is likely that genetic vulnerability plays an even greater role in childhood-onset bipolar disorder. The environment, and its powerful effects on what genes get expressed, can also have major influences. In many instances, gene-environment interactions have been shown to be important in the onset or progress of affective illnesses.

THE GENETICS OF
BIPOLAR ILLNESS

The genetic vulnerability associated with bipolar illness is most evident from studies of identical twins compared with fraternal twins. Identical twins share the same genes and thus should have the same illnesses, to the extent that there are genetically mediated factors. Identical twins are moderately concordant for bipolar illness (both having the illness between 40% and 80% of the time, a rate higher than other psychiat-

ric illnesses), whereas the concordance is lower for fraternal twins, who do not share the same genes but do share the same environment.

These data in identical twins are supported by familial studies indicating that when there is a positive family history of bipolar illness in first-degree relatives, risk in their offspring increases considerably from about 1–3% of the normal population to about 10–20%. Thus, one in five offspring are likely to develop bipolar illness based on this type of vulnerability. However, when there is bipolar illness on one side of the family and either unipolar or bipolar illness on the other side, the risk of the offspring developing some type of affective illness (either unipolar or bipolar) then increases to about a 70% lifetime incidence. This rate increases because the risks appear to be additive or multiplicative, based on what is thought to be a very complex and polygenic (multiple causes) basis of the hereditary vulnerability, as well as influences from the environment. Thus, several vulnerability genes may come from the paternal lineage and converge with several other vulnerability genes from the maternal side of the family.

Not only is the genetic risk evident from these family studies, but it is also apparent when one studies first-degree relatives of children with early onset bipolar disorder. In this instance, there is a much greater incidence of bipolar illness in family members than in individuals with a later onset of bipolar illness in adolescence and adulthood. This further suggests that a greater background of genetic vulnerability is associated with the increased risk of earlier (childhood) onset bipolar illness.

Year of Birth or Cohort Effect

In recent years there has been discussion of what is technically called the *cohort effect* in bipolar illness, meaning that each generation born since World War I appears to have an increased incidence, as well as an earlier onset, of both unipolar and bipolar illness than the previous generation. There has been much speculation about the potential mechanisms involved in such an increased incidence and earlier onset of affective disorders in the general population. These potential explanations have included collapse of the multigenerational family structure, the increased divorce rate, population density, the increasing incidence of substance abuse, and increasing physical or sexual abuse in most Western countries. It is noteworthy that in cultures such as that in Puerto Rico, where the family structure has remained more intact, there is little evidence of a cohort effect.

Some have wondered whether the increased recognition of rapid fluctuations in mood in children, if not the clear oscillations characteristic of adult bipolar illness, are partially attributable to increasing use of psychomotor stimulants for the treatment of ADHD. This is of some concern because many investigators have noted that there is a high comorbidity of ADHD with bipolar illness, and that ADHD cannot be treated adequately until the bipolar illness is first treated with a mood stabilizer. If one treats this comorbidity only with stimulants, it might be associated with exacerbation of mood fluctuations in those vulnerable to bipolar illness.

Generational or Anticipation Effect

Anticipation refers to the finding in some genetic illnesses that the age of onset of illness in offspring may occur much earlier than in the parental generation. This anticipation effect in

bipolar illness leads to an average age of onset about 10 years younger. A genetic basis of anticipation has been found in several single gene neurological illnesses such as Huntington's chorea, spinocerebellar degeneration, and the fragile X syndrome. In the case of Huntington's chorea, it was found that the defect that causes this illness (associated with progressive dementia and involuntary motor movements) occurs in a protein called huntingtin. The DNA for this protein has multiple triple-repeat sequences coding for the amino acid glutamine. If an individual has less than 38 of these triple-repeat sequences in a row in the coding area for this protein, Huntington's chorea does not occur. If there are 42 or more, the individual will develop Huntington's chorea late in life. However, with a very large number of triple repeats, say 60 or 70, the illness may be associated with a very early onset (even in childhood), as occurs in rare instances.

When the sperm and egg cells of individuals with the Huntington's chorea gene reproduce themselves, there is some tendency for the number of triple-repeat sequences in the DNA to expand. Thus, an individual who might be destined to develop Huntington's chorea relatively late in life (around age 65) because he or she was born with approximately 50 triple-repeat sequences may have offspring with 60 to 70 triple repeats in a row, rendering the huntingtin protein highly dysfunctional and causing a much earlier onset of the illness.

While it is far from clear, several investigative groups have suggested that there are triple-repeat sequences associated with bipolar illness that could then expand. In bipolar illness, there is more clear evidence across multiple studies that offspring with the illness may have an average age of onset of bipolar illness as great as 10 years earlier than the parent with the illness. Whether this anticipation effect is genetically or environmentally mediated is uncertain.

Searching for Genetic Vulnerability Factors

Over the past decade, there has been a very substantial effort to identify the genetic changes that may increase vulnerability to bipolar illness. One of the most promising leads has been found on the short arm of chromosome 18 with initial findings of Berrettini and colleagues (1994), which were replicated and extended by DePaulo's group at Johns Hopkins (McMahon et al., 1997). Both of these groups noted that inheritance on chromosome 18 was associated with bipolar II illness on the father's side of the family and that the common maternal transmission of the illness was not associated with this region of chromosome 18. Many other potential vulnerability loci have been found on other chromosomes, and investigators have begun to search in these hot spots in order to precisely identify the nature of the molecular alteration involved. However, even when the area of chromosome 4 was discovered to convey vulnerability to Huntington's chorea (which shows a much simpler pattern of genetic inheritance involving a single gene), it still required approximately a decade before the actual huntingtin protein defect was found, and now, another decade later, there is still no treatment based on this single gene defect that conveys the vulnerability.

Thus, in the case of bipolar illness, it is likely to take as long or longer for the precise gene defect on chromosome 18 and others to be discovered, and it is highly likely to be only one of a great many vulnerability factors that each contribute a small effect, much like that now evident in diabetes, heart disease, or even cancer. For example, in the development of colon cancer (Figure 10.1, top), there are initial stages of increased proliferation and cell multiplication before a full-blown adenoma (polyp) is developed. With further evolution and progression of the tumor, an adenocarcinoma may develop in a single location characterized by more aggressive cell types that clearly are abnormal upon microscopic examination. In later stages, the tumor cells may break away from the primary site and metastasize at a distance, and with this transition become even more resistant to treatment. Each of the stages of this progression involves a series of additional somatic mutations in the cells involved, some of which further turn on new mechanisms of cellular proliferation, while others disable remaining tumor suppressor factors. If an individual is born into a family that already has a genetic vulnerability based on a loss of one or more tumor suppressor factors, he or she may be at particularly high risk for earlier onset or more aggressive course of colon cancer, because fewer new somatic mutations would be necessary to produce the full-blown illness.

We believe that analogous stages of illness progression occur in bipolar illness, with each involving a number of alterations in gene expression rather than somatic mutations (Figure 10.1, bottom). Some of them occur based on heredity and another group based on environmental factors, such as stresses, the occurrence of episodes themselves, and substances of abuse. However, instead of these environmental events causing irreversible mutations as in cancer, they would only cause transient and potentially reversible biochemical alterations based on what genes are expressed and to what degree.

Therefore, as the hereditary genetic vulnerability factors for bipolar illness are ultimately identified (such as the *val66val* allele of brain-derived neurotrophic factor, BDNF, noted below), they will likely interact with environmental events in relation to illness onset and progression. Moreover, genetic vulnerability factors are not likely to provide the definitive kind of information that comes with knowing whether or not one has inherited the single gene defect causing Huntington's chorea. In that case, one knows with a fair degree of certainty whether or not one will eventually get the illness.

In contrast, in the case of multigene-determined illnesses with many vulnerability factors, the presence of a given susceptibility gene would not necessarily mean that an individual will become ill. However, although such an identification would help to understand the mechanisms involved in the illness and possibly develop new targeted treatments, it is even more likely that the array of multipe common gene variants called single nucleotide polymorphisms (SNPs, pronounced snips) will help direct the choice of current therapeutic strategies and rapidly become part of the screening process that helps one to initiate treatment at the very earliest onset of symptoms, in order to attempt to prevent the development of more full-blown affective illness.

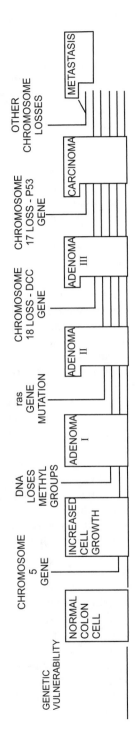

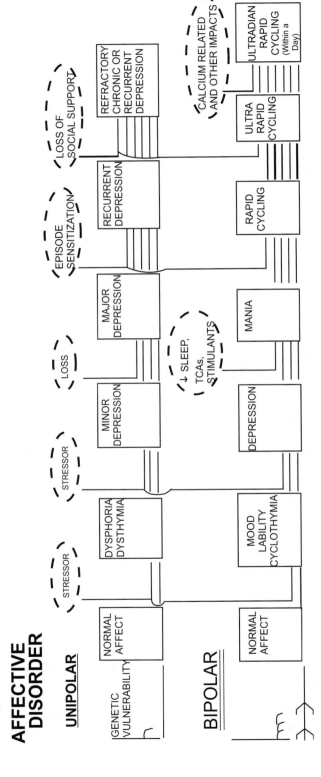

Figure 10.1 Similarities between the accumulation of somatic mutations in gene expression underlying carcinogenesis and of environmental/experiential alterations in gene expression observed in unipolar and bipolar affective disorder. TCA, tricyclic antidepressant.

THE NEUROCHEMISTRY OF AFFECTIVE ILLNESS

The Indoleamines: Serotonin and Its Transporter

Coppen, Prange, Sourkes, and van Praag have been most closely associated with the serotonin-permissive hypothesis of affective illness (Coppen, Prange, Whybrow, & Noguera, 1972). Serotonin is one of many transmitters that helps to convey messages from one cell to the next across a synapse; that is, an electrical impulse (when the cell fires) releases chemical transmitters such as serotonin into the area (synapse) between cells. Serotonin binds to a receptor site on the second cell (the postsynaptic site), which then is associated with activation and firing of the second neuron. A deficiency of serotonin was postulated as a vulnerability factor in the development of recurrent affective illness and by Marie Asberg et al. (1976) in the increased impulsivity associated with suicide attempts and completed suicide.

This serotonin-permissive theory has had much support with the development of selective serotonin reuptake inhibitor (SSRI) antidepressants, which increase serotonergic tone in the synapse by preventing the reuptake or inactivation of serotonin, thus making it more available for action at the postsynaptic side of the synapse. Serotonergic mechanisms have most recently been clearly implicated in unipolar depression with a tryptophan depletion test. When patients who have responded to a serotonin-active antidepressant are given a diet of amino acids deficient in tryptophan (the precursor to serotonin), their mood is transiently worsened for a period of several hours because of the drop in brain serotonin synthesis.

The SSRIs inhibit serotonin reuptake by blocking the serotonin transporter (5HT-T). There are two common genetic variants or single-nucleotide polymorphisms of the serotonin transporter, a short (s) form and a long (l) form, which are less or more active, respectively. Caspi et al. (2003) showed that among those patients with a childhood history of physical or sexual abuse, reexposure to a stressful life event in adulthood led to marked increases in depression only in those with the $5HT\text{-}T_{SS}$ variant. Those with the $5HT\text{-}T_{LL}$ form were relatively invulnerable. This is an elegant documentation of a gene-environment interaction pertinent to the onset of unipolar depressive illness. It also validates and extends the stress-sensitization model that early life adversities and increase the responsivity to subsequent stressors, in this case more of less depending on ones genetic inheritance.

The Catecholamines Dopamine and Norepinephrine: Postulated Deficiency in Depression, Excesses in Mania

Two other transmitters called catecholamines (dopamine, DA; and norepinephrine, NE) are in different cells in the brain stem and midbrain, and have now been postulated to be deficient in depression and excessive in mania. A modicum of evidence supports this viewpoint from the biochemical perspective, and in terms of the mechanism of action of drugs, there is considerable support for such a theory. For example, the antipsychotic drugs (major tranquilizers or neuroleptics) that block DA's action at the DA receptor are all antimanic agents, as well as the traditional treatment of choice for the psychosis of schizophrenia. In addition, inhibition of the synthesis of DA and NE has been associated with antimanic effects as well. The postulated excesses in NE have been directly observed in the spinal fluid of manic patients.

Hints from the Mechanism of Action of Lithium Carbonate

With the recognition that the lithium ion was effective in the treatment of bipolar illness, it was hoped that an understanding of its mechanism of action would rapidly lead to a clarification of the pathological mechanisms involved in bipolar illness. Unfortunately, this has not proven to be such an easy shortcut since lithium (as described in Chapter 9) has a multiplicity of biochemical effects, and which of these is most important to its therapeutic effects has not been adequately defined.

In addition, the absence of a suitable animal model for manic-depressive illness has clearly hampered such an investigative route. With a variety of mood-stabilizing anticonvulsants now available such as carbamazepine, valproate, and perhaps a second-generation agent such as lamotrigine, one can further hope to identify convergent mechanisms of action and thus have assistance in uncovering the biochemical alterations involved in the illness.

Hypersecretion of the Adrenal Stress Hormone Cortisol

Ed Sachar, rapidly followed by a number of other investigators, demonstrated that depressed patients consistently secreted too much of the adrenal stress hormone cortisol (Figure 10.2)

during depressive episodes, and this normalized with recovery (Sachar et al., 1973). Barney Carroll (1978) and many others found that if one gave a synthetic steroid such as dexamethasone to normal volunteers, it completely suppressed cortisol production, because of the body's feedback messages that there were high levels of the circulating synthetic steroid dexamethasone. However, in approximately 50% of severely depressed patients, given the same dose that suppressed cortisol in normal volunteers, dexamethasone failed to suppress cortisol. This has now become one of the most widely replicated findings in the clinical neuroscience of depression, and suggests that there is an increased activity or drive in the hypothalamic-pituitary-adrenal (HPA) axis that controls cortisol secretion. When patients recover from their depression, if their lack of suppression of cortisol persists, they are at a high risk for relapse.

There is some direct evidence that corticotro-

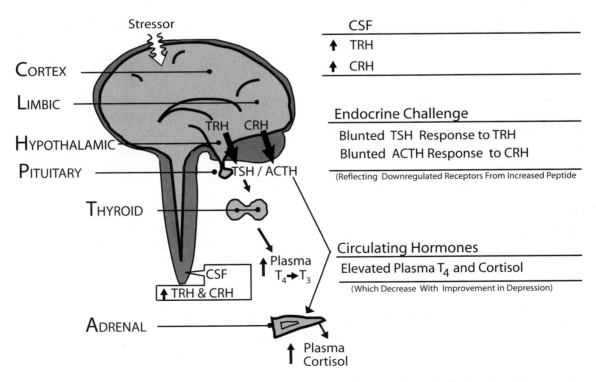

Figure 10.2 Increased cortico-limbic hypothalamic-pituitary-adrenal and hypothalamic-pituitary-thyroid axes in depression. CSF, cerebrospinal fluid; TSH, thyroid-stimulating hormone; TRH, thyrotropin-releasing hormone; CRH, corticotropin-releasing hormone; ACTH, adrenocorticotropic hormone.

pin-releasing hormone (CRH), located in the hypothalamus, is hypersecreted in depression, as measured indirectly in the spinal fluid of depressed patients. Thus, an increased amount of CRH would increase release of adrenocorticotropic hormone from the pituitary, which in turn causes the release of cortisol from the adrenal gland (Figure 10.2). When this happens in Cushing's disease (associated with an adrenal tumor), the hypersecretion of cortisol into the blood (hypercortisolemia) is associated with fatigue, cognitive impairment, and depression in a high percentage of patients.

In a similar manner, the functional endocrine disturbances that occur with depression are thought, at least in part, to be related to such hypercortisolemia driven by increases in CRH. It is noteworthy that many of the effective antidepressant agents do, in fact, exert mechanisms that reverse this hypersecretion of cortisol. They increase the amount of two types of cortisol receptors (mineralocorticoid receptor, MR; and glucocorticoid receptor, GR) that help turn off the excess cortical secretions. It is noteworthy that evidence of deficient GRs is found on lymphocytes of depressed patients and that MRs are decreased in the frontal cortex of bipolar patients compared with controls (studied at autopsy). The MR deficiency is one of many deficits found in the frontal cortex of bipolar patients that might be relevant to some of the dysfunction seen in the illness.

The Balance of "Good Guys" Versus "Bad Guys" in Illness Recurrence and Remission

In addition to CRH, there is also evidence of increased secretion of thyrotropin-releasing hormone (TRH), another peptide localized in the hypothalamus, that releases thyroid-stimulating hormone (TSH) from the pituitary and allows the thyroid gland to release its quadra-iodinated thyroid hormone T_4 (Synthroid) as well as the triiodinated form T_3 (Cytomel). Depressed patients also tend to hypersecrete these thyroid hormones, which normalizes with improvement in depression (Figure 10.3). Such hypersecre-

tion is evidenced by a blunted TSH response to an intravenous injection of TRH (presumably because the TSH receptor is downregulated because of the ongoing hyperactivity in this pathway).

In contrast to CRH, which is thought to be intimately involved in the pathophysiology of depression (a chemical bad guy), TRH hypersecretion may actually represent one of a whole host of the body's mechanisms that attempt to restabilize the system and act as an internal (endogenous) antidepressant (a good guy; Figure 10.3). We think that this is the case because many studies using intravenous TRH, compared with placebo, have suggested that it has antidepressant effects. Moreover, one study that consisted of directly injecting TRH into patients' spinal fluid in order to have sufficient quantities to reach the brain (avoiding the blood-brain barrier), also found that TRH had antidepressant, antianxiety, and antisuicidal effects compared with a sham procedure in a small group of treatment-refractory patients studied at the NIMH.

Thus, because these two peptides (CRH and TRH) with apparently opposite effects on depressed mood and behavior are both increased during depressive episodes, it is thought that their relative ratio might account for the periods of illness or well intervals between episodes (Figure 10.3). In other words, while CRH and other pathological factors are increased out of proportion to compensatory mechanisms, the bad guys predominate and depression occurs. However, when good guys, such as TRH and company, predominate, periods of wellness may ensue. It is postulated that these two peptides are merely representative of a whole host of chemical changes that are related to either the primary pathology of depression (like CRH) or endogenous adaptive factors (like TRH).

This formulation not only helps to conceptualize why the illness may spontaneously fluctuate with periods of illness and recovery between episodes, but also provides a new set of targets for therapeutics. Not only would one want to inhibit the bad guys (such as the CRH hypersecretion and its downstream hypercortisolemia), but one might also attempt to enhance certain other abnormalities associated with the illness

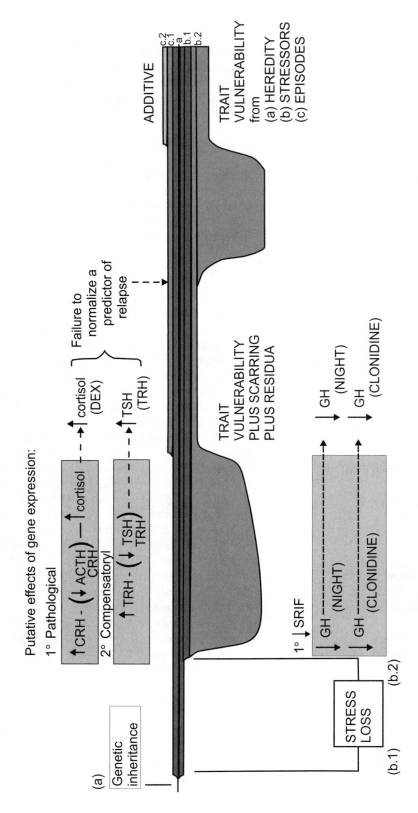

Figure 10.3 Accumulating experiential genetic vulnerability in recurrent affective illness. Schematic of how initial stressors may leave behind trait vulnerabilities (at the level of alterations in gene expression). With appropriate reactivation by stress of relevant neurobiological systems, the threshold for neuropeptide and hormonal changes associated with a depressive episode may be exceeded. These episode-related alterations may be normalized with the termination of episode but in some instances may persist and add further trait vulnerabilities toward recurrence (c) in addition to the genetic (a) and stressor (b) changes. CRH, corticotropin-releasing hormone; ACTH, adrenocorticotropin-releasing hormone; TRH, thyrotropin-releasing hormone; TSH, thyroid-stimulating hormone; DEX, dexamethasone; SRIF, somatostatin; GH growth hormone. (See details in Post, 1992).

that may be good guys, like TRH. Some effort in this direction of boosting TRH is being pursued by Andy Winokur and associates at the University of Connecticut (Gary et al., 2003); other endogenous adaptive mechanisms may be amenable to enhancement in the future once they are adequately identified and discriminated from the pathological ones.

Somatostatin Deficits in Depression

There is also evidence that the peptide somatostatin (SRIF, somatotrophin release inhibiting factor) is decreased during periods of depression and returns to normal with recovery (Figure 10.3). This finding is of considerable interest, because SRIF is decreased in the brains of patients with Alzheimer's disease in proportion to the severity of cognitive impairment. Thus, it is possible that some of the cognitive difficulties that depressed patients transiently experience could be related to alterations in this and other critical chemicals involved in normal cognition, learning, and memory, such as dopamine and norepinephrine.

However, in contrast to Alzheimer's disease, in which cells are permanently damaged and lost, the deficit in SRIF in depression is transient, and SRIF levels return to normal when the patient recovers. Thus, SRIF gene expression is turned down during depression, while in recovery the DNA for SRIF is activated, more mRNA coding its synthesis is produced, and more SRIF is synthesized and released. It is of interest that the calcium channel blocker nimodipine increases brain SRIF (as reflected in the spinal fluid) and has some positive effects on memory in Alzheimer's dementia, as well as on mood in those depressed patients who have the lowest levels of SRIF in their CSF at baseline (see Chapter 32).

Increased Calcium Influx into Cells

Another highly consistent finding in affective illness is increased calcium in white cells and platelets of patients with depression compared with healthy volunteers. The molecular mechanisms responsible for this alteration are not known for certain, but it is hoped that their identification in peripheral cells (those circulating in blood) might lead to identification of similar mechanisms that could be involved in increased intracellular calcium in brain cells (neurons). There is some evidence that the defect in intracellular calcium is a trait marker for the illness, since it has been identified in bipolar patients whose cultured macrophages have undergone immortalization and multiple replications outside of the body. This is evidence that the defect in calcium regulation persists independent of mood state or circulating factors in blood.

These intracellular calcium increases are also interesting because of observations that many agents effective in the treatment of bipolar illness block calcium influx into neurons by a variety of mechanisms. These drugs include not only the direct L-type (L for long opening time) calcium channel blockers, such as nimodipine (Nimotop), isradipine (Dynacirc), and amlodipine (Norvasc), but also the mood stabilizers such as lithium, carbamazepine, valproate, and lamotrigine (see Chapter 9).

Chris Hough and collaborators (1993) at the NIMH have observed that, like carbamazepine, lithium, and lamotrigine inhibit calcium influx through the NMDA receptor as well. It is an excess of this type of calcium influx that has been associated with increased amounts of pre-programmed or apoptotic cell death. Lithium also prevents the spreading of the area of dead cells after a stroke and moderates the associated neurological dysfunction.

NEUROPHYSIOLOGY OF DEPRESSION: BRAIN IMAGING

Dramatic new technical developments have allowed us to examine functional brain activity in a fully awake individual. Positron emission tomography (PET) can measure metabolism with fluorine-18 deoxyglucose, or blood flow with a heavy isotope O^{15} water, and convey precise information about regional brain activity during depression and normal states.

Hypofunction of the Prefrontal Cortex

A large number of studies have indicated that depressed patients have decrements in blood flow metabolism in the frontal cortex, often in proportion to the severity of depression as rated on the Hamilton depression scale (Figure 10.4). In many instances this deficit is reported to normalize on recovery from depression. However, in the case of treatment with electroconvulsive therapy, successful treatment appears associated with further decrements in frontal hypoactivity rather than its normalization.

Beyond the absolute or relative decrements in brain metabolism in patients with bipolar illness compared with controls noted above, Benson and associates (2002) have found pathological alterations in regional brain functional connectivity or associativity independent of clinical state or severity of depression (Figure 10.4, far right). In a correlational analysis, normal volunteers were found to have a variety of reciprocal relationships between, for example, frontal cortex and cerebellum and a rough balance of the number of brain areas positively and inversely associated with thalamic activity. However, in patients with bipolar illness, the balance of associativity was dramatically shifted toward positive correlations only, and few areas showed the normal degrees of inverse associativity.

In bipolar patients, the frontal cortex had lost its normal reciprocal or inhibitory interactions with cerebellum and amygdala. In addition, because the thalamus is a major way station for the modulation of incoming sensory information and is part of a series of critical frontal-basal ganglia-thalamic loops described by Alexander, Crutcher, and Delong (1990), the loss of balanced positive and negative associativities of this area could prove important to the behavioral and emotional imbalance and dyscontrol in bipolar illness. These preliminary data begin to suggest the importance of the functional balance of neuronal activity and the modulatory interrelationships among different areas of the brain as

being important in the affective disorders (Figure 10.4, right), in addition to absolute increases or decreases in regional neural activity and chemical levels compared with controls (Figure 10.4, left side).

Limbic Hyperactivity

There is also considerable evidence linking affective disorders with alterations in the size and activity of structures in the medial part of the temporal lobe, such as the amygdala, hippocampus, and parahippocampal gyrus that are thought to be intimately involved in modulation of emotion and cognition. Thus, modern brain imaging techniques are beginning to provide confirmatory evidence of frontal cortex and limbic dysfunction, which has long been postulated based on indirect data from humans or more direct data in laboratory studies of emotion in animals.

Papez (1937) first suggested that the limbic circuit (amygdala, hippocampus, hypothalamus, and related structures) was associated with emotion modulation. This concept has been propelled further by Paul MacLean (1973) and many others, suggesting that dysfunction in limbic areas of the brain may be associated with alterations in affective modulation. If this part of the brain is stimulated directly with depth electrodes in patients with epilepsy, a variety of emotional and experiential phenomena are induced, including considerable degrees of anxiety.

The local anesthetic procaine has been shown to be a relatively selective activator of the amygdala and its outflow pathways into the insula, anterior cingulate gyrus, and orbital frontal cortex. When given to normal volunteers, procaine is associated with either euphoric or dysphoric effects, further supporting the concept of limbic modulation of emotional function. Bipolar depressed patients have altered limbic responsivity to procaine compared with normal volunteers.

Alterations have also been reported in amygdala size and composition. Four groups have reported an increased size of the amygdala in adults, with one finding the size correlated with the number of prior hospitalizations for mania. However, studies of children and adolescents

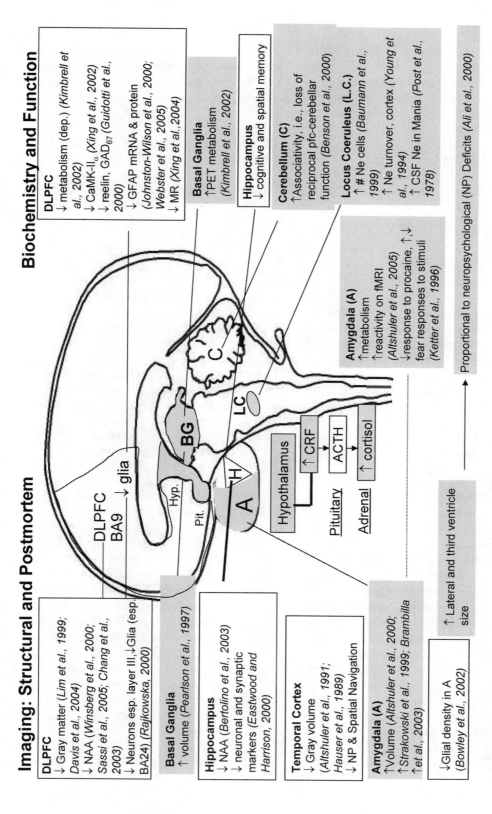

Imaging: Structural and Postmortem

DLPFC
→ Gray matter (*Lim et al., 1999; Davis et al., 2004*)
→ NAA (*Winsberg et al., 2000; Sassi et al., 2005; Chang et al., 2003*)
→ Neurons esp. layer III, ↓Glia (esp. BA24) (*Rajkowska, 2000*)

Basal Ganglia
↑ volume (*Pearlson et al., 1997*)

Hippocampus
→ NAA (*Bertolino et al., 2003*)
→ neuronal and synaptic markers (*Eastwood and Harrison, 2000*)

Temporal Cortex
↓ Gray volume (*Altshuler et al., 1991; Hauser et al., 1989*)
↓ NP & Spatial Navigation

Amygdala (A)
↑Volume (*Altshuler et al., 2000; Strakowski et al., 1999; Brambilla et al., 2003*)

↓Glial density in A (*Bowley et al., 2002*)

Biochemistry and Function

DLPFC
→ metabolism (dep.) (*Kimbrell et al., 2002*)
→ CaMK-II_α (*Xing et al., 2002*)
→ reelin, GAD₆₇ (*Guidotti et al., 2000*)
↓ GFAP mRNA & protein (*Johnston-Wilson et al., 2000; Webster et al., 2005*)
↓ MR (*Xing et al., 2004*)

Basal Ganglia
↑PET metabolism (*Kimbrell et al., 2002*)

Hippocampus
→ cognitive and spatial memory

Cerebellum (C)
↑Associativity, i.e., loss of reciprocal pfc-cerebellar function (*Benson et al., 2000*)

Locus Coeruleus (L.C.)
↑ # Ne cells (*Baumann et al., 1999*)
↑ Ne turnover, cortex (*Young et al., 1994*)
↑ CSF Ne in Mania (*Post et al., 1978*)

Amygdala (A)
↑metabolism
↑reactivity on fMRI (*Altshuler et al., 2005*)
↓response to procaine, ↑,→ fear responses to stimuli (*Ketter et al., 1996*)

Proportional to neuropsychological (NP) Deficits (*Ali et al., 2000*)

↑ Lateral and third ventricle size

Figure 10.4 Convergence of structural, biochemical, and functional abnormalities in bipolar illness. DLPFC, dorsolateral prefrontal cortex; NAA, *N*-acetyl-aspartate; BA24, Brodmann's area 24; fMRI, functional magnetic resonance imaging; CaMK-II, calcium calmodulin kinase II; GAD 67, glutamate decarboxylase 67; GFAP, glial fibrillary acidic protein; MR, mineralocorticoid receptors; PET, positron emission tomography; Ne, neurones; CSF, cerebrospinal fluid; CRF, corticotropin-releasing factor; ACTH, adrenocorticotropin-releasing hormone; Hyp., hypothalamus; Pit., pituitary gland. (Detail references are found in Post et al., 2003.)

and those earlier in their course of illness have a reduced size of the amygdala, suggesting that it may change in size over the course of the illness. Multiple functional brain imaging studies indicate that in bipolar illness, the amygdala is hyperactivated on PET in response to a variety of probes, particularly those involving recognition of facial affect. Most recently, it has been found that there are reductions in the number of glial cells, not only in the frontal cortex, but also in the amygdala and related areas of the brain, such as the anterior cingulate gyrus.

NEUROCHEMISTRY FINDINGS FROM AUTOPSY STUDIES

E. Fuller Torrey, Mike Knable, and associates have made available the brains of individuals who died with a diagnosis of schizophrenia, unipolar depression, bipolar illness, or no diagnosis (15 in each category) for biochemical analysis in a variety of laboratories throughout the world (Knable, Torrey, Webster, & Bartko, 2001). Preliminary findings have already begun to reveal a host of interesting possible molecular alterations in bipolar illness (Figure 10.4, far left).

Deficits in Reelin and GABA Interneurons

Guidotti and associates (2000) have reported decreases in reelin in patients with bipolar illness (and schizophrenia), and they have replicated these findings in both the prefrontal cortex and in the hippocampus of patients with bipolar illness (Figure 10.4). Reelin is an important compound for neural development and is secreted from one type of GABAergic interneurons across the synapse to cortical and hippocampal pyramidal cells. Guidotti and associates have found up to 50% reductions in reelin in patients with bipolar illness and schizophrenia, in association with selective decrements in a marker for GABAergic neurons, glutamic acid decarboxylase (GAD) 67. This loss of GABA interneurons would likely result in decreased inhibition of pyramidal cells leading to uncontrolled

increased firing and possibly even to cell death, which could be one mechanism for some of the cell losses found in bipolar illness and schizophrenia.

CaMK-II, Necessary for Long-Term Cortical Memory, Is Reduced

Xing and associates (2002) have found decreases in calcium calmodulin kinase-2 (CaMK-II) in the prefrontal cortex of bipolar patients (Figure 10.5). This finding is of particular interest because CaMK-II is a critical calcium-sensing enzyme (Figure 10.6), which is necessary for the development of either synaptic enhancement (long-term potentiation necessary for learning and memory) or synaptic suppression (long-term depression; Figure 10.7). A deficit of such a critical modulator of signal transduction could account for some of the prefrontal neuropsychological and neurocognitive defects observed even in euthymic bipolar patients. In animals, deficits in cortical CaMK-IIα of a magnitude similar to that observed in bipolar illness have been linked to deficits in cortical long-term, but not short-term, memory (Figure 10.8).

Glial Numbers and Activity Are Reduced

In addition to the decreased numbers of glial cells in the cortex, cingulate, and amygdala, there is also evidence of decreased glial cell activation in bipolar illness, documented by findings of decreases in both the mRNA and protein levels of glial fibrillary acidic protein, a marker of glial activity in the prefrontal cortex (Figure 10.4). Since glial cells produce a variety of neurotrophic factors and are also important protectors of neurons by taking up excess glutamate (which in overabundance can kill cells), it is possible that deficits in glial numbers or function could indirectly lead to neuronal dysfunction and, potentially, even cell death via an excess in glutamate (Figure 10.6). This glial-based neuronal dysfunction then could be further enhanced by the deficit in specific subtypes of in-

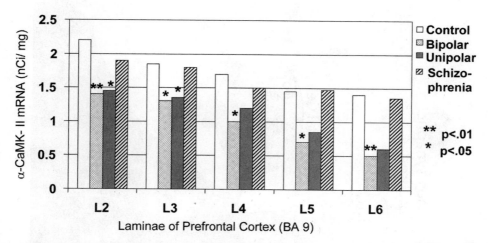

Figure 10.5 Decreased CaMK-II₄ mRNA in cortical laminae 2–6 of prefrontal cortex in bipolar illness. BA9, Brodmann's area 9. (From Xing et al., 2002.)

hibitory GABAergic interneurons noted above, which would allow neurons to fire more rapidly and release more glutamate.

Limbic Abnormalities

Eastwood and Harrison (2000) have found a number of markers of synaptic function that are decreased in the cingulate cortex and hippocampus of autopsy specimens of patients with bipolar illness compared with controls. These markers included decrements in synaptophysin, complexin I mRNA, and complexin II mRNA, which were inversely correlated with the duration of bipolar illness, suggesting a relationship to illness duration and severity. Others, however, have found (paradoxically) that an increased size of the hippocampus was associated with the number of prior episodes and the degree of neurocognitive deficit in patients with bipolar disorders.

OVERVIEW: POTENTIAL CLINICAL CORRELATES OF NEUROBIOLOGICAL ABNORMALITIES

Thus, as summarized in Figure 10.4, there appears to be a series of findings that implicate multiple areas of the brain and neuropeptide systems in the neuropathology and pathophysiology of bipolar illness. There is evidence for HPA hyperactivity in depressive phases and some evidence of thyroid dysfunction, not only noted above but also in the increased proportion of bipolar patients who have antithyroid antibodies compared with other illnesses or healthy volunteer controls.

In the prefrontal cortex, deficits are evident in neural and glial density, measures of glial activity and neuronal integrity, discrete biochemistry (i.e., decreases in reelin, CaMK-II, GAD 67, and MR mRNA), hypoactivity on functional brain imaging, as well as hyperconnected relationships with other areas of the brain. These frontal cortical deficits in conjunction with increases in amygdalar, ventral striatal, and cerebellar function could account for many of the aspects of disturbed regulation of emotional, behavioral, and endocrine function observed in the illness.

Amygdala overactivity at baseline and altered amygdala responsiveness, depending on the type of neuropsychological task, is seen on PET. Alterations are also observed in the nucleus accumbens (ventral striatum), an area that has been implicated in the modulation of emotion, psychomotor activity, drug self-administration, and hedonic reward, all of which appear

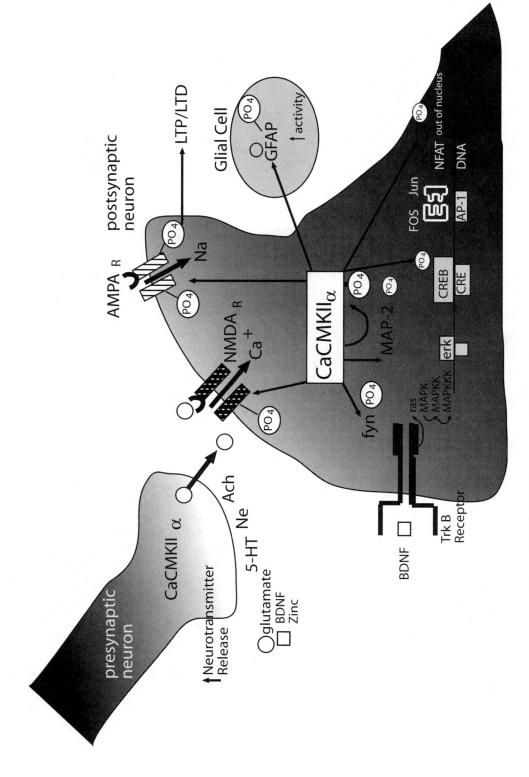

Figure 10.6 CaCMK-II$_\alpha$: A key calcium sensor for neuroplasticity and long-term memory.

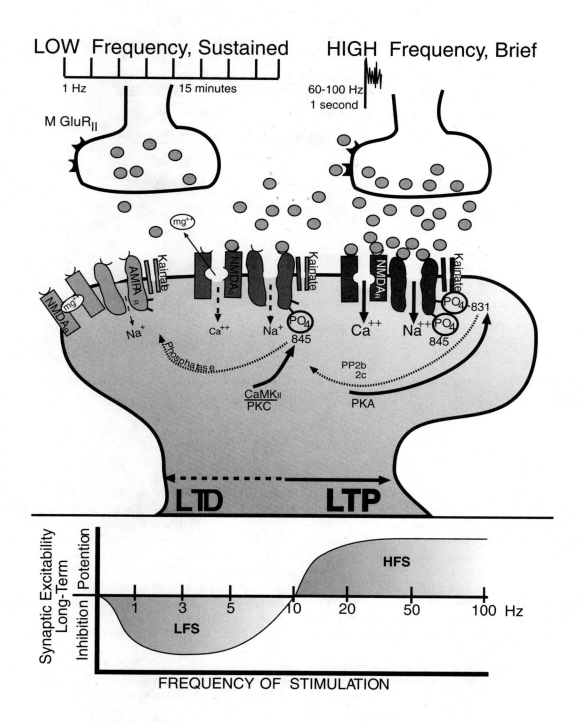

Figure 10.7 Bidirectional modification in synaptic excitability as a function of frequency of stimulation (top and bottom) and putative cellular components (middle) of long-term depression (LTD) and long-term potentiation (LTP). LTD occurs following low-frequency (LFS; e.g., 1 Hz for 15 minutes, top left) and may involve increased phosphatase activity leading to dephosphorylation of the AMPA receptors. LTP occurs following brief high-frequency stimulation (HFS; e.g., 100 Hz for 1 second, top right) and involves relatively large increases in calcium flux through the NMDA receptor and increases in kinase activity leading to increased phosphorylation of the AMPA receptors. The bottom illustrates the frequency dependence of these two phenomena with LFS (1–5 Hz) producing relative synaptic inhibition and HFS (20–100 Hz) producing potentiation. (Modified from Dudek, Bear, et al., 1991; Li et al., 1998; and Malenka, 1995.)

Null Mutation αCaMKII:	Heterozygous αCaMKII +/-	Homozygous αCaMKII +/+
	50% Depletion	100% Depletion
Hippocampal LTP	Normal	Blocked
Learning (Intensive Training)	Normal	Blocked
Short-Term Memory* 1-3 days	Normal	
Long-Term Memory* 10-50 days (Interm. training 3x, 8x)	Impaired	
Spatial Memory	Impaired	
Cortical LTP (both in visual & temporal cortex)	Impaired	

Figure 10.8 Behavioral and physological effects of αCaMK-II knockouts. CaMK-II, calcium calmodulin kinase II; LTP, long-term potentiation. (From Frankland, O'Brien, Ohno, Kirkwood, and Silva, 2001.)

altered in bipolar illness. The evidence from PET scans of relative cerebellar hyperactivity in unipolar and bipolar depression compared with normal volunteers is of considerable interest in relation to the observations of Schmahmann and Sherman (1998) of affective as well as motor dysregulation in patients with cerebellar lesions.

Each of these biochemical, structural, and functional neuroanatomical abnormalities have plausible relationships to the signs and symptoms of bipolar illness and deserve further direct exploration and confirmation. Much work remains in better defining which abnormalities relate to state (depression- and mania-related) abnormalities and which may be trait or illness vulnerability changes, either as an underlying cause or as a consequence of episodes and chronic illness. Moreover, it will be important to separate which changes are primary (pathological) versus secondary (adaptive). Is hyperactivity of a given area of the brain a pathological process that needs to be ameliorated, or an adaptive one that should be enhanced? Some evidence may be derived on this point from procedures which can alter the activity of specific areas of brain,

such as those that can be achieved with repetitive transcranial magnetic stimulation (rTMS) of the brain (Chapter 57). It appears possible to differentially modulate the activity of different areas of the brain. Andy Speer found that high-frequency rTMS increases, and low-frequency rTMS decreases, neural activity in a moderately long-lasting fashion after a series of 10 daily rTMS treatments (Speer et al., 2000). Thus, such changes in a given neural pathway induced by rTMS may help to elucidate whether an illness-related abnormality needs to be augmented or inhibited in order to produce clinically relevant therapeutic effects.

Etiological Pathways

Given this emerging picture of diverse biochemical, functional, and structural alterations in the brains of patients with bipolar illness compared with controls (Figure 10.4), the question arises as to what are their causes and mechanisms. In addition to changes based on heredity, early environmental and experience-based alterations in gene expression are also likely involved both as long-lasting vulnerability factors and as short-term perturbations related to episode occurrence and recovery. For example, studies of single and repeated episodes of maternal deprivation in the neonatal rat pup have revealed persisting alterations in biochemistry (increases in CRH and corticosterone) and behavior (anxiety) extending into rodent adulthood.

These data suggest that environmental events, as modulated by a host of environmental contingencies, could produce alterations in gene expression in neural systems important in emotion regulation. It is of interest that one day of neonatal maternal deprivation acutely decreases BDNF and CaMK-IIα in the rat pup and increases the number of cells dying from apoptosis (preprogrammed cell death; Figure 10.9). Repeated maternal separations and related stressor lead to decreases in cortical BDNF which persist into adulthood in laboratory animal studies. Normal volunteers who have the common variant of BDNF val66met that works slightly less efficiently than the usual val66val allele of BDNF have decrease in the volume of areas in their prefrontal cortices, (as well as decreases in hippocampal volume in association with minor deficits in episodic memory). Thus, either genetic vulnerabilities in these systems, environmentally mediated changes in gene expression, or (most likely) their interaction could account for the many abnormalities observed in bipolar illness.

Neurological and Psychiatric Overlaps

As we move into the 21st century, we are beginning to have an understanding of some of the alterations in physiology and biochemistry that accompany major fluctuations in mood (Figure 10.4). The data on genetics and the well-replicated findings of peptide, endocrine, and calcium alterations in the illness and alterations in frontal cortex and limbic system activity all place bipolar illness in a position similar to other medical disorders, with not only distinct mood, motor, and vegetative symptoms but also an increasingly well-delineated neurobiology.

Whereas neurology has typically been the area of interest to physicians in studying structural alterations in the brain, it is clear that the epilepsies are more functional and obviously connected to alterations in biochemistry and physiology that eventually produce a seizure disorder. Likewise, the margins between psychiatry and neurology are beginning to blur as physiological, biochemical, and microstructural changes are observed in the major psychiatric illnesses.

Thus, while neuronal dysregulation or the "functional" lesions of psychiatry have often been referred to as somehow less robust or less well documented than those in most of neurology (where there is usually clear neuronal loss and defective nerve circuits and reflexes), the information on the fundamental neurobiology of bipolar illness (and schizophrenia) is beginning to alter this perspective and unequivocally place these illnesses in the realm of brain disorders similar to many other neurological disorders. Given the growing evidence for glial as well as neuronal deficits in bipolar illness and schizophrenia, perhaps the term "mental" illness, with its pejorative connotations of imagined or existing only in the mind, should be changed to neuroglia illness instead.

It is important to remember that while the functional nature of the psychiatric illnesses suggests that they may be somewhat more complex and more difficult to understand, many psychiatric illnesses are currently more amenable to treatment than those in neurology, where the major cell losses or excesses of strokes, tumors, parkinsonism, and Alzheimer's cannot yet be easily remedied. The brain not only houses 10 billion neurons (each of which has about 100,000 synapses) and perhaps 80 to 100 billion glial cells yielding an almost infinite number of points of cellular contact, but it is extremely plastic, adaptive, and constantly changing (Figure 10.10). Its complexity is thought to enable uniquely human attributes such as self-awareness, abstract reasoning, and planning for the future. Its complexity may also relate to both the vulnerability to affective disorders and the ability to overcome a host of insults and stressors, particularly with the help of drug and psychotherapeutic treatments.

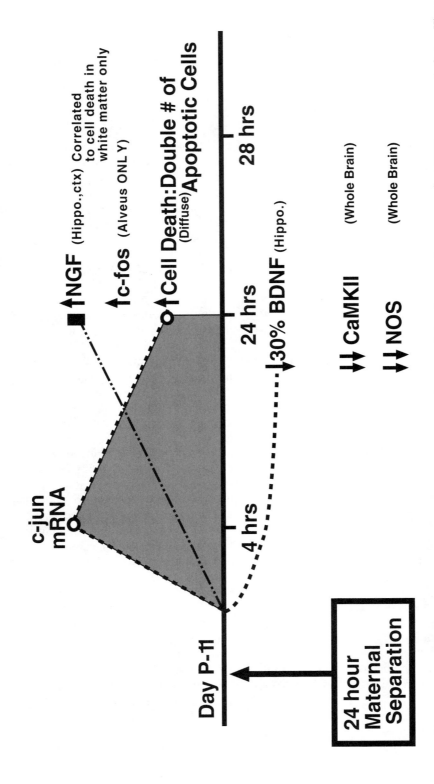

Figure 10.9 Effects of maternal separation in neonatal rat pups on neurotrophins, transcription factors, and gene expression. NGF, nerve growth factor; Hippo., hippocampus; ctx., cortex; BDNF, brain-derived neurotrophic factor; CaMK-II, calcium calmodulin kinase II; NOS, nitric oxide synthase. (From Zhang et al., 2002.)

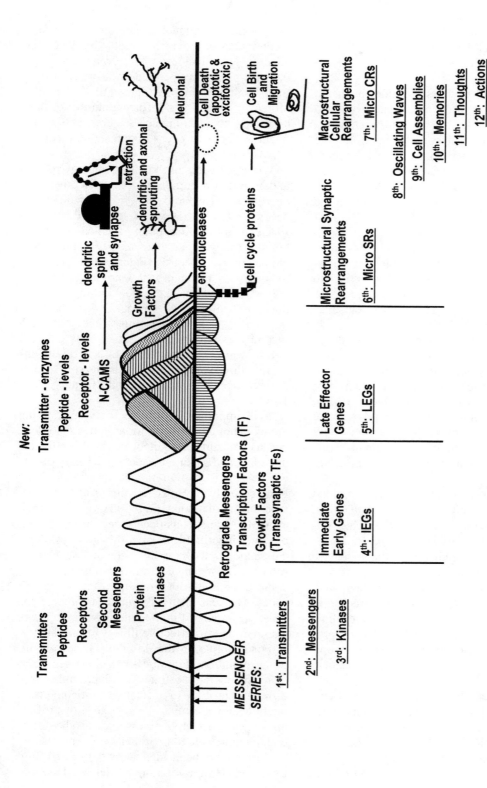

Figure 10.10 Remodeling the central nervous system based on experience. Figure portrays an evolving cascade of messenger systems, each with its own complex regulatory mechanisms and cross-talk with other systems (not illustrated). In addition to showing immediate early genes (IEGs) and late effector genes (LEGs), this figure suggests that environmental stimulation can engage mechanisms that change the connectivity of the brain on a biochemical as well as microstructural basis, including cell sprouting, cell migration, or even cell death. These synaptic changes may ultimately be reflected in larger functional units (eighth and ninth messengers) that encode thoughts, memories, and preparation for action. N-CAMs, neural cell adhesion molecules.

Environmental Vulnerabilities in the Onset and Progression of the Recurrent Affective Disorders

Kraepelin observed that first episodes of mania or depression were often precipitated by psychosocial stresses, but that with sufficient numbers of recurrences, episodes begin to emerge more spontaneously and autonomously (Figure 10.3). These observations are now supported by a substantial controlled literature validating this concept. We refer to this phenomenon under the name *stress sensitization*, based on the findings that animals can show increased reactivity to some repeated intermittent stressors over time. This finding would parallel the clinical observation that patients become more sensitive to stressors to the point at which minor stressors or no stressors at all can trigger affective episodes (Figures 10.3 and 10.11).

Kraepelin was also among the first to document that the well interval between the first and second episodes tended to be longer than the interval between successive episodes (i.e., there tends to be cycle acceleration; Figure 10.11). This, too, has also now been generally validated in the literature. However, this does not imply that the tendency for progression cannot be arrested upon institution of successful prophylactic drug therapy.

Kessing and associates (1998) have provided the best documentation of episode sensitization, that is, that episodes beget episodes. They observed that in both unipolar and bipolar hospitalizations, the best predictor of the incidence and time to relapse was the number of prior hospitalizations (Figure 10.12). These data were observed in 20,250 patients carefully tracked in the Danish case registry, confirming Kraepelin's original formulation. This likely reflects a process of episode sensitization in which each episode increases the vulnerability to a subsequent one.

We have linked stress sensitization and episode sensitization together, because each increases the vulnerability to future episodes, and discuss both in relationship to another process, kindling, that grows over time with repetition. In typical kindling, repeated electrical stimulation of one area of the brain (such as the amygdala) for 1 second each day, which initially produces few effects (Figure 10.13, top left), eventually evokes full-blown seizures to what was previously a subthreshold stimulus (Figure 10.13, middle). Moreover, following a sufficient number of these triggered amygdala-kindled seizures, untriggered seizures begin to occur spontaneously (Figure 10.13, top right).

We use this seizure kindling analogy to help understand how parallel processes in other neural systems related to behavior (not seizures) may become stimulus (stressor) sensitized and episode sensitized to the point at which (as in real kindling) they occur more readily, rapidly, and ultimately spontaneously (Figure 10.11). The neurobiology of the neuronal learning process in amygdala kindling (i.e., the kindling memory trace) is beginning to be revealed at the level of changes in neurotransmitters, receptors, and second messengers, as well as effects on gene transcription and downstream effects on the microstructure of the brain involving cell sprouting, cell retraction, and cell death (Figures 10.10, 10.14).

It is important to realize that the kindling model is not a literal one for affective disorders, because seizures do not occur in the affective disorders and seizure episodes are vastly different from affective in the behaviors and time frames involved. However, the progressive development of behavioral seizures and their eventual spontaneous occurrence provides a set of easily identifiable behavioral and physiological endpoints for examining the analogous neurobiological mechanisms in other systems that could underlie the progression of affective episodes. One can then ask whether some of the principles revealed in the kindling paradigm are also pertinent to affective illness progression.

For example, in the different phases of kindling evolution (Figure 10.13), there are very-different neural substrates involved and a very different profile of effective anticonvulsant pharmacology. Similarly, we believe that different stages of affective illness may also be differentially amenable to treatment interventions, but this has not yet been adequately delineated (Figure 10.15). In the kindling model, we have ob-

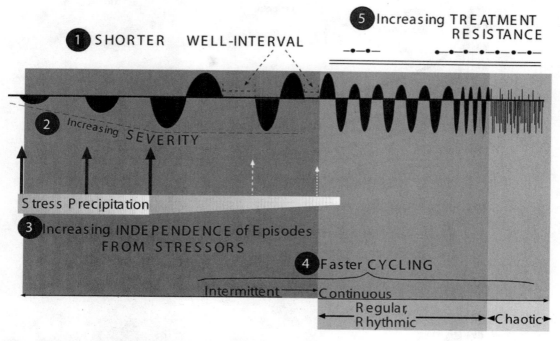

Figure 10.11 Sensitization in affective illness. Evidence of the tendency for the illness to progress is based on a variety of observations, including: (1) increases in episode frequency; (2) increases in episode severity, quality, or complexity; (3) early episodes precipitated by psychosocial stressors, but later ones occurring more spontaneously; (4) transition from intermittent to continuous to chaotic cycling patterns; and (5) possibly increasing treatment resistance, especially to lithium.

served that animals treated earlier in the course of the seizure are less likely to lose responsivity via a tolerance mechanism to a given course of treatment than animals treated later in their course of illness (Chapter 9). Higher and steady doses of drugs are more effective in preventing kindled seizures than lower doses or use of marginally effective agents.

These predictions from the kindling model need to be tested in the clinic for their ultimate applicability to affective illness progression. However, a considerable number of studies (at least nine) indicate that lithium is less effective if treatment is initiated later, after many affective episodes have occurred, than when it is started earlier in the course of illness (Figure 10.15). These empirical data and the kindling theoretical formulation both raise the question of whether early intervention with effective

treatment at the first onset of symptoms could prevent many of the adverse consequences and course of bipolar illness, or even prevent the entire syndrome from developing into a full-blown illness.

It is possible (as the kindling model predicts) that effective early treatment intervention could prevent the development of subsequent vulnerabilities to recurrence (Figure 10.16), prevent illness morbidity and mortality, and actually change the predicted course of illness. Adolescents and young adults are recognized to be at substantial risk for suicide in the context of severe affective disorders, and this is a population in which suicide is rising rapidly. Moreover, particularly in adolescents and young adults, bipolar illness is an enormous risk factor for the acquisition of problems with substance abuse.

Each substance of abuse has its own effect

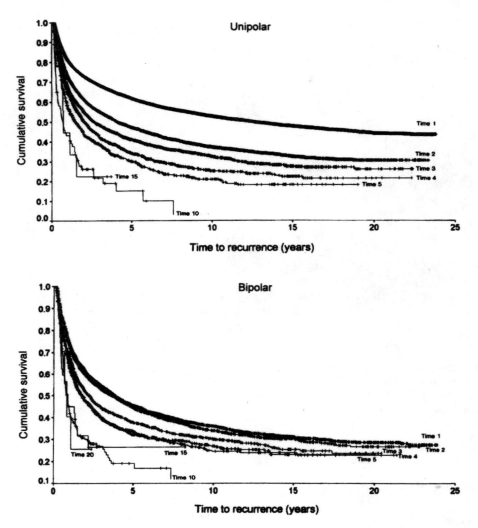

Figure 10.12 Cumulative survival (probability of remaining well) was calculated usng the Kaplan-Meier method for estimation with censored observations. Eight different index admissions (1, 2, 3, 4, 5, 10, 15, and 20) represent the number of prior hospitalizations. For both unipolar (top) and bipolar (bottom) patients, incidence of and latency to relapse varied as a function of the number of prior depressions. (From Kessing et al., 1998.)

on gene expression, which can interact with and compound some of those of the illness itself, and thus greatly complicate treatment. In this fashion, juvenile and adolescent bipolar illness should be carefully diagnosed and considered for early intervention, not only to attempt to treat and prevent future affective episodes, but also to prevent some of the secondary consequences of the illness, such as drug and alcohol abuse, and the possibility of greater degrees of

biological change that correlate with either number of episodes or illness duration (Table 10.1).

Summary and Clinical Implications

New finding on BDNF help place these concepts in a more concrete perspective. Not only do stressors in animals decrease BDNF in the

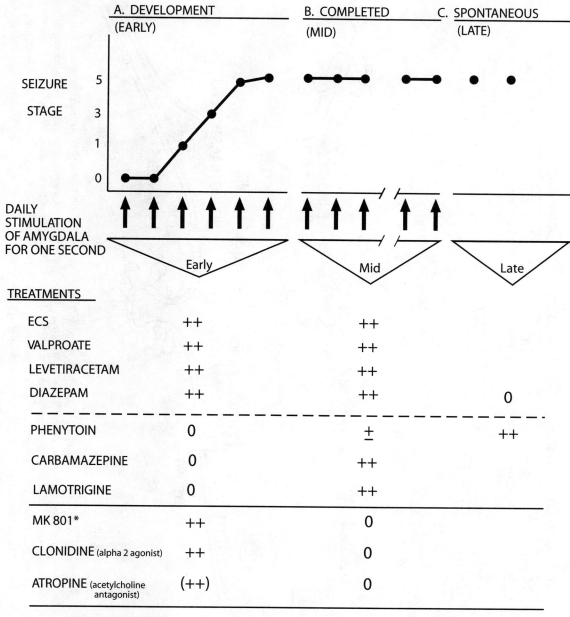

Figure 10.13 Pharmacological responsivity as a function of stage of kindling. Top: Schematic illustration of the evolution of kindled seizures. Initial stimulations (development) are associated with progressively increasing afterdischarge duration (not shown) and behavioral seizure stage. Subsequent stimulations (completed) produce reliable generalized motor seizures. Spontaneous seizures emerge after sufficient numbers of triggered seizures have been generated (usually over 100). Bottom: Amygdala- and local anesthetic–kindled seizures show differences in pharmacological responsivity as a function of kindled stage (++, very effective; ±, partially effective; 0, not effective; parentheses indicate inconsistent data). The double dissociation in response to diazepam and phenytoin in the early versus the late phases of amygdala kindling, as described by Pinel, is particularly striking. Note also that carbamazepine is effective in inhibiting the developmental phase of local anesthetic but not amygdala kindling, whereas the converse is true for the completed phase. ECS, electroconvulsive seizure. *Glutamate *N*-methyl-D-aspartate antagonist.

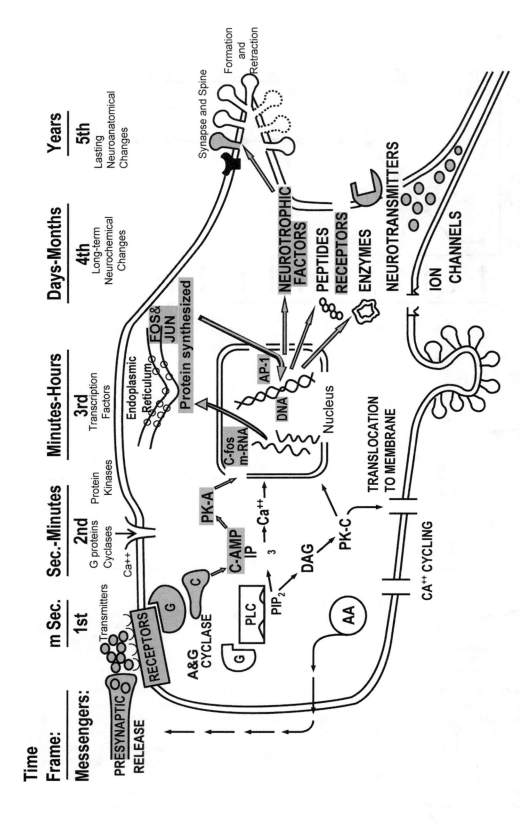

Figure 10.14 Neural mechanisms of synaptic plasticity and short- and long-term memory. This schematic of a cell illustrates how transient synaptic events induced by external stimuli can exert longer-lasting effects on neuronal excitability and the microstructure of the brain via a cascade of effects involving alterations in gene transcription. Neurotransmitters activate receptors and second-messenger systems, which then induce IEGs, such as c-fos and c-jun. Fos and jun proteins are synthesized on the endoplasmic reticulum (ER) and then bind to DNA to further alter the transcription of late effector genes (LEGs) and other regulatory factors, the effects of which could last for months or years. PLC, phospholipase C; PIP₂, phosphatidyl inositol 4,5-biphosphate; AA, arachidonic acid; DAG, diacylglycerol; PK-C, protein kinase C; AP-1, activator protein 1 (binding site on DNA); PK-A, protein kinase A.

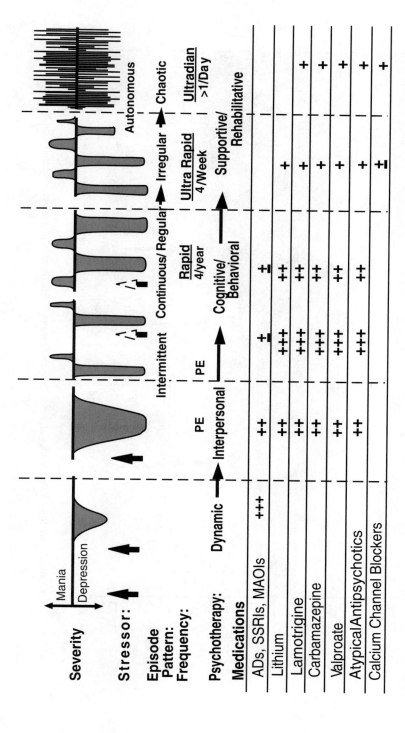

Figure 10.15 Phases in the evolution of mood cycling; potential relationship to treatment response. In an analogous fashion to kindling, episodes of affective illness may progress from triggered (arrows) to spontaneous and show different patterns and frequencies (top) as a function of the stage of syndrome evolution. Although systematic and controlled studies have not examined the relationship of the illness phase to treatment response, anecdotal observations provide suggestive data that some treatments may be: +++, highly effective; ++, moderately effective; +, possibly effective; or ±, equivocal; as a function of course of illness. Note that the pharmacological dissociations in the nonhomologous model of kindling are different from those postulated in mood disorders; nonetheless, the principle of differential response as a function of stage may be useful, and deserves to be specifically examined and tested. PE, psychoeducation; ADs, antidepressants; SSRIs, selective serotonin reuptake inhibitors; MAOIs, monoamine oxidase inhibitors.

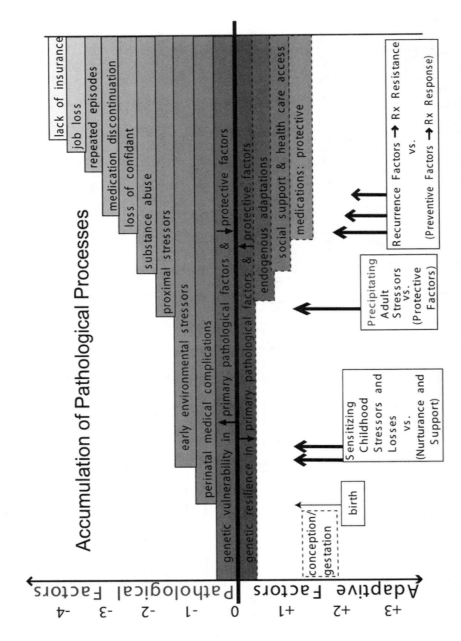

Figure 10.16 Ratio of pathological versus adaptive factors in determining illness episodes and well intervals.

Table 10.1 *More Episodes or Longer Duration of Illness Could Drive Neurobiological Abnormalities*

Finding	UP/BP	Episodes	Duration	Authors
Subgenual Pfc.	UP	#*		Kimbrell et al., 2002
Hippocampus				
Volume decreased (MRI)	UP	#*[a]	—*[a]	MacQueen et al., 2003
Decreased volume (MRI)	UP		—*	Sheline et al., 1999
Decreased synaptic markers (autopsy)	BP		—*	Law et al., 2004
Neurocognitive				Denicoff et al., 1999
Dysfunction and disability	BP	#*		Balanza-Martinez et al., 2005
Risk of dementia	UP/BP	#*[b]		Kessing et al., 2004
Increased amygdala volume	BP	#*		Altshuler et al., 1988
		(manias)		
Endocrine				
Increased dex. escape	UP		—*[c]	Coryel al., 1985
Increased Dex-CRH response	UP/BP	#*[c]		Kunzel et al., 2003

a = exponential; b = doubles after ≥ 4; c = also relates to risk of relapse in euthymic patients.
Original references in Post et al., 2003.

hippocampus, but each episode of affective illness in people is associated with decreased in BDNF in serum. In both manic and depressive episodes, the BDNF decreases occur in proportion to the severity of symptoms (Figure 10.17). In addition, each episode is associated with an increase in oxidative stress which produces free radical toxins that damage cells. Thus, each episode appears to endanger cells, both by reduced amounts of neuroprotective factors such as BDNF and by increased toxic factors.

In an animal model of depression, depressive-like behaviors caused by repeated bouts of defeat stress, the BDNF changes are essential to the behaviors manifest. In this model, BDNF decreases in the hippocampus and increases in the dopamine pathway from the VTA to the nucleus accumbens. If either of these BDNF changes are prevented, depressive behaviors do not occur (Tavaskova et al., 2006; Berton et al., 2006). Cocaine, like defeat stress, also increases BDNF in the VTA/accumbens pathway, and if the BDNF changes are prevented, cocaine induced behavioral sensitizaton does not occur.

Thus, BDNF may be one link between the effects of stressors, drugs of abuse like cocaine, and affective episodes. Each can predispose to the other. Moreover, each can show increased responsivity to its own repetition, i.e. stress sen-

sitizaton, cocaine sensitization, and episode sensitization. The BDNF decreases in the hippocampus and increases in the VTA/accumbens may be one common element is these progressive changes and in their cross sensitization to the other forms of sensitization.

Each of these types of sensitization appears to have learned or conditioned components, and it is of interest that BDNF is not only involved in synaptogenesis and cell survival, but is necessary for long term memory. BDNF is co-released with glutamate in the hippocampus and with dopamine in the accumbens, and is thought to help cement events modulated by these areas into long term memory. The hippocampus could be conveying contextual and spatial information, while the VTA/accumbens pathway provide information on reward value, motivation, activity, and hedonic mechanisms that are involved in stress reactivity, drug abuse, and affective episodes,

In this fashion, repetition of affective episodes could affect the brain in two ways. Passively by endangering cells with neurotrophic factor decrements and increased in oxidative stress, and actively by learning and memory based mechanisms involving BDNF in hippocampus and accumbens. Since many mood stabilizers increase BDNF and other neurotrophic factors

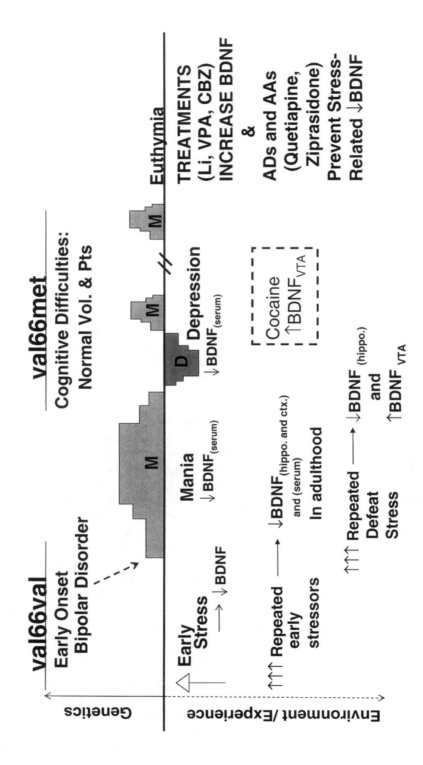

Figure 10.17 BDNF is involved in: genetic (top) and environmental (bottom) vulnerability to bipolar illness. During each manic and depressive episode, BDNF decreases (in proportion to symptom severity). Stressors early in life decrease BDNF in the hippocampus (hippo.) and cortex (ctx.) and in the serum of humans. Both defeat stress experiences and repeated cocaine use increase BDNF in the dopamine pathway from the VTA to N. Accumbens likely reflecting the learned components of these behaviors. Conversely, the psychotropic drugs increase BDNF in the hippocampus and/or prevent its decrease by stress.

directly, or would do so by preventing episode-related decrements in BDNF, these new data should facilitate illness and treatment reconceptualizations that should have a major impact on the assessment of the risk/benefit ratio long term prophylactic treatment, We always knew that affective episodes are associated with enormous suffering, but now they also are likely bad for the brain. Effective treatments, while they convey some side effects, prevent episodes and therefore help ameliorate or prevent the progression of the neurobiological alterations underlying bipolar illness. The bottom line is long term prophylactic treatment may protect the brain.

Part IV

RESPONSE TO
MOOD STABILIZERS

Lithium

11

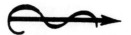

An Excellent Response to Lithium

CASE HISTORY

This case describes a 38-year-old bipolar woman with rapidly recurrent severe depression interrupted by brief periods of full-blown psychotic mania (requiring seclusion) (Figure 11.1). These episodes first alternated with periods of mute depression with catatonic elements (such as waxy flexibility). She showed an excellent response to lithium (in 1975) and achieved an essentially complete remission for 15 years (Figure 11.2).

Periodically, she would call the first author (RMP) to renew communication and ask whether he thought it was a good idea or not to stop her lithium. Following two such yearly telephone calls and despite advice to the contrary, she decided to discontinue her medication and did so with a careful self-initiated lithium taper (in 1988) over about 1 month. She indicated that she wanted to try this because while feeling stabilized, she thought that lithium had slightly lowered her exciting "edge" and "creative glitter."

She subsequently relapsed into a hypomania and then moderately severe depression that persisted despite the reinstitution of lithium and a variety of other treatment augmentation strategies (Figure 11.2, right side). In contrast to several other patients we have seen with this phenomenon (Chapter 13), she eventually regained her original level of excellent lithium responsiveness. However, this renewed response required 2 to 3 years to achieve, caused considerable discomfort and at times despair, and necessitated the use of additional medications (Figure 11.2).

BACKGROUND LITERATURE

This patient illustrates a number of points of considerable interest in relationship to lithium prophylaxis. The patient possessed a number of illness characteristics, some of which predicted lithium response, and a number of others that have been associated with a poorer response to the drug in the literature (Table 11.1).

John Cade reported on the first clinical series of patients indicating the antimanic effects of lithium. This series was followed by the pioneering studies of Baastrup and Schou and their colleagues in Denmark (Baastrup & Schou, 1967). After a considerable delay, the use of lithium began in the United States in the late 1960s and early 1970s. At this time it was the treatment of choice for the acute and long-term management of bipolar illness, often with adjunctive use of antidepressants for breakthrough depressions, and antipsychotics for breakthrough mania (Schou, 2001).

Although initial clinical studies suggested 50–80% acute and prophylactic responsivity, it is now recognized that a variety of common features of bipolar illness predict lesser degrees of acute and prophylactic response to lithium. We have generated a schematic or rule of thumb that differentiates the patients in the excellent (70%) response group from those in the poorer (30%) response group.

Predictors of excellent response to lithium appear to be a positive family history of bipolar illness in first-degree relatives; a positive family

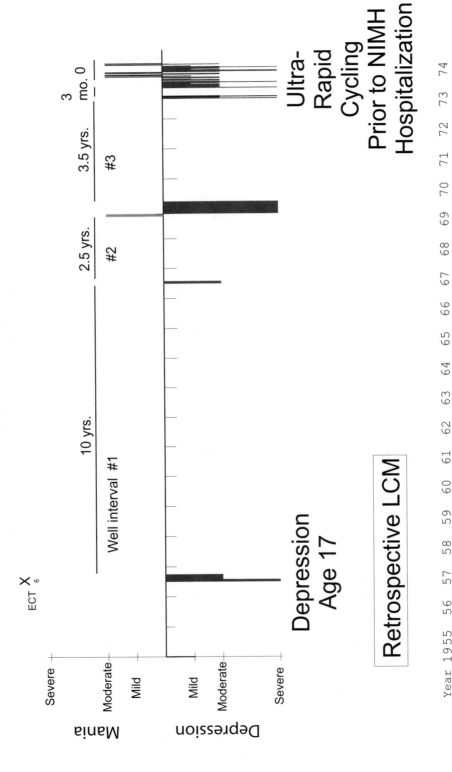

Figure 11.1 Retrospective course of illness shows an almost 10-year interval between the first and second depression, 2.5 years between the second and third depression, and 3.5 years between the third and fourth depressions; ultrarapid cycling began in 1973 and continued into 1975 (as seen in Figure 11.2).

112

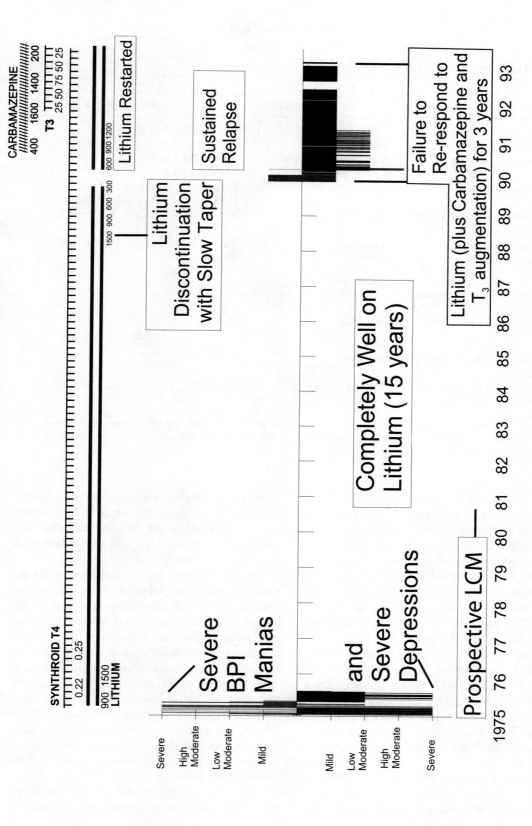

Figure 11.2 Despite an ultrarapid cycling course between extremes of psychotic mania and almost catatonic depression within days to weeks, this patient showed an excellent and complete response to lithium prophylaxis (with T₄ augmentation), which was sustained for more than 15 years. Even with an extremely slow taper of lithium over 9 months, she relapsed off drug and did not completely restabilize for several years.

Table 11.1 *Correlates of Relative Good versus Poor Responsiveness*

Factors	Good Response Rates (About 60–80%)	Low Response Rates (About 20–40%)	Strength of Evidence
Episode Characteristics			
1. Rapid or faster cycling	No	Yes	+++(12)
2. Episode contiguity	Intermittent, i.e., with a well interval (I)	Continuous, i.e., no well interval (I)	+
3. Sequence pattern	Mania → depression → I M-D-I	Depression → mania → I D-M-I	+++(4)
4. Number of episodes prior to starting prophylaxis	3 or fewer	4 to 10 or more	+++(9)
5. Quality of mania	Euphoric	Dysphoric	+++(4)
6. Insight/compliance	Good	Poor	+
Comorbidities			
7. History (Hx) of substance abuse	Negative	Positive	+
8. Hx of anxiety disorder	Negative	Positive	++
Genetic Background			
9. Family history of anxiety disorder	Negative	Positive	++
10. Family Hx of bipolar illness and especially lithium response	Positive	Negative	+++

+, Reported by several clinician observers; ++, reported in several studies; +++, well-documented (# = approximate number of supportive studies in literature).

history of lithium response; classic euphoric mania; beginning prophylaxis relatively early in the course of illness; good treatment adherence and compliance; lack of comorbid alcohol and substance abuse; lack of comorbid anxiety disorder or other comorbid personality disorder; and a history of not having rapid or continuous cycling course of illness (Aagard & Vestergaard, 1990; Bowden, 1995; Calabrese, Fatemi, Kujawa, & Woyshville, 1996; Post, Frye, Denicoff, et al., 1998; Goodwin & Jamison, 1990). In addition, five studies in the literature have noted that the pattern of mania, followed by a depression, followed by a well interval (M-D-I pattern) is much more likely to be lithium responsive than patients with the D-M-I pattern (Faedda, Baldessarini, Tohen, Strakowski, & Waternaux, 1991).

This patient has a number of positive lithium-responsive illness characteristics, including a lack of comorbid substance abuse, anxiety dis-

order, or personality disorder; however, characteristics of her illness that might be less responsive to lithium would include her ultrarapid course of illness and lack of a family history in first-degree relatives.

This patient was highly compliant with her medications, but complained of a too tight constriction of her affective range and loss of her normal exuberance and joie de vivre. This is not infrequently cited as a problem for patients maintaining lithium adherence and in many instances can be circumvented with more aggressive treatment of an underlying depression or with thyroid augmentation (whether or not thyroid values are in the abnormal range). Other lithium side effects such as tremor, gastrointestinal distress, weight gain, and increased urination are often cited as additional reasons for lithium discontinuation.

Lithium's side effects and some potential approaches to their management are indicated in

Table 11.2 *Common Lithium Side Effects and Their Management*

Side Effect	Possible Approaches (Most Not Based on Strong Evidence)	
Tremor (C); usually worse under social scrutiny	Lower dose ++; use beta blocker or such as propanolol 10 mg Q.I.D. ++; Consider mysoline as alternative +	
	Replace some of lithium dose with dihydropyridine calcium channel blocker	+
Gastrointestinal distress (O)	Lower dose	+
	Switch lithium preparations	±
	Replace some of lithium dose with a calcium channel blocker	±
Weight gain (O)	Warn and treat in advance	±
	Avoid nondiet sodas	+
	Consider weight loss adjuncts	++
Cognitive impairment (UC)	Treat residual depression	+
	Check thyroid	
	Even if euthyroid: consider treating with T_3	+++
Increased urination (C) (diabetes insipidus, i.e., blockage of vasopressin receptor response at level of decreased production of C-AMP)	If extreme or functionally impairing, treat with thiazide diuretics or ameloride; Switch to other mood-stabilizing agents	
	Carbamazepine will not cause diabetes insipidus, but will not correct lithium-related diabetes insipidus	
Kidney function impairment (UC)	Reduce dose	±;
	Monitor closely	
	Discontinue drug if rise in creatine is consistent	±
	Replace with other mood stabilizers	+
Psoriasis (O)	Omega-3 fatty acid supplementation may help suppress Li effect	+
Acne (O)	Retinoic acid only for women not of childbearing age or men	++
	Tetracycline; clindamycin	+
Hypothyroidism (O)	Replace with T_4	++
	Use T_4 and T_3 combination if mood remains low	+

VC, very common; C, common; O, occasional; UC, uncommon; VR, very rare; D, dose related; I, idiosyncratic; S, sensitivity may cross to other drugs; +++, well supported, controlled data; ++, many case reports; +, likely works; ±, questionable or hypothetical.

Table 11.2. These side effects should be treated diligently to minimize the inconvenience and discomfort of taking lithium and thus enhance compliance. However, in our experience, the desire to discontinue lithium after short to extended periods of stability occurs with a substantial number of patients, even in the virtual absence of side effects. New data on the likelihood of relapse, the small but possible chance of failing to reresspond to lithium once it is restarted, the increased incidence of suicidality and completed suicide off lithium, the glial and neuronal deficits of bipolar illness, and the convergent therapeutic effects of lithium in enhancing neurogenesis and inhibiting cell death all reinforce the importance of continuing effective lithium prophylaxis. The enormously creative and heroic life of a Kay Jamison and countless others, who maintain or enhance their creativity and enjoyment of life thanks to the mood stabilizing effects of lithium, provide inspiring examples.

PRINCIPLES OF THE CASE

STRENGTH OF EVIDENCE

1. Sustained long-term complete response to lithium monotherapy occurs in a small to moderate percentage of patients.   +++

2. Predictors of a less robust response to lithium include those

with rapid-cycling illness, dysphoric mania, comorbid anxiety disorders and substance abuse, increased numbers of episodes prior to initiating prophylaxis, a lack of family history with bipolar illness in first-degree relatives, and the D-M-I pattern. +++

3. Despite these general categorizations, many patients with these negative predictors still have an excellent response to lithium. ++

4. Long-term lithium treatment decreases the rate of suicide in patients with recurrent affective disorders. ++

5. Discontinuation of lithium is associated with an approximately 7- to 20-fold increase risk of suicide. ++

6. Lithium reduces the excess medical mortality that patients with unipolar or bipolar recurrent depression experience because of other medical illnesses such as heart attack and stroke. +

7. In discussing the risk-to-benefit ratio of continuing versus stopping lithium treatment, patients should be aware of the following:

   a. Specific risks of relapse (such as 50% in the first 5 months off of lithium treatment, and 90% by 18 months). ++

   b. Lithium's potential neurotrophic and neuroprotective effects, which have not yet been directly linked to its mechanism of action in bipolar illness, but are nonetheless likely to be positive attributes, and ones that could account for the reduction in the excess medical mortality in patients who do remain on long-term treatment. ++

   c. No guarantee that the same degree of response will be achieved again if they stop their lithium and experience relapses. +

8. Recent controlled studies reconfirm the efficacy of lithium monotherapy in the prevention of recurrent episodes of manic and depressive illness. +++

9. Several of these studies indicate that lithium's prophylactic antimanic effects are superior to those of either carbamazepine or lamotrigine. ++

10. A 1-year prophylaxis study (Tohen et al., 2004) reported the superior efficacy of olanzapine compared with that of lithium in the prevention of mania. +

11. In the face of an excellent response to lithium, one should be extremely reluctant to recommend going off this medication. +++

12. If a lithium discontinuation period is absolutely required, it should be achieved with an extremely slow taper, as this may help reduce, but not remove, the otherwise high relapse rate. +

TAKE-HOME MESSAGE

When bipolar illness is under control with lithium, one should continue full-dose pharmacoprophylaxis, because there are considerable risks in stopping treatment, which could include relapse, hospitalization, suicide attempt, and failure to rerespond as well as previously.

12

Development of Treatment
Resistance (via Tolerance) to the
Prophylactic Effects of Lithium

CASE HISTORY

The patient had a brief episode of depression at age 5 followed by more persistent periods of depression in 1961–1962. Depressions began to increase in frequency and manias in severity during his teenage years, when he engaged in considerable alcohol and substance abuse. In 1973 he was hospitalized for a severe mania (Figure 12.1). Despite stopping use of alcohol and substances of abuse, another severe manic episode occurred in 1977 that required hospitalization and was followed by a severe depression. The full-blown nature of this patient's manic psychosis was revealed during one of his manic episodes when he attempted to smash the Liberty Bell in Philadelphia with a sledgehammer.

In 1979, his illness was stabilized on lithium prophylaxis, and he maintained good compliance with this treatment. Despite lithium continuation, after approximately 5 years he began to show breakthrough mild and moderate episodes of depression and then manias of increasing severity and frequency (Figure 12.1, third row).

BACKGROUND LITERATURE

This patient shows the classic Kraepelinian progression of illness, with 6 years between the first and second episode, 2 to 3 years between the next two, and subsequent continuous cycling from 1973 to 1975. Some 40% of bipolar patients have additional problems with alcohol or substance abuse (Sonne & Brady, 1999; Suppes et al., 2001), and this patient was typical of this substantial subgroup. It is unknown to what extent the severe mania in 1974 was exacerbated by the use of substances, although this is highly likely. However, the patient would meet criteria for primary (rather than substance-induced) bipolar I mania, because in 1977 another episode occurred in the absence of substance abuse, a progression that is not atypical.

Episodes initially precipitated by the occurrence of substances of abuse may reveal the vulnerability to bipolar episodes, as the illness subsequently becomes manifest spontaneously. This transition may reflect another element of the sensitization phenomena beyond those of episode sensitization and stress sensitization, that is, substance-related sensitization. This might occur with exogenous substances, or even those produced endogenously by the endocrine or gonadal organs. For example, it is not uncommon for a woman with an initial episode of postpartum depression or mania to then go on to have a more classic spontaneous course of bipolar illness independent of endocrine and hormonal correlates.

Substantial lithium responsiveness in this patient is revealed despite the findings that a history

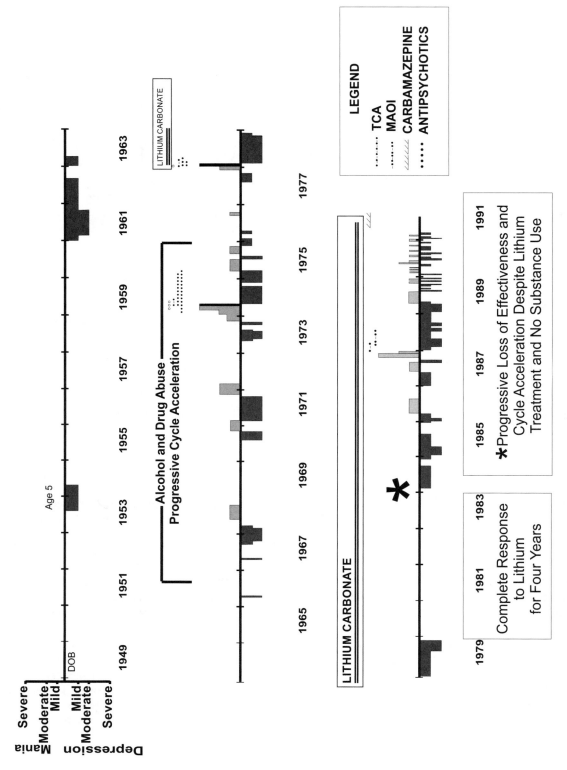

Figure 12.1 Development of tolerance to lithium's therapeutic effects. This patient showed an increase in manic severity and an acceleration of episode frequency during his teenage years when his illness was comorbid with alcohol and substance abuse (1966–1975). Following a second severe mania in 1977 requiring hospitalization, lithium treatment was instituted, and the patient subsequently had an excellent response. He was almost completely well for approximately 5 years and then began to show the same progressive increases in episode severity and frequency, despite good compliance with lithium and the absence of alcohol and substance abuse.

118

of prior alcohol or substance abuse is usually associated with a less robust response to lithium as compared with the anticonvulsant mood stabilizers (Bowden, 1995; O'Connell, Mayo, Flatow, Cuthbertson, & O'Brien, 1991). This patient had an excellent response from mid-1979 to the beginning of 1984 without any mood fluctuations. However, he began to show periodic emergence of depressions of mild to moderate severity and mild to moderate manic episodes with an increasing intensity, cyclicity, and persistence. This pattern appears consistent with the development of treatment resistance or tolerance as episodes begin to emerge with increasing frequency, severity, and duration despite the maintenance of previously adequate lithium levels (Post, Leverich, et al., 1993).

Of the patients coming to our clinical research unit at the NIMH with a history of lithium refractoriness, 43% appeared to acquire this via the process of tolerance development (Post, Leverich, et al., 1993). Again, a much lower rate of tolerance development would likely occur in the general population not selected for treatment resistance. However, a variety of other investigators in other clinical settings also have noted phenomena consistent with a tolerance process. In particular, Maj et al. (1998) examined patients who were complete responders to lithium for a period of at least 2 years and then followed them for another 5 years. A substantial number of these patients began to have breakthrough episodes despite close monitoring for adequate lithium levels. Koukopoulos et al. (1995) has also reported similar phenomena.

The mechanisms responsible for this progressive emergence of breakthrough episodes after a good initial treatment response is unknown. However, based on our model of tolerance to the anticonvulsive effects of carbamazepine as discussed in Chapter 19, we believe episode reemergence through medications follows many of the same principles that account for the initial illness recurrence off medications. In Chapter 10, we discussed the possibility that episodes of illness and their spontaneous remission might be related to the relative predominance of primary pathological factors (driving periods of illness) and secondary compensatory or endogenous antidepressant and mood-stabilizing factors (driving periods of remission) (Post & Weiss, 1992, 1996). In the well period of this patient from 1979 to 1984, some of these positive endogenous factors would not be induced, potentially leading to the vulnerability to illness reemergence despite the presence of lithium's (exogenous) mood-stabilizing mechanisms.

With episode breakthrough, we would also postulate that lithium might attenuate some of the episode-driven adaptations (similar to those observed for carbamazepine) leading to increasing episode emergence and finally complete loss of efficacy. Perhaps this patient was more prone to tolerance development because of the large number of prior episodes occurring before the beginning of lithium treatment, which has previously been shown to relate to the rapidity of tolerance development in the kindled seizure model (Chapter 10). At least nine studies in the literature have indicated that those with a greater number of episodes prior to using lithium are less likely to respond to lithium. This patient and the one in the previous chapter did show an excellent initial response to lithium, however, again indicating that there are often many exceptions to the general observations.

In addition to the failure to induce endogenous adaptive factors, tolerance could also be related to a progression of the underlying illness (even in the absence of episodes). This would be similar to tolerance during illness progression of Parkinson's disease that occurs with L-dopa treatment, where adequate initial treatment response is eroded by continued loss of dopamine cells (Nutt, 1995). However, in contrast, in bipolar illness there is currently no strong evidence that the mechanisms underlying illness vulnerability progress in the absence of the occurrence of breakthrough symptoms and episodes.

PRINCIPLES OF THE CASE   **STRENGTH OF EVIDENCE**

1. As observed by Emil Kraepelin, untreated illness tends to

show progression with shortening well intervals between episodes and at times increasing frequency or severity.   ++

2. Alcohol or substance abuse often are comorbid with bipolar illness and may exacerbate its manifestations and presentations.   +++

3. Substance-related manias are also likely to subsequently occur spontaneously (as they did in 1977 in this patient).   ++

4. The predictors of lithium responsiveness in the literature are only relative, as demonstrated by the patient's excellent response for approximately 5 years that occurred despite a variety of characteristics that would have predicted nonresponsiveness, including a history of substance abuse, rapid cycling, and many episodes prior to beginning lithium prophylaxis.   ++

5. During tolerance development, episodes of increasing frequency, severity, or duration tend to reemerge.   ++

6. In the face of such loss of efficacy to lithium via a tolerance process, one can recommend a variety of options, although none of them have been systematically tested for their relative efficacy. These include the following:
   a. Augmentation with a mood-stabilizing anticonvulsant such as carbamazepine, valproate, or lamotrigine.   ++
   b. Use of an atypical antipsychotic.   ++
   c. A period of time off a drug in the face of loss of re-

sponsiveness via tolerance development; it is not recommended in the case of lithium for several reasons, including increase in suicidality; difficulty in evaluating the efficacy of a new agent in the face of possible worsening of the illness off lithium; and loss of lithium's likely beneficial neurobiological effects, which include increases in neurogenesis and neurotrophic factors such as BDNF and Bcl-2. This loss could lead to accelerated loss of neurons and glia and loss of the increases in cortical gray matter that lithium induces, as revealed on the MRI.   +

7. The possibility of the eventual development of tolerance adds another reason to the importance of maintaining long-term full-dose prophylaxis, as both theory and a modicum of clinical observations suggest that treatment with marginal doses of a drug is more likely to be associated with tolerance development than more adequate doses.   +

8. Thus, if patients reduce the dose of an adequate prophylactic regimen, they may be putting themselves at increased risk for breakthrough episodes and the eventual loss of response via tolerance.   +

9. If this patient had had an earlier treatment intervention with lithium (e.g., in 1961 or 1962), one can only wonder what would have been the subsequent course of illness. Would earlier treatment have

prevented the onset of alcohol and substance abuse as well as the subsequent progression to full-blown bipolar I illness?   ±

10. The long lags from the first episodes meeting diagnostic thresholds (in 1961 for major depression with dysfunction, and in 1968 for hypomania) to the first treatment (in 1974) or the first sustained treatment (in 1978) allowed the emergence of multiple recurrent depressions and full-blown psychotic manias that may have resulted in a more difficult-to-treat course of illness.   +

TAKE-HOME MESSAGE

A good initial and sustained response to lithium is an excellent prognostic sign for long-term continuous illness prevention but, as illustrated in this case, it is still not an absolute guarantee that symptoms will not reemerge and require additional pharmacotherapy.

13

Loss of Previous Responsiveness to Lithium Following Its Discontinuation and Subsequent Episode Recurrence

CASE HISTORY

Case I: Failure to Respond After a Second Lithium Discontinuation

This 44-year-old male, a patient of G. M. Goodwin in England, experienced two severe depressions in his mid-20s, each requiring electroconvulsive therapy (ECT), and a severe mania at age 28 that responded well to the institution of lithium. Lithium treatment, however, was discontinued after 2 years (Figure 13.1, Arrow 1). A severe depressive relapse and suicide attempt 1.5 years later necessitated rehospitalization and treatment with ECT. Following reinstitution of lithium, the patient remained entirely trouble-free in terms of mood dysregulation for the next 10 years.

When the patient decided to discontinue his lithium treatment a second time (Figure 13.1, Arrow 2), he relapsed within 6 months into a severe depression with a suicide attempt. Despite restarting lithium immediately, his illness, with severe depressions (three requiring hospitalization) and intermittent hypomanias, had now become unresponsive to lithium. After 2 years of continued and disabling mood instability, the patient committed suicide. Thus, in a patient who

had demonstrated a sustained and completely successful prophylactic response to lithium, the second (but not the first) discontinuation of this effective treatment led to nonresponse in this patient.

It is important to note that this pattern of lithium discontinuation-induced refractoriness is entirely different from the pattern of tolerance development to lithium (i.e., loss of treatment response while on the treatment), which is discussed in Chapter 12. In the above case, it is highly unlikely that the patient's illness would have run this refractory course spontaneously, if not for lithium discontinuation, because the 10 entirely trouble-free years on lithium represent a substantially longer well interval than would have been expected from his previous course of illness.

Case II: Failure to Rerespond After the First Lithium Discontinuation

We have seen a number of other patients illustrating the phenomenon of lithium discontinuation-induced refractoriness. One of these is portrayed in Figure 13.2, which we constructed with a patient who had come to the NIMH for

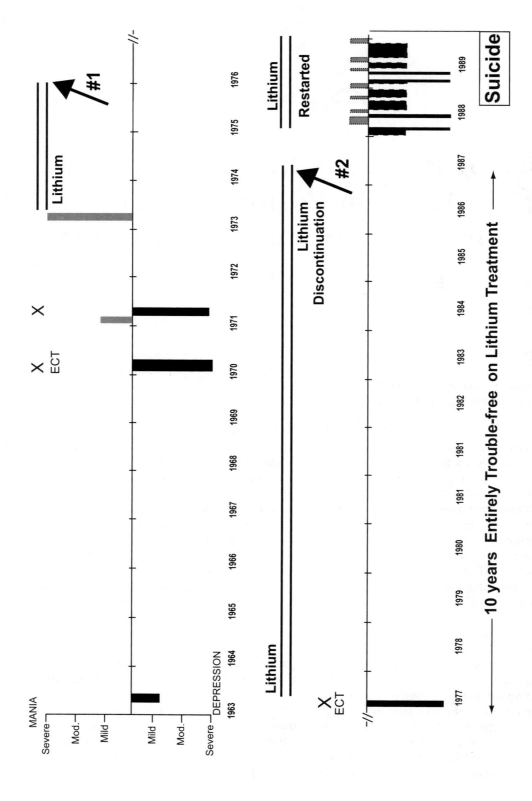

Figure 13.1 Loss of drug responsiveness following lithium discontinuation. First lithium discontinuation (Arrow 1): severe relapse after 17 months; patient reresponds to lithium maintenance treatment for 10 years after the first discontinuation (bottom row). The second lithium discontinuation (Arrow 2) was associated with another severe relapse, this time after only 6 months, leading to a severe depression and suicide attempt. Despite renewed treatment with lithium at doses similar to those previously effective, severe depressions recurred continuously in 1988–1989 with an ultimately tragic outcome.

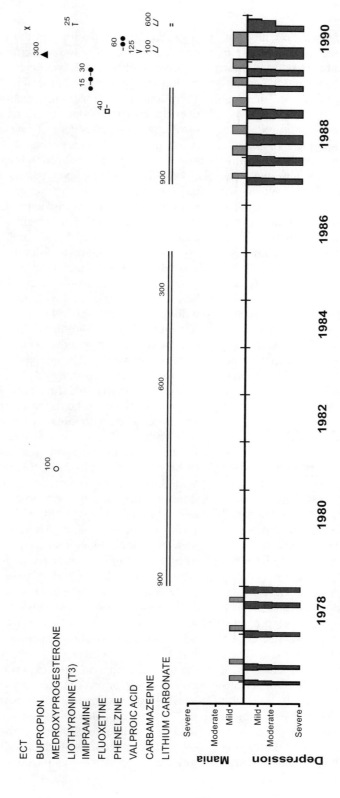

Figure 13.2 Lithium discontinuation-induced refractoriness. After more than 7 years of good functioning during lithium treatment, this patient eventually discontinued her lithium with an extremely slow taper. Despite the 3-year taper, she relapsed about 18 months later into a severe depression. Although she immediately restarted her lithium and eventually augmented it with many different treatments, even after more than a decade later (not illustrated) she did not fully regain her original degree of response.

an evaluation of her very refractory course of bipolar illness. She had done very well for a number of years, after treatment with lithium had been instituted in 1979 following the occurrence of a series of five severe, 2- to 3-month-long disabling depressions followed by mild hypomanias. After 7 years of good and productive functioning with renewed enjoyment of her life and family, she eventually discontinued her lithium (with a slow taper), thinking that long-term treatment was no longer necessary. When she relapsed 18 months later with a severe depression, she immediately restarted lithium at the previously effective dose and subsequently at higher doses, but did not reresponed and remained unresponsive to other medications for a great number of years. Again, it is highly unlikely that her illness would have run this refractory course had she stayed on lithium maintenance treatment. The patient herself has since become an outspoken advocate for staying on long-term effective lithium maintenance treatment, attempting to warn others of this rare but potentially catastrophic liability.

BACKGROUND LITERATURE

Although there is increasing recognition that significantly fewer bipolar patients respond adequately to lithium than had previously been believed—only 30–50% of patients rather than the earlier assumed 80% are lithium responsive (Aagaard & Vestergaard, 1990; Denicoff et al., 1997; Maj et al., 1998)—it has usually been believed that responsiveness to lithium prophylaxis, once demonstrated, could always be obtained or regained. In studies establishing the efficacy of lithium by looking at relapse rates after lithium discontinuation (Baastrup et al., 1970; Cavanagh, Smyth, & Goodwin, 2004; Suppes, Baldessarini, Faedda, & Tohen, 1991), patients generally responded to lithium reinstitution (even though a relapse itself following lithium discontinuation can be a critical problem with potentially serious sequelae). However, 50% of patients relapse within 5 months of stopping lithium and 90% relapse within 18 months (Sup-

pes et al., 1991), pointing to the continued underlying vulnerability to recurrence of the illness regardless of the duration and quality of the treated well interval (Chapter 11).

Systematic life chart construction and review of many patients' prior course of illness led us to what we now consider to be an important and newly discovered phenomenon that we call lithium discontinuation-induced refractoriness. Guy Goodwin in England, upon hearing of our presentation of cases illustrating this new potential adverse effect of lithium discontinuation, was kind enough to share one of his tragic clinical experiences with us in which the same phenomenon of lack of reresponse to lithium had occurred after the patient discontinued his effective lithium maintenance treatment and had a relapse. The first life chart of this patient, constructed with Goodwin's input and review, illustrates the potential hazard of lithium discontinuation in a patient who has responded well.

It is noteworthy that the patient reresponded to lithium when he relapsed 2 years after discontinuing lithium the first time (Figure 13.1, Arrow 1). However, he did not respond the second time, when he relapsed after only 6 months off the drug (Figure 13.1, Arrow 2). This latter failure to respond suggests that the appearance of an additional episode at this point could be something analogous to crossing a vulnerability threshold (i.e., one episode too many), thus conceivably engendering additional changes at the level of gene expression. These could occur either by episode-driven increases in neurobiology or by loss of lithium-induced long-term positive adaptations. Either or both of these could potentially contribute to the patient's lack of response to lithium. It may be somewhat unpredictable and unique for each patient when this one episode too many occurs, depending possibly on one's genetic vulnerability and prior environmental alterations in gene expression.

The observations reported here raise the possibility in some patients that periodic and repeated noncompliance with lithium over time may lead to multiple subsequent relapses that could eventually engender self-induced lithium refractoriness in a patient who would otherwise be highly lithium responsive. Careful reconstruction of some patients' life charts has shown a pattern consistent with this proposition.

Together, these observations strongly suggest the importance of not discontinuing lithium maintenance treatment when a good preventive response has been achieved. The possible increases in illness-related suffering and dysfunction (morbidity) are high, and the less likely but real possibility of episode recurrence, progression, and the induction of treatment nonresponsiveness or even loss of life by suicide should not be discounted as potential consequences of stopping otherwise effective lithium treatment.

Lithium discontinuation-induced refractoriness, although uncommon, is not entirely a rarity and can have severe consequences, as we have seen in many of the patients illustrated here and those whom we have observed on our unit. The incidence is likely about 10–15% in a population of patients with high episode frequencies and proneness to treatment resistance, although it probably is lower in the general population of those with more benign and less recurrent illness (Post, Leverich, et al., 1992, 1993).

The discontinuation phenomenon deserves further study and investigation, not only as it pertains to lithium but perhaps to some other pharmacological interventions as well. We have some cases in which loss of responsiveness to previously effective antidepressant medications in recurrent unipolar depression seems to indicate a potentially parallel phenomenon with many of the same difficult personal consequences (Chapter 37). We want to alert both patients and physicians to the inherent dangers potentially accompanying the discontinuation of effective maintenance treatments in bipolar illness. Although discontinuation-induced refractoriness has not been systematically observed with other prophylactic treatments, any decision to discontinue effective preventive treatment should be made with very careful weighing of the risks and benefits.

Although there are no good predictors as to who might become refractory to lithium following its discontinuation and reinstitution after relapses have occurred, it is possible that merely the appearance of new affective episodes (with their decrements in BDNF) makes the occurrence of subsequent episodes even more likely (with or without treatment; Figure 10.12).

Another related possibility is that the lithium discontinuation period is associated with an off-drug neurobiology that is a particularly fertile ground for an episode. Thus, despite appearing behaviorally similar to previous episodes, the biochemical consequences could be more severe. For example, since lithium both increases neurogenesis and cell survival factors Bcl-2 and BDNF and decreases cell death factors Bax and p53 (Chen et al., 1999; Chen & Chuang, 1999; Fukumoto, Morinobu, Okamoto, Kagaya, & Yamawaki, 2001), the absence of these potentially restorative effects on the neurobiology of bipolar illness could yield increasing levels of episode-related neuropathology. Such changes could render the illness less responsive upon attempts at retreatment.

As noted in Chapter 10, there is considerable evidence for neuronal or glial cell loss in various areas of the cingulate gyrus and prefrontal cortex of patients with affective disorders. It is not clear whether some of these are developmentally mediated vulnerabilities or whether some may reflect changes that are associated with illness progression. To the extent that episodes of illness do generate neurobiological mechanisms that could be detrimental to the survival of existing neurons and normal replacement of new neural and glial elements in areas of the brain (such as the hippocampus through neurogenesis), it is conceivable that the new episode in the absence of lithium's protective effects could generate further neural dysfunction at the level of both biochemistry and brain microstructure. The new findings that each episode of depression or mania is associated with decreases in serum BDNF in proportion to the severity of symptoms and increases in oxidative stress are entirely consistent with this proposition. This formulation also raises the possibility that a recurrence of an episode in the absence of lithium could have more severe consequences than an episode occurring as a breakthrough during ongoing lithium prophylaxis, and its maintained neurotrophic and neuroprotective effects. Whatever the mechanistic explanation, the clinical occurrence of lithium discontinuation-related refractoriness in a small number of patients should give one pause when adding this possibility to the range of liabilities potentially associated with stopping a successful treatment.

PRINCIPLES OF THE CASE	STRENGTH OF EVIDENCE
1. Discontinuation of effective lithium prophylaxis can lead to relapse, for example, 50% relapse in first 5 months, 90% by 18 months (Suppes et al., 1991).	+++
2. Long-term response to effective lithium maintenance (even after 15 or more years) does not preclude relapse if lithium is discontinued (the underlying illness vulnerability is not reset by lithium).	++
3. Discontinuation of effective lithium prophylaxis can lead to reduced responsiveness when the drug is restarted.	++
4. If a patient reresponds the first time, it does not guarantee a response following subsequent discontinuations (see Case I).	±
5. A slow taper of drug may lower the risk of relapse to some extent but does not necessarily prevent discontinuation-induced refractoriness (see Case II).	+
6. Repeated discontinuation of other effective pharmacotherapies (with associated repeated relapses) could lead to lack of response; we have seen this with antidepressants in several unipolar patients.	+
7. Relative treatment nonresponsiveness can lead to noncompliance, for example, "What's the use in taking these drugs anyway? They aren't helping." However, the cases in this chapter also suggest the opposite is possible. Noncompliance can lead to treatment refractoriness, meaning that people who repeatedly stop taking lithium could be lessening its effectiveness.	+
8. Lithium has antisuicide effects in those who remain on it for maintenance treatment.	++
9. The antisuicide effects of lithium may be independent of its primary efficacy on episode prevention.	±
10. Lithium normalizes the excess medical mortality that occurs with recurrent affective disorder (depressed patients are at increased risk of dying from causes other than suicide, such as heart attack or stroke.	++
11. Discontinuation of lithium is associated with an approximately 7- to 20-fold increase in the risk of suicide (Tondo, Hennen, & Baldessarini, 2001).	++
12. If one does decide to discontinue lithium, one should taper the dose extremely slowly over a period of a month or more, and watch carefully for early signs of symptom re-emergence.	+++
13. A slow taper may not only decrease the risk for relapse somewhat but also allows early intervention if minor symptoms begin to return during the taper.	++
14. Lithium increases the generation rate of new neurons (neu-	

rogenesis) and glial cells, as well as cell survival factors.   +++
15. Thus, lithium may help reverse or prevent some of the neurobiological changes in the brain associated with bipolar disorder.   +

TAKE-HOME MESSAGE

When lithium treatment works well, stay the course; keep the illness under control. Consider effective lithium treatment the same as vitamin B$_{12}$ for pernicious anemia, insulin for diabetes, or digitalis for congestive heart failure. Stopping these treatments risks more than a relapse—it may be disabling and life threatening.

ADDENDUM: HOW TO STOP LITHIUM IF NECESSARY

As summarized above, lithium discontinuation carries potentially severe consequences. There are some instances, however, when lithium discontinuation may be required for medical reasons or intolerable side effects, or the decision may have been reached with the treating psychiatrist to stop lithium treatment because of pregnancy. In all of these instances, the issue of discontinuing an effective medication needs to be carefully discussed and the risk-to-benefit ratio reviewed. While discontinuing ineffective medications should be less of a problem, in some instances the same principles may apply. The following guidelines may assist in reducing the potential hazards associated with medication discontinuation.

Tapering Medication Dosage

The first rule is to go slowly; that is, do not stop the medication abruptly, but taper the dosage carefully. The advantages of tapering are as follows:

1. Avoid withdrawal symptoms.

2. Lessen psychological symptoms (i.e., worry over the possible consequences of discontinuing medications).

3. Decrease psychiatric symptoms (decrease the incidence or severity).

4. If early symptoms emerge while tapering, one is able to increase the dose and add other medications if necessary to institute more aggressive treatment.

5. If discontinuation is planned not due to a medical emergency or other urgent reasons, it might be advisable to look at the patient's retrospective course of illness using the Life Chart Method (see Appendix 3) to elucidate when the patient's history suggests that he or she may be the least vulnerable to a relapse. It would be prudent to plan and institute, whenever possible, a slow taper during these periods of lessened illness vulnerability if they are readily identifiable.

Early Warning System

The establishment of an early warning system is relevant in the discontinuation of both effective and ineffective maintenance medications. It is important to recognize the very first symptoms of an impending breakthrough (on or off medications) so that early and aggressive treatment can be reinstituted to prevent the emergence of a full-blown episode.

The patient and clinician together should establish a symptom checklist that includes the typical symptoms of an impending episode for that individual patient (such as decreased need for sleep, increased energy, increased social activity, religiosity, etc.) as possible precursors of a manic episode; or decrease in sociability, lack of interest, lack of motivation, increased need for sleep, and so on, as possibly heralding the emergence of a depressive episode. Although key symptoms will vary considerably among different patients, they generally are consistent over time for an individual. Knowledge and recognition of these typical early symptoms will alert both the patient and the physician to the possibility of an emerging episode and will promote and facilitate treatment intervention.

Contingency Contracts

It is often very useful to make specific and explicit contingency contracts about the process and procedures to follow if a certain level of symptoms emerge. For example, one may write: (a) if sleep drops off 1–2 hours, increase dose of a benzodiazepine, gabapentin, or atypical antipsychotic; (b) for greater degrees of insomnia, call MD; (c) if typical paranoia returns, add a dose of atypical antipsychotic; (d) if extremely agitated or potentially violent, go to emergency room. This type of explicit instruction will help a patient to not ignore symptoms in hopes they will just go away between visits.

Lithium Discontinuation During Pregnancy

A careful judgment with regard to use of lithium during pregnancy should be made by the patient, spouse, and physicians. Data based on retrospective and prospective studies indicate that the risk of cardiac anomalies and transposition of the great vessels (Ebstein's anomaly) is less than previously thought, and only slightly greater than in control patients not exposed to lithium and in the normal population (Altshuler et al., 1996; Viguera, Cohen, Baldessarini, & Nonacs, 2002). The risk is about 1 in 20,000 in normal controls and only about 10 in 20,000 (i.e., 1 per 2,000) in patients on lithium.

When considering the substantial risk of relapse following lithium discontinuation and the serious consequences and potential effects on the subsequent course of illness, these new data should promote a reevaluation of whether or not lithium should be discontinued in women wishing to become pregnant. In the case of continued lithium treatment, careful monitoring with level II ultrasound and fetal echocardiography should be considered to further monitor normal development of the fetus. In the case of a major malformation, one could then terminate the pregnancy if that is the agreed-upon contingency plan.

Carbamazepine

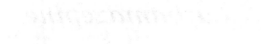

14

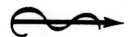

Early Example of a Prophylactic Antimanic Response to Carbamazepine

CASE HISTORY

This patient's course of illness in 1974 and 1975 was mapped from detailed case notes after an almost continuous hospitalization in a state institution. Her recurrent manic episodes were extremely severe and occurred relentlessly, despite treatment with lithium and high-dose antipsychotics, and sometimes with intervening tricyclic antidepressants for her immobilizing depression (Figure 14.1). Thus, this patient exemplifies the general problem of treatment-resistant illness as it existed prior to the advent of the use of carbamazepine and related mood-stabilizing anticonvulsants such as valproate and lamotrigine, and the atypical antipsychotics.

When she was admitted to the NIMH for double-blind clinical trials of carbamazepine in 1977, she was among the first cohort of patients studied in a double-blind fashion with this agent in the world. A double-blind trial with carbamazepine in acute mania was published by Okuma and colleagues in 1979 following his open observations suggesting efficacy in 1973 (Okuma, Inanaga, Otsuki, & Sarai, 1979; Okuma, Kishimoto, Inoue, Matsumoto, & Ogura, 1973). This patient's initial response to blind carbamazepine was described in our first publication (Ballenger & Post, 1978b).

During her outpatient follow-up period, she was able to continue on carbamazepine mono-

therapy. Her relapse into mania in 1979 could have occurred on the drug (a) as part of the tolerance phenomenon, or (b) may have been attributable to missing doses because of noncompliance. In any event, she remained in need of continuous state hospitalization for intractable mania when she was again treated with the existing typical antipsychotics, but was able to resume her outpatient status each time when carbamazepine was substituted. Her more traditional antipsychotic treatment occurred in part because carbamazepine was not a well-accepted treatment in the general community at this time (in the late 1970s) and was not considered for use in most state hospital settings.

BACKGROUND LITERATURE

Necessary Use of Off-Label Treatments in Bipolar Illness

When carbamazepine began to be used in a state hospital in Virginia, the local newspapers wrote a highly negative and inflammatory article suggesting patients were receiving inappropriate, unconventional, and experimental treatment (i.e., anticonvulsants when they did not have a seizure disorder) and that its use was unwarranted and should be curtailed. Apparently, continuing to insist on treating patients with an FDA-approved

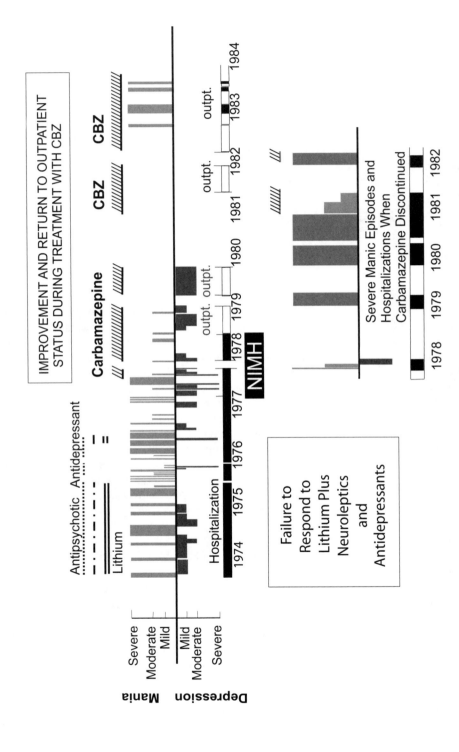

Figure 14.1 Efficacy of carbamazepine in a lithium nonresponder. This patient required continuous state hospitalization while on lithium, antipsychotics, and antidepressants, despite a course of electroconvulsive therapy (not illustrated). When admitted to the NIMH in 1977, she had a good response to carbamazepine, as documented in an off-on-off-on fashion, but then experienced breakthrough loss of efficacy. However, she reresponded to carbamazepine in 1979, 1980, and again in 1981, each time with a considerable period without severe mania and was able to function as an outpatient for the first time in many years. CBZ, carbamazepine; outpt., outpatient. The insert on the second line illustrates the manic recurrences and hospitalization that occurred each time CBZ was stopped.

134

drug (lithium) that did not work was preferable to using one that might be effective in this treatment-resistant population.

Similarly, physicians in another state hospital system (to which this patient returned when her mania became severe) were either not aware of the efficacy of carbamazepine in general or not convinced of its effectiveness in this patient. However, each time carbamazepine was reintroduced upon our suggestion, it stopped her periods of intractable mania, which were also completely unresponsive to the more traditional treatment of high-dose antipsychotic agents.

Whereas the off-on-off-on trial at the NIMH in early 1978 was performed in a double-blind, placebo-controlled fashion in conjunction with formal approval for the protocol by the NIMH Investigational Review Board, the subsequent on-off-on-off periods of carbamazepine treatment in 1979, 1980, and 1981 illustrated in the life chart were unintended, and occurred in part because physicians were unappreciative of her clear prior responsivity to carbamazepine and reverted to the FDA-approved treatments at that time (antipsychotics and lithium).

This patient thus clearly demonstrates an early but ongoing liability in the treatment of patients with bipolar disorder. As discussed in Chapter 9, until recently almost all of the drugs used for bipolar disorder were off-label, that is, not FDA approved for the specific indication of bipolar illness. Most of these off-label drugs are FDA approved for use in unipolar illness (antidepressants) or schizophrenia (antipsychotics), or in the treatment of patients with epilepsies (the anticonvulsants). Thus, if one adheres only to FDA-approved indications, this may have severe consequences for treatment-refractory patients, such as this individual, as it resulted in prolonged hospitalizations for severe mania in 1980 and 1981. Although 18 controlled studies in acute mania indicated efficacy of carbamazepine in acute mania (1978 to 2004), it was not until 2005 that a long-acting formulation of carbamazepine (Equetro) was finally FDA approved for acute mania.

To the extent that this patient began to break through in a full-blown manic episode, leading secondarily to her stopping carbamazepine treatment in 1979, it would suggest a potential loss of efficacy of short-term carbamazepine via a tolerance process. If this were the case, her reresponsivity in late 1979 and 1980, and again in 1981 after periods of time off the drug, would conform to the principles illustrated in more detail in Chapters 19 and 24, which describe reresponsivity to an agent after a period of time off drug if there has been a loss of prior efficacy via tolerance. If the breakthrough occurred, rather, because she stopped her carbamazepine in 1979 and 1980, her life chart would nonetheless illustrate the point of consistent renewal of responsivity to carbamazepine each time treatment was instituted. Thus, whether the patient was becoming tolerant to carbamazepine in 1979 and 1980, and this was contributing to her manic relapses or not, her very consistent responsiveness to this agent is demonstrated.

Research Design Controversies in Bipolar Illness

This last point is important from an academic as well as a personal perspective. An editorial and a meta-analysis were published about the lack of robust evidence of the prophylactic efficacy of carbamazepine (Dardennes, Even, Bange, & Heim, 1995; Murphy, Gannon, & McGennis, 1989). Although there had been multiple trials of carbamazepine prophylaxis in comparison to lithium, and trials using a mirror image or off-on-off design, the authors of those articles were critical of the lack of a randomized parallel-group placebo design. They emphasized that one group of patients should be treated with carbamazepine alone (for a year) and the other with placebo (for a year). This is also the FDA standard for approval of a drug for long-term prophylaxis, and it is because of the difficulty of performing such trials, both from an ethical and financial perspective, that few other drugs besides lithium and lamotrigine are currently approved for long-term prophylaxis in bipolar illness. Yet the key to good treatment of bipolar disorder is effective long-term prophylaxis.

In response to the editorial criticism noted

above, we cited the very considerable literature (Post, Denicoff, Frye, & Leverich, 1997) using other research designs such as mirror image and off-on-off designs that document the unequivocal response of at least some patients with bipolar illness to carbamazepine (Chapters 15, 16, and 18). Disappointingly, there have been few NIMH-sponsored single-center or multicenter prophylactic trials in bipolar illness since the early studies of Prien and associates (Prien, Caffey, & Klett, 1972; Prien, Klett, & Caffey, 1973), which yielded the data that helped lead to the approval of lithium. The only exception of which we are aware is the study of Calabrese, Bowden, et al. (2003), comparing the addition of either lamotrigine or placebo as an adjunct to lithium and valproate treatment in those who were not responsive to the combination.

Given the 30-year gap in the funding by NIMH of such long-term prophylactic trials in bipolar illness, it appears even more imperative to consider other treatment designs in the initial investigation of potentially effective treatments for this illness. We have written an extensive review article (Post & Luckenbaugh, 2003) suggesting a variety of alternative designs that could facilitate the initial and secondary phases of drug assessment for bipolar illness. We continue to argue that a patient such as this, and those in Chapters 32 and 33 for the calcium channel blocker nimodipine, represents strong evidence of individual responsivity to a drug, and what remains more important for the field now is to assess potential clinical and biological predictors of who may be within that responsive subgroup. If a better initial choice of the best medicine for individual patients could be achieved, the long periods of sequential clinical trials now often required to find an effective prophylactic treatment might be avoided.

It is also noteworthy that a true clinical response to treatment in a placebo-controlled, parallel-group design cannot be clearly ascertained in any given patient. Such a design can only find that the magnitude or incidence of response to the active agent exceeds that of placebo. Since some patients will have a response to placebo (as high as 25–40% in some studies; Keck, Welge, McElroy, Arnold, & Strakowski, 2000;

Keck, Welge, Strakowski, Arnold, & McElroy, 2000), it will also be unclear which patients in the active treatment group actually responded to the active drug and which merely had the placebo response expected to occur in a proportion of the patients. In contrast, using off-on-off-on designs (as illustrated for this patient) presents clear evidence of individual responsivity (see also Chapter 32). These kinds of response confirmation data that identify individual responsiveness to a given agent will also facilitate the elucidation of the clinical and biological markers that predict clinical response (Post & Luckenbaugh, 2003).

From the patient's own perspective, one would not necessarily need to have such off-on-off confirming trials. If a true clinical response to a given agent were highly suggested by the lengthening of time between episodes (i.e., much longer than that seen previously prior to the new treatment), one could begin to infer with increasing certainty as the time well increases that a real drug response has likely occurred. When the period of time well markedly exceeds that of previous interepisode intervals (such as in 1978 and 1979 in this patient, compared with any other previous 2-year period), one can be relatively confident that the improvement was not a spontaneous course of illness variation.

When a good prolonged response occurs in the usual clinical treatment context (as opposed to the research context), one is usually merely pleased to continue with such therapeutic success and not require a further confirmation of efficacy by a period of time off drug (associated with a loss of effect) and another period on drug (with a renewal of improvement). In the patient described here, the later discontinuations occurred in a naturalistic and unintended fashion, which added to the considerable weight of the evidence for a real response to carbamazepine already demonstrated by the initial double-blind off-on-off-on clinical trial.

In some instances in which the initial positive effectiveness of a drug is more ambiguous, and some risk of side effects is present, the patient and physician may elect to pursue further confirmatory evidence of efficacy by such a closely monitored off-on-off trial in clinical practice.

| | STRENGTH OF |
| PRINCIPLES OF THE CASE | EVIDENCE |

1. Prior to the 1970s, the only available treatments for patients with bipolar illness (lithium, antipsychotics, and tricyclic and MAOI antidepressants) left many patients (such as this one) with incapacitating degrees of recurrent illness.   +++

2. Since lithium was the only FDA-approved drug for long-term prophylaxis of manic-depressive illness until lamotrigine's approval in 2004, the appropriate treatment for the large group of lithium-nonresponsive patients has been, by necessity, off-label.   +++

3. If a patient shows a good response to a given (especially unconventional) agent, it may be very useful to have this documented with a mood chart graphic representation of this response; it may help convince subsequent physicians who may be dubious about this approach in general, and in a given patient in particular, that a clear response (even if only partial) has occurred and the patient should be continued on that agent.   +

4. Conversely, if clear periods of nonresponsivity to conventional or other agents are noted despite good doses, blood levels, and durations of treatment (as in 1974 and 1975 in this individual), having a mood chart documentation of this lack of responsivity may also help facilitate the process of exploring and finding new and more effective treatment regimens.   ++

5. Carbamazepine is an effective acute antimanic and prophylactic compound for some individuals, even though in some studies lithium appears more efficacious than carbamazepine for patients with classic presentations.   +++

6. Despite unequivocal evidence from double-blind, placebo-controlled off-on-off-on trials and mirror image studies in otherwise treatment-resistant (refractory) patients such as this one, carbamazepine did not become a widely used and accepted agent until the mid to late 1980s (about 15 years after our studies and those of Okuma).   ++

7. This drug and several others in the same category remained available to physicians and patients off-label, because carbamazepine was FDA approved only for trigeminal neuralgia and seizure disorders until 2005. Even then, FDA approval was granted for only one preparation (i.e., long-lasting Carbatrol as named for epilepsy, or Equetro as named for mania), and only for acute mania and not prophylaxis.   +++

8. The pharmaceutical industry is often not willing or able to bear the expense of doing the extensive and costly clinical trials necessary for FDA approval for a new indication. This is especially true when the drug is off patent and available in generic preparations; the many millions of dollars required for the clinical trials would not be recouped with generic formulations.   ++

9. Some expensive trials may fail for methodological reasons, even when the drug is known to work based on information from other designs, which happened with the Bowden et al. (2000) study, where valproate did not show statistical significance on the main outcome measure. Thus, valproate is not

yet FDA approved for prophylaxis even though it is widely used for this indication.   +

10. This individual, who had years of continuous hospitalization for severe recurrent manias, had a good, confirmed response to a novel intervention and resumed a much more normal life in a residential setting.   ++

11. Patients and families should continue to search for effective treatment approaches, whether or not they are currently FDA approved for bipolar disorder.   +++

12. Many different agents that are currently available and widely used for treatment of bipolar illness are not yet and perhaps never will be FDA approved for a bipolar indication.   ++

13. It is often only with careful retrospective (past history) and prospective (current and future) life charting that a pattern of drug responsivity in a given individual can be elucidated with clarity; without a life chart or some other systematic form of record keeping, one may miss critical areas of change indicating subtle to substantial treatment response or nonresponse.   ++

14. Proceeding to treat severe or rapidly recurrent illness without a good monitoring system is like being stranded in a forest without a compass; you do not know which way to go or whether you have been there before.   +

TAKE-HOME MESSAGE

Careful evaluation of the effectiveness of non-FDA-approved (or even FDA-approved) drugs may be invaluable in making the best treatment decisions for each patient. FDA documentation of efficacy of a drug for the general population of patients with bipolar disorder does not necessarily translate to effectiveness of that drug for a given patient.

15

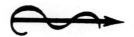

Selective Response to Carbamazepine, but Not Valproate, Phenytoin, or Lithium

CASE HISTORY

This patient was a 55-year-old single woman at the time of admission to NIMH in 1979, following an essentially continuous hospitalization at a state facility from 1955 to 1979 (Figure 15.1; Post, Berrettini, Uhde, & Kellner, 1984). In that institution, she was unresponsive to treatment with high doses of antipsychotics used alone or in combination with intermittent administration of lithium carbonate and other adjunctive psychotropic treatments, including tricyclic antidepressants. There was no family history of psychiatric illness. Except for the presence of tardive dyskinesia, her neurological examination was normal; an EEG, CAT scan, and lumbar puncture also were within normal limits.

The patient's illness was characterized by rapid, sometimes almost instantaneous, switches from mania into depression. Mania was severe and characterized by marked and incessant pressure of speech, hyperactivity, and aggressive irritability or grandiose euphoria. During manic periods, the patient required either intermittent or continuous seclusion, as she was unable to respond to limit setting and unable to control her aggressive outbursts. During periods of mania, she was psychotic, delusional, and at times apparently hallucinating. She was unable to carry out activities of daily living and at times became extremely regressed and incontinent.

Even during periods of relatively mild mania, she remained delusional about being married to a staff member (RMP) and often manifested confabulatory responses.

During periods of depression, the patient exhibited extreme psychomotor retardation, maintaining a given position in her chair for long periods of time, essentially mute. This patient showed state-dependent exacerbation of her tardive dyskinesia, which worsened during depression and improved during mania (Cutler & Post, 1982; Cutler, Post, Rey, & Bunney, 1981).

The patient's severe mania was attenuated shortly after she received moderate doses of carbamazepine, resulting in blood levels in the 6 to 12 µg/ml range. As illustrated in Figure 15.2, during two instances of dose reduction or discontinuation of carbamazepine, severe manic psychotic symptoms rapidly reemerged. Symptoms were quickly attenuated by increasing the dose or restarting treatment with active carbamazepine on a double-blind basis.

Clear evidence of dose-related response to carbamazepine during treatment of the patient's initial severe episodes is illustrated in Figure 15.2. Both mania and psychosis ratings were markedly elevated on the 15-point Bunney-Hamburg scale in the periods on placebo, prior to initiation of active carbamazepine treatment or following its discontinuation. With increasing doses of carbamazepine, particularly those over

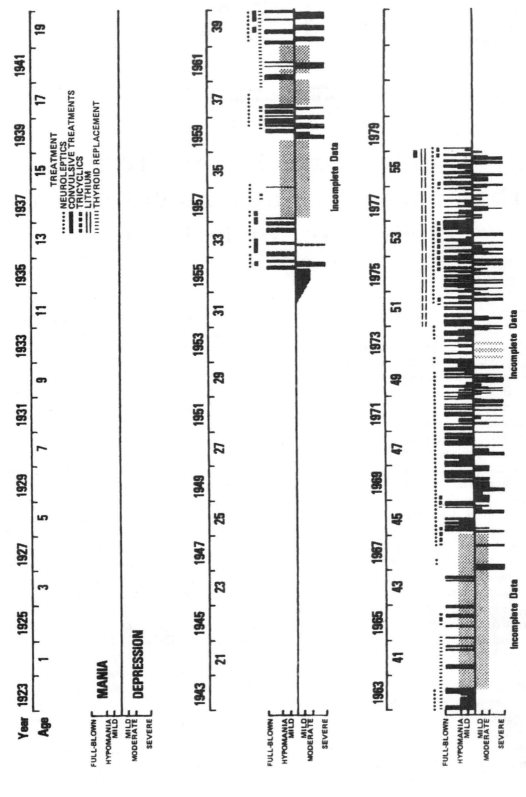

Figure 15.1 Retrospective life chart of a medication-resistant, rapidly cycling manic-depressive patient who was hospitalized continuously from 1955 to 1979 and then subsequently responded to carbamazepine.

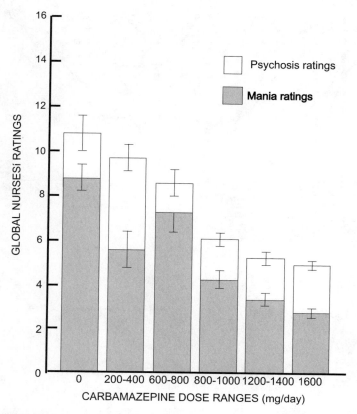

Figure 15.2 Dose-dependent therapeutic effects of carbamazepine during a prolonged manic episode.

800 mg/day, the patient showed a remarkable improvement in both manic and psychotic components of her illness. On 1,600 mg/day of carbamazepine, there was substantial reduction in these symptoms and the patient was able to participate in the regular activities of the unit.

The relatively selective antipsychotic response to carbamazepine treatment of two manic episodes compared with two episodes observed during placebo administration, and manic episodes treated with phenytoin and valproic acid, are illustrated in Figure 15.3A. Compared with these placebo-treated episodes, a notable acute and sustained antimanic and antipsychotic response to carbamazepine was shown by this patient. In contrast, during treatment with phenytoin up to 600 mg/day, achieving blood levels of 19.8 ± 2.2 μg/ml, the patient showed no evidence of clinical response and required essentially continuous seclusion.

As illustrated in Figure 15.3B, mania ratings during treatment with phenytoin were substantially higher than those observed during either carbamazepine or placebo treatment. During treatment with valproic acid up to 2,000 mg/day, achieving blood levels of 88.8 ± 2.4 μg/ml, the patient again showed little evidence of clinical response and again required seclusion for long periods of time.

The degree of carbamazepine-induced prophylaxis is indicated by a 24% reduction in the number of severe manic days and an 85% reduction in depressed days during treatment with carbamazepine (=800 mg/day) compared with the number of days severely ill during placebo treatment. There was also a 129% increase in the number of improved days during carbamazepine treatment compared with placebo.

Evidence of the substantial impact of carbamazepine on this patient's severe, rapid-cycling,

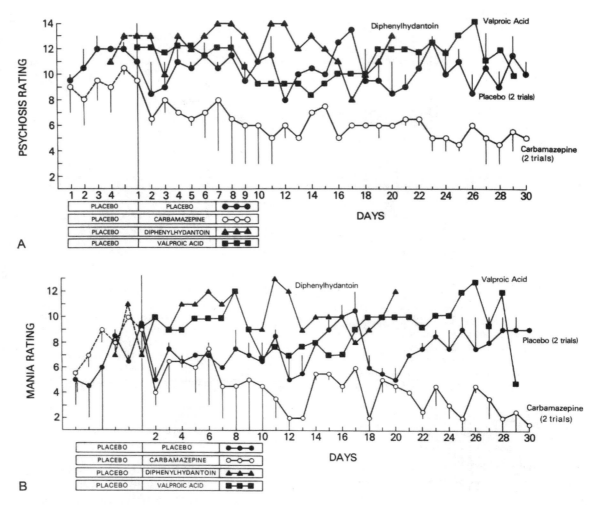

Figure 15.3 Selective antimanic response to carbamazepine but not valproate or phenytoin. (A) Carbamazepine, but not diphenylhydantoin (Dilantin) or valproic acid (Depakene, Depakote), decreases manic psychosis in a patient with recurrent manic illness. (B) Antimanic response to the anticonvulsant carbamazepine but not to diphenylhydantoin or valproic acid in a manic-depressive patient.

drug-refractory bipolar illness is illustrated in Figure 15.4. This figure illustrates the percentage of time the patient required seclusion for protection of herself and staff members during treatment with various psychotropic and anticonvulsant medications on a double-blind basis. Decisions about seclusion were made by nurses who were blind to medication status. Percentage of time in seclusion was calculated on an hourly basis for each 24-hour day the patient was treated with a given drug regimen. As indicated, this patient's severe psychotic illness, which was previously nonresponsive to long-term and high-dose treatment with antipsychotics and lithium, continued to be severe, requiring seclusion 25.8% of the time during periods off medication.

During at least four separate trials of 540 days on carbamazepine administration, the need for seclusion was reduced to just 4%. In con-

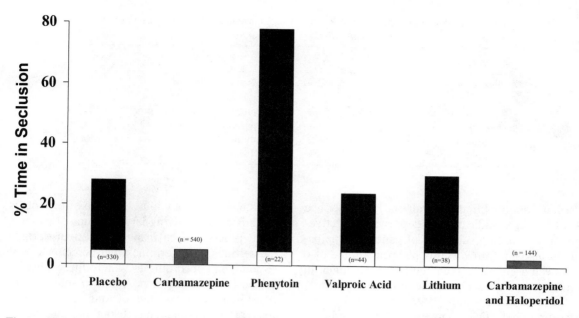

Figure 15.4 Selective long-term response to carbamazepine in a patient unresponsive to lithium, valproate, and phenytoin. Carbamazepine alone and with haloperidol (Haldol) decreased time in seclusion, while valproate had little effect and phenytoin exacerbated her illness.

trast, the patient needed almost continuous seclusion during the 22 days of treatment with phenytoin (76.9% of the time in seclusion). While treated with valproic acid, the percentage of time in seclusion (21.5%) was similar to that during placebo administration. Consistent with the previous retrospective history of lithium carbonate nonresponse, the patient also required seclusion 29.8% of the time during the 38 days of prospective, double-blind lithium administration (at doses between 1,200 and 1,500 mg/day), achieving blood levels of 1.3 ± 0.2 mEq/L.

When carbamazepine was administered in combination with haloperidol (16 mg/day) in order to maximize the antimanic and antipsychotic effects, further improvement was achieved, as evidenced by the reduction in the need for seclusion to 1.6% of the time. It is of clinical interest that these brief periods of seclusion occurred during times of psychosocial stress on the unit, particularly around discharge of fellow patients (Chapters 6 and 7).

BACKGROUND LITERATURE

On a clinical research unit of the NIMH, we began studying carbamazepine in the mid-1970s and early 1980s. Because we did not use a traditional parallel group, placebo-controlled design, many investigators in academia did not accept the unequivocal evidence of responsiveness to carbamazepine in this patient and the many others studied in a similar fashion, using an off (placebo)-on (drug)-off-on design. However, over the next several decades, more than 19 controlled studies using the more conventional placebo-controlled parallel group design have further documented the acute antimanic efficacy of carbamazepine, as summarized in Table 15.1.

What has been less well documented in the literature is carbamazepine's acute antidepressant efficacy. In a group of 10 patients who showed an initial positive antidepressant response to carbamazepine and who then relapsed off the drug, their renewed response during a

Table 15.1 *Summary of Response Rates of Carbamazepine and Oxcarbazepine in 20 Controlled Studies in Acute Mania*

Monotherapy		Adjunctive Therapy	
Placebo	22%	Placebo (add-on)	42%
versus		versus	
Carbamazepine/oxcarbazepine	55%	Carbamazepine/oxcarbazepine	69%
Comparators		*Comparators (add-ons)*	
Lithium	68%	Lithium	66%
Typical antipsychotics	68%	Typical antipsychotics	50%

second double-blind clinical trial, as described in Chapter 9, indicates antidepressant effectiveness in at least a subgroup of patients. This patient also conforms to this perspective and also showed a greater percentage of improvement in time depressed compared with time manic.

Greil and associates (1997) found better long-term prophylactic response to carbamazepine (in contrast to lithium) in those with schizoaffective illness. Not only did this patient exhibit a major psychotic component to her manic and depressive episodes, but she would also meet most criteria for schizoaffective illness; even during periods of marked improvement in mood (virtual euthymia), she still had persistent delusions that she was married to one of the ward staff members.

More than 15 studies, all of which at least partially controlled, indicate the prophylactic efficacy of carbamazepine, usually demonstrated in randomized comparisons to lithium carbonate (Post & Frye, 2005). This patient provides even more convincing evidence of the prophylactic efficacy of carbamazepine, because of the marked clinical improvement achieved each time she was placed on the drug on a blind basis. Moreover, this improvement did not occur with other presumptively active treatments, such as lithium or the anticonvulsants valproate or phenytoin.

We have made the argument elsewhere (Post, Denicoff, Frye, et al., 1997; Post, Denicoff, & Leverich, 2000; Post & Luckenbaugh, 2003) that a series of patients with documented clinical efficacy of a given drug in an off-on-off-on design can provide a highly reliable indication of clinical efficacy, at least in a subgroup of pa-

tients. Once efficacy in a subgroup of patients is demonstrated, studying larger groups of patients could proceed, even using less formal designs and settings, to determine what percentage will respond, and according to which illness characteristics. In this way, one could to some extent avoid many clinical trials of long-term prophylaxis in bipolar patients, using the traditional parallel group design with one group receiving only placebo.

Moreover, in the initial studies designed to examine the potential efficacy of a drug, one would not have to use placebo substitution in nonresponders. Instead, as in the present case, only patients who are apparently responsive to the drug would require a brief period of placebo reexposure to document that their initial improvement was not a result of the natural course of their illness or other nonspecific aspects of the study, such as increased medical interest, observation, and attention.

This sequence—of individual intensive studies followed by larger, less controlled ones to assess percentage or likelihood of response, possible predictors, and overall tolerability—would also appear to be a more efficient way to proceed when exploring new drugs for the group of treatment-refractory patients (such as this one). In the intensive design, evidence of efficacy could be preliminarily assessed with a high degree of reliability in a relatively small number of patients. Ineffective agents could rapidly be discarded with little need for placebo exposure (as most patients would be nonresponders). In contrast, the traditional parallel group design is often highly inefficient in bipolar illness, requir-

Table 15.2 *Carbamazepine Decreases Serum Concentrations of Some Other Drugs Also Metabolized by 3A4*

Antidepressants	*Anticonvulsants*	*Immunosuppressants*
Bupropion	Carbamazepine*	Cyclosporine (?)
Citalopram	Ethosuximide	Sirolimus
Mirtazapine	Felbamate	Tacrolimus
Tricyclics	Lamotrigine*	*Muscle Relaxants*
Antipsychotics	Oxcarbazepine	Doxacurium
Aripiprazole	Phenytoin	Pancuronium
Clozapine	Primodine	Rapacuronium
Fluphenazine (?)	Tiagabine	Rocuronium
Haloperidol*	Topiramate	Vecuronium
Olanzapine	Valproate*	*Steroids*
Quetiapine (?)	Zonisamide	Estrogen in hormonal contraceptives*
Risperidone	*Analgesics*	Dexamethasone*
Thiothixene	Alfentanil	Mifepristone
Ziprasidone	Buprenorphine	Prednisolone
Antiolytics/Sedatives	Fentanyl (?)	*Stimulants*
Alprazolam (?)	Levobupivacaine	Methylphenidate
Buspirone	Methadone	Modafinil
Clonazepam	Tramadol	*Others*
Midazolam	*Anticoagulants*	Bepridil
Zopiclone(?)	Dicumarol (?)	Oxiracetam (?)
	Phenprocoumon	Paclitaxel
	Warfarin*	Quinidine
	Antimicrobials	Remacemide(?)
	Caspofungin	Repaglinide
	Doxycycline	Theophylline*
	Antivirals	Thyroid hormones
	Delavirdine	
	Protease inhibitors	

*Clinically most important. (?) = ambiguous, inconsistent, or small magnitude of effect.

ing both very large numbers of subjects and one half or one third of these automatically exposed to placebo.

For example, four large multicenter trials were conducted to examine topiramate monotherapy for the treatment of acute mania, before the drug was deemed ineffective compared with placebo. Many hundreds of patients were studied on the drug and on placebo at the cost of many millions of dollars. One can ask whether this unfortunate occurrence could have been prevented by initial findings of a lack of true and confirmed responders to topiramate in a small series of off-on-off-on trials.

The viewpoint enunciated above is not currently widely held by investigators in search of novel treatments for bipolar illness, and many continue to feel that the only truly reliable and valid study design is one using a parallel placebo group. However, given the tremendously heterogeneous presentation of bipolar illness with depression, mania, mixed states, multiple comorbidities, and a variety of cycling frequencies within and among patients, other approaches to the traditional randomized controlled clinical trial that requires patient homogeneity are needed. Even a drug as widely used and accepted as the antidepressant fluoxetine (Prozac) had many large failed trials in homogenous groups of depressed subjects that did not show statistically significant degrees of antidepressant effectiveness over placebo when they used the placebo-

Table 15.3 *Drugs That Increase Serum Concentrations of Carbamazepine by Inhibiting the Induction of 3A4*

Antidepressants	Calcium channel
Fluoxetine*	blockers
Fluvoxamine*	*Diltiazem***
*Nefazodone**	*Verapamil***
Antimicrobials	(but not nifedipine
*Isoniazid***	or nimodipine)
Quinupristin/dalfopristin	Hypolipidemics
Macrolide antibiotics**	Gemfibrozil
*Clarithromycin***	Nicotinamide
*Erythromycin***	Others
*Flurithromycin***	Acetazolamide
*Josamycin***	Cimetidine (*)
*Ponsinomycin***	Danazol
*Triacetyloleandromycin***	Omeprazole
	d-Propoxyphene*
	Ritonavir**
	Ticlopidine

Anticonvulsant
    Valproate** increases carbamazepine effects by inhibiting the conversion of the active-10,11-epoxide metabolite to the inactive diol

Note. Italics = potential for toxicity; (*) = weak effect; * = mild to moderate; ** = important or severe effect.

controlled parallel group design. Thus, even when a drug does work, this traditional design may not yield consistent results.

DOSING AND KINETICS

Pharmacokinetics refers to how a drug is handled, metabolized, and excreted and how drug levels are affected by other drugs. Carbamazepine has clinically important interactions with both components. It is metabolized by liver enzymes of the CYP-3A4 subtype. Carbamazepine itself induces this 3A4 enzyme, such that its own blood levels on a given dose decrease after 2 to 3 weeks of treatment.

Thus, blood levels of other drugs metabolized by 3A4 will be reduced in the presence of chronic carbamazepine. This includes haloperidol, estrogen in birth control pills, and a variety of other compounds (Table 15.2). In contrast, if another drug inhibits the induction of the 3A4

enzyme, the blood levels of carbamazepine will markedly increase; these drugs include erythromycin and verapamil, among many other commonly used drugs (Table 15.3).

Carbamazepine is metabolized to an active intermediate compound, carbamazepine-10,11-epoxide, which has active anticonvulsant effects and can also cause side effects. As illustrated in Figure 15.5, valproate blocks the conversion of the -10,11-epoxide to its inactive diol, thus building up total active blood levels (carbamazepine plus the -10,11-epoxide) and potentially causing side effects. The dose of carbamazepine is thus usually reduced when valproate is added (Chapter 49).

PRINCIPLES OF THE CASE	STRENGTH OF EVIDENCE
1. Prior to the availability of the mood-stabilizing anticonvulsants and atypical antipsychotic agents, many patients suffered for long periods of time with treatment-resistant bipolar illness.	+
2. This patient, despite being in a state hospital for more than 20 years, was still able to show a remarkable degree of response to the novel treatment carbamazepine.	+++
3. The patient clearly demonstrated the principle that some lithium and typical antipsychotic nonresponders will show a good response to the anticonvulsant carbamazepine.	++
4. The patient clearly illustrates that response to one anticonvulsant does not predict a response to another, since this patient showed little evidence of response to valproate and worsened on maximally tolerated doses of phenytoin.	+++

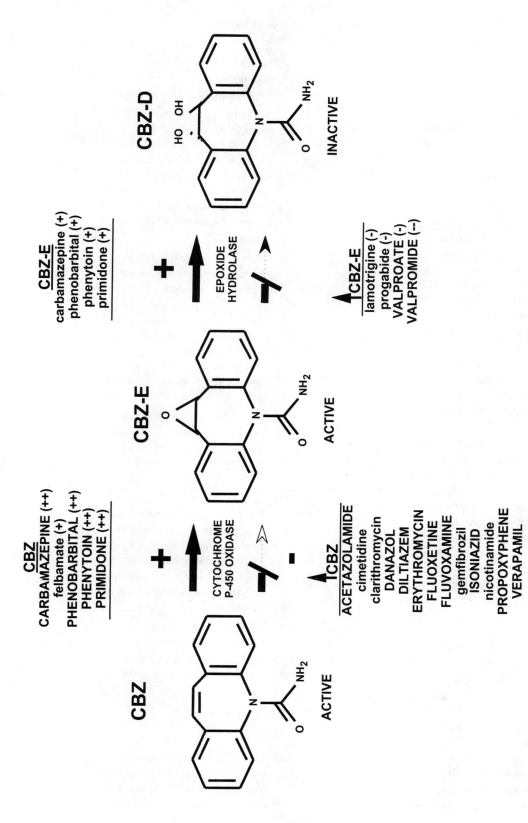

Figure 15.5 Pathways of carbamazepine metabolism; carbamazepine-10,11-epoxide (CBZ-E; middle) is an active metabolite and the dihydroxy metabolite (CBZ-D, right) is inactive. CBZ, carbamazepine. Other drugs enhancing conversion are illustrated on top, while those inhibiting enzymatic conversion are listed below.

5. The lack of valproate response in some carbamazepine-responsive patients would be expected based on their different mechanisms of action and range of clinical effects in the epilepsies.   ++

6. Phenytoin, like carbamazepine, is a potent blocker of sodium channels and has a similar range of clinical effects in the epilepsies. Thus, the lack of response to this agent suggests that sodium channel blockade is not a sufficient explanation of carbamazepine's antimanic effects.   +

7. Not only are not all anticonvulsants mood stabilizers, as illustrated in Chapter 25 for gabapentin, but within patients, responsivity among the widely accepted anticonvulsants can differ dramatically.   ++

8. Consistent with this case observation, Greil et al. (1997) found that patients with schizoaffective presentations, particularly in the depressed phase, may show a better response to carbamazepine than to lithium. This patient fits that profile to some extent and clearly showed a dose-related responsivity to carbamazepine in both antimanic and antipsychotic components.   ++

9. There is great individual variability in carbamazepine doses that patients tolerate and to which they show an adequate response. Some patients may not tolerate doses much higher than 400–600 mg/day, whereas 1,600 mg/day was used here without any side effects.   ++

10. One should individualize doses to side effect tolerability rather than try to achieve a preset absolute dose or blood level range of carbamazepine.   +++

11. Sometimes an antipsychotic is required to augment the mood-stabilizing and antipsychotic effects of an anticonvulsant such as carbamazepine, as illustrated in the further improved response to the combination of carbamazepine and haloperidol.   +++

12. Currently, atypical antipsychotics are recommended over the typicals because of fewer motor side effects and a lower risk of tardive dyskinesia. This patient is representative of the 20–40% of bipolar patients treated with the older drugs who did develop tardive dyskinesia.   ++

13. Her tardive dyskinesia was much more prominent when she was depressed and virtually absent when she was manic (Cutler et al., 1981).   +++

14. Carbamazepine is a potent inducer of hepatic enzymes and these are likely sufficient to drop the blood levels of haloperidol to about half their original value; despite this, the patient improved markedly on the combination.   ++

15. A carbamazepine-induced drop in blood levels of the estrogen components of birth control pills can also occur, and one needs to take a higher dosage form of estrogen to have adequate pregnancy protection.   +++

16. The need for higher doses of estrogen in oral contraceptives also extends to the anticonvulsants oxcarbazepine (Trilep-

tal), topiramate (Topamax), phenytoin (Dilantin), and primidone (Mysoline). ++

17. Other drugs (such as valproate, erythromycin, and some calcium channel blockers) can raise carbamazepine levels and potentially cause toxicity. These other drugs are discussed in Chapter 49, on carbamazepine and valproate combination treatment. ++

18. Ginsberg and Lawrence (2006) have reported extensive open experience with the extended release preparation (Equetro) with good effects in both children and adult with once daily (nighttime) dosing. ++

TAKE-HOME MESSAGE

Even a patient with the most severe and apparently treatment-resistant form of bipolar illness can show dramatic and sustained clinical response to selected new treatment interventions.

16

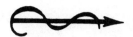

ECT-Sparing Effects of Carbamazepine Prophylaxis in a Patient With Recurrent Psychotic Depression: Predictors of Carbamazepine Response

CASE HISTORY

We present the case of this patient with unipolar recurrent psychotic depression in order to illustrate five distinct points:

1. Multiple courses of ECT, although highly acutely effective in terminating psychotic depressive episodes, were not effective in preventing recurrences.

2. Appropriate institution of pharmacoprophylaxis, in this instance with carbamazepine with minimal adjunctive antipsychotics, markedly reduced the need for hospitalization and ECT. Eight hospitalizations had occurred in the 5 years prior to starting carbamazepine treatment, while none occurred in the next 5 years.

3. This effective prevention of psychotic unipolar depressions may be pertinent to the effectiveness of carbamazepine in bipolar depression as well (Dilsaver et al., 1996; Neumann, Seidel, & Wunderlich, 1984; Schaffer, Mungas, & Rockwell, 1985).

4. Although lithium is often effective in the prevention of recurrent unipolar as well as bipolar depression, this patient did not experience a prophylactic response to lithium (see 1975 in Figure 16.1). Carbamazepine was highly effective, indicating differential responsivity between these two mood stabilizers within different patients.

5. As discussed more extensively in Chapter 19, episodes can begin to break through effective pharmacoprophylaxis with carbamazepine, sometimes in a progressive tolerance-like pattern, and ways of approaching this problem are noted under Principles of the Case.

BACKGROUND LITERATURE

The effectiveness of acute ECT for episodes of psychotic depression has not been exceeded by any single psychopharmacological agent (Fink, 2001b). Combination therapy with lithium, an atypical antipsychotic, and an antidepressant has often been recommended for such patients.

In the ECT follow-up studies of Sackeim, Haskett, and colleagues (2001), they found that

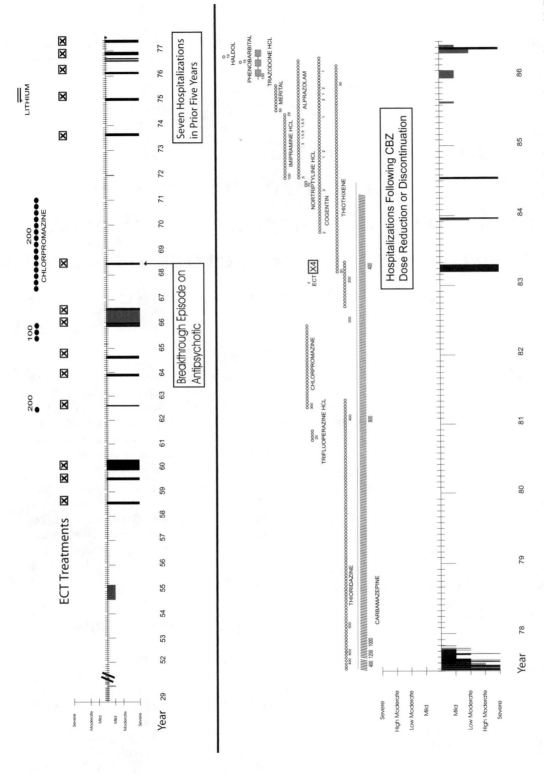

Figure 16.1 This patient demonstrated an increased frequency of psychotic depressions (top line), each requiring hospitalization despite acute interventions with ECT and attempts at prophylaxis with lithium from 1975 to 1977. Treatment with carbamazepine (bottom line) and minimal adjunctive doses of antipsychotics reduced the number of hospitalizations from eight in the previous 5 years to zero in the next 5 years (1978–1983), although two depressions requiring rehospitalization did occur in 1983 as well as two more after carbamazepine was discontinued. Note change in time scale in top versus bottom timeline. CBZ, carbamazepine.

when patients were randomized to nortriptyline plus placebo or lithium, long-term prophylaxis was significantly better maintained on the combination, although, in many instances, patients still demonstrated relapses. The data in this patient support the view that an alternative anticonvulsant mood stabilizer may be capable of exerting substantial prophylactic antidepressant effects, even in an individual clearly not responsive to lithium carbonate (Barker & Eccleston, 1984; Cullen et al., 1991; Post, Speer, Obrocea, & Leverich, 2002; Stuppaeck, Barnas, Miller, Schwitzer, & Fleischhacker, 1990).

These observations are consistent with the case report of Kobayashi, Kishimoto, and Inagaki (1988) wherein long-term carbamazepine administration was associated with a minimal time depressed, and off-drug periods were associated with major relapses. That pattern appears unequivocal in demonstrating that the patient in question with recurrent unipolar depression was also clearly a responder (Post, L'Herrou, et al., 1998; Post & Luckenbaugh, 2003).

Carbamazepine would appear to have made a substantial personal and economic impact in the case presented here. Using the 5 years following carbamazepine institution compared with the 5 years prior to its use in a mirror image design, one can see not only the avoidance of eight separate hospitalizations but also at least five courses of ECT with the associated need for anesthesia. Thus, the actual monetary savings would be extraordinary, in addition to the invaluable savings to the patient suffering from a profoundly incapacitating psychotic depression.

In a mixed population of unipolar and bipolar depressed patients with highly treatment-refractory affective disorders, we found initial responsivity to carbamazepine on a double-blind basis in about one third of patients (Post, Uhde, Roy-Byrne, & Joffe, 1986). In 10 of these patients the improvement on drug was subsequently replicated during a second blind trial of carbamazepine after patients had relapsed off drug (see Chapter 18, indicating unequivocal responsiveness in at least a subgroup of patients.

It is interesting that the response in this patient with recurrent unipolar depression is remi-niscent of some of the characteristics that predicted response in Greil, Kleindienst, Erazo, and Muller-Oerlinghausen's (1998) randomized trial comparing lithium and carbamazepine prophylaxis in bipolar patients. They found that lithium was most effective in patients with classical bipolar I illness without mood-incongruent delusions and other comorbidities. In contrast, carbamazepine tended to have a better effect in patients with bipolar II and NOS, mood-incongruent delusions, and other comorbidities (Greil et al., 1998). This patient's depression presented with extreme anxiety and marked delusional components (most of which were mood congruent, however). A consistent predictor of lithium nonresponsiveness is high levels of anxiety and panic, and this patient clearly demonstrated this characteristic.

Other possible correlates of carbamazepine response in depression include:

- Greater acuity and severity
- Frontal and paralimbic (especially left insula) hypermetabolism on positron emission tomography
- History of alcoholism
- Comorbid PTSD
- Low cerebrospinal fluid homovanillic acid, a dopamine metabolite
- Higher ratio of the 10,11-epoxide to carbamazepine levels
- Degree of T_4 and free T_4 decrease during carbamazepine treatment

Correlates for carbamazepine response in prophylaxis include:

- Lack of family history of bipolar illness in first-degree relatives
- Lack of prior rapid cycling
- Nonclassical presentations, such as bipolar II, noneuphoric mania, schizoaffective (especially depressive with mood-incongruent delusions), and comorbidities
- Comorbid trigeminal neuralgia
- Chronic alcohol-related dysphoria

Some of these predictors of response may not be selective to carbamazepine since valproate (Chapter 23) and lamotrigine (Chapter 25) also appear effective in some patients with recurrent depression of psychotic proportions.

PRINCIPLES OF THE CASE	STRENGTH OF EVIDENCE
1. Carbamazepine may be effective in preventing recurrent psychotic depressions of either the unipolar (as in this case) or bipolar type.	+
2. Patients can respond to carbamazepine when they have clearly failed to respond to lithium prophylaxis.	++
3. Carbamazepine may be particularly useful in depressed patients with a history of alcoholism (which, however, this patient did not have.).	+
4. ECT is highly acutely effective for even the most severe psychotic depressions, but does not appear to have any long-lasting impact on the course and recurrence of illness, and other treatment modalities in follow-up are required.	++
5. Lithium is often ineffective in bipolar patients in the face of extreme levels of anxiety or panic, as in this patient.	++
6. Carbamazepine produced dose-related decreases in anxiety in four studies of patients with epilepsy and comorbid anxiety.	+++
7. Whereas carbamazepine was effective in preventing all episodes for the first 5 years after NIMH hospitalization, two hospitalizations were required in 1983. This could have been in	

part due to the progressive carbamazepine dose reductions in 1981 and 1983. Some patients begin to lose carbamazepine response after 3 to 5 years of good response even on the same doses and blood levels of carbamazepine.   +

8. If this type of loss of efficacy via tolerance occurs, a variety of manipulations could be considered in order to renew efficacy:

a. The dose of carbamazepine could be increased if the patient was below his or her side effects threshold.   +

b. If the psychotic components of the illness persisted, use of an atypical antipsychotic would also likely prove effective.   +++

c. A conventional unimodal antidepressant might be added.   ++

d. Lithium augmentation might be helpful, even in the face of nonresponse to lithium monotherapy.   ±

e. Other anticonvulsants that might be considered for augmentation strategies if the recurrent depressions persisted would include lamotrigine and valproate (although each has the potential problem of cross-tolerance with carbamazepine in epilepsy models).   +

f. With episodes beginning to occur through multiple antidepressants, antipsychotics, and anxiolytic medications in this patient in 1985 and 1986, a renewed trial of carbamazepine might also be indicated. Other strategies are noted in Chapters 38–41.   +

TAKE-HOME MESSAGE

Acute interventions with ECT for recurrent or refractory persistent psychotic depression may be highly effective, but finding adequate long-term pharmacoprophylaxis (drug treatment, in this case with carbamazepine) may save the patient from some of the great psychological and monetary costs of recurrent depressions requiring hospitalization, general anesthesia, and ECT.

17

Acute and Prophylactic
Carbamazepine: Management
of Side Effects

CASE HISTORY

This woman is a 35-year-old mother of several children. She had a history of severe manias unresponsive to lithium prophylaxis plus adjunctive treatments, which resulted in a series of hospitalizations (Figure 17.1). She was referred to the NIMH for further evaluation and study. Another manic episode was observed, and carbamazepine administered on a double-blind basis resulted in dramatic amelioration of her manic symptoms (Figure 17.2). In order to ascertain whether this was a spontaneous remission, placebo was substituted, and because the patient had a recurrence of her mania, double-blind carbamazepine was reinstituted with an excellent response.

There was ongoing discussion about whether the patient had been compliant with her lithium regimen, and she was discharged to outpatient status with close monitoring of her lithium in order to achieve levels greater than or equal to 0.8 mEq/L. Despite good lithium compliance, a third manic episode occurred in 1978, she was readmitted, and for the third time rapidly responded to the blind institution of carbamazepine (Figure 17.2).

Following moderate depression on carbamazepine monotherapy, her outpatient treatment managed by others was augmented with lithium with an excellent result. The patient discontinued her medication in 1991, with the exception of tricyclic antidepressants that had been started at the end of 1980 for a mild depression. A full-blown manic episode occurred and the patient was rapidly restarted on a lithium-carbamazepine combination with a good response. Because of some ongoing mood lability through these two treatments, she was coadministered tricyclic antidepressants and low-dose antipsychotics throughout most of her subsequent treatment.

BACKGROUND LITERATURE

A variety of studies summarized by Vestergaard (1992) and others indicate that lithium treatment in community and clinical samples is often less than adequate for mood stabilization. This patient clearly demonstrates this phenomenon with a lack of response to lithium, both on a retrospective basis and then confirmed on a prospective basis when the patient was maintained on blinded medications and followed closely in the outpatient clinic. Despite the maintenance of good blood levels and excellent compliance, she suffered a relapse that then responded to the initiation of carbamazepine treatment for a third time. However, as noted, she continued to have periods of mood instability on lithium and carbamazepine, and outpatient therapists felt that this regimen needed further augmentation with

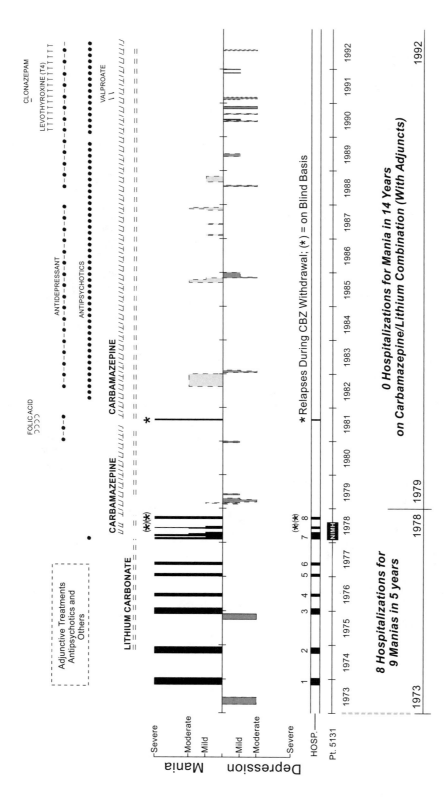

Figure 17.1 Confirmed acute and prophylactic response to carbamazepine in a lithium nonresponder. Five hospitalizations (3–6 and 8) for mania occurred despite lithium and other agents. Carbamazepine augmentation dramatically reduced this need. * = manic relapses when off carbamazepine.

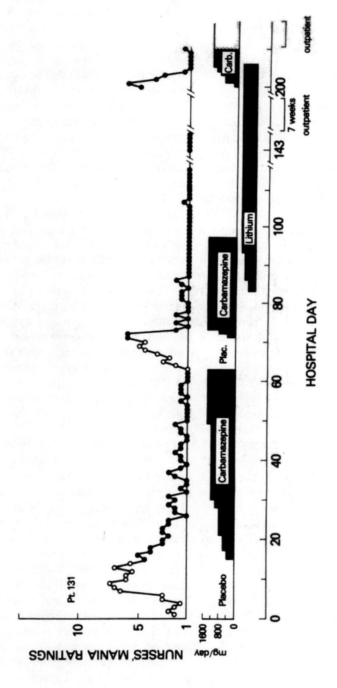

Figure 17.2 Amelioration of manic symptoms with administration of carbamazepine. Detailed illustration of 1978 hospitalization demonstrating an unequivocal response to carbamazepine under double-blind conditions on 3 separate occasions, including the last when a manic episode occurred despite carefully monitored lithium administration.

antidepressants and antipsychotics through most of her course of illness after 1982. Thus, there was a dramatic reduction in frequency of hospitalizations from the precarbamazepine to postcarbamazepine treatment phases.

These data are convergent with a moderate number of controlled clinical trials of patients, conducted on a blind or randomized basis, reporting good response rates (approximately 50%) to carbamazepine monotherapy or in combination with previous ineffective regimens. In addition, a large series of patients studied in an open fashion with adjunctive use of carbamazepine also shows an excellent response in 320 (51%) of 629 patients, as reviewed elsewhere (Post, Denicoff, Frye, et al., 1997).

Lithium and carbamazepine share some mechanisms of action, such as (a) the ability to decrease the second messenger systems via inhibition of G proteins, adenylate cyclase, and inhibit the inositol transporter; (b) decrease DA turnover; (c) decrease calcium influx through the glutamate NMDA receptor; and (d) increase substance P levels in the striatum and decrease $GABA_B$ receptors in the frontal cortex of animals with chronic but not acute administration. However, there are a multitude of differences as well, with lithium and carbamazepine having opposite effects on the inositol phosphatases, for example. In addition, carbamazepine acts as an adenosine A1 antagonist, a peripheral-type benzodiazepine receptor agonist, and a blocker of sodium channel influx. Thus, it is unclear whether some shared mechanisms of carbamazepine and lithium account for their similar range of positive effects in affective illness, or whether differential properties of these compounds account for differences in response within individual patients, or combine to make a more robust response than either agent alone, as suggested in the current life chart (Post, Chalecka-Franaszek, & Hough, 2002; Post, Weiss, et al., 2000).

There are relatively few clinical or biological markers that predict who might show an excellent response to carbamazepine. Since carbamazepine is an anticonvulsant with mood-stabilizing properties, we thought that the ability of carbamazepine to dampen activity in the limbic areas of the brain may be important to its ac-tions. We assessed limbic hyperactivity indirectly by asking patients whether they had many psychosensory symptoms and distortions (such as déjà vu and olfactory illusions), particularly since these are experienced by patients with temporal lobe epilepsy (i.e., complex partial seizures of the amygdala and hippocampus and related structures of the medial temporal lobe). Our affectively ill patients without seizures did show a high incidence of these psychosensory symptoms, but surprisingly, those with the highest levels were better responders to lithium and there was no prediction for carbamazepine (Silberman, Post, Nurnberger, Theodore, & Boulenger, 1985).

However, more recently, Ketter, Kimbrell, and associates (1999) reported that depressed patients who are responsive to carbamazepine tend to have hypermetabolism, particularly in the frontal and temporal lobes and insula, and that this is decreased by treatment with carbamazepine (Chapter 18). In contrast, nonresponders are those who have initial hypometabolism at baseline on positron emission tomography (which carbamazepine further exacerbates). The depressed patients with initial hypometabolism at baseline are the majority of patients, and these patients appear to be more responsive to the calcium channel blocker nimodipine and perhaps lamotrigine as well.

Our data (Denicoff, Smith-Jackson, Disney, et al., 1997) and those of Okuma (1993) suggest that carbamazepine, like most other prophylactic agents, works less well in rapid cyclers than in nonrapid cyclers. In terms of acute response, it is interesting to note that those with greater severity of depression responded best, and paradoxically, the patients with the largest decrements in T_4 and free T_4 on the drug were the best responders (Post, Uhde, et al., 1986). Lithium also decreases thyroid indices but increases thyroid-stimulating hormone and is associated with clinically relevant impairment of thyroid function, and occasionally hypothyroidism; these clinically relevent thyroid problems almost never occur during carbamazepine treatment. The decrements in T_4 and free T_4 observed on carbamazepine are not associated with clinical hypothyroidism or changes in basal metabolic rate and usually do not require T_3 or T_4 augmentation.

SIDE EFFECTS AVOIDANCE AND MANAGEMENT

Management of side effects is displayed in Table 17.1, based on discussion in Post and Frye (2005), and Post et al. (2007).

Dizziness, Ataxia, Diplopia

Careful individualized dose titration is important with carbamazepine, as individual patients will begin to have side effects at low doses and others will tolerate very high doses. Moreover, the use of single nighttime dosing with the long-acting CBZ-ER preparations may help avoid dizziness, ataxia, and diplopia. However, patients who arise during the night when plasma concentrations of carbamazepine are high with bedtime dosing need to be vigilant for dizziness, ataxia, and diplopia.

Rash

Benign maculopapular rash, often associated with itchiness, was a relatively common side effect of older carbamazepine preparations. Even with rapid dose titration with the CBZ-ER preparation in more recent studies of acute mania, the rate of rash and associated itchiness was low and relatively similar to that observed on placebo. Selected patients experiencing a widespread but benign rash on carbamazepine (i.e., one that rapidly disappears on drug discontinuation with or without diphenhydramine treatment and does not progress) can be considered for cautious rechallenge with the drug under the cover of systemic prednisone therapy without experiencing renewal of rash.

It is not recommended that steroids (such as prednisone) be used in someone who has experienced a more fulminant rash reaction such as Stevens-Johnson syndrome or toxic epidermal necrolysis wherein rechallenge, even with steroids, may not be successful. However, in the presence of a benign rash (but not a severe one), one could consider crossing the patient over to the keto-analog of carbamazepine, oxcarbazepine, where in 70% of cases the rashes will not recur.

Patients should be informed that a rash on the palms of the hands, soles of the feet, or canker sores or bullae (large blisters) in the mouth should lead to immediate drug discontinuation, followed with a call to the treating physician. Similarly, any rash associated with vesicles, blebs, or bullae should lead to immediate drug discontinuation, because these are more likely precursors of the more severe forms of rash.

Hematological Monitoring

The experience of severe hematological dysfunction on carbamazepine is rare. It is estimated that the incidence of agranulocytosis (lack of white cells) is 1 per million patients, and of aplastic anemia (lack of production of all blood cells, including red blood cells and platelets) is 5.2 per million patients, per year of exposure. The background rate of aplastic anemia is thought to be in the range of 2 per million in the general population, and therefore one can see that the increased risk on carbamazepine is severalfold higher, but the likelihood is still quite small.

Rather than intensive monitoring, which is largely acknowledged as neither useful nor cost effective, one should advise patients that if any worrisome signs develop, they should immediately contact their physician and obtain a complete blood count. The presence of a fever or sore throat (that would most likely be associated with a viral infection or the flu) needs to be differentiated from a bacterial infection secondary to insufficient numbers of white cells requiring drug cessation. However, if petechiae (tiny broken capillary blood vessels) or evidence of bleeding occurs, which may be related to the suppression of platelets, the drug should be immediately discontinued and ongoing medical management and monitoring should begin.

Carbamazepine treatment is typically associ-

Table 17.1 *Some Carbamazepine Side Effects and Their Possible Management*

Side Effect (Frequency, Type)	Possible Approach (Strength of Evidence or Practice)	Comment
Dizziness, ataxia, diplopia (C,D)	Reduce peak dose effects by ↓dose (+++); Switch to all H.S. sustained-release formulation (+)	Will occur 2–3 hours after IR dose if patient near side effect threshold (+++)
Fatigue, sedation (C,D)	Switch more of IR dose to H.S. (+++) or all of ER dose to H.S. (+); ↓Dose or wait for adaptation or autoinduction (++)	Start with low H.S. dose; given wide individual variability in side effects threshold, titrate slowly to clinical effect or to side effects (+++)
Benign rash (VC,I)	Discontinue drug (+); antihistamines (+); steroids (+)	Possible switch to oxcarbazepine, 2/3 no rash (++); or can restart slowly under coverage of prednisone (++)
Severe rash (R,I,S)	Discontinue drug (+++)	Obtain medical/dermatological consultation (+++); rechallenge not recommended (even with steroids)
Benign WBC suppression (VC,D) versus	Lower dose (+); add lithium (+++)	Lithium increases C.S.F. (+++) whereas CBZ suppresses C.S.F. (+++); 2,500 to 3,000 WBC lower limit of tolerability (±)
Agranulocytosis (VR,I)	Discontinue drug (+++)	Medical support and consultation required (+++)
Aplastic anemia (VR,I)	Discontinue drug (+++)	Medical support and consultation required (+++)
Weight gain (UC,I)	Consider topiramate or zonisamide augmentation (++) or switch to weight-neutral drug such as LTG, OXC (+)	Rarely a problem
Hyponatremia (O,D)	↓Dose (++); add lithium (++); add demeclomycin (++);	Women, older age, and use of higher doses are vulnerability factors (+++)
Thyroid hormone suppression (VC,D)	None needed as ↓T_4 may correlate with better response (++)	No ↑TSH; no change BMR with CBZ (+); thyroid supplements rarely needed (+++); ↓T_4 and ↓T_3 may be additive with lithium (++)
Tremor (R,D)	↓Dose (+)	Check ammonia levels when combined with VPA if tremor is coarse (or flappy) (±)
Teratogenic (O,D) Spina bifida ~1% Cranial facial abnormality	Pretreat with ↑folate (+)	Avoid combination Rx if possible, especially with VPA (+); minor developmental delays do not persist
Hepatitis (R,I)	Discontinue if enzymes ↑ to 3× normal (++) Discontinue if patient is symptomatic (+++)	
Memory disturbance (UC,D)	↓Dose (+); switch to all H.S. with long-acting preparation (±)	CBZ potentiation of vasopressin receptors may prevent memory loss

Note. Frequency: VC, very common; C, common; O, occasional; UC, uncommon; VR, very rare; Type: D, dose related; I, idiosyncratic; S, sensitivity may cross to other anticonvulsant; Evidence: +++, well supported, controlled data; ++, many case reports; +, likely works; ±, questionable or hypothetical; Abbreviations: ↑, increase; ↓, decrease; IR, immediate release; ER, extended release; H.S., at night; CBZ, carbamazepine; WBC, white blood cell; LTG, lamotrigine; OXC, oxcarbazepine; VPA, valproate; T_4, levothyroxine; T_3, triiodothyronine; Rx, treatment; C.S.F., colony stimulating factor which increases WBCs and platelets.

ated with an inconsequential mild to substantial white blood cell (WBC) suppression, usually leaving the patient's WBC count within the normal range. Conventional guidelines suggest that a WBC count of 2,500 or 3,000 WBC/mm^3 with an absolute neutrophil count of 1,000–1,500 WBC/mm^3 should be sufficient to continue to fight infections. If the WBC count on carbamazepine begins to drift toward these lower levels, dose reduction or the addition of lithium could be considered.

Carbamazepine is thought to inhibit a factor that stimulates WBC and platelet production (colony-stimulating factor), whereas lithium has the opposite effect, and lithium will often normalize a low WBC count on carbamazepine. This strategy should not be used in the presence of a more severe or broad suppression of all cellular elements. For example, if aplastic anemia were developing, lithium is unable to stimulate the production of red cells, in contrast to its positive effects on both WBCs and platelets by enhancing colony-stimulating factor.

Hepatitis

Asymptomatic liver enzyme elevation up to three times normal is common with most of the anticonvulsants. However, patients should be instructed to consult their physicians in the presence of malaise, right upper quadrant pain, cola-colored urine, fever, vomiting, or jaundice. If liver enzymes exceed three times normal or the above symptoms occur, the drug should be discontinued.

Hyponatremia (Low Serum Sodium)

Hyponatremia is a relatively uncommon side effect of carbamazepine estimated to occur in about 1% of patients; risk factors include being in the older age range and use of higher doses of the drug. Carbamazepine dose reduction often sufficiently resolves this side effect, but if it is more problematic, one could consider cotreatment with the antibiotic demeclomycin or lith-

ium, both of which have been reported to treat or prevent the development of carbamazepine-induced hyponatremia.

The mechanism of this effect is not precisely known, but carbamazepine appears to indirectly enhance the actions of arginine vasopressin (another name for antidiuretic hormone) at or near the level of the receptor. Thus, blocking the efficacy of arginine vasopressin actions by inhibiting adenylate cyclase with lithum or demeclomycin would decrease fluid overload, the cause of hyponatremia. In instances of carbamazepine-induced hyponatremia, switching a patient to oxcarbazepine would not appear warranted since there is an even higher incidence of hyponatremia with this closely related compound than with carbamazepine itself.

Cholesterol

Carbamazepine appears to increase total cholesterol levels by about 18 to 20 points from baseline. This includes both positive increases in high-density lipoproteins and unwanted increases in the low-density lipoprotein fraction, such that the ratio (one of the main correlates of cardiovascular risk in the Framingham study) does not change in most studies. The eventual clinical consequence of this alteration, in the absence of major changes in triglycerides, has yet to be specifically explored and addressed. However, for those at high risk for cardiovascular problems derived from current marginal or high levels of circulating cholesterol, one may want to directly address this potential problem in advance with statins and other lipid-lowering approaches.

Thyroid

Another area of interest is the effect of carbamazepine on thyroid function. Like lithium, carbamazepine can decrease levels of T_3 and T_4, but unlike lithium, is rarely associated with increases in thyroid-stimulating hormone or subclinical or clinical hypothyroidism that require treatment. In fact, we reported that the degree of decrease in T_4 and free T_4 levels on carbamazepine was associated with the degree of improvement in depression.

Pregnancy and Breast-feeding

Carbamazepine is teratogenic (pregnancy category D) and is associated with low birth weight, craniofacial deformities, digital hypoplasia, and, in about 2% of women, spina bifida. For the last group, it is unclear whether folate supplementation may attenuate the risk, but high-dose pretreatent is nonetheless recommended. Fetal ultrasound studies may allow early detection of this potentially devastating anomaly. The risk of spina bifida on carbamazepine appears to be about one half the risk on valproate. In rare patients with severe mood disorders refractory to other drugs, clinicians may determine in consultation with a gynecologist that the benefits of treating with carbamazepine outweigh the risks as compared with other treatment options. Carbamazepine is present in breast milk, at concentrations about half those in maternal blood, but may not accumulate in fetal blood. Clinicians and patients may, nonetheless, prefer to avoid putative risks of exposing infants to carbamazepine in breast milk and discourage breast-feeding in women taking carbamazepine.

PRINCIPLES OF THE CASE	STRENGTH OF EVIDENCE
1. Many patients, even in the subgroup most likely to respond to lithium, that is, women with euphoric manias and high compliance rates, do not always show a response to this traditional treatment.	+++
2. Carbamazepine is effective in the treatment of acute mania, as documented in more than 19 controlled studies in the literature, and its long-acting preparation (Equetro) is FDA approved for acute mania.	+++
3. Carbamazepine appears highly effective in prophylaxis, including in a subgroup of patients not responsive to lithium, such as is illustrated in this case.	+++
4. Although there was a dramatic improvement in this patient's illness and a complete reversal of the need for hospitalizations for mania during carbamazepine cotreatment with lithium, other adjunctive measures are often still necessary for more minor breakthrough episodes.	++
5. Carbamazepine and lithium both share and show differential mechanisms of action; how these are eventually related to their similarities and differences in neurobiological responsiveness in manic-depressive illness remains to be delineated.	+++
6. In contrast to the small subgroup of patients who gradually demonstrate loss of efficacy during long-term treatment with regimens involving carbamazepine, this patient was among the larger group who show sustained moderate to marked degrees of clinical response. The combination of carbamazepine and lithium prevented further hospitalizations for mania for the 14 years illustrated in Figure 17.1, and for an additional 15 years to the present time (data not illustrated).	+
7. Nonresponse to lithium does not predict nonresponsivity to the other agents such as carbamazepine or valproate.	++

8. This patient's case makes a very important point about treatment response:
   a. Several studies report that lithium is more effective in large groups of subjects than carbamazepine in the prevention of mania. ++
   b. Despite this, there are many patients such as this one and the patient in Chapter 15 who are complete nonresponders to lithium but are highly responsive to carbamazepine. +++
   c. While group data give some rough estimate of likelihood of clinical response, it cannot provide confirmation of a clinical response in any individual, and it cannot predict with much certainty responsiveness of any other individual. +++
9. The bottom line is that evidence of individual responsivity, especially when it is confirmed (such as in this and many other patients in this volume) trumps all generalities about efficacy or relative efficacy in the literature. +++
10. Patients and most clinicians know this, but, sadly, many academicians, regulatory authorities, and lawyers do not. ++
11. In the 1970s there was good reason to keep on trying lithium with antipsychotic adjuncts because that was all that was available at the time. In contrast, now that many different alternatives are available, one should not stay with a regimen that repeatedly does not work, but should begin to systematically explore other options whether or not they are FDA approved. ++

TAKE-HOME MESSAGE

Many patients with severe bipolar I illness, not responsive to lithium carbonate, will respond to another mood stabilizer such as carbamazepine, used either alone in the treatment of acute mania (this patient, 1978) or adjunctively in the long-term prevention of affective episodes (1979 to the present).

18

Excellent Response to Carbamazepine but Not Nimodipine: Possible Prediction From Baseline PET Scans and Other Biological Markers

CASE HISTORY

Using functional brain imaging with positron emission tomography (PET), this patient showed the atypical pattern of prefrontal hypermetabolism at baseline compared with age- and gender-matched controls (Figure 18.1). Usually, depressed patients are hypometabolic; that is, they have reduced frontal neuronal activity (Baxter et al., 1989). Thus, this case is an example of the future possibility of better assigning the most effective type of treatment based on assessment of the pattern of cerebral metabolism or blood flow at baseline.

This patient's life chart is also of interest because it illustrates an initial apparently excellent response to treatment with lithium in conjunction with antidepressants (from 1985 to 1990) but followed by progressively severe depressive breakthroughs (in 1988, and in 1991 and 1992 requiring hospitalization) despite ongoing lithium and other adjunctive treatment. We have observed that 35% of bipolar patients referred to the NIMH because of lithium nonresponse showed this pattern of loss of response (toler-

ance) to lithium prophylaxis over time (see Chapter 12).

In this and other instances, the patients indicated that they maintained good compliance. Thus, this type of loss of efficacy does not appear to be based on pharmacokinetics (i.e., related to low blood levels or stopping treatment) but may be related to a loss of drug effectiveness in inhibiting illness episodes that begin to break through what was previously an adequate treatment.

This patient is representative of the possible positive outcome of switching to a different drug such as carbamazepine, which has many mechanisms of action that are quite different from those of lithium carbonate (see Chapters 9 and 17 for details).

As indicated in the bottom right of Figure 18.1 (in a detailed view of this individual's daily mood ratings at the NIMH), a double-blind trial with the calcium channel blocker nimodipine (Chapters 32 and 33) was not effective for the patient's depression and may have exacerbated his affective dysregulation with increased periods of dysphoric hypomania in the

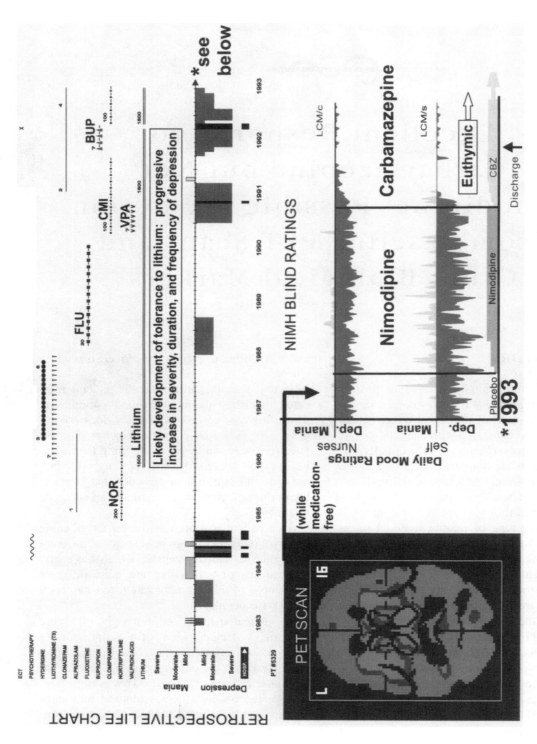

Figure 18.1 Good response to carbamazepine but not nimodipine in a bipolar II patient with paralimbic hyperactivity on PET scan. The retrospective life chart illustrates a progressively more difficult course of depressive illness despite lithium and antidepressants prior to NIMH (top). The depression in 1990–1991 may even have been exacerbated by valproate. The patient ultimately showed excellent response to double-blind administration of carbamazepine after a poor response to a double-blind clinical trial with nimodipine (bottom right). The darker areas in this patient's PET scan are those that show 2 to 3 standard deviations more regional metabolic activity than a large group of age- and gender-matched controls; that is, these areas are much more overactive than they should be (bottom left). FLU, fluoxetine; NOR, nortriptyline; CMI, clomipramine; BUP, buproprion; VPA, valproic acid; LCM/c, life chart method, clinician rated; LCM/s, self-rated.

evening. In contrast, remarkable mood stabilization was achieved soon after he was switched on a blind basis to carbamazepine, and this improvement persisted for several years following his discharge from the NIMH.

BACKGROUND LITERATURE

There is substantial evidence from more than a dozen studies that patients with depression have increased intracellular calcium in their blood elements (either lymphocytes or platelets). On the basis of these and other data implicating calcium dysregulation in the affective disorders, Dubovsky pioneered the use of the calcium channel blocker verapamil for the potential treatment of mania, with some success (Dubovsky, Franks, Lifschitz, & Coen, 1982). Given the apparent inadequacies of verapamil in the treatment of the depressed phase of the illness, however, we began to pursue the possible better efficacy of another calcium channel blocker, nimodipine, which has some actions that are different from verapamil despite their shared ability to block voltage-dependent calcium channels.

It is of considerable interest that this patient was extremely anxious and secondarily unable to focus and attend to tasks necessary for maintaining any type of employment. He had lost so many jobs prior to hospitalization that most staff members believed that he had an intractable personality disorder that would not respond to treatment. However, once he showed a dramatic response to carbamazepine, his level of anxiety was markedly reduced, he was able to focus, and he immediately began to prepare for discharge and look for new employment. These observations highlight the issue that many symptoms and dysfunctions attributable to personality disorders may remit when the appropriate treatment for the primary mood disorder is achieved.

Figure 18.1 (bottom left) illustrates the general pattern of baseline hypermetabolism on the PET scan of this patient compared with age- and gender-matched normal volunteer controls. It is evident that there is increased metabolism in a variety of brain structures, including medial parts of the left and right temporal lobes, basal ganglia, and thalamus, as well as smaller areas in anterior and posterior cingulate gyrus. The increased activity may reflect dysfunction in these areas intimately involved in mood regulation and cognition. This patient was extremely anxious, highly disorganized, and incapable of focused attention during his periods of affective dysregulation, which were accompanied by considerable cognitive deficits on formal and informal neuropsychological testing. Yet, when he was placed on an appropriate medication, in this case carbamazepine, he sustained a remarkable improvement not only in his mood disorder but also in his cognitive function and was able to return to active employment. Carbamazepine typically reduces hypermetabolism in the brains of most patients with affective illness as well as those with epileptic disorders (Ketter, Kimbrell, et al., 1999).

Prediction of Differential Clinical Response

While some patients clearly respond to nimodipine (Pazzaglia, Post, Ketter, George, & Marangell, 1993; Pazzaglia et al., 1998), as documented in an on-off-on design, this patient did not respond in terms of either the severity of his depression or his mood lability with dysphoric hypomanias, which tended to occur in the evenings. In contrast, he showed a rapid onset of complete response to carbamazepine, achieving symptom amelioration in all of the realms affected. This differential and divergent response to these two agents raises the issue of whether such responsiveness can be predicted in advance, potentially saving patients from many weeks or months of a clinical trial that will not be effective (Figure 18.1).

Use of PET Scans to Image Baseline Brain Activity

A small data set is beginning to accumulate suggesting that neural activity as imaged in patients with PET scans may eventually help in directing therapeutic strategies. This patient was part of the cohort presented by Ketter, Kimbrell, et al. (1999) indicating that there was an overall positive response to carbamazepine in those who had baseline hypermetabolism, but that none of the patients with the more typical pattern of baseline hypometabolism of depression responded to this drug. Conversely, the nimodipine responders tended to be drawn from those with the more classic pattern of baseline hypofunction in concert with their depression.

Sackeim and colleagues have observed that those with the best responses to electroconvulsive therapy (ECT) have a pattern of baseline frontal hypofunction, and this hypofunction is further exacerbated by ECT in the best clinical responders (Nobler et al., 1994). In contrast, many of the serotonin-selective and other antidepressants appeared to normalize patterns of altered cerebral metabolism or blood flow compared with pretreatment (Little et al., 2005).

As noted in Chapter 57, we have preliminary evidence that those with the classical pattern of prefrontal hypofunction at baseline may respond best to high-frequency (20 Hz) repetitive transcranial magnetic stimulation (rTMS), which tends to increase neural activity (Speer et al., 2000), whereas those with baseline hyperactivity (such as this patient) would tend to respond best to low-frequency (1 Hz) rTMS, which tends to dampen neural hyperexcitability.

From the clinical perspective, PET scans are not available to the general community and are currently performed only in the context of specific clinical research studies. However, a number of other functional brain imaging techniques are in use, such as single photon emission computed tomography scans and functional magnetic resonance imaging for regional blood flow, and even assessment of a variety of biochemical substances in the brain using magnetic resonance spectroscopy (MRS).

These procedures are much less expensive than PET scans and eventually are likely to be widely available in the general community. Thus, we are suggesting the future possibility that baseline levels of neural activity or brain biochemical markers with MRS may ultimately be able to assist in the choice of optimal treatment agents. The data currently are not strong

enough to support such a clinical application and, clearly, baseline PET scans are not diagnostic in the way that they can be for ascertaining which patients do or do not have, for example, Alzheimer's disease, Parkinson's disease, or Huntington's chorea.

Opposing Neurochemical Effects of Carbamazepine and Nimodipine

The present case clearly documents the general principle that among the putative mood-stabilizing agents there are marked individual differences in responsiveness, and it is of interest to consider some of the differences in mechanisms of action of carbamazepine and nimodipine (Table 18.1). While a modicum of data suggest that carbamazepine may exert some blockade of calcium influx through L-type calcium channels, this primary effect is not as strong as it is for nimodipine. Conversely, while carbamazepine is a potent and widely used anticonvulsant, the anticonvulsant properties of nimodipine are relatively limited and this drug is not used clinically for epilepsy (Post, Pazzaglia, et al., 2000). In fact, it is only marketed for use in subarachnoid hemorrhage, which is part of the reason it is so expensive. Other dihydropyridine L-type calcium channel blockers may also be useful instead of nimodipine (Chapter 32).

It is also of interest that carbamazepine and nimodipine exert opposite effects on measurements of somatostatin concentration in the cerebrospinal fluid (CSF) of our patients with affective disorders. Carbamazepine decreases somatostatin, while nimodipine has the novel action of increasing it (Pazzaglia, George, Post, Rubinow, & Davis, 1995). Since somatostatin is one of the peptides that is reduced in Alzheimer's disease, we wondered whether the ability to increase somatostatin could be related to initial reports of nimodipine's efficacy in moderately ill patients with Alzheimer's.

In addition, because depressed patients have significantly lower baseline levels of CSF somatostatin compared with normal volunteers, we asked whether those with the lowest CSF somatostatin levels might be among those who responded best. Preliminary evidence from Frye,

Table 18.1 *Comparative and Opposite Effects of the Anticonvulsant Carbamazine and the Dihydropyridine Calcium Channel Blocker Nimodipine*

Findings	Carbamazepine	Nimodipine
Blockade of Ca++ influx	Via ligand-gated NMDA receptor	Via voltage-gated L-type Ca++ channel
Ca++ channel blockade	Weak	Strong
Anticonvulsant	Potent	Weak (not used clinically)
Somatostatin in CSF	Decreased	Increased[a]
Memory	Unchanged	Enhanced
Dopamine	Turnover reduced[b]	Cocaine-induced dopamine overflow decreased
Cocaine hyperactivity	Little effect	Inhibition
Left insula metabolism on PET scan	Hypermetabolism predicts good response	Hypometabolism predicts good response
Correlation with antidepressant response	$r = +.516$ ($df22, p < .02$)	$r = -.519$ ($df16, p < .005$)

[a]Better response to nimodipine in those with low CSF somatosatin at baseline.
[b]Better response to carbamazepine in those with low versus high baseline CSF homovanillic acid, the major metabolite of dopamine.

Pazzaglia, and colleagues (2003) suggested that this is the case, but the predictive validity and potential clinical utility of somatostatin as a marker of response will require further study. Although nimodipine worked better in those with low versus high somatostatin, there was considerable overlap in values between the two groups. Whether this patient's poor response to nimodipine is attributable to his already high baseline levels of somatostatin (Figure 18.2, lower right arrow) and not needing even higher levels of somatostatin is a matter of speculation.

It is also of interest that this patient had the highest concentration of the dopamine metabolite homovanillic acid in his spinal fluid (Figure 18.2, lower left) and among the highest levels of corticotropin-releasing factor (top right). Carbamazepine is known to decrease dopamine turnover (reflected in patients by low homovanillic acid in CSF) and to decrease release of CRH from the hypothalamus. Thus, any of these effects (or others) could have been important to this patient's dramatic responsiveness to carbamazepine, although any direct links remain to be more systematically studied (Post, Pazzaglia, et al., 2000). Brain levels of many chemical substances are now available from MRS, and we present these CSF measures with the hope that these or MRS assessments can soon be used to help predict a patient's likelihood of response to a given agent.

Future Prediction of Response and Side Effects With SNPs

Many investigators have predicted that modern assessment of single-nucleotide polymorphisms (SNPs) will eventually be able to help choose the most appropriate medication (Semple, Morris, Porteous, & Evans, 2000). In contrast to mutations, which are by definition rare, SNPs are common genetic variations that exist in the general population. For example, some people inherit a short (s) variant of the serotonin transporter (5HT-T), which functions relatively less efficiently than the long (l) form of the transporter. These 5HT-Tss individuals are at higher risk for depression with recent adult stressors than those with the 5HT-T$_{ll}$ form (when both groups also have a history of childhood trauma as well; Caspi et al., 2003). In many, but not all, studies, unipolars with the 5HT-Tss are less likely to respond to SSRI antidepressants, and bipolars with this allele are more likely to switch into mania. How the SNPs val66val BDNF associated with early onset bipolar illness and the val66met associated with cognitive dysfunction

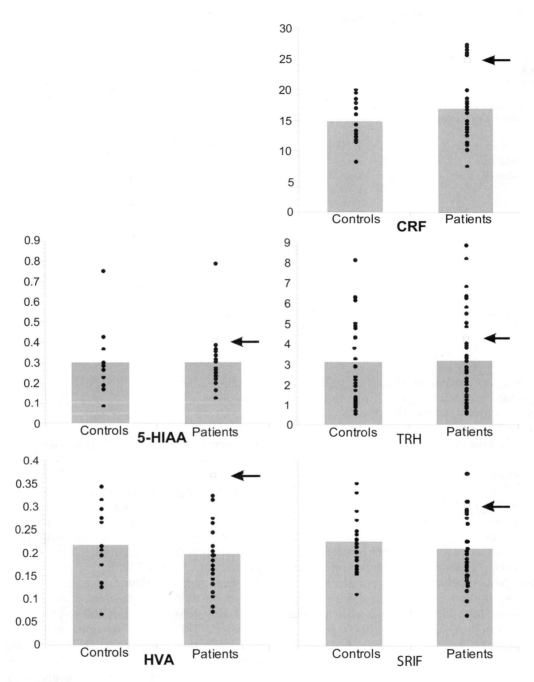

Figure 18.2 Evidence of neurotransmitter and peptide dysregulation in a bipolar male. This figure shows how this patient's profile of spinal fluid biochemical measures (open square and arrow) compares with other patients and normal volunteer controls. CRH (corticotropin-releasing hormone) releases pituitary adrenocorticotropic hormone, which drives adrenal cortisol. This patient's CRH value was the fifth highest among the patients and much higher than any control, perhaps consistent with severity of dysphoria and anxiety and prior history of abuse. 5-HIAA (5-hydroxyindoleacetic acid) is a serotonin metabolite, and this patient's 5-HIAA value was second highest among all patients. HVA (homovanillic acid) was higher in this patient than in all others or controls, suggesting dopaminergic hyperactivity. TRH (thyrotropin-releasing hormone), which releases pituitary thyroid-stimulating hormone and drives thyroid secretion, was normal in this patient. SRIF (somatostatin), which is usually low in depression, was high in this patient.

in bipolars relate to treatment response would be of great interest.

It is currently estimated that there are approximately 100,000 SNPs, and clinicians are speculating that a percentage of these will soon be able to be assessed in individual patients at relatively low cost. Currently, it costs about $1 per SNP, making routine SNP screening cost prohibitive. However, if one ascertained a profile of a small group of high-priority SNPs in those who responded to a given agent compared with those who did not, one might eventually be able to use this SNP pattern to better predict both clinical responsiveness and the potential for serious adverse drug reactions.

Interestingly, this use of the pattern of a series of SNPs could even be done in the absence of knowledge of the function of a given SNP, rendering this technology and methodology likely to become clinically relevant in a relatively short period of time. The elucidation of the function of a gene and the pathological significance of a given mutation or common polymorphism may take decades. In contrast, the appropriate combination and pattern of SNPs predicting clinical response to a given treatment could be discovered and immediately used clinically without knowing how each of the SNPs affected CNS function.

It is hoped that, in addition to helping predict clinical response, one could also use an SNP profile to avoid use of a given drug if the profile suggested that a patient might be particularly prone to having a serious drug side effect. For example, there may be a specific SNP profile of those who have a serious rash on lamotrigine. If this profile is shared by a patient who is being considered for lamotrigine treatment, this might weigh heavily in favor of choosing other medications.

PRINCIPLES OF THE CASE

STRENGTH OF EVIDENCE

1. While this is not a very clear example (see Chapter 12), many patients will show apparent good initial responses to lithium but subsequently begin to have breakthrough episodes in a pattern consistent with the development of tolerance to long-term prophylaxis. ++

2. One should be very wary about attributing even very chronic symptoms and areas of dysfunction to personality or character disorders; these may be linked to the presence of untreated affective illness and may be ameliorated with adequate treatment of the primary mood disorder. +

3. This patient subsequently failed to respond to the addition of valproate to lithium and desmethylimipramine in 1991, yet responded dramatically to another anticonvulsant (carbamazepine) even in monotherapy. This highlights the idea revealed in Chapters 15 and 22 that response to one putative mood-stabilizing anticonvulsant does not necessarily hold positive or negative predictive value toward response to another. ++

4. The same principle may be true for the dihydropyridine calcium channel blocker nimodipine and the anticonvulsant carbamazepine, because highly differential response to these two agents was revealed in this instance. +++

5. As reported in the series studied by Ketter, Kimbrell, et al. (1999), this patient was representative of the group who showed a baseline pattern of relative brain hyperactivity on PET scan and who responded to carbamazepine. ++

6. While the identification of clinical and biological correlates of response to the whole range of putative mood-stabilizing agents used in the treatment of bipolar patients is a major goal for the future, relatively few robust or well-replicated

predictors of response so far have been discovered. Thus, the clinician and patient are generally required to pursue a sequential clinical trials methodology in finding the best drug for any given patient. ++

7. However, as preliminarily summarized in Chapter 9 and in Table 18.1, there are a number of tentative predictors that may be used in the initial choice and sequencing of medication trials. We alert the reader to the fact that in many instances, these are highly preliminary and have not yet been replicated, but list them in the hope that they may ultimately be proven useful and so other investigators can study these possibilities more systematically. +

8. This patient had a traumatic early life and we can wonder whether anxiety and PTSD-like symptomatology, including marked sleep disturbance and ultrarapid mood fluctuations, might also be added to this list of correlates of response to carbamazepine. +

9. In addition to case studies and the relatively meager published literature on correlates of differential drug responsiveness, the patient and clinician may wish to choose among agents based on a variety of other principles including: (a) targeting residual symptomatology with drugs known to work against that symptom in other illnesses; (b) the most and least appropriate side effects profile for a given patient; and (c) using drugs with highly different and nonoverlapping mechanisms of action. +++

10. If a patient such as this individual were to experience new breakthrough episodes on his current regimen of carbamazepine monotherapy, further treatment approaches could include:

a. The addition of lithium, to which the patient initially showed some apparent responsiveness +++

b. A reconsideration of another trial of an SSRI antidepressant in light of the potential positive response to fluoxetine in 1989, and a possible negative response to stopping the drug prior to the severe depression in 1991 ++

c. A clinical trial of lamotrigine, given the patient's profile of severe depressions with high levels of anxiety +

d. Possibly an augmenting trial with an agent such as gabapentin for anxiety, mood, and sleep, instead of clonazepam, which did not have a good effect when used in much of 1992 and 1993 +

e. Augmentation with an atypical antipsychotic such as quetiapine which has shown potent antianxiety as well as antidepressant effects. ++

11. Carbamazepine may show excellent antidepressant and antianxiety effects in some individuals with bipolar I, II, NOS, and even unipolar presentations. This patient appeared to respond to this mood stabilizer without the need for added antidepressant augmentation. ++

TAKE-HOME MESSAGE

Response among the putative mood stabilizers (lithium, valproate, lamotrigine, and carbamazepine) may be highly divergent in different individuals, and lack of response to one does not predict positive or negative response to another. Assumptions about a patient's possible personality disorder and substantial cognitive disabilities should be withheld until the patient has recovered from the primary affective disorder; these supposedly long-term traits may disappear with appropriate treatment.

19

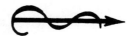

Loss of Response to Carbamazepine and Lithium Combination Treatment via Tolerance: Reresponse After a Period Off Drug

CASE HISTORY

This is the early course of illness of the patient who had a complete response to complex combination therapy, as described in Chapter 50. Each time she was started on the combination of carbamazepine with lithium, there was evidence of initial antidepressant response (in 1986, late 1987, and then again in 1988), but breakthrough depressive episodes reemerged each time. The retrospective chart was created from detailed notes and records, and from recollections independent of any idea about carbamazepine tolerance and reresponse, which only became clear after the chart was completed.

The patient's depression presented with dramatic psychomotor slowing to the point at which she had difficulty getting out of bed, speaking, dressing herself, or maintaining adequate hygiene. She rapidly became unable to work at her job, which involved much outdoor activity. The depression was complicated by guilt, social withdrawal, low self-esteem, and much self-doubt and indecisiveness. Initially, her depressions were characterized by a marked increase in sleeping, while in the late 1980s this switched to a more agitated presentation with not only early morn-

ing awakening but multiple awakenings throughout the night with a high degree of anxiety.

She complained of extreme memory loss, being unable to recall recent events and visits with friends or vacations that she knew must have occurred. This extreme degree of memory loss is not uncharacteristic of severe depression, and it is sometimes labeled pseudodementia because of its profundity. The patient also had such marked slowing of mentation that she would often have a delay from 10 to 30 seconds in responding to even the most simple question. The delay was at times so long that it was not clear whether she had forgotten the original question altogether. Her hypomanias were of the irritable variety, as noted in Chapter 50.

It is noteworthy that the continuous course of cycling between severe depression and hypomania began after her initial treatment with tricyclic antidepressants in 1984. This patient, and those noted in Chapters 34 and 35, are examples of clinical reasons that many treating physicians are wary of using antidepressants either with or without concurrent mood stabilizers. In early 1986, with the onset of concomitant treatment with carbamazepine and lithium (which had previously been ineffective in moderating the severity of her depression), she experienced a substantial decrease in depressive severity and even some days of euthymia. There was also some moderation of the severity of her hypomania. However, toward the end of the year, depressions of increasing frequency and severity began to break through with a parallel increase in manic severity as well.

After a brief period of time off medications in 1987, she was reexposed to the lithium-carbamazepine combination for a second time and appeared to have a number of months without depression, before again starting to have a depression following the discontinuation of lithium and persistence of carbamazepine. After several months off both drugs in early 1988, her third reexposure to carbamazepine with lithium was again associated with minimal depression in the first half of 1988. With the appearance of some breakthrough episodes, fluoxetine was added in an attempt to abort them, without success.

The patient had begun thyroid supplementation in 1985 because of apparent lithium-related hypothyroidism. In 1990 her thyroid status was reevaluated at the NIMH and a diagnosis of Hashimoto's thyroiditis was made, and it was decided to treat her with a combination of T_3 and T_4 because of several case reports suggesting the utility of this approach. During the period of time indicated by the triangles in Figure 50.1, the patient had a double-blind clinical trial of nimodipine (see Chapters 32 and 33), which did not ameliorate the severity of her recurrent depressions. However, it is noteworthy that the patient felt during this time that her mind was clearer and that her memory was substantially improved. This effect is of interest in relation to the observations that nimodipine can increase brain somatostatin and has shown some positive effects in Alzheimer's disease, which were not of sufficient magnitude for the pharmaceutical company to pursue further when they initially noted these effects in their controlled studies.

With the resumption of another new severe depressive episode on nimodipine and valproate, a brief retrial of carbamazepine augmentation was attempted without effect. Her illness remitted completely in 1991 on the combination of lithium, valproate, bupropion, T_3, and T_4, as described in detail in Chapter 50.

BACKGROUND LITERATURE

In this chapter, we focus particularly on the issue of loss of clinical responsivity during long-term prophylaxis with carbamazepine-lithium combination treatment. This kind of loss of effectiveness after a period of good initial responsivity is not entirely rare (Frankenburg, Tohen, Cohen, & Lipinski, 1988; Koukopoulos et al., 1995; Maj et al., 1989; Post, Leverich, et al., 1993). We note this can occur on lithium (Chapter 12), on carbamazepine as described here, and on valproate (Chapter 24). In fact, loss of efficacy via a tolerance mechanism has been noted to occur in the long-term use of antidepressants and monoamine oxidase inhibitors in the prophylaxis of recurrent unipolar depression as well. Preliminary observations suggest that some patients may show a tolerance phenomenon to lamotrigine and gabapentin, suggesting that a wide variety of treatment agents may be prone to this loss of effectiveness over time.

In the late 1970s and early 1980s, when we were using carbamazepine as the major intervention for lithium nonresponsive patients, we had the opportunity to observe the long-term treatment response to carbamazepine prophylaxis in apparent acute responders or in those who were started on the drug for potential prevention in between episodes (Post, Denicoff, Frye, et al., 1997; Post, Leverich, et al., 1990). Forty-four patients were followed prospectively for a mean duration of 6.9 years after their discharge from NIMH. Twenty-nine of these (65.9%) showed initial evidence of a clinically relevant moderate to marked improvement as rated on the CGI scale. Although the majority of these patients ($n = 16$; 55.2%) maintained their initial degree of responsiveness over a number of years, a substantial group ($n = 13$; 44.8%) showed a pattern of gradual loss of efficacy consistent with tolerance development. The beginning of this loss of efficacy occurred after an average of 2.8 ± 1.9 years. It should be noted that this was a unique patient population drawn only from those with

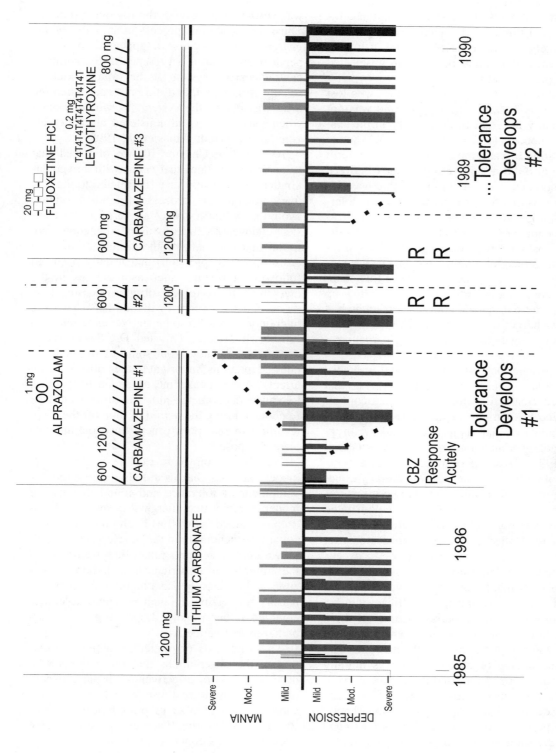

Figure 19.1 Tolerance and reresponse (RR) to the antidepressant effects of carbamazepine (CBZ). Initial partial response to carbamazepine on three occasions, followed by the development of manic and depressive episodes of increasing severity (Tolerance #1) and increasing severity of depression (Tolerance #2). There are two instances of reresponse when carbamazepine was restarted after a period of time off the drug.

the most treatment-refractory illness in the community, and this rate of tolerance development is not likely to reflect the percentage of loss of effectiveness that might occur in an unselected clinical practice setting.

The dose of carbamazepine in those who lost efficacy was $1,092 \pm 287$ mg/day and was not significantly different from the dose in the sustained responders ($1,173 \pm 337$ mg/day). Whether or not lithium was employed in the long-term regimen also did not differ significantly between the two groups. The one difference that was significant was that the patients who became tolerant had a greater number of prior hospitalizations for mania (5.0 ± 4.7) compared with the 16 who sustained their response (2.1 ± 2.4 prior hospitalizations for mania; $p < .001$). The patient illustrated in the current case in this chapter was not included in that long-term follow-up study, because it included only patients who had been discharged from the NIMH with a good response using regimens involving carbamazepine.

We became increasingly interested in potential tolerance phenomena after observing that tolerance clearly developed to the anticonvulsant effects of carbamazepine in the prevention of amygdala-kindled seizures induced by amygdala-kindling stimulation on a daily basis (Weiss et al., 1995). Over a period of 3 days to a week, a dose of carbamazepine that was initially effective in preventing amygdala-kindled seizures became entirely ineffective. We demonstrated that this was not a pharmacokinetic effect, because animals that received carbamazepine after a seizure occurred for many days to weeks never became tolerant to the anticonvulsant effects of carbamazepine when it was given before the seizure in order to test efficacy.

Interestingly, after a period of time off drug, the previously tolerant animals reresponded to the anticonvulsant effects of carbamazepine with the same degree of efficacy that was initially observed, but upon repeated pretreatment eventually lost responsiveness again (also seen in the patient described in this chapter). Remarkably, even a period of time when animals continued to get the same dose of once-daily carbamazepine, administered after a seizure had occurred, was sufficient to reverse the tolerance process. Thus, we named this process in animals *contingent tolerance* because it appeared to be dependent on the drug's presence in the animal's central nervous system at the time of kindled seizure stimulation, and did not occur when the drug was out of the system (as would happen when the drug was administered after the seizure had occurred; Weiss et al., 1995).

As noted in Chapter 10, we observed that some of the changes that occur with amygdala-kindled seizures appear to be related to the primary pathological process of kindled seizure evolution, while a subset appeared to be transient endogenous anticonvulsant adaptations. We found that a variety of these changes in gene transcription (expression) that usually occurred following a seizure, such as increases in the messenger RNA for thyrotropin-releasing hormone, failed to occur in the animals that were tolerant to carbamazepine and yet experienced a full-blown seizure. This led Dr. Susan Weiss and me to speculate that some of the endogenous adaptations important to the anticonvulsant effects of carbamazepine might be lost during tolerance phenomena and that these would be reinduced during the period of time off the drug, resulting in reresponsiveness once the animals were reexposed.

We also attempted to explore in the animal model variables that would slow down the development of tolerance and found that use of moderate rather than marginal doses of carbamazepine helped, as well as beginning carbamazepine treatment early in the development of full-blown kindled seizures rather than waiting until the animals had experienced a plethora of seizures and apparently had a highly ingrained propensity for seizing. In such instances, tolerance emerged rather rapidly despite high-dose carbamazepine treatment.

This finding is of particular interest in relation to the observations that the patients who developed loss of effectiveness in our prospective follow-up were those who had a significantly greater number of prior hospitalizations for mania, suggesting that their illness may have been later in its course or more severely developed compared with the patients who had fewer hospitalizations for mania and sustained their good responsivity. These data are also relevant to the observation that patients with a greater number of episodes, but prior to beginning lithium prophylaxis, are at greater risk for initial lithium nonresponse (Swann, Bowden, Calabrese, Dilsaver, & Morris, 1999). In addition, we have also observed that patients with a greater number of prior unsuccessful clinical trials and a greater number of hospitalizations for depression were the ones who responded least well to lamotrigine (Obrocea et al., 2002; Chapter 25). The observations about tolerance development to carbamazepine in long-term follow-up are somewhat different from the two examples above in that the patients in our carbamazepine series did, in fact, show a good initial response but then lost it over time. In contrast, the lithium and lamotrigine response data related to the number of prior episodes are linked to an initial lack of drug responsiveness. In either case, greater number of prior episodes appears to be a risk factor for poorer response to a variety of treatments used in the naturalistic treatment of patients with bipolar illness (Post et al., 2003; Nolen et al., 2004).

In the animal model, we also observed that the combination of carbamazepine with valproate (at marginally effective doses) was more effective than either agent alone in delaying tolerance development. In addition, if the animals were stimulated more intensely (i.e., at a current considerably above their seizure threshold) as compared with less intensely, they were more likely to develop tolerance rapidly. Thus, the intensity of the inducing stimulus, or intensity of illness drive, appears to be a factor that relates to the likelihood and rapidity of tolerance developing.

These preclinical observations in the laboratory model of tolerance (to the anticonvulsant effects of carbamazepine) deserve to be systematically explored for their potential relevance to the clinical context of treating patients with affective disorders (Post & Weiss, 1996). The laboratory principles may not translate to the clinic because of the very different treatment end points (seizures versus affective episodes) and the very different temporal domains (days to lose effi-

cacy in the laboratory compared with years to lose it, if at all, in the clinical situation of affective illness).

Since it is possible that very different biochemical effects of carbamazepine are involved in its anticonvulsant compared with its mood effects, one should further be cautious about immediately translating laboratory observations to the clinic. Nonetheless it is of interest that carbamazepine is a treatment of choice for the severe recurrent lightning (paroxysmal) pains of trigeminal neuralgia. While there is an 80% initial response rate, a substantial number of patients lose efficacy over long-term treatment, also via an apparent tolerance mechanism. Thus, tolerance phenomena appear relevant to a variety of episodic neuropsychiatric syndromes treated with carbamazepine and related compounds.

Despite the reservations noted above, it is of considerable interest that many of the predictions that would be made from the contingent tolerance laboratory model appear pertinent to the clinical situation in affective illness (Table 19.1). As illustrated by the patient in this chapter, a period of time off drug, as in the animal model, did appear to be associated with reresponsivity on three occasions (Pazzaglia & Post, 1992). The prediction of rapid tolerance development in those with greater numbers of prior fully kindled seizures would also appear pertinent to the observations that increased numbers of prior hospitalizations for mania are a risk factor for clinical tolerance development in affectively disordered patients. These empirical findings, along with the theoretical formulation drawn from the kindling model, strongly suggest that early intervention is very much in a patient's best interest. This might give the patient a better chance not only for response to lithium and lamotrigine (where number of prior episodes is a factor in nonresponse) but also in sustaining response to an agent such as carbamazepine in long-term prophylaxis.

It should be noted that even if these tolerance observations and theoretical predictions are not supported with further data, the importance of early institution of effective long-term prophylaxis would nonetheless appear to stand on its own merit. Avoiding episodes of mania and de-

Table 19.1 *Clinical Predictions on Approaches to Tolerance Development to Be Explored Based on Observations From the Preclinical Model of Amygdala-Kindled Seizures*

Preclinical Study Findings on Factors Affecting Loss of Efficacy via Tolerance	*Future Studies to Assess Predictive Validity for Clinical Tolerance in Affective Illness*
Tolerance to Anticonvulsant Effects Slowed By:	Would Tolerance Be Slowed By:
Higher doses (except w/LTG)	Maximum tolerated doses rather than minimally effective doses?
Not escalating doses	Stable dosing?
More efficacious drugs (VPA > CBZ)	Valproate compared with carbamazepine?
Treatments initiated early in course of kindled seizures	Early institution of lithium treatment (which does appear more effective than late)?*
Combination treatment (CBZ + VPA; LTG + GPN)	Combination treatment better than monotherapy?
Reducing illness drive (stimulation intensity)	Treatment or prevention of comorbidities and concomitant stressors?
Treatment Response in Tolerant Animals Is Restored By:	Would Treatment Response Be Restored By:
Period of drug discontinuation, then reexposure to previously effective drug	Period of time off CBZ (randomized study of discontinuation and reexposure needed)?
Agents with different mechanisms of action, i.e., no cross-tolerance	Are anticonvulsant cross-tolerances clinically predictive of cross-tolerance in affective illness?

Note. VPA, valproic acid; CBZ, carbamazepine; LTG, lamotrigine; GPN, gabapentin.
*Supported by multiple clinical studies (see Table 11.1).

pression has many benefits in its own right; not only is the associated suffering avoided, but also the potential for loss of educational or employment opportunities, the risk of substance abuse, the development of other comorbidities, and the possibility of further exacerbating illness-related brain abnormalities.

In the case of tolerance development, on the basis of our very preliminary and unsystematic set of case observations, we would recommend increasing the dose or adding or switching to agents with different mechanisms of action that are not likely to show cross-tolerance phenomena. Moreover, consistent with the observations in the current case, one might want to consider a period of time off the drug and then reinstitution of it later to attempt to regain some degree of responsivity for a period of time if other maneuvers failed.

In the example in Chapter 24, a period of time off appeared to be sufficient to regain and maintain responsivity, although, in our current example, breakthrough episodes rapidly redeveloped in each instance of retreatment. Thus, a variety of other strategies should be considered,

including approaching the illness from multiple novel mechanistic perspectives simultaneously and considering other augmentation strategies, such as low-dose thyroid or even the suprathreshold doses of synthroid recommended by Bauer and associates (2003). However, in this instance, we are not aware of any patient in these series sustaining a good long-term response to high-dose T_4 in instances of prior loss of efficacy via tolerance, as opposed to treatment resistance.

These observations on the potential development of loss of efficacy are in particular contrast to the emerging evidence of the opposite pattern with vagus nerve stimulation in which, over the first months to years of treatment, the degree and number of responsive patients appears to increase over time (Chapter 58). One can hope that this pattern of progressive improvement further indicates the effectiveness of vagus nerve stimulation.

In the medical literature concerning multimodal treatment of patients with AIDS, when eventual loss of effectiveness of triple antiviral therapies takes place (as evidenced by increased viral load and decreased white cell elements), the recommendation is to rather radically change several of the major components of the treatment regimen rather than making only small modifications. This approach may also have merit in a patient with bipolar illness who has lost responsivity via tolerance development, and it appears to be consistent with the observations in the current patient, where an entirely new regimen based on lithium, valproate, bupropion, and thyroid augmentation eventually was effective in achieving and maintaining remission as described in Chapter 50.

As noted in the patient described in Chapter 2, there is some evidence that anticonvulsant tolerance on carbamazepine can cross to that of valproate, and it is interesting that this either did not occur in the current case or was ameliorated by the fact that a period of time off carbamazepine had taken place. Cross-tolerance seen in the anticonvulsant model (Weiss, Post, Sohn, Berger, & Lewis, 1993) may or may not cross to other medications for bipolar illness.

PRINCIPLES OF THE CASE	STRENGTH OF EVIDENCE
1. Even the hardest working people can get incapacitating depressions and bipolar illness.	+++
2. Some 25% of women in the United States and 12% of men will suffer major depression at some point in their lifetime.	+++
3. Half of bipolar illness begins with a depressive episode as opposed to a first presentation with mania.	+++
4. Initiation of the illness with depressions may predispose to greater number of episodes and rapid cycling.	±
5. The role of tricyclic antidepressants in the initiation of this patient's rapid and continuously cycling pattern is not known. However, in patients with documented bipolar depression, meta-analyses suggest that the older tricyclic antidepressants are more prone to cause switches than the newer second-generation antidepressants such as the SSRIs or bupropion.	++
6. Tolerance can occur in a subgroup of patients with a good initial response to carbamazepine alone or in combination with other agents.	++
7. If tolerance occurs, adding or switching to drugs with different mechanisms of action (that do not show cross-tolerance to the initial drug) should be considered if dose increases are not sufficient or possible.	++
8. When loss of efficacy via tolerance does occur, it may be related to the phenomenon of contingent tolerance, and a period of time off the original medicine might be associated with renewed responsivity, albeit not necessarily likely to be sustained.	+
9. Treating patients earlier in their course of illness and instituting long-term effective prophylaxis may help prevent initial treatment resistance or its eventual development via a tolerance process.	++
10. Early treatment is a good thing in its own right; it will help prevent future episodes.	+++
11. The eventual emergence of tolerance in some initially responsive patients is another reason to maintain individuals on full-dose prophylaxis. Decreasing the dose may cause breakthrough episodes and facilitate	

the rapidity of tolerance development. +

12. If combination treatment is effective and the side effects are benign, one should consider continuing with the combination treatment that caused improvement initially, because even maintenance on full-dose combination treatment is not a guarantee that episodes will not reemerge. +

13. Even in the face of severe recurrent and incapacitating episodes of depression, one should not give up hope and should continue to search for an effective treatment regimen, which this patient found (Chapter 50). This patient has remained well since 1991. +++

14. The severity of cognitive impairment can mirror a profound dementia and look like Alzheimer's disease. Despite its severity, the patient should be counseled that poor memory is a typical symptom of severe depression and will remit along with the depressive episode. ++

TAKE-HOME MESSAGE

A careful charting of mood may reveal previously unsuspected patterns of illness and treatment response, and will eventually facilitate finding an optimal treatment regimen.

20

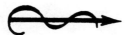

Oxcarbazepine (Trileptal): A Close Structural Relative of Carbamazepine

CASE HISTORY

Hummel, Walden, et al. (2002) exposed patients with moderate to severe mania to oxcarbazepine. Over the first 3 weeks, they titrated the dose up to a range of 300 to 2,100 mg/day. Drug discontinuation on Days 14 to 21 was associated with relapses in five of the six responders, and reresponse was seen in those who were reexposed to oxcarbazepine. In this small series, mild to moderately ill patients responded, while those with full-blown severe or psychotic mania did not (Figure 20.1). Five of the 12 patients discontinued the trial because of side effects; 3 (25%) with the typical mild anticonvulsant side effects such as fatigue, excessive perspiration, vertigo, ataxia, headache, nausea, or increased appetite, and 2 (17%) because of severe side effects (one patient with strong vertigo in combination with severe ataxia and excessive perspiration, and another patient with strong nausea, repeated vomiting, and slight hyponatremia).

BACKGROUND LITERATURE

Oxcarbazepine has been more widely available in some European countries for the last several decades, but it only received FDA approval in the United States in 2000 for the treatment of complex partial seizures, either adjunctively or in monotherapy. Oxcarbazepine is structurally very similar to carbamazepine except that a keto oxygen group is attached to the middle ring instead of the double bond in the middle ring with carbamazepine (Ketter, Wang, & Post, 2004; Figure 20.2). This change makes for a very distinctive difference in the pattern of hepatic metabolism compared with carbamazepine, which is a potent inducer of the hepatic p450 enzyme 3A4.

In contrast, oxcarbazepine and its active monohydroxy metabolite are only very weak inducers of hepatic enzymes, and thus oxcarbazepine is not subject to autoinduction or the wide range of clinically important drug-drug interactions that can occur with carbamazepine (Ketter et al., 2004). The only interaction of significance is that oxcarbazepine still accelerates the metabolism of estrogen, so that women using low-dose estrogen in their birth control pills should shift to a higher dosage formulation to ensure efficacy (Fattore et al., 1999; Rattya et al., 2001).

The dose equivalency of oxcarbazepine to carbamazepine is approximately 1.5, such that 800 or 1,200 mg/day of carbamazepine would be approximately equal to 1,200 or 1,800 mg/day of oxcarbazepine. It is wise to increase the dose of oxcarbazepine slowly to avoid typical anticonvulsant side effects of dizziness, ataxia, sedation, or diplopia. Since there is no autoin-

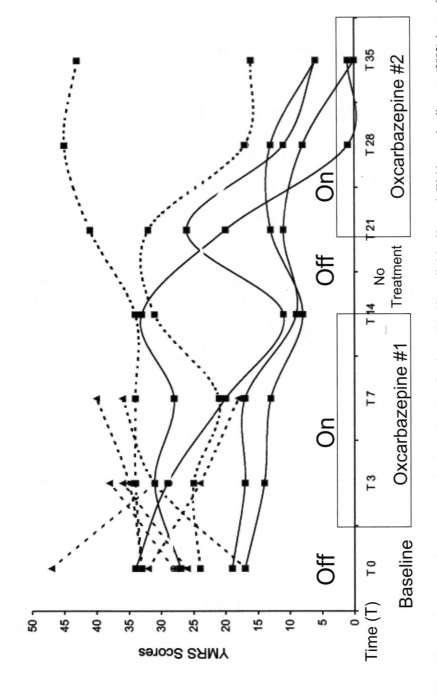

Figure 20.1 Efficacy of oxcarbazepine in acute mania. A small series of patients (*N* = 12) studied by Hummel, Walden, and colleagues (2002) in an off-on-off-on design illustrates the possible acute antimanic efficacy of oxcarbazepine in moderate mania. Many of the most severely ill patients did not respond (dots at top of figure). The five who improved in the first weeks of treatment showed exacerbations during the week off medication (Days 14–21), and a reresponse in four of the five reexposed to the drug (solid lines; Days 22 to 35).

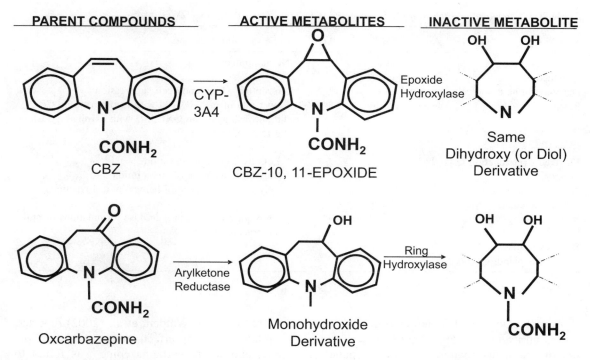

Figure 20.2 Structural similarity of carbamazepine (top) and oxcarbazepine (bottom). Carbamazepine has a double bond in the middle ring and looks a little like the tricyclic antidepressant imipramine. Oxcarbazepine has an oxygen molecule there instead. CBZ, carbamazepine.

duction with oxcarbazepine (Isojarvi, Pakarinen, Rautio, Pelkonen, & Myllyla, 1994), subsequent dose increases would not likely be needed once a suitable therapeutic dose has been achieved (Ketter et al., 2004).

The only side effect that is more prominent with oxcarbazepine than with carbamazepine (Bennett et al., 1996) is hyponatremia (Isojarvi, Huuskonen, Pakarinen, Vuolteenaho, & Myllyla, 2001; Nielsen, Johannessen, & Bardrum, 1988), where the incidence rate is reported to be approximately 3% but may be higher in some vulnerable populations such as older patients at higher doses (Table 20.1). Unlike carbamazepine, there is no black box warning for the rare occurrence of aplastic anemia or agranulocytosis, and thus hematological monitoring is not required for oxcarbazepine. The incidence of rash also appears somewhat lower with oxcarbazepine than with carbamazepine and, in many instances, patients who have had a rash on car-

bamazepine will not have another rash if crossed over to oxcarbazepine (Friis et al., 1993). However, in the case of severe dermatological reactions such as Stevens-Johnson syndrome, cross-sensitivity between the two compounds has been reported by the manufacturer.

The mechanisms of action of carbamazepine and oxcarbazepine are thought to be closely related (Ambrosio, Soares-da-Silva, Carvalho, & Carvalho, 2002; Samia, Joca, Skalisz, Maria Aparecida, & Vital, 2000). A primary effect of oxcarbazepine is the blockade of sodium channels. In addition, some calcium channel blocking properties have been reported, which could account for a slightly different spectrum of efficacy in the two drugs. For example, it has been reported that a substantial proportion of patients who had failed to respond to carbamazepine for trigeminal neuralgia had a positive response to the keto analog oxcarbazepine (Zakrzewska & Patsalos, 1989).

Table 20.1 *Comparative Effects of Carbamazepine (CBZ) and Oxcarbazepine (OXC)*

Side Effects	CBZ	OXC	Comment on OXC
Hepatic enzyme 3A4 induction	+++	+	No autoinduction
Decrease white blood cells	+++	±	No routine white blood cell suppression
Rash	6.5%	2.5%	Lower rate of rash: 83/106 with benign rash on CBZ did not rash again on OXC; 3/3 with exfoliating rash did re-rash, however
Hyponatremia	+	++	
Elevated liver function tests	+	±	? Less liver enzyme elevation
Teratogenic	++	?	Likely less incidence of spina bifida
Agranulocytosis	1/10,000 to	?	Likely lower incidence of hematological reactions
Aplastic anemia	1/100,000		
Reduces estrogen levels	++	+	Both require higher estrogen dose formulations of oral contraceptives
Reduces testosterone or dehydroepiandrosterone	+	0	

Emrich, Dose, and Von Zerssen (1984) reported an average of 50% improvement in mania during acute mania trials in six patients. Four of the seven trials showed moderate to marked improvement with doses ranging from 1,800 to 2,100 mg/day. Randomized comparisons of oxcarbazepine to both haloperidol and lithium carbonate in separate studies showed evidence of equivalent efficacy in each instance (Emrich, 1990). Therefore, it is likely that oxcarbazepine will share at least some of carbamazepine's psychotropic profile (Ghaemi, Ko, & Katzow, 2002). However, in contrast to carbamazepine, controlled studies of oxcarbazepine in acute depression and in long-term prophylaxis have not yet been performed. Moreover, Wagner, Kowatch and Findling (2005) reported that oxcarbazepine was no more effective than placebo in the treatment of child and adolescent mania.

Thus, with these highly preliminary data suggesting some but not complete comparability of carbamazepine and oxcarbazepine, and in the absence of data to the contrary, one could consider initiating treatment with oxcarbazepine rather than carbamazepine if a patient is not willing to risk the known rare side effects of carbamazepine (Table 20.1). A possible exception might be for full-blown manic psychosis,

where Hummel, Walden, et al. (2002) reported a relative lack of effectiveness of oxcarbazepine, and where carbamazepine was found to be highly effectve (Post, Uhde, Roy-Byrne, & Joffe, 1987).

We have seen patients who responded to carbamazepine when they had failed to respond to valproate (Chapter 15; Post, Berrettini, et al., 1984) and vice versa (Chapter 21). To the extent that oxcarbazepine's profile of efficacy is relatively similar to that of carbamazepine in bipolar illness, one might also expect dissociations in response between oxcarbazepine and other anticonvulsants within individual patients, but this remains to be directly explored.

Thus, if a given patient fails to respond to lithium and valproate or cannot tolerate their side effects, oxcarbazepine or carbamazepine remain treatment options to be considered, particularly because some aspects of the side effects profiles of the latter drugs differ considerably from those of lithium or valproate, where weight gain, tremor, and gastrointestinal upset are occasionally problematic. Oxcarbazepine, like lamotrigine, is thought to be relatively weight neutral and thus represents another option when the potential for weight gain becomes a major factor in treatment choice. However, if a patient tolerated but did not respond to adequate doses of carbamazepine, a clinical trial of oxcarbazepine would not be a high priority option.

PRINCIPLES OF THE CASE	STRENGTH OF EVIDENCE
1. Oxcarbazepine and carbamazepine have structural similarity and share a positive therapeutic profile in trigeminal neuralgia and complex partial seizures, and perhaps in some bipolar patients as well.	+++
	+
2. Carbamazepine is a potent inducer of the hepatic p450 enzyme of the 3A4 type and oxcarbazepine is not.	+++
3. Oxcarbazepine thus has fewer drug-drug interactions than carbamazepine.	++
4. Higher dose forms of estrogen should be used in birth control pills because oxcarbazepine also lowers estrogen levels.	+++
5. While valproate increases and carbamazepine decreases the bioactivity of androgen, oxcarbazepine is neutral in this regard.	++
6. The side effects profile of oxcarbazepine is generally more benign than carbamazepine, with the exception of a higher incidence of low serum sodium (hyponatremia).	++
7. Signs of hyponatremia include weakness, confusion, dizziness, disorientation, and seizures, although most cases are asymptomatic and low sodium levels are often only detected with blood tests of serum electrolytes.	+
8. It is not known whether lithium and demeclomycin (which can treat or prevent hyponatremia on carbamazepine) will also do so for oxcarbazepine.	±
9. Oxcarbazepine does not have an FDA black box warning and does not require hematological monitoring.	+
10. The dose equivalency of oxcarbazepine is approximately 1.5 times that of carbamazepine, for example, 1,200 mg/day of carbamazepine equal 1,800 mg of oxcarbazepine.	++

TAKE-HOME MESSAGE

Oxcarbazepine looks like an easier-to-use version of carbamazepine because of fewer drug-drug interactions. Whether its psychotropic profile will precisely match that of carbamazepine remains to be seen.

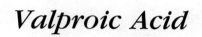

Valproic Acid

21

Prophylactic Response to Valproate in a Nonresponder to Lithium and Carbamazepine: Approaches to Side Effects

CASE HISTORY

As depicted in the life chart in Figure 21.1, the patient's illness started in her early teens with a persistent mild hypomania that lasted 7 years. The illness progressed with the initial emergence of a mild depressive episode in 1972, followed within a year by a severe depression requiring hospitalization and ECT in 1973. As the illness advanced to continuous cycling without any period of euthymia or level mood, in 1981 she was hospitalized and treated with an antipsychotic (haloperidol) for a manic episode that had apparently been exacerbated by treatment with a monoamine oxidase inhibitor (MAOI) antidepressant. She was then started on a therapeutic trial of lithium and had no further severe manic episodes, until she was again treated with desipramine and then an MAOI, which also appeared to induce ultrarapid cycling despite the presence of lithium.

When another anticonvulsant, valproate (or divalproex sodium, Depakote), was recommended by her physician in New York City in the fall of 1987 (i.e., about 9 years prior to the approval of divalproex for acute mania), the patient responded not only acutely with an essentially complete remission of her mania and depres-

sions but continued to remain well with the exception of occasional minor mood swings. Thus, prior to valproate, this patient was mildly to severely ill almost continuously for 23 years and hospitalized eight times, whereas during treatment with valproate over 18 years she required no hospitalizations except when she went off her medications.

BACKGROUND LITERATURE

Despite therapeutic levels of lithium instituted in late 1981, the patient essentially continued to cycle within the mild to moderate range of depressive and hypomanic episodes, thus falling into the large group of patients who are not adequate lithium responders. There is increasing recognition that only a subgroup of patients respond well to lithium, rather than the earlier assumed 80% of patients (Gelenberg et al., 1989; Harrow, Goldberg, Grossman, & Meltzer, 1990; Maj et al., 1998; Prien & Gelenberg, 1989; Vestergaard, 1992). Lithium nonresponders are overrepresented in the subgroup of patients who are rapid cyclers (Denicoff, Smith-Jackson, Disney, et al., 1997; Dunner & Fieve, 1974; O'Connell et al., 1991); who have experienced more

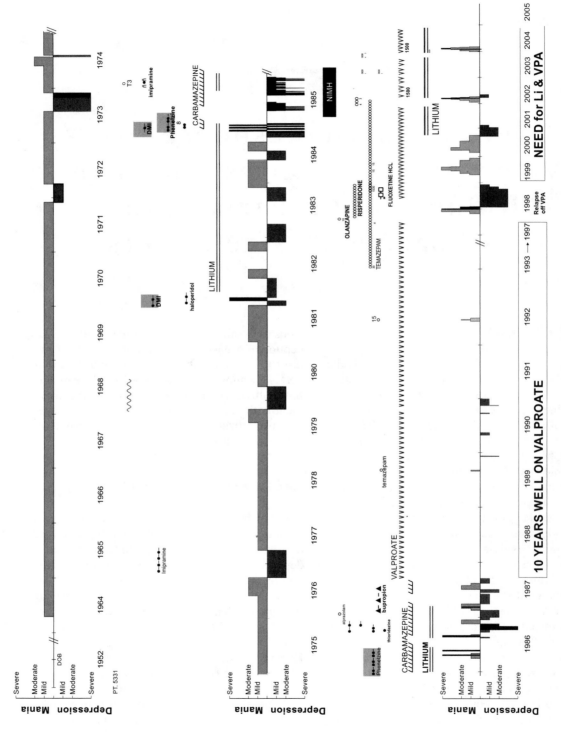

Figure 21.1 Prophylactic efficacy of valproate in a poor responder to lithium with and without carbamazepine. Severe depressions emerged in 1973, 1974, and 1984. Despite concurrent lithium, treatment with antidepressants at the end of 1984 was correlated with an increase in cycle frequency from rapid cycling to ultra rapid cycling and exacerbations in the severity of the manic phases occurred then and again in 1986. The patient experienced a sustained remission on valproate for 10 years except for a few hypomanic episodes. She relapsed after stopping VPA in 1997, and re-responded with difficulty and apparent need for lithium augmentation. Breakthrough episodes occurred off drug in 1998, 2002, and 2004.

than three affective episodes prior to the institution of lithium (Gelenberg et al., 1989); who have comorbid substance abuse; or who have dysphoric or unhappy mania (Himmelhoch & Garfinkel, 1986; Post, Rubinow, et al., 1989; Prien, Himmelhoch, & Kupfer, 1988). The use of the mood-stabilizing anticonvulsants (carbamazepine and valproate) in the treatment of mood disorders in the last two decades of the 20th century as adjuncts or alternatives to lithium has substantially increased treatment options. This case continues to illustrate the theme that different patients are differentially responsive to these two anticonvulsant drugs (see Chapters 15 and 18).

The availability of a series of anticonvulsant compounds, such as carbamazepine and valproate for the treatment of acute mania, and lamotrigine for the prevention of depression, has created multiple options for the lithium nonresponsive, partially responsive, or side effects-intolerant patient. The efficacy of carbamazepine was discussed in the preceding chapters. Carbamazepine has potent effects inhibiting limbic excitability; that is, carbamazepine has preferential effects in blocking the amygdala- compared with cortical-kindled afterdischarges (Albright & Burnham, 1983). Phenytoin is not prominent in this limbic ratio, but there are two positive studies in bipolar disorder (Mishory, Winokur, & Bersudsky, 2003; Mishory, Yaroslavsky, Bersudsky, & Belmaker, 2000), although this needs to be further investigated (Dreyfus, 1981). Valproate is second among the anticonvulsants in its effect on limbic excitability, which may account for part of its psychotropic efficacy.

An early review (McElroy, Keck, Pope, & Hudson, 1992) found that at least 16 uncontrolled studies supported the acute and long-term mood-stabilizing efficacy of valproate in approximately 50% of patients, and a large clinical literature supports its utility in a variety of clinical practice settings (Calabrese, Woyshville, & Rapport, 1994; McElroy, Keck, Pope, & Hudson, 1988, 1989, 1992; McElroy, Pope, Keck, & Hudson, 1988; Post, 1990; Schaff, Fawcett, & Zajecka, 1993). Some nonresponders to lithium and carbamazepine (even using complex augmentation strategies) may dramatically respond to valproate, as demonstrated by the patient in this chapter.

Valproate is now FDA approved for the treatment of acute mania, but not for long-term prevention (prophylaxis). A collaborative study representing one of the largest placebo-controlled trials in acute mania showed a significant antimanic effect of valproate and lithium when compared with placebo (Bowden et al., 1994). However, only half the patients experienced 50% improvement in their mania rating scales on either drug, again highlighting the need for adjunctive medications for many patients.

Schaff et al. (1993) reported an 81% response rate in rapid-cycling patients when valproate was added to their previously ineffective lithium or carbamazepine. A number of studies suggest good response to valproate in dysphoric mania (McElroy, Keck, Pope, & Hudson, 1988, 1992; Swann, 1995), and possible predictors of prophylactic response to valproate include nonpsychotic mania, a pattern of prior stable or decreasing cycle frequencies in rapid cyclers, and absence of comorbid personality disorder (Bowden, 1995; Calabrese, Fatemi, et al., 1996; Calabrese, Woyshville, Kimmel, & Rapport, 1993).

Open studies in acute depression suggest some degree of response in about 25% of the patients (Calabrese, Woyshville, & Rapport, 1994; Davis et al., 1996; Lambert, 1984; McElroy, Keck, Pope, & Hudson, 1988; Winsberg, Degolia, Strong, & Ketter, 2001), and several smaller controlled studies suggest efficacy over placebo (Davis, Bartolucci, & Petty, 2005; Gyulai et al., 2003). We observed a good prophylactic response against depressive recurrence in 50% (and against mania in 67%) of patients that had an initially positive acute response and then were followed during naturalistic treatment. These response rates are more similar to those of Calabrese et al. (1994) but are not reflected in the one well-controlled, long-term study of valproate versus lithium versus placebo (Bowden et al., 2000) which failed to show prophylactic efficacy on the main outcome measure (time remaining in the study prior to dropout for the occurrence of a manic episode) for either lithium or valproate compared with placebo. That

Table 21.1 *Some Valproate Side Effects and Their Potential Management*

Side Effect (Frequency)	Potential Treatment	Support	Comment
GI distress (O)	Switch to enteric coated preparation	++	Effect may be additive with lithium
	Add H2 blocker	+	
	Give with meals or all H.S.	+	
Tremor (O)	↓Dose	+	Additive with lithium?
	Propranolol	±	
Weight gain (O)	Prophylactic diet and exercise instructions	+	Additive with lithium?
	Augment with topiramate, zonisamide	++	
Alopecia (hair loss) (UC)	Prophylaxis with zinc and selenium supplements	+	Straight hair may grow back curly
Thrombocytopenia (low platelets) (UC)	Discontinue valproate	+	Monitor for bleeding
PCO syndrome (UC)	Preventive treatment with oral contraceptives	++	Menstrual irregularities may precede use of VPA and may increase on VPA
	Switch to lamotrigine	++	Testosterone not ↑ in 4 of 5 studies
Hepatitic enzyme (O) elevation < 3x normal	Monitor direction of change		Caution patient to advise you if RUQ pain, fever, malaise, fatigue, colored urine, or jaundice occurs
Hepatitis (VR)	Discontinue VPA		
Pancreatis (VR)	Discontinue VPA, monitor amylase		Patient to advise you if severe GI pain, nausea, vomiting occurs
Metabolic:			
a. Asymptomatic ↑ ammonia (UC)	↓Dose, add l-carnitine	±	Is there a history of urea cycle abnormalities in the patient or family?
b. Coarse, "flapping" tremor (UC)	↓Dose, add l-carnitine	±	
c. Encephalopathy (VR)	Discontinue VPA or add l-carnitine		
d. ↑homocysteine (C)	Add folate	+	VPA may also lower folate levels
e. ↓carnitine and ↑acylcarnitine?			
Teratogenicity	Avoid pregnancy	+++	Avoid VPA and especially other anticonvulsants in combination
a. Neural tube defects such as spina bifida (several percent of exposed fetuses)	Use birth control pill, other methods	+++	
b. Developmental delay (mild to severe)	Use folate, B_6, and B_{12} prophylactically in women of childbearing age on VPA	+	

Note. VC, very common; C, common; O, occasional; UC, uncommon; VR, very rare; D, dose related; I, idiosyncratic; S, sensitivity may cross to other anticonvulsant; +++, well supported; controlled data; ++, many case reports; +, likely works; ±, questionable or hypothetical; RUQ, right upper quadrant; PCO, polycystic ovary; H.S., at night; GI, gastrointestinal; CBZ, carbamazepine; VPA, valproate.

study apparently recruited a subgroup of highly stable patients, where few relapsed even on placebo, and thus there was an apparent floor effect so that further improvement could not readily be detected. Nonetheless, valproate in that study was more effective than placebo (or lithium) in the prevention of depressive episodes.

Differential response among the anticonvulsants appears to be the rule in some bipolar patients. In Chapter 18 we observed response to carbamazepine but not to valproate or phenytoin. Conversely, this patient, and another in Chapter 21, responded well to valproate after failing on lithium and carbamazepine, similar to the observations of McElroy, Keck, Pope, and Hudson (1988, 1992), Calabrese et al. (1994), and Schaff et al. (1993). In the case of treatment nonresponse, switching to a medication with a different mechanism of action may be helpful (as in the current chapter).

It is noteworthy that although the anticonvulsants are all FDA approved for long term treatment of seizure disorders, only lamotrigine is approved for long term prophylaxis in bipolar disorder, and valproate and carbamazepine are only FDA approved for acute mania. Once again, this case supports the proposition that treatment of bipolar illness only in accordance with FDA guidelines (as they existed at the time and as they currently stand) is often substandard. In this patient, treatment without valproate might have been catastrophic and she might have lost many years of wellness and good functioning.

The differential response to the anticonvulsants illustrated here also reemphasizes the importance of eventually delineating clinical or biological markers of treatment response, so that treatments can be targeted more effectively and expeditiously. Careful retrospective and prospective life charting helps in the evaluation of the major mood stabilizers and assists in formulating a sequential and rational pharmacological approaches to the illness. In this case, the life chart method provides almost incontrovertible evidence of MAOI precipitation of more severe mania or cycle acceleration because it regularly occurred on the MAOI and dissipated off the drug. Some common to rare side effects of valproate are summarized in Table 21.1.

PRINCIPLES OF THE CASE	STRENGTH OF EVIDENCE
1. Bipolar illness often has an onset in childhood or adolescence (about 50% to 66% of the time in the United States).	++
2. Antidepressant treatment was likely associated with increased severity of mania in this patient in 1981, in 1984, and twice in 1986, that is, the only times in her life with severe mania when she was on antidepressants.	++
3. In many other instances, antidepressant-induced hypomanias or manias may be milder than the spontaneous type (Stoll et al., 1994).	++
4. Heterocyclic and MAOI antidepressants may have been involved in this patient's cycle accelerations in 1984, 1986, and 1987, and this occurred despite the presence of lithium or two mood stabilizers (lithium and carbamazepine).	+
5. Nonresponse to lithium is more likely to occur with more than three episodes prior to starting prophylactic treatment with lithium.	++
6. Lithium is less effective in continuous and rapid cyclers than in intermittent and nonrapid cyclers.	++
7. About 50% of rapid cyclers respond to the lithium-carbamazepine combination; the other half, as illustrated by this patient, must seek other approaches.	++
8. This patient (prior to valproate) illustrates the difficulty that confronts patients when it comes to the use of antidepressants; although antidepressants may be sought for treatment of depression, they can trigger mania or cycle acceleration.	++
9. If this patient were not a good responder to valproate, other approaches might include:	
a. Use of lamotrigine rather than an antidepressant	++
b. Adjunctive use of an atypical antipsychotic with one mood stabilizer	+++
c. Triple mood stabilizer therapy prior to adding an antidepressant (preferably now a second-	

generation antidepressant rather than a tricyclic antidepressant or an MAOI)   ++

d. T$_3$ 25μg–37.5 μg augmentation (Chapter 51)   ±

e. High-dose T$_4$ augmentation (200–400 μg/day after discontinuing T$_3$)   +

f. Use of the "atypical" atypical aripiprazole, if a regular atypical (such as olanzapine, quetiapine—which has the best data for antidepressant efficacy—or ziprasidone) was not an effective adjunct for depression on its own or in preventing antidepressant-induced switches   +

g. Clozapine as a treatment component, because it appears highly effective in rapid cycling, dysphoric mania, (although weekly blood monitoring is required) and its antidepressant efficacy is not established   ++

h. Maintenance ECT, despite the minimal evidence of efficacy in prophylaxis (there are no systematic, comparative trials in bipolar illness of maintenance ECT, although it is used by some experts)   ±

10. This patient showed a dramatic response to the anticonvulsant valproate even though she did not achieve a full response to lithium, carbamazepine, or the lithium-carbamazepine combination.   ++

11. In bipolar illness, differential response to different mood stabilizers, even within the anticonvulsant class, is often observed, necessitating a long series of sequential clinical trials in many patients (it took 5 years for this patient to find the right drug).   ++

12. While the natural course of bipolar

illness often tends to be an accelerating one, this patient clearly illustrates that effective treatment at any time in the illness course can still arrest this process; that is, the concepts of sensitization and kindling (Chapter 10) are only pertinent to the untreated illness or a subset of patients who have not yet responded to treatment.   +++

13. Although response to a single mood stabilizer, such as lithium or valproate monotherapy, can last for a lifetime, such complete responses to monotherapy are relatively unusual, and most patients treated in academic centers require some form of augmentation or combination treatment to achieve and sustain remission.   ++

14. A study reported decreased alcohol intake in bipolar patients with comorbid alcoholism during treatment with valproate versus placebo (Salloum et al., 2005).   ++

15. Valproate is FDA approved for the prevention of migraine.   +++

16. Single nighttime dosing (even of the regular preparation) may help with tolerability and compliance.   +

17. Valproate should not be used during pregnancy, as it is associated with both the major untreatable malformation of spina bifida and a greater degree of developmental delay than other anticonvulsants.   +++

TAKE-HOME MESSAGE

Despite a long and accelerating course of illness and a lack of adequate response to two major mood stabilizers (lithium and carbamazepine) and confounded by antidepressant-induced cycling, a sustained and complete remission can still be achieved with an alternative medication approach such as valproate.

22

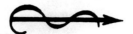

Prophylactic Antimanic Response to Valproate in a Lithium and Carbamazepine Nonresponder

CASE HISTORY

This 32-year-old white female was admitted to NIMH in 1985 with a bipolar I disorder inadequately responsive to lithium treatment. As delineated in her life chart, her illness began in the form of depression at age 11 complicated by concomitant anorexia nervosa, which continued until age 16, for which she was treated with weekly psychotherapy (Figure 22.1). Her depression, after a brief period of remission, reoccurred at age 14, and at age 16 her depression deepened significantly with suicidal thoughts, social withdrawal, continued anorexia, and poor self-care. She was hospitalized for 10 months with a diagnosis of borderline schizophrenia. After discharge from the hospital medication free and able to graduate from high school 10 months later, the patient started using alcohol excessively. During a 3-month period of further substance abuse in 1972, which included mescaline, LSD, and amphetamines (speed), she experienced the sudden onset of a delusional mania.

Her illness reemerged after the birth of a child in 1979, when mild depression was followed by an abrupt switch into a brief moderate mania, a severe untreated depression of several months' duration, and a subsequent severe psychotic mania requiring commitment treatment in 1979. Lithium was instituted with good response but was discontinued by the patient after dis-

charge. She relapsed into another psychotic mania a year later and responded well to lithium reinstitution. However, 2 years later in 1982, while apparently still taking lithium, the patient experienced breakthrough manic symptoms and went off her lithium, and her mania became more severe.

She again responded well to a quick restart of lithium for her mania in 1982 but then relapsed into depression, for which she admitted herself to a hospital. She remained moderately depressed after discharge while continuing on lithium. The addition of carbamazepine for subsequent depressions in 1985 was discontinued after 2 months due to severe headaches. Another delusional mania while continuing on lithium necessitated a further hospitalization with an increase of lithium and requiring the addition of thiothixene. Shortly thereafter she was admitted to NIMH mildly depressed on lithium and thiothixene.

At the NIMH, a retrial of carbamazepine was discontinued after 8 weeks due to a lack of significant amelioration in her increasing depression and her inability to tolerate more than 600 mg/day due to side effects.

Lithium was reinstituted with some improvement in her depressive symptoms, but after 2 weeks the patient rapidly switched into a delusional mania with religious and grandiose themes and lack of sleep despite increasing doses of

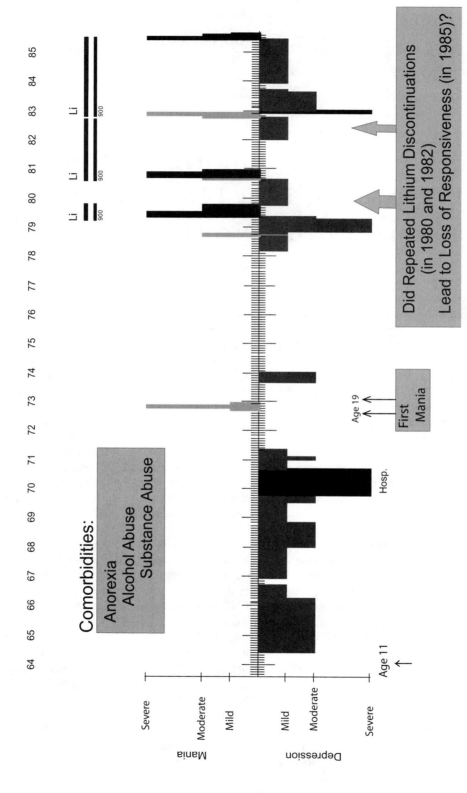

Figure 22.1 Early onset illness (at age 11) with depression and multiple comorbidities and ultimate failure to respond to lithium in 1985 after several apparent responses on drug and relapses off.

lithium. This reconfirmed in a closely monitored setting that lithium was no longer effective in controlling the patient's manic episodes, and therefore valproate was added to lithium in a blinded fashion as an experimental treatment in 1986 (i.e., 8 years prior to its FDA approval for mania). Within 2 weeks after the initiation of valproate, the mania subsided without any recurrence during her stay at NIMH (Figure 22.2). The patient continued to experience some mild to moderate depressions, alternating with well intervals (euthymia), following the addition of valproate to lithium.

After discharge and ongoing treatment with lithium and valproate in the community, the patient continued to experience mild to moderate depressions. She was able to start and maintain full-time work, however. Augmentation with levothyroxine for the depressive symptoms was ineffective and in 1988 the monoamine oxidase inhibitor (MAOI) antidepressant phenelzine was initiated. After initial improvement but subsequent recurrence of depression, phenelzine was increased to 45 mg/day, but manic symptoms emerged. Phenelzine was first decreased, then discontinued. Her mania subsided, and she continued on the combination of valproate and lithium alone.

After more than a year symptom free, recurrences of depressive symptoms were interfering with the patient's ability to function. Fluoxetine, a selective-serotonin reuptake inhibitor (SSRI), was initiated in 1990 at the low dose of 10 mg/day while continuing the mood stabilizers lithium and valproate. Following an increase to 20 mg/day of fluoxetine, the patient again quite rapidly began to experience symptoms of mania. Fluoxetine was discontinued and again her mania rapidly decelerated and ended.

The patient discontinued lithium in 1990, believing that the side effects of lithium outweighed its therapeutic efficacy for her. A brief spontaneous hypomania in 1991 responded well to an increase in the dose of valproate from 750 mg/day to 1,000 mg/day. She linked her depressive exacerbations to her menstrual cycle and took the highly unusual approach of using a series of leuprolide acetate injections to suppress menstruation. This worked in 10 of 18 patients

in one series (Schmidt, Nieman, Danaceau, Adams, & Rubinow, 1998), but was less impressive in another (West & Hillier, 1994). In light of other menstrual complications and her positive response to leuprolide acetate, a hysterectomy was performed, followed by hormone replacement therapy. This appeared to help ameliorate her depressive symptoms as hoped, but since her depressions had waxed and waned with periods of euthymia in the past, such an inference could not be drawn unambiguously. Although valproate did not eliminate her depressive recurrences, she has not been hospitalized for a manic episode since the institution of valproate in 1986, compared with four hospitalizations for mania (and seven manic episodes) in the prior 6 years.

BACKGROUND LITERATURE

As illustrated in this patient's life chart, onset of her illness in adolescence (and lack of appropriate treatment) may likely have contributed to alcohol abuse and subsequent multiple substance abuse in an effort to treat her depression. Epidemiological studies have shown that bipolar disorder, of all the major psychiatric disorders, has the highest rate of comorbidities (Kessler et al., 1997; Regier et al., 1990), including substance abuse. McElroy et al. (2001) found that in a cohort of 288 patients with primarily bipolar I disorder who participated in the Stanley Foundation Bipolar Network, 65% had at least one comorbid lifetime Axis I disorder, with 42% having a substance use disorder. Frye, Altshuler, et al. (2003) additionally found that the odds of having comorbid alcoholism were almost eight times greater in women with bipolar disorder when compared to the general population as opposed to men with bipolar disorder, where the increase over the general population was only by a factor of about 2.7. As in this case, women with more prior depressions were particularly at risk for alcohol abuse, presumedly as a form of self medication.

This patient's affective disorder remained essentially untreated for 15 years until 1979, when lithium was administered for her severe delu-

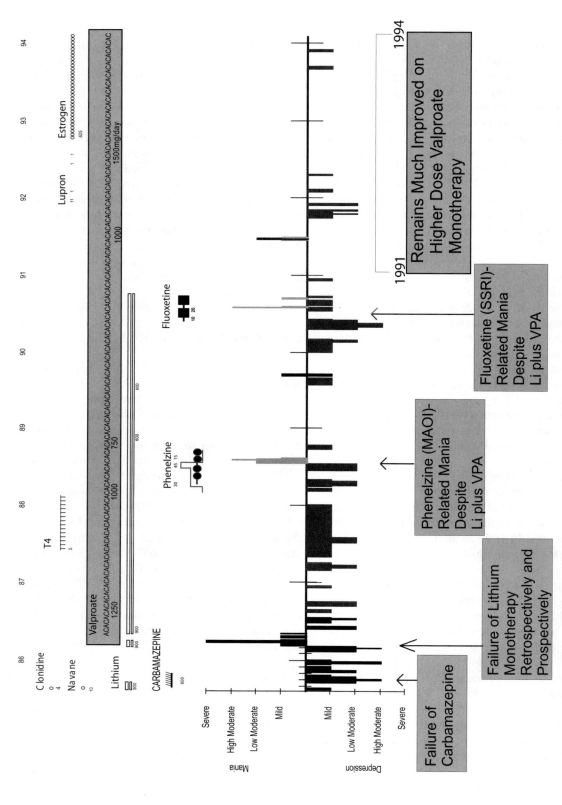

Figure 22.2 Good prophylactic response to valproate. As illustrated in her prospective LCM, after discharge from NIMH on the combination of lithium and valproate and on valproate monotherapy since 1990, the patient had no further hospitalizations for mania (from 1986 to the present), but occasional depressive recurrences. Note the two antidepressant-related manias despite lithium plus valproate prophylaxis.

sional mania (Baastrup & Schou, 1967). A 10-year lapse from illness onset to first treatment has also been observed in studies by Egeland, Blumenthal, Nee, Sharpe, and Endicott (1987), in the Stanley Foundation Bipolar Network (Suppes et al., 2001), and in a subgroup in the survey of the National Depressive and Manic-Depressive Association (Hirschfeld, Lewis, & Vornik, 2003; Lish, Dime-Meenan, Whybrow, Price, & Hirschfeld, 1994).

The patient had a good response to lithium during her first and second hospitalization for mania, yet she discontinued lithium shortly after she was discharged (which is not uncommon), and she relapsed into mania within a year. She appeared to rerespond to lithium in 1981, but not thereafter. Other patients described in Chapter 13 are much clearer examples of those who relapse after discontinuing lithium after many years of complete remission and then fail to rerespond.

While some studies have suggested a moderate response to valproate for depression in 25% of patients (see review in Chapter 23), the questions as to what constitutes the best treatment approaches to bipolar depression breaking through a mood stabilizer are understudied and remain largely unanswered (Bowden, Lawson, Cunningham, Owen, & Tracy, 2002; Kowatch, DelBello, & Findling, 2002; Post, 2002; Post, Denicoff, et al., 2002; Sachs et al., 2007). In a 1-year prospective follow-up of 258 patients with daily life charting in the Stanley Foundation Bipolar Network, we found that patients experienced three times as many days depressed as days manic despite expert treatment in naturalistic follow-up (Post, Denicoff, et al., 2003).

As delineated in this patient's life chart, in addition to her severe manic episodes, she experienced prolonged and then briefer periods of depression, which interfered with her ability to function optimally in occupational settings as well as with her quality of life outside of work. The patient became manic with the addition of two different classes of antidepressants, an MAOI in 1989 and an SSRI in 1990, despite continuing on double mood-stabilizing treatment (lithium and valproate). When the antidepressants were reduced or discontinued, in both instances, the mania subsided. This patient's life chart provides good evidence of valproate's prophylactic efficacy in preventing her severe hospitalized manias over time and also illustrates the difficulties that arose when trying to address her breakthrough depressive recurrences despite the presence of two mood stabilizers.

PRINCIPLES OF THE CASE / STRENGTH OF EVIDENCE

1. Bipolar illness can begin with depressions (50% of the time), have an early onset, and have co-occurrence of other syndromes (anorexia nervosa here). +++

2. Lack of early effective interventions for adolescent-onset depression or mania may lead to the development of other comorbidities such as alcohol and substance abuse. ++

3. The rate of alcohol and substance abuse is very high in outpatients with bipolar disorder (about 40%). +++

4. Repeated discontinuations of an apparently effective treatment (lithium) may lead to relapses and eventual loss of its effectiveness (see Chapter 13 for clearer examples). +

5. Nonresponse to lithium and carbamazepine does not preclude response to other agents with different mechanisms of action (e.g., valproate). ++

6. This patient had a good response to the anticonvulsant valproate for mania, but depressive episodes recurred (especially premenstrually). ++

7. The menstrually associated exacerbation of depressive symptoms is not uncommon in bipolar illness, but consistent linkage of the

timing of distinct episodes to
menses is rare.   ±

8. The treatment of bipolar depression with unimodal antidepressants can lead to switches into hypomania despite cotreatment with
two mood stabilizers.   ++

9. Dose increases of two different
classes of antidepressants (MAOI
and SSRI) were likely associated
with a switch into mania for this
patient, and dose decreases were
associated with symptom abate-
ment.   ++

10. The risk-to-benefit ratio of the
use of antidepressants in bipolar
disorder needs to be further studied in bipolar disorder and assessed for the individual patient.   +

11. Mood charting can help uncover
the consistency of previous
switches on antidepressants and

lead to the formulation of differ-
ent options.   ++

12. Options might include the addition of:

a. Lamotrigine instead of an antidepressant   +

b. An atypical antipsychotic instead of an antidepressant   ++

c. Combinations of mood stabilizers and atypical antipsychotics prior to starting the antidepressant   +

TAKE-HOME MESSAGE

One should not stop treatments that are working
well, because relapses are common. However,
even then, one can almost always find effective treatment options when many others have
failed.

23

Prophylactic Response to Valproate Augmentation of Lithium in Bipolar I Recurrent Psychotic Depressions

CASE HISTORY

The patient whose life chart is presented in this chapter had an onset of her illness with a severe psychotic postpartum depression in 1964 (not illustrated). After initial unsuccessful treatment with antipsychotics, she responded acutely to a course of ECT and remained well for the next 12 years, performing at a very high level as an academician. Her illness recurred in 1977 (not illustrated) in the form of a severe manic episode followed by two depressive episodes, which were each again acutely responsive to ECT (Figure 23.1). On lithium prophylaxis, she remained well for 5 years.

Four years after discontinuing lithium treatment, her illness reemerged unrelentingly in 1986 in the face of significant life stressors. The episodes were now unresponsive to the reinstitution of lithium, adjunctive antipsychotics, and minor tranquilizers. One can only speculate how long she might have remained well if she had stayed on her lithium prophylaxis, as discussed in Chapter 13. Further, one can wonder whether buspirone, added for her depression and anxiety, may have contributed to the onset of 3 years of continuous cycling between moderate manias and severe depressions, a phenomenon that is

more closely associated with typical tricyclic antidepressants in approximately one fifth of bipolar patients and is seen in Chapter 34.

When this patient was admitted to the NIMH, she had experienced 5 years of continuous cycling between manias that included increased energy, decreased sleep, grandiosity, and spending sprees, and depressions that were profound, psychotic, and completely disabling. She felt she should be burned in hell for her sins and at times required restraints, seclusion, and tube feeding for total anorexia. A trial of carbamazepine, briefly alone and then in combination with lithium, instituted during her NIMH hospitalization, was effective in reducing the amplitude of the manias but had no impact on the severe, recurrent, delusional depressions the patient was experiencing.

Following the discontinuation of carbamazepine, valproate was added to the lithium and the patient started to get better. The remaining hypomanias and her profound depressions improved dramatically and she soon experienced a complete and sustained remission for the first time in 5 years. The small dose of a concomitant antipsychotic was unlikely to have been important to this pattern, because when antipsychotics were used with lithium in 1987 and 1988, they

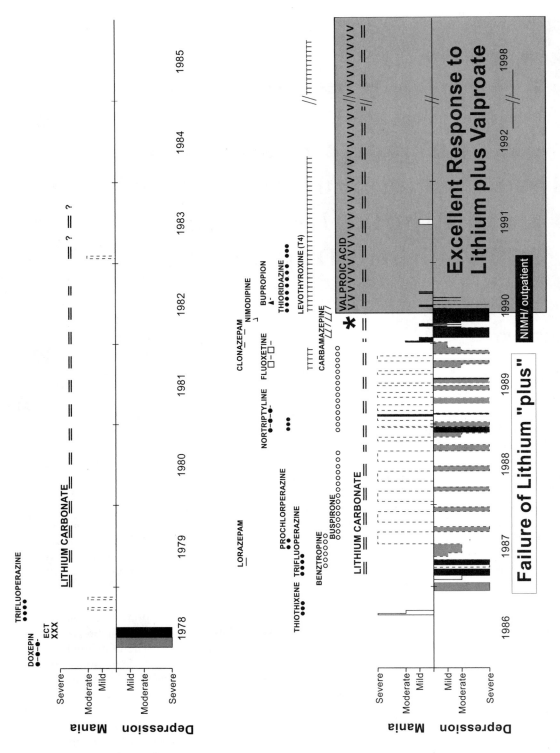

Figure 23.1 Valproate augmentation in a lithium-refractory bipolar patient with profound recurrent psychotic depression. Reemergence of the illness in 1986 was unresponsive to the reinstitution of lithium, buspirone, a variety of antidepressants, adjunctive antipsychotics, and minor tranquilizers. Carbamazepine, alone and in combination with lithium, was effective in reducing the amplitude of the manias (see *, 1990) but had no impact on the patient's severe, psychotic, delusional depressions. When carbamazepine was discontinued and valproate was added to lithium, the patient soon started to improve and reached a complete and sustained remission for the first time in 5 years.

204

were ineffective. She was discharged on valproate, lithium, T$_4$, and a small dose of trifluoperazine (1.5 mg), which was discontinued shortly thereafter. She has continued to do well from mid-1990 until the present. She slowly resumed work, first as a volunteer, then on a part-time basis, and has now returned to full-time employment in a highly rewarding position consistent with her past high level of education.

This patient's course of illness again illustrates that the illness can progress from first episodes far apart (13 years and 9 years in the first and second intervals, respectively) to periods of continuous cycling. The approach of combination therapy with two mood stabilizers (lithium and valproate) without concomitant use of unimodal antidepressants (even for incapacitating depressive episodes) may have helped reduce and control this patient's continuous cycling, which also had persisted on the combination of lithium, antipsychotics, and carbamazepine. Similarly, lithium with adequate trials of nortriptyline and with fluoxetine had not been effective. The efficacy of valproate in acute mania is well recognized and FDA approved, although the potential efficacy of valproate for acute and long-term intervention in the psychotic depression component of this illness is less appreciated, but highlighted by this life chart.

BACKGROUND LITERATURE

A number of studies have noted valproate's efficacy in the open treatment of rapidly cycling bipolar patients who were refractory to lithium and carbamazepine (Calabrese, Markivitz, Kimmel, & Wagner, 1992; Schaff et al., 1993). The literature review of 16 uncontrolled studies using valproate (McElroy, Keck, Pope, & Hudson, 1992) and other reports (Bowden et al., 2002; Keck, McElroy, Tugrul, & Bennett, 1993) suggests that it may be an effective agent in the treatment of mania, especially dysphoric mania, rapid cycling, and in some psychotic disorders. The FDA approved valproate for the treatment of acute mania based on a series of double-blind studies demonstrating that valproate had antimanic efficacy approximately equivalent to lithium (Bowden et al., 1994; Pope, McElroy, Keck, & Hudson, 1991).

Valproate's efficacy for the acute treatment of bipolar depression has been studied in a controlled fashion in just a few studies, which suggest positive effects (Davis et al., 2005). In another study (Gyulai et al., 2003), adding valproate, lithium, or placebo to an SSRI resulted in a lower dropout rate for depression with valproate (9.8%) than for lithium (28.6%) or placebo (45%). Some open studies suggest that valproate may be more effective in depression prophylaxis than in the acute treatment of depression, but response may still be less robust in depressed compared with manic episodes (Calabrese et al., 1992; McElroy, Keck, Pope, & Hudson, 1992). These observations are consistent with our findings at the NIMH in a smaller subgroup of patients (Post, 1999).

Sharma, Persad, Mazmanian, and Karunaratne (1993) reported on a small open study of nine refractory patients who had failed to respond (or had only achieved partial responses) to a great number of pharmacological interventions, including combination therapy with carbamazepine and lithium (i.e., similar to the patient illustrated here). Valproate in combination with lithium was effective in the treatment of bipolar depression for all of the patients in that study. In addition, approaching the treatment of bipolar depression with two mood stabilizers rather than antidepressants may offer greater protection against cycle acceleration or a switch into mania, potential liabilities of antidepressants for a subset of patients who appear more vulnerable to these occurrences (Chapters 34–36). This recommendation is even stronger given the recent evidence that augmentation with antidepressants was no more effective than placebo (Sachs et al., 2007)

The percentage of antimanic responders to valproate is similar to that of lithium, but valproate appears to have a different, and perhaps a broader, spectrum of efficacy in those with rapid cycling, comorbid anxiety, substance abuse disorders, or dysphoric rather than euphoric mania. In this fashion, valproate is also emerging as a promising treatment for childhood-onset or adolescent-onset bipolar disorder (Kowatch et al., 2000) with its marked mood lability and dysphoric manias.

In the study of Denicoff, Smith-Jackson, Bryan, et al. (1997), 24 outpatients with bipolar disorder, who had 2 years of prophylactic non-response to lithium or carbamazepine (patients were crossed over to the other drug after 1 year) and whose third year on the combination had been inadequate, were offered an additional fourth year on the combination of lithium and valproate. As a result, 33% of these highly treatment-refractory patients had a moderate to marked clinically relevant prophylactic response to valproate when used with lithium.

In Bowden and colleagues' (2000) maintenance study comparing valproate, lithium, and placebo as prophylactic therapy, the treatments did not differ significantly in time to recurrence to a manic episode during the maintenance therapy period, but valproate was superior to lithium in producing a longer duration of time before the occurrence of depressive symptoms.

In addition to its demonstrated efficacy in acute bipolar and schizoaffective episodes (McElroy, Keck, Pope, & Hudson, 1992), valproate has prophylactic efficacy against migraines (valproate is FDA approved for migraine prevention) and other types of headaches (Balfour & Bryson, 1994). Valproate can increase plasma concentrations of some other anticonvulsants such as phenytoin and carbamazepine, so their doses should be reduced. Valproate doubles the levels of lamotrigine and increases the risk of a serious lamotrigine-related rash. The dose of lamotrigine should accordingly be half (i.e., 12.5 mg/day) if it is started during valproate treatment.

In the epilepsies, valproate is also a broad-spectrum drug (similar to lamotrigine), effective in the treatment of petit mal (absence, or spike and wave), partial complex seizures (temporal lobe epilepsy), and major motor (grand mal) seizures. Valproate's diverse effect in enhancing brain GABA, the major inhibitory neurotransmitter, is thought to contribute to some aspects of its psychopharmacological and anticonvulsant profile. However, since two other potent agents in increasing brain GABA (gabapentin and tiagabine) do not appear to be antimanic or

mood stabilizers, it is likely that valproate's efficacy lies elsewhere, as discussed in Chapter 9.

PRINCIPLES OF THE CASE / STRENGTH OF EVIDENCE

1. The first episode of bipolar illness may be heralded by postpartum depression. ++

2. In this case, lithium was apparently effective from 1978 to 1984, but following lithium discontinuation and relapses in 1986 and 1987, it was no longer effective (see Chapter 13 for more definitive examples of this type of treatment resistance. ±

3. Buspirone may deserve to be added to the list of more traditional antidepressants that can cause cycle acceleration. ±

4. Rapid cycling and psychotic depression are predictors of relative lack of response to lithium, as observed here. ++

5. Nonresponse to one anticonvulsant, such as carbamazepine, does not preclude response to another (such as valproate), as observed here and in the two previous chapters. ++

6. About one half of the rapid-cycling outpatients do not respond to the lithium-carbamazepine combination. ++

7. Only about 25% of rapid cyclers respond even acutely to the combination of lithium and valproate (Calabrese, Shelton, et al., 2005). +

8. It is unclear whether valproate and lithium together were truly necessary in this patient

or whether valproate alone would have been successful (as in the previous chapter).   ±

9. The only way to ascertain whether the combination was needed would be to discontinue the lithium. This has many potential liabilities, as discussed in Chapter 13, and the patient elected not to risk them.   ±

10. Only about 12.5% of rapid cyclers in Calabrese's latest study (2005) responded to either lithium or valproate in monotherapy. This low response rate in this subgroup is another reason to consider lithium and valproate in combination from the onset.   ++

11. Lithium appears to have antisuicide effects, and its discontinuation increases suicide risk some 8- to 18-fold (Tondo, Hennen, & Baldessarini, 2001).   ++

12. This chart helps reinforce the message that even a 3.5-year-long phase of recurrent, incapacitating bipolar episodes with psychotic depressions does not preclude a complete response to the institution of the appropriate combination of mood stabilizers in the acute and long-term treatment of bipolar disorder.   +

TAKE-HOME MESSAGE

With appropriate treatment, remission can occur in even the most incapacitating forms of fulminant recurrent bipolar depressive illness. While carbamazepine is found to treat psychotic symptoms in some patients with bipolar illness, valproate may be another alternative.

24

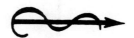

Gradual Loss of Responsiveness to the Long-Term Prophylactic Effects of Valproate: Tolerance and Reresponse

CASE HISTORY

This patient is a 62-year-old married white male with a long history of extremely dysphoric manic episodes requiring hospitalization despite lithium treatment (Figure 24.1, 1979–1981). The patient's first manic episode occurred at age 21, which responded only to 48 insulin shock treatments. He was well for 8 years until he was hospitalized, this time for a severe depression. Subsequently, manic episodes occurred with increasing frequency and severity, totaling 15 prior to NIMH admission (not illustrated). The last five of these hospitalizations for dysphoric mania, which occurred despite lithium (average blood levels 0.9 mEq/L) and adjunctive neuroleptic treatment, are illustrated in Figure 24.1.

During his NIMH hospitalization initiated for depression, a manic episode was observed to be associated with extreme dysphoria and panic attacks in the context of a full-blown dysphoric manic psychosis. The patient was delusional and had to be placed in seclusion, during which time he disrobed and screamed, and was anxious, irritable, tearful, paranoid, and suicidal. This episode did not respond adequately to carbamazepine (up to 1,400 mg/day) on a double-

blind basis or to lithium augmentation of this treatment.

Haloperidol was associated with increased panic attacks, with the patient feeling that he was going to die or lose control. However, when valproate (up to 1,375 mg/day) was added to lithium (900 mg/day), which had previously been ineffective alone or in combination with carbamazepine, dramatic improvement of his full-blown dysphoric manic symptoms was observed, and the patient rapidly became ready for discharge. Medical and neurological workups were unexceptional except for idiopathic basal ganglia calcification (not related to hyperparathyroidism) and a history of alcoholism.

Following his discharge from the NIMH, he was euthymic but reported intermittent periods of mild depression (1984) or mild hypomania (1985), which were associated with minimal dysfunction or disruption in his life. However, by the fourth and fifth years post-NIMH discharge (1986–1987) some of these episodes assumed a larger magnitude and were associated with some functional incapacity. Seven years after discharge from NIMH on the lithium-valproate combination (1989) he experienced a full-blown manic episode that required hospitalization in a city in the northeast.

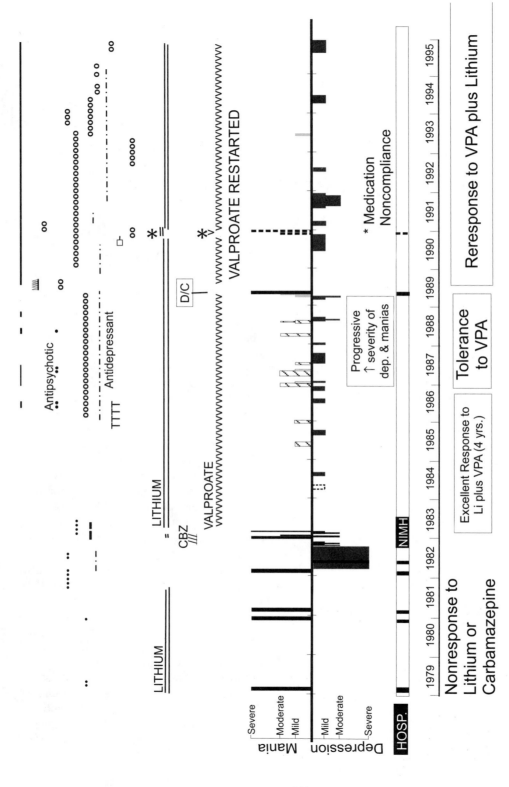

Figure 24.1 Tolerance and reresponse to the prophylactic effects of valproate. This kind of progressive loss of response (from 1983 to 1989) to valproate in combination with previously ineffective lithium is consistent with a pattern of development of treatment resistance via tolerance. In this instance, the patient showed a good renewed response to valproate added to lithium after a brief period of time off valproate in 1989. VPA, valproic acid or divalproex-sodium. A brief manic episode occurred in late 1990 when the patient stopped taking his medications (see *).

210

During that hospitalization the patient's valproate was discontinued because the staff was unaware that it had worked so well, and it was not FDA approved at that time. He was treated with lithium and adjunctive neuroleptics, without much of a response. Following receipt of the patient's NIMH life chart (like the one illustrated), clearly illustrating that the patient was not a good responder to lithium alone, valproate treatment was reinstituted with good effect. Since 1989 he has remained well without a further hospitalization. Thus, in someone who showed a progression from mild to moderate to severe breakthrough episodes associated with complete loss of responsivity to valproate (in combination with lithium) in what appeared to be a tolerance pattern, a period of time off the drug may have been associated with the renewal of response to valproate.

BACKGROUND LITERATURE

Gradual loss of efficacy while maintaining the same doses and blood levels of a drug (i.e., tolerance) can develop during long-term prophylaxis with any of the major mood stabilizers such as lithium (Koukopoulos et al., 1995; Maj et al., 1989; Peselow, Fieve, Difiglia, & Sanfilipo, 1994; Post, Leverich, et al., 1993), carbamazepine (Frankenburg et al., 1988; Post, Leverich, et al., 1990), or valproate (Post, Ketter, et al., 1993), as illustrated in the current case. In a series of excellent and complete responders to lithium during the first 2 years of treatment, Maj et al. observed that when these patients were followed another 5 years, several began to develop episodic breakthroughs in a pattern consistent with tolerance.

Similarly, in one third of our selected group of patients referred because of lithium refractoriness, retrospective mood charting showed that their refractoriness had developed via an apparent tolerance route. That is, lithium initially had a good effect in preventing recurrent episodes, but then it gradually and progressively lost efficacy. Another 43% of this selected group were lithium nonresponsive from the outset, however

(Post, Leverich, et al., 1993). A subgroup of patients have shown gradual loss of efficacy to regimens involving carbamazepine by an apparent tolerance process during long-term prophylaxis as well (Post, Leverich, et al., 1990; Chapter 19).

Since loss of efficacy via tolerance has only recently been recognized as a potential problem during long-term prophylactic treatment, the best approaches to this type of treatment resistance are not well delineated. Using an additional mood stabilizer with a different mechanism of action would appear to make the most sense, although the empirical basis for this course of action is not well defined. Switching to a drug with a different mechanism of action also has both a theoretical and an empirical rationale based on treatment strategies in epilepsy (Post, Denicoff, et al., 1999; Post, Frye, Leverich, & Denicoff, 1998; Post & Weiss, 2004).

In a preclinical model of tolerance to the anticonvulsant effects of carbamazepine (or valproate or lamotrigine) on amygdala-kindled seizures in the rodent, we have observed that a period of time off the previously effective medication, that now no longer works at all, may be associated with a renewal of responsivity (Post & Weiss, 1996; Weiss et al., 1995). In addition, tolerance developed more slowly to the combination of carbamazepine and valproate than to either drug alone, and the utility of combination treatments in the prevention of tolerance deserves further prospective systematic clinical evaluation, particularly in those patients at high risk for tolerance development.

Although predictors are not available for which patients might become tolerant, in our clinical carbamazepine studies we found that patients with the most rapidly accelerating courses in the years prior to carbamazepine treatment were at the greatest risk for tolerance development (Post, Leverich, et al., 1990). These data are convergent with those from our preclinical model in which tolerance developed more readily in animals with high illness drive (increased intensity of amygdala-kindled stimulation) or low-dose treatment (Weiss et al., 1995). These data suggest that, in patients at high risk for illness based on a prior severe course of affective illness (or a high genetic loading), one might consider using the highest possible optimal dose or combination strategy from the outset in order to avoid episodic breakthroughs that may herald a complete loss of efficacy.

Findings derived from this model system also suggest that tolerance may be associated with the loss of endogenous adaptive mechanisms that normally occur with seizure or affective episodes (Post & Weiss, 1996; Weiss et al., 1995), and that the reinduction of these adaptive mechanisms during a new episode that occurs in the medication-free period would theoretically be associated with renewed responsivity, as may have occurred in the current case when he was taken off his valproate treatment and as reported in another case in the literature (Pazzaglia & Post, 1992). It is of particular interest that this patient experienced a fortunate natural clinical experiment when valproate was discontinued in 1989. If valproate had not been discontinued, one would predict that he would have remained tolerant and maintained his treatment resistance to the valproate/lithium combination. More systematic studies are required to assess whether this prediction of a reresponse after a period of time off the drug to which a patient has become tolerant that is based on observations in the amygdala kindled seizure model has parallels in the affective disorder clinic as suggested by this case report.

It is again emphasized that this potential treatment approach to loss of efficacy via tolerance is completely opposite to the situation when a patient is well-maintained on long-term prophylaxis (Chapter 11). In those instances of a persistently good long-term response, a period of treatment discontinuation then may, unfortunately, be associated with the appearance of new episodes, furthering the primary pathological illness process to a new level of virulence and increasing the potential for nonresponse to renewed treatment. Thus, as in the current case, it is only when the illness has already fully broken through a previously effective treatment (complete tolerance) that one might consider the discontinuation option.

PRINCIPLES OF THE CASE

STRENGTH OF EVIDENCE

1. Patients such as this one with markedly dysphoric mania (see years 1979–1981) are less likely to be lithium responsive than those with pure euphoric mania.   +++

2. Lack of response to one anticonvulsant is not predictive of lack of response to another; for example, this patient failed to respond to carbamazepine (in combination with lithium), but was an excellent responder to valproate (as in the three previous chapters). Conversely, some patients respond to carbamazepine and not valproate (see Chapters 15 and 18).   ++

3. Patients may require combinations of mood stabilizers (lithium plus valproate) for full remission. Although this was not "proven" by observing breakthrough episodes during a period on valproate alone in this individual, we have seen many patients in whom this is well documented. Moreover, the patient eventually developed increasingly severe breakthrough episodes even on the combination of valproate plus lithium; this likely would have happened even sooner with valproate alone.   ++

4. Lithium and valproate each have both shared and separate mechanisms of action that likely convey their neuroprotective effects in animals, and the combination may have additive effects in some individuals.   ±

5. Excellent response to a prophy-

lactic regimen in the first several years is a good predictor of longer term response but is not a guarantee against eventual episodic breakthroughs. ++

6. Minor breakthroughs often presage more major ones. ++

7. This case emphasizes the importance of attempting to maintain as stable an illness course as possible. This can often be achieved by careful charting of mood and building a good two-way working relationship of patient and physician so that early symptoms will be addressed and treated rather than ignored. ++

8. Subtle medication adjustments combined with good psychotherapeutic approaches to stress coping strategies may head off further minor or more major recurrences. Perhaps this is why the patient remained largely well after 1980. ++

9. In the face of complete loss of previous effectiveness via tolerance development one might consider:

a. Adjunctive treatments ++
b. Alternative drugs with different mechanisms of action ++
c. A period of time off the primary medication in order to see whether renewed responsivity may be achieved, as was likely the case in the current patient +

TAKE-HOME MESSAGE

The differential treatment implication of the prior course of illness as it interacts with treatment response is encapsulated under the general rubric that if things are going well, remain conservative and do not change the treatment regimen; and, conversely, in the face of inadequate response, engage in more aggressive and sometimes radical treatment approaches in an attempt to restabilize the illness. Valproate treatment was somewhat radical in 1983, about 12 years before it was FDA approved for acute mania. The valproate discontinuation was inadverant, but may have been associated with the renewed response to the valproate treatment to which this patient had become tolerant.

Lamotrigine

25

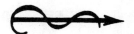

Selective Response to Lamotrigine but Not Gabapentin or Placebo in Refractory Depression

CASE HISTORY

This patient was a 40-year-old lawyer with an extraordinarily long period without treatment (Figure 25.1), a recent history of refractory bipolar depression, and a serious suicide attempt. The patient had been incapacitated by his severe depressive illness in 1996 and had had to withdraw from his legal practice. He remained moderately to severely depressed despite treatment with carbamazepine, valproate, desipramine, and benzodiazepines (including alprazolam and clonazepam) as needed for extreme anxiety.

At the NIMH, he remained moderately to severely depressed and was entered into the repetitive transcranial magnetic stimulation (rTMS) protocol as augmentation to valproate (Chapter 57) with no response to Phase I (sham), partial response to Phase II (20-Hz rTMS), and substantial but incomplete response to phase III (20-Hz rTMS extension). Despite increasing the dose of 20-Hz rTMS over the left frontal cortex by giving it twice daily, the patient slid into a more severe depression and this clinical trial was discontinued; the patient then entered another ongoing NIMH double-blind, randomized clinical trial of lamotrigine, gabapentin, and placebo.

As illustrated in Figure 25.2, the patient, while moderately to severely depressed, began

Phase I studies (which, after unblinding, turned out to be lamotrigine). Lamotrigine was initiated at 25 mg for 1 week and 50 mg for the second week, and then a titration to a dose of 250 mg/day. The patient reported substantial improvement in mood for the first time in many months and also reported a notable decrement in his profound anxiety.

With the patient's entry into Phase II of the trial, this substantial clinical improvement dissipated and he returned to his more severe depressive phase. After unblinding, Phase II was found to be placebo. With the switch to Phase III, the patient showed an initially substantial improvement in mood but remained extremely anxious (Phase III was gabapentin). Moreover, his mood was highly labile with swings from moderate depression to a profound sense of hopelessness with extreme anxiety and suicidality. At the highest doses of gabapentin (4,800 mg/day), the patient experienced several days of dysphoric mania with extreme discomfort, with the internal sense of pressure, anxiety, and agitation.

It was particularly noteworthy in this patient that the brief periods of extreme depression occurring suddenly (from a baseline of mild to moderate depression) were accompanied by a sense of permanence and absence of hope, even though the patient had just been feeling substantially better, and, based on his prior pattern of

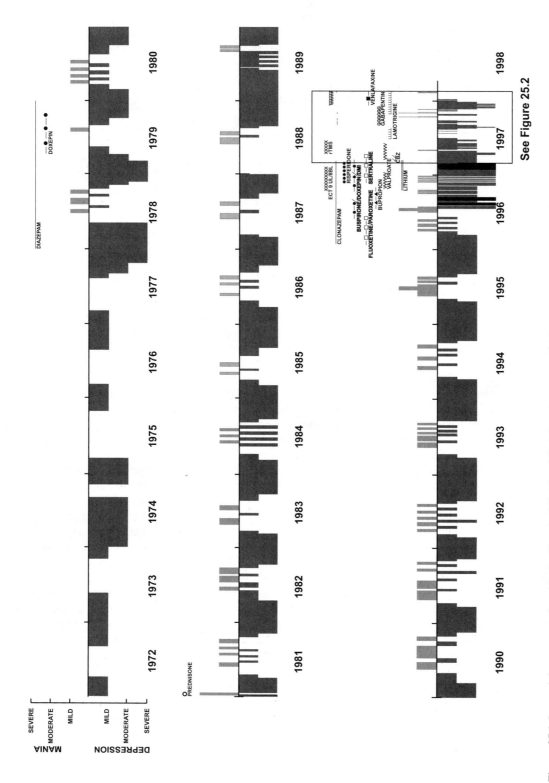

Figure 25.1 Lamotrigine response in a bipolar II male following failed first-line mood stabilizer and antidepressant regimens. Recurrent major depression began in the early 1970s and remained essentially untreated (see 1978–1979) until 1996, during which time the patient was able to remain productive. In 1996 the depressions became more severe and did not respond to multiple antidepressants, benzodiazepines, lithium, valproate, and nine unilateral and eight bilateral treatments with ECT.

218

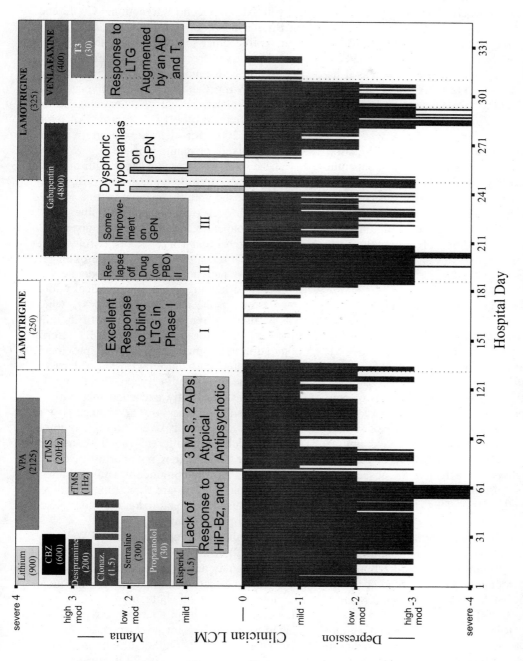

Figure 25.2 Response to lamotrigine and augmentation with venlafaxine and T₃. The patient entered the hospital severely depressed despite desipramine (for noradrenergic effects), sertraline (for serotonergic effects), clonazepam (for sleep and anxiety), risperidone (for agitation), lithium (for antidepressant augmentation), and the later addition of carbamazepine (for mood, anxiety, and sleep). Repetitive transcranial magnetic stimulation (rTMS) and valproate are discussed in the text. On blind lamotrigine (Phase I) the patient's depression remitted, but with the lamotrigine taper he relapsed. Phase II was shortened because of his worsening depression. Phase III was gabapentin, which was associated with some improvement in depression and anxiety, but manias became more dysphoric. The Phase I medication was blindly added back, but a severe depression ensued. Augmentation with venlafaxine and T₃ resulted in essential euthymia. CBZ, carbamazepine; GPN, gabapentin.

illness, would likely experience this improved level within hours or the next day. The patient was eloquent in his description of the "timelessness" and horror of even these brief depressive bursts, which achieved the only reality with which the patient could relate. For him the immediate past and future were nonexistent; it was as if he had been pulled into a "black hole" and there was no hope of achieving "a new event horizon."

A return to the blind Phase I medication (which he and we did not then know was lamotrigine) for double-blind, response confirmation in combination with lower doses of gabapentin resulted in substantially improved mood again for several weeks, but some fading of the improved mood occurred with a return of moderate depression. These residual symptoms responded well to the addition of venlafaxine and, later, T_3 augmentation.

BACKGROUND LITERATURE

Lamotrigine was approved in 1997 as an adjunctive treatment for refractory epilepsy. It showed dose-related improvement in seizure disorders, with higher response rates at 400–500 mg/day than 100–200 mg/day. It is of considerable interest that lamotrigine has a broad spectrum of efficacy across a number of seizure subtypes, suggesting that it may have unique mechanisms of action beyond those of carbamazepine (which is not effective in absence or atonic seizures and may even exacerbate them; Choi & Morrell, 2003). This potentially wider spectrum of efficacy in seizure disorders could relate to the fact that lamotrigine may also act on other neurochemical systems, making it effective for some patients' mood stabilization, even when carbamazepine or another broad-spectrum anticonvulsant (such as valproate) is not (Ketter, Manji, and Post, 2003).

Calabrese, Rapport, Shelton, Kujawa, and Kimmel (1998) reported a series of patients in whom lamotrigine was used as an open adjunct for refractory depression and cycling. He found a very substantial improvement rate (approximately 60%) in depression without problematic

induction of mania, and some evidence that the drug might have concomitant antimanic effects as well. At the Second International Conference on Bipolar Disorder (in Pittsburgh, June 1997), four or five other investigative groups also reported positive effects of lamotrigine in bipolar depression and rapid cycling. These early findings, following the first two positive case reports of Weisler, Risner, Ascher, and Houser (1994), anticipated the FDA approval of lamotrigine in 2003 for the prevention of a depressed, mixed, or manic episode.

These data are also consistent with our own double-blind, controlled data with a design similar to that used with this patient, with a planned 6 weeks on each treatment phase, either lamotrigine, gabapentin, or placebo administered in a randomized order (Frye, Ketter, Kimberly, et al., 2000; Obrocea et al., 2002). Approximately 51% of the patients responded moderately or markedly to lamotrigine on the Clinical Global Impressions Scale for Bipolar Illness, which was particularly remarkable in light of the high treatment refractoriness of the NIMH referral population (i.e., most patients had previously failed lithium, carbamazepine, and valproate). Lamotrigine response for overall illness and for depression significantly exceeded that with either gabapentin or placebo. The average dose of lamotrigine was slightly over 200 mg/day in our series, which is parallel to the dose used in many other studies. It is noteworthy that if lamotrigine is used in conjunction with carbamazepine, the blood levels are approximately halved, and if it is used with valproate, the blood levels are approximately doubled.

Our results match closely those of Calabrese et al. (1999), who reported that lamotrigine at both 50 mg/day and at 200 mg/day was significantly more effective than placebo in the monotherapy treatment of acute bipolar depression. However, 4 subsequent attempts to replicate the Calabrese study did not produce stastically significant results. Nonetheless, a meta-analysis of these 4 studies (with or without the original Calabrese study) was positive. In addition, a recent double-blind study of Van der Loos and colleagues (2007) found lamotrigine highly significantly more effective than placebo in augmentation of ongoing lithium treatment in acute bipolar depression (despite the need for a slow titration).

Calabrese, Bowden, et al. (2003) and Bowden et al. (2004) completed two separate 1.5-year studies of patients randomized to either placebo, lamotrigine, or lithium. One study population consisted of patients who were recently manic, and the second population was patients who were recently depressed and fairly well stabilized on other treatments. Lamotrigine was added to the treatment regimen on an open basis and the other drugs slowly tapered off. Those patients who remained well were eligible for the randomization to lamotrigine (mostly 200 mg/day), lithium in the usual dose levels and blood level ranges, or placebo. The time until the need for additional clinical intervention for breakthrough manic or depressive symptoms was the primary outcome measure.

When these two studies are combined, the results are particularly striking in that lithium was a significantly superior antimanic prophylactic agent compared with either lamotrigine or placebo, although lamotrigine did appear to exert some preventive effects against mania in this combined analysis (Calabrese et al., 2002). Most intriguingly, the efficacy of lamotrigine exceeded both lithium and placebo in the time required for a necessary intervention for depression. These data are thus consistent with those from shorter term studies suggesting the acute antidepressant effects of lamotrigine. Importantly, the rate of switching into mania in the acute and long-term studies was no greater than that for placebo, and in the long-term studies less than placebo, again suggesting that lamotrigine was exerting substantial acute and prophylactic antidepressant effects in the absence of the usual risks of the unimodal antidepressants for inducing additional switches into mania. These data would thus appear to change clinical treatment algorithms considerably, and this change was reflected in the American Psychiatric Association guidelines ("Practice Guideline," 2002) even prior to FDA approval. The guidelines suggested lamotrigine as a first-line agent for bipolar depression along with the more traditional approach of an antidepressant supplementation of a mood stabilizer.

The possible development of a serious rash on lamotrigine requires close monitoring and a very slow dose titration (increase) schedule (Guberman et al., 1999). It is recommended that one 25-mg pill of lamotrigine be administered daily for the first 2 weeks and then two pills for the next 2 weeks with an approximate 25 mg/week increase thereafter. However, if the patient is concomitantly being treated with carbamazepine (which halves lamotrigine levels), doses of lamotrigine can be doubled. Conversely, if the patient is concomitantly treated with valproate (which doubles lamotrigine levels), the doses of lamotrigine should be halved, that is, the patient is only given one half a pill (12.5 mg/day for the first 2 weeks). A benign rash (red, itchy, but not progressive) occurs in approximately 5–8% of subjects. In 1 in 5,000 adults and 1 in 2,500 children, a severe and potentially life-threatening rash can occur where the skin begins to sluff off (exfoliate) or vesicles or bullae (blisters) form; lesions in the mouth or on the palms of the hand or soles of the feet may be a precursor. A series of medical complications can ensue that usually require hospitalization, intravenous steroids, and other attempts to reverse the rapid progression and prevent infection. Risk factors for the serious rash on lamotrigine are: (1) too high a starting dose, too rapid a titration, or too large a dose increase once on steady levels; (2) a history of prior severe rashes on other drugs; (3) younger age; and 4) taking valproate concurrently.

If a patient gets through the first month or two on the drug, there is a markedly reduced chance of the serious rash occurring, and the side effects of lamotrigine appear to be generally very benign. Some dizziness, ataxia, and the like can be observed, but lamotrigine is generally slightly activating rather than sedating like carbamazepine. For some, it should be dosed in the morning if it interferes with sleep.

The exact mechanism of action of lamotrigine in seizure and affective disorders is not known, but like carbamazepine, the drug is a potent blocker of sodium channels and it is by this mechanism that it is thought to decrease release of the excitatory amino acid glutamate (Fitton & Goa, 1995). However, it is likely that other effects of lamotrigine are important to its psychotropic profile, as illustrated in this patient, who was a nonresponder to carbamazepine and a responder to lamotrigine. Biochemical effects that are not shared between the two drugs would be expected, such as lamotrigine blockade of N-type calcium channels (Wang, Huang, Hsu, Tsai, & Gean, 1996).

There appear to be few established predictors of clinical response based on clinical or biological characteristics of patients. Alda and colleagues (2002) in a small patient series found correlates of lamotrigine response included a family history of anxiety and substance abuse disorders, as well as a continuous course of cyclic illness. In contrast, lithium responders had an intermittent illness course with distinct well intervals and a family history for primary affective disorder in first-degree relatives. Work in our group suggests that patients who have hypoperfusion of the frontal cortex as assessed with O^{15} water positron emission tomography scans may be among the best responders to the drug. In contrast, lamotrigine nonresponders showed unremarkable baseline blood flow during their depression. Preliminary data also suggest better response in bipolar than unipolar depressive illness, in males versus females, and in those with fewer prior medication trials and hospitalizations for depression (Obrocea et al., 2002).

We are hopeful that eventually clinicians may be able to use clinical characteristics, single-nucleotide polymorphism profiles (Chapter 10), and different brain imaging techniques at baseline to assist in the pursuit of optimal treatment (Chapter 18). The biological predictors are not currently clinically available, and a systematic clinical trials approach in individual patients appears to be required. Nonetheless, a clinical trial of lamotrigine in the refractory depressed or rapid and ultrarapid-cycling patients (Calabrese et al., 2000) may be effective in the absence of a good response to a variety of other treatment agents, as illustrated in the current patient. It is also noteworthy that many aspects of

Table 25.1 *Lamotrigine's Profile: An Ideal Match for Bipolar Depression*

Bipolar Depression Characteristics	Lamotrigine Properties
1. Recurrent episodes	1. Prevents new depressions
2. Liability to manic switch	2. Antidepressant with no increased switch liability over placebo
3. Low energy, fatigue	3. Slightly activating
4. Hypersomnia	4. Nonsedating
5. Appetite and weight gain	5. No weight gain
6. Sexual dysfunction	6. No sexual impairment
7. Menstrual irregularities	7. No endocrine abnormalities
8. Anxiety comorbidity	8. Especially effective with anxiety comorbidity and positive family history of anxiety disorder
9. Teratogenic concerns with many other medications	9. Little evidence in approximately first 1,000 pregnancies in 4 of 5 case registries

lamotrigine's efficacy and side effects profile are a particularly good fit to act on many of the chief characteristics of bipolar depressive illness, as schematized in Table 25.1.

PRINCIPLES OF THE CASE	STRENGTH OF EVIDENCE
1. Lamotrigine may have acute antidepressant effects in monotherapy of bipolar depression.	+
2. Lamotrigine has prophylactic antidepressant effects that exceed not only those of placebo but also those of lithium.	+++
3. Lamotrigine may have some mood-stabilizing effects because it increased time to intervention for a manic episode over that of placebo in a combined analysis of the two largest randomized studies.	+

4. Lithium was superior to lamotrigine as a prophylactic antimanic agent, however. +++

5. Lamotrigine may be effective even in some instances when lithium, carbamazepine, valproate, and gabapentin are not. ++

6. The rate of switch into hypomania or mania was no greater on lamotrigine than on placebo. ++

7. Tolerance may develop to the effects of prophylactic lamotrigine. ±

8. High-potency benzodiazepines (alprazolam and clonazepam), while helpful adjuncts, are usually insufficient alone as antimanic agents. +

9. Lamotrigine blocks glutamate release by Na+ channel blockade, as does carbamazepine, but may also affect N-type calcium channels. ++

10. As described for carbamazepine in Chapter 19, it is possible that loss of effectiveness to lamotrigine in long-term treatment can occur. Cross-tolerance may develop between lamotrigine and carbamazepine (as observed in kindled seizure prevention in animals). ±

11. A serious, potentially life-threatening rash may occur in 1 in 5,000 adult patients and 1 in 2,500 children. +++

    a. Very slowly increasing the dose appears to decrease the incidence of serious rash. ++

    b. Valproate doubles lamotrigine blood levels and increases risk of serious rash, so that the rate of lamotrigine titration should be halved on the combination. ++

    c. Carbamazepine halves lamotrigine levels, so the starting dose of lamotrigine may be 50 mg/day. ++

    d. Lamotrigine is not generally recommended for children under age 16 because of the rash risk, but it has recently been FDA approved for use in children with refractory seizures. ++

    e. Other rash risk factors (in addition to age, valproate use, initial dose, and rate of titration) include a history of prior serious rash on other drugs. +

    f. The dose of lamotrigine should not be increased by more than 25 mg/week even after the initial upward titration has been achieved. ±

12. Lamotrigine provides a first-line alternative to the older typical approach to bipolar depression (i.e., adding an antidepressant to a mood stabilizer). ++

13. The combination of lithium and lamotrigine in prophylaxis (although not well studied) could have significant potential because lithium's superior antimanic effects would be combined with the superior antidepressant effects of lamotrigine. ±

14. No specific teratogenic effects of lamotrigine have been reported, but experience with the drug in pregnancy is still small, about 1,000 pregnancies. In 1 of 5 different pregnancy regrestries, a signal for lamotrigine increasing the incidence of cleft lip and cleft palate was seen that was not replicated in the other series so the reliability of these observations remain to be further clarified. What is clear is that the risk of major fetal malformations, such as spina bifida, seen with valproate and to a lesser extent carbamazepine have not been observed with lamotrigine despite exposure of about

1,000 women in the various registries.   +

15. If a woman becomes pregnant, this increases the clearance of lamotrigine (>65%), so that higher doses may be required to maintain blood levels.   ++

16. The need for better recognition and earlier treatment of severe depression is a major public health problem that accounts for a great amount of suffering and dysfunction.   +++

17. One can ask whether the lack of treatment of this patient's prior 20 major depressions contributed

to his extreme treatment refractoriness in the 2 years prior to NIMH admission.   +

TAKE-HOME MESSAGE

The mood-stabilizing anticonvulsant lamotrigine may be helpful particularly for depression when other anticonvulsants (carbamazepine, valproate, and a host of antidepressants) are not. While only FDA approved for prevention of particularly depressive, but also manic and mixed episodes, some data support its acute antidepressant efficacy, and starting lamotrigine early in a depression given its need for slow dose titration, would appear appropriate and expedient.

26

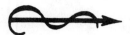

Lamotrigine and Gabapentin Combination Therapy

CASE HISTORY

Retrospective Course

As illustrated in the life chart, this 44-year-old male patient had recurrent and mild bouts of (winter) depression from 1960 until 1971, when they became more severe and disabling (Figure 26.1, top). The course of his illness changed in 1975 to more continuous hypomania, followed by severe depressions of many months' duration beginning in 1981 (Figure 26.1, middle). Treatments with antidepressants in 1983 (amitriptyline and maprotiline) without a concomitant mood stabilizer were associated with the induction of a more severe mania than had previously been observed, but no further manic episodes occurred despite a variety of subsequent antidepressant clinical trials with or without mood stabilizer coverage.

The antidepressants amitriptyline and nortriptyline were inadequate for preventing depressions in 1987 and 1989, the latter of which did not remit until the combination of desipramine and fluoxetine was instituted. With the onset of another depression in 1991, the MAOI phenelzine in combination with lithium was instituted without success, and only a partial response to ECT was observed in 1994. The serious depression of 1996 did not respond to treatment with two mood stabilizers (lithium and valproic acid), the addition of the antidepressant amoxapine, augmentation with the psy-

chomotor stimulant methylphenidate, and thyroid hormone (T_4).

Inpatient Double-Blind Trial

The patient was admitted to the NIMH and gave written, informed consent for participation in a double-blind, randomized, 6-week clinical trial comparing lamotrigine, gabapentin, and placebo with two subsequent crossovers to the other agents. As illustrated (Figure 26.1, bottom), the patient was minimally worse (CGI-E) in Phase I, which was revealed to be placebo administration, but in Phase II had a substantial, but partial, response to lamotrigine (i.e., a rating of B, or much improved on the CGI scale). Then, in Phase III, he showed some loss of response during gabapentin administration (resulting in a CGI rating of C, or minimally improved). In Phase IV for response confirmation, the Phase II drug was reinitiated on a double-blind basis (later revealed to be lamotrigine), although in this instance the response was not as robust as previously observed (CGI scale score C, minimally improved). At this juncture, gabapentin was added to lamotrigine, which resulted in rapid, substantial improvement to a virtual symptom-free baseline (i.e., CGI scale score A, very much improved).

Although we highlight this case as a potential clinical response to lamotrigine and gabapentin in the presence of only partial responses to mon-

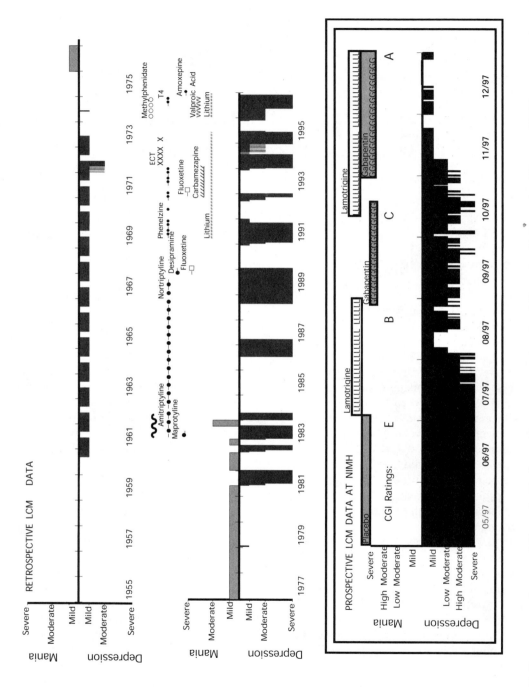

Figure 26.1 Twenty years of untreated illness; ineffective antidepressant monotherapies; failure of multiple mood stabilizers and ECT; response to the combination of lamotrigine and gabapentin after partial response to blind lamotrigine monotherapy on two occasions.

otherapy, the data conveyed and inferences that can be drawn from this life chart are not unambiguous. It appears that a partial response to lamotrigine was converted to a more complete one with the addition of gabapentin. However, it is also possible that this improvement resulted from a natural cycling out of a depressive episode, as might be expected on the basis of prior durations of depression. It is noteworthy that the time frame on the time line or date line is changed on the bottom row of the life chart, so that months rather than years are illustrated (i.e., 5/97–12/97).

The patient continued in remission from November 1997 to July 1998, but a moderate depressive episode ensued (not shown) despite continuing prophylaxis with both lamotrigine and gabapentin at the same doses previously utilized. Although the depression was less severe than observed in previous episodes, the failure of lamotrigine and gabapentin to prevent the onset of the next episode further supports the possibility that the presumptive response to the addition of gabapentin to lamotrigine was related to the natural course of illness.

BACKGROUND LITERATURE

Despite the ambiguity (noted above), we present this case for discussion for a number of reasons. Several other partial responders to lamotrigine appeared to benefit from the addition of gabapentin. The two drugs have very different mechanisms of action, which could result in additive effects. That is, gabapentin increases the levels of the major inhibitory neurotransmitter in brain, gamma-aminobutyric acid (GABA), and inhibits a subtype of the L-type calcium channel blocker. In contrast, lamotrigine is thought to act in part by decreasing the release of the excitatory amino acid glutamate in the brain (via blockade of sodium and N-type calcium channels) and also limiting its postsynaptic effect by decreasing the amount of Ca^{++} entering the cell through glutamate's N-methyl-D-aspartate (NMDA) receptor (Post, Chalecka-Franaszek, et al., 2002). In addition, the two drugs have very different mechanisms of anticonvulsant effects

on amygdala-kindled seizures. Gabapentin increases the threshold for seizures, and lamotrigine inhibits the spread of seizures without changing the threshold.

As noted in other chapters (27 and 28), two double-blind clinical trials of gabapentin have failed to reveal superiority to placebo (Frye, Ketter, Kimbrell, et al., 2000; Pande, Crockatt, et al., 2000). Nevertheless, a considerable literature of open-label gabapentin augmentation of other mood stabilizers continues to suggest its potential utility for some subgroups of bipolar patients (Chapter 28). This utility is convergent with the other documented effects of gabapentin, such as efficacy in anxiety and social phobia syndromes, as well as in paroxysmal pain syndromes, each of which has a moderately high incidence of comorbidity with bipolar illness. Gabapentin also does not have many pharmacokinetic interactions with other drugs, because it is secreted largely unchanged in the kidney. In addition, its side effects profile is generally relatively benign when used in combination with other agents.

Brodie and Yuen (1997) and others in the neurological literature suggest the excellent efficacy and tolerability of the lamotrigine-valproate combination. However, because of the increased risk of serious rash when lamotrigine and valproate are used in combination, this may not be a high-priority treatment option for some patients. To the extent that gabapentin shows some biochemical effects similar to valproate (i.e., it increases brain GABA levels), it is possible that some of the potentiating effects observed for lamotrigine (inhibiting glutamate overexcitability) and valproate (increasing GABA inhibition) could also extend to the lamotrigine-gabapentin combination.

This proposition remains to be more systematically explored in formal clinical trials. However, at present, it would appear that gabapentin monotherapy has little place as a primary mood stabilizer in bipolar illness, but its use as an adjunct may be associated with substantial clinical improvement and, occasionally, a complete remission, as occurred at least transiently in this patient, and in the patient in Chapter 27. The current case at least raises the possibility and rationale of combining these two drugs with very different mechanisms of action in order to achieve a more complete response than with either alone.

PRINCIPLES OF THE CASE

1. The addition of gabapentin for incomplete responders to lamotrigine may be associated with clinically useful therapeutic effects. Gabapentin monotherapy was not effective in this or other patients compared with placebo.   ++

2. This patient was a partial but unequivocal responder to lamotrigine based on his: (a) failure to respond to placebo, and subsequent improvement on lamotrigine; and (b) worsening off lamotrigine and partial reresponse once the drug was reinstituted (i.e., an off, on, off, on design).   +++

3. The literature is now highly supportive of lamotrigine's preventive effects on bipolar depression with some evidence of acute antidepressant efficacy as well. However, when response to it is not complete, the literature is unclear as to what might be the best augmentation strategy. In this case, gabapentin appeared effective as a representative of a differently acting class of anticonvulsants that increase brain GABA levels: ±

   a. Gabapentin has definite antianxiety properties and may be useful when one wishes to avoid benzodiazepines.   ++

   b. While lithium or valproate might also represent excellent options to augment the partial effect of lamotrigine, these were

unsuccessful on their own in 1996 in this patient and were thus not the first choice for utilization.   ++

   c. ECT was also an unlikely candidate because in 1994, this patient failed to sustain his response to ECT, and a retrial of ECT in 1995 was not effective.   +++

4. This patient showed a pattern of increasing severity of depression; mild depressive episodes recurred from 1961 to 1971, with a moderate episode in 1972 and then recurrent incapacitating depressions lasting from several months to a year or more. Would earlier, more effective treatment with mood stabilizers rather than antidepressants have prevented this progression?   +

5. The antidepressant-related mania in 1983 (more severe than previous spontaneous switches) appears to be the exception rather than the rule in this individual. Repeated antidepressant trials either with or without mood stabilizers (such as in 1989 with nortriptyline, desipramine, and fluoxetine) did not result in manic inductions.   +

6. This and other patients suggest that, particularly in non-rapid-cycling patients (such as this individual), use of antidepressants in conjunction with mood stabilizers may not consistently be associated with the induction of mania, and one such antidepressant-related switch should not necessarily rule out use of antidepressants as adjunctive treatment.   +

7. In the face of this patient's subsequent moderate depression breaking through the lamotrigine-gabapentin combination treatment, one would consider the option of:

a. Adding lithium to the combination (despite the previous failure to respond to it in combination with other agents) +

b. Adding an atypical antipsychotic ++

c. Adding an antidepressant to the regimen, either before or after lithium augmentation ±

d. If needed, augmentation with T_3 +

8. Once this patient was stabilized, it would appear critical to encourage him to maintain long-term, full-dose prophylaxis given the previous history of relentless recurrence of incapacitating depressions. +++

9. Although the response to the combination was complete, only the persistence of response well beyond the length of the typical or immediately prior well interval (not seen here) would reassure one that a real drug response rather than a variation in course of illness has occurred. The 8 months of remission were not substantially longer than remission seen previously on other regimens. ±

10. Gabapentin and lamotrigine would appear to be a combination strategy in need of further systematic exploration in light of their differential mechanisms of action, complementary side effects profile, and lack of pharmacokinetic interaction. For some patients, lamotrigine may be mildly activating, and this might be usefully countered by gabapentin (or another, more sedating, mood stabilizer). Gabapentin helps patients with insomnia, as well as with agitation and anxiety. +

11. Any quality managed care or health maintenance program should encourage regular visits for a patient such as this without requiring frequent treatment plans or other justifications. This patient has a severe, life-threatening, chronic medical condition which, like many other chronic medical conditions such as heart disease, diabetes, and arthritis, is acknowledged (without repeated treatment plans) to need lifelong medical intervention and follow-up. +++

12. One is often forced into combination strategies with newer agents when combination treatments with a variety of more traditional mood stabilizers, antidepressants, and ECT have not been effective, and response to the novel agent (such as lamotrigine) is not complete. A primary therapeutic task with this patient was just beginning in December 1997 as, with the remission of the acute episode, prevention of further episodes became the primary focus of therapeutics. ++

13. Clear, but partial, responses to lamotrigine and other agents are common. +++

14. While gabapentin on its own was ineffective, it appeared highly effective when added to lamotrigine. +

15. Gabapentin has definite anxiolytic properties that may be useful when benzodiazepines are to be avoided (as in those with a history of alcohol or sedative abuse). ++

TAKE-HOME MESSAGE

While lamotrigine often has acute antidepressant effects, it may need to be augmented with other agents with different symptomatic efficacy profiles, mechanisms of action, or side effect profiles in order to achieve and maintain a full remission.

Part V

OTHER ANTICONVULSANTS

27

Potential Antidepressant Response to Gabapentin in a Lamotrigine Partial Responder

CASE HISTORY

This patient had a history of repeated severe manic episodes and immobilizing psychotic depressions. During the depressive episodes, he showed a profound psychomotor retardation, to the point that he was unable to manage the simplest activities of daily living. He had previously failed to respond to lithium, valproate, carbamazepine, and a variety of antidepressants and antipsychotics.

As illustrated in Figure 27.1, his manic symptoms on admission decreased in severity and, after several depressive bursts lasting 1 to 2 days, ended in a profoundly retarded depression characteristic of his previous episodes. After giving appropriate oral and written informed consent for admission to a research ward and involvement in protocols, he was entered into a 6-week randomized comparison of lamotrigine, gabapentin, and placebo (Frye, Ketter, Kimbrell, et al., 2000). He showed a partial response (CGI scale score B, much improved) in the lamotrigine phase, minimal worsening on placebo, and marked improvement (CGI scale score A, very much improved) during the course of gabapentin treatment, with virtually complete clearing of his depression by the end of the trial.

While not floridly hypomanic, he continued to show evidence of poor social judgment toward females on the unit. Because of this symp-

tomatology in the continuation phase of gabapentin treatment, valproate (for hypomania) and then topiramate (for weight loss) were added to his regimen prior to discharge.

Thus, while the patient showed a complete antidepressant response during the phase of blinded gabapentin treatment and an amelioration of his usual severe manic symptomatology in the continuation phase, it is not certain that gabapentin caused the improvement in his depression. This could have occurred spontaneously as a function of his expected prior course of illness and usual spontaneous cycling out of depressive episodes. This interpretation is supported by the observation that the duration of this depression was not substantially shorter than the typical length of his previous depressive episodes. However, his onset of improvement was temporally consistent with a real therapeutic effect, and the subsequent hypomania on gabapentin was much less severe than expected based on previous episodes.

Thus, the overall clinical importance of gabapentin to the treatment of this patient's recurrent depressive episodes and his general course of illness appeared good, but the need remains for clinical confirmation with the extension of the drug trial and gabapentin's subsequent ability to prevent future episodes of depression. If the patient did have depressive recurrences, resuming the addition of lamotrigine, to which he had been

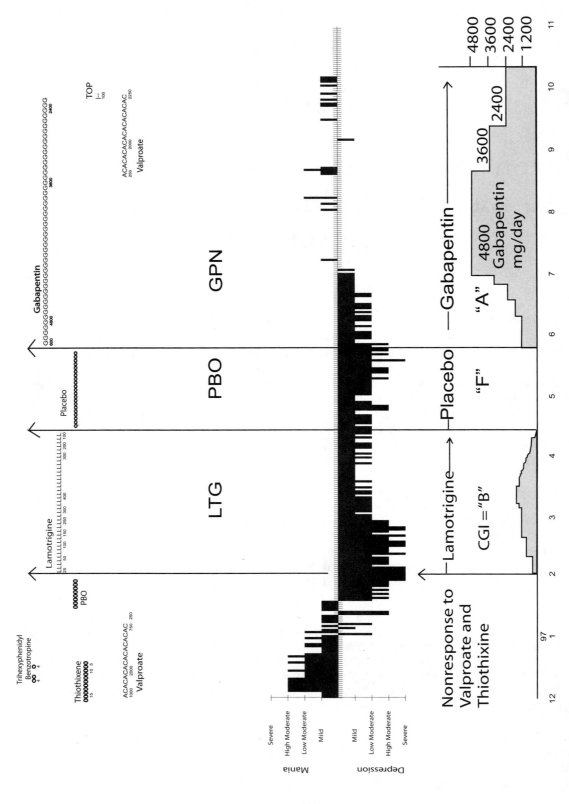

Figure 27.1 This 45-year-old bipolar I patient with a profound psychotic depression showed a partial response to lamotrigine, slight worsening on placebo, and an apparent excellent response to high doses of gabapentin. CGI, Clinical Global Impression scale: B, much improved; F, worse; A, very much improved.

a partial responder, might be a high-priority option.

BACKGROUND LITERATURE

Double-blind controlled studies fail to indicate a primary antimanic or mood-stabilizing effect of gabapentin, whereas studies suggest utility of the drug as an adjunct in open studies in inadequately responsive bipolar patients on other regimens. Consistent with this view, a placebo-controlled study suggests the utility of adjunctive prophylactic gabapentin (compared with placebo) in patients inadequately responsive to other agents (Vieta et al., 2006).

The primary antidepressant efficacy of gabapentin monotherapy has not been systematically explored in controlled studies in bipolar illness beyond the study of Frye, Ketter, Kimbrell, et al. (2000). In that study (in which this patient participated), patients were titrated up to maximum doses of 4,800 mg/day, and doses averaged 3,987 mg in the 6-week evaluation. Despite these relatively high doses in monotherapy, the degree of efficacy in depression was not superior to placebo and was statistically inferior to that of lamotrigine (Frye, Ketter, Kimbrell, et al., 2000). Yet younger patients on gabapentin with shorter durations of illness and lower weight at baseline were among those who responded best (Obrocea et al., 2002).

Further controlled studies of gabapentin in children and adolescents would appear indicated, based on this initial small study of possible clinical correlates of positive response (younger age) in highly treatment-refractory affectively ill patients. Gabapentin not only increases brain GABA by effects that are thought to involve alterations in amino acid transport but also blocks calcium influx through the L-type calcium channel (via actions at an alpha-2 δ subunit). Thus, it is possible that these GABA-enhancing and calcium-blocking actions of gabapentin are more helpful in younger individuals or as additions to the effects of other mood-stabilizing agents than they are in monotherapy. Open and, in a few cases, controlled studies suggest the potential usefulness of gabapentin in helping to treat many of the comorbidities that are common in bipolar patients, including sleep, pain syndromes, and anxiety disorders.

PRINCIPLES OF THE CASE	STRENGTH OF EVIDENCE
1. Controlled studies suggest gabapentin is not a primary antimanic agent nor a mood stabilizer (Frye, Ketter, Kimbrell, et al., 2000; Pande et al., 1999).	++
2. Yet gabapentin's utility as an add-on (adjunctive) therapy has been widely reported as positive in uncontrolled studies and now in one controlled study (Vieta et al., 2006).	++
3. Gabapentin's use as an add-on treatment could be related to its effectiveness in many conditions with which bipolar illness is often comorbid.	±
a. Pain syndromes (widely used in neurology)	+++
b. Anxiety and social phobia (each confirmed in respective double-blind studies)	+++
c. Obsessive-compulsive disorder (one positive open, one negative controlled study)	±
d. Sleep disorder (including restless leg syndrome)	+
e. Alcohol withdrawal (possible alternative to benzodiazepines; one positive, one negative study	±
f. Parkinson's syndrome	±
4. The potential antidepressant effects of gabapentin in monotherapy were not supported, but its efficacy in combination therapy remains to be further explored.	+
5. Predictors of individual responsiveness to gabapentin, such as	

in younger individuals, need to
be further studied.   +

6. Gabapentin has a wide margin
   of safety.   +++

7. Small doses, 100–300 mg at
   night (H.S.) may help sleep,
   anxiety, and mood, while very
   high doses (2,400–4,800 mg/
   day) can often be well toler-
   ated, as observed here.   ++

8. After more than 800–1,200 mg
   are given in a single dose at
   night, the drug should be given
   in divided daytime doses because gabapentin has a short duration of action ($T_{1/2}$ or half-
   life) and will inhibit its own re-
   absorption and transport into
   the blood if all of it is given in
   a single high dose.   ++

9. A close analogue of gabapentin,
   pregabalin, has been FDA approved for adjunctive treatment
   of adults with epilepsy who have
   partial-onset seizures; how pregabalin will mimic or differ
   from gabapentin in patients
   with mood and anxiety disorders remains for further study.
   Since the antipain effects of gabapentin are thought to be related to actions on the alpha-2
   δ subunit of the L-type calcium
   channel, and pregabalin is more
   potent on this subunit than gabapentin, very good antipain effects would also be expected.   ++

TAKE-HOME MESSAGE

Gabapentin may play an important adjunctive
role in the treatment of many comorbidities occurring in bipolar illness, but it is not an antimanic or mood-stabilizing drug in monotherapy.

28

Apparent Tolerance to Gabapentin Augmentation in an Ultrarapid-Cycling Patient

CASE HISTORY

The patient illustrated here is a 50-year-old single male with a 30-year history of bipolar disorder. His illness course had shown a general pattern of accelerating episode frequency. After the first biphasic episodes of hypomania and severe depression, the following eight episodes were isolated and intermittent, but his illness course progressed to rapid cycling in the late 1970s and ultrarapid cycling in the 1990s.

A substantial number of mood fluctuations continued to occur, reaching moderate levels of severity for both mania and depression despite a variety of long-term treatment interventions including lithium monotherapy, carbamazepine monotherapy, the combination of lithium and carbamazepine, the combination of lithium and valproate, and triple therapy with lithium, carbamazepine, and valproate. In each phase, he was also treated for breakthrough manic and depressive episodes with adjunctive medication, including thioridazine and perphenazine and the antidepressant nortriptyline, respectively.

The patient showed a pattern of increasing severity of both mania and depression despite triple therapy (Figure 28.1, left side) until gabapentin was added in May 1997. With the addition of gabapentin to carbamazepine and lithium combination treatment, an approximately 9-month remission was achieved. However, with continued drug administration, episodic depressions of mild and more moderate severity began to break through and continued to do so in this pattern despite a gabapentin dose increase from 1,500 mg/day to 2,100 mg/day.

BACKGROUND LITERATURE

The controlled study of Pande, Crockatt, Janney, Werth, and Tsaroucha (2000) comparing gabapentin with placebo as adjunctive treatment for acute mania revealed that gabapentin was not an effective acute antimanic agent. These findings were confirmed in the study of Frye, Ketter, Kimbrell, et al. (2000) in which we did not find gabapentin to be an effective mood stabilizer in monotherapy in highly treatment-refractory patients; with high doses, gabapentin appeared to exacerbate either the dysphoric components of mania or increase ultrarapid cycling frequencies (Chapter 25).

Yet gabapentin is widely used for a variety of indications in bipolar and other neuropsychiatric illnesses. Why is this the case despite two negative controlled trials? A large number of studies suggest the utility of gabapentin when it is used adjunctively in the treatment of incompletely responsive bipolar illness (Altshuler et al., 1999;

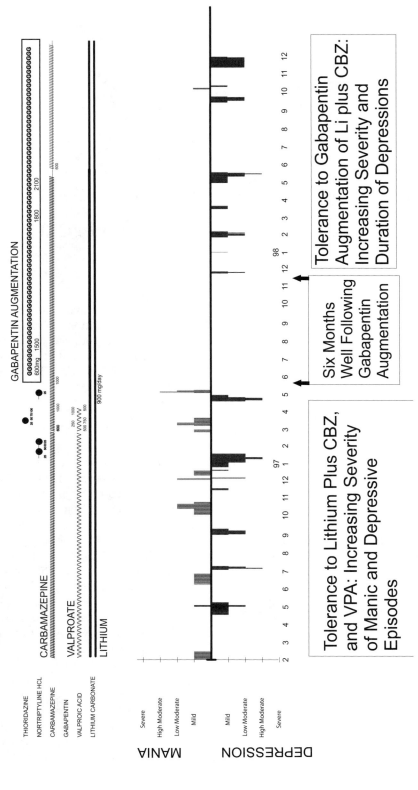

Figure 28.1 Apparent response to gabapentin augmentation of carbamazepine plus lithium: loss of prophylactic antidepressant effect. Gabapentin augmentation of lithium and carbamazepine was associated with the absence of hypomanic or full-blown depressive episodes for approximately 9 months. The effect on hypomania was sustained, but depressive episodes of increasing duration began to reemerge after 6 months, suggesting a partial loss of efficacy, likely related to a tolerance mechanism. CBZ, carbamazepine; VPA, valproate; Li, lithium.

Cabras, Hardoy, Hardoy, & Carta, 1999; Erfurth, Kammerer, Grunze, Normann, & Walden, 1998; Knoll, Stegman, & Suppes, 1998; Mauri et al., 2001; McElroy, Soutullo, Keck, & Kmetz, 1997; Young, Robb, Patelis-Siotis, MacDonald, & Joffe, 1997). Either these open, uncontrolled, adjunctive studies are in error or there is some other explanation for the discrepancy between these uncontrolled add-on studies and controlled observations of Pande and Frye and associates.

One possibility may be that the drug is useful as an adjunct to other partially effective agents, whereas it is not effective in acute severe mania or as a mood stabilizer in monotherapy in highly treatment-refractory patients. Another potential explanation is that it helps with many of the co-morbid diagnoses and symptoms with which bipolar patients struggle. For example, placebo-controlled studies indicate that gabapentin has antianxiety effects in both panic and social phobia (Pande et al., 1999; Pande, Pollack, et al., 2000), and some 40% of patients with bipolar illness have a comorbid anxiety diagnosis (McElroy, Altshuler, et al., 2001). An open study suggested the utility of gabapentin augmentation in obsessive-compulsive disorder (Cora-Locatelli, Greenberg, Martin, & Murphy, 1998), but a more recent controlled study was negative (Sporn et al., 2001). Preliminary observations suggest gabapentin effectiveness in some of the sleep and anxiety components of PTSD (Hamner, Brodrick, & Labbate, 2001).

Gabapentin is also widely used in a variety of neuropsychiatric and other medical conditions because of its robust antipain effects (Mellegers, Furlan, & Mailis, 2001). To the extent that somatic complaints and medical comorbidity are prominent in bipolar illness (which they are), these antipain effects may be particularly helpful as well. Gabapentin, because of its anti-anxiety effects and positive effects in restless leg syndrome, appears to improve sleep duration and possibly sleep quality (Garcia-Borreguero et al., 2002), thus possibly facilitating treatment response secondary to improvement in other areas of bipolar symptomatology, including depressed mood, because of the positive effects on sleep and anxiety.

This patient and several others in our open case series suggests that tolerance may develop to the therapeutic effects of gabapentin, even when it is used initially and highly effectively as an adjunct. Tolerance development has been preliminarily and anecdotally reported with the use of gabapentin for its anticonvulsant and antipain effects, and further systematic long-term follow-up studies are required in order to ascertain whether this example of apparent gabapentin tolerance occurs in a substantial number of bipolar patients. Some loss of efficacy via tolerance might be expected in apparent gabapentin responders, because this phenomenon has been reported in 25–40% of our highly treatment-refractory patients initially responsive to regimens employing lithium (Chapter 12), carbamazepine (Chapter 19), or valproate (Chapter 24) as the major mood stabilizer.

The pharmacological characteristics of gabapentin itself make it particularly attractive for adjunctive treatment. In addition to its potential spectrum of efficacy noted above, it is not metabolized by hepatic enzymes and is largely excreted unchanged in the urine, making it easy to use with other compounds because there are few drug-drug interactions (Ketter, Frye, Cora-Locatelli, Kimbrell, & Post, 1999). It has an extremely wide effective dose range, with some people improving on 100 mg/day or less and others both tolerating and requiring 3,600 to 4,800 mg/day or higher for a good response. No particularly dangerous or life-threatening side effects have been identified, so that the drug can be rapidly titrated to clinical efficacy or general side effects tolerability.

Gabapentin's one potential difficulty relates to its relatively short half-life of 5 or 6 hours, requiring multiple dosing over the course of a day with dose administration two, three, or four times per day. Another reason that large doses cannot be given all at once is that gabapentin inhibits its own transport into the body. Thus, if large total daily doses are desired, they must be given in a divided fashion so that gabapentin can be adequately absorbed and taken up into the brain.

	STRENGTH OF EVIDENCE
PRINCIPLES OF THE CASE	

1. As reported widely in the open literature, the addition of gabapentin to previously ineffective mood-stabilizing regimens appears to have positive effects in some bipolar patients. +

2. This patient, who was in a phase of increasing severity of both manic and depressive episodes prior to the initiation of gabapentin augmentation, went into a period of complete remission for 6 months, greatly exceeding the duration of previous well intervals, suggesting that it was the drug contributing to the clinical improvement rather than a spontaneous remission. +

3. However, with continued drug administration, depressions gradually began to break through with a general pattern of increasing severity or duration of episodes, highly suggestive of a pattern of loss of efficacy due to development of treatment resistance to gabapentin via a tolerance mechanism. +

4. Treatment approaches to tolerance development may include the following (discussed in more detail in other chapters):

   a. Increased dose of drug. +

   b. Adding a drug with a different mechanism of action. +

   c. Switching to a drug with a different mechanism. +

   d. After a period of time off the original effective drug (to which the patient has now developed tolerance), renewed effectiveness of the original drug. ±

   e. If such a response is achieved, tolerance is likely to recur at a rate equivalent to or faster than that originally observed, however. ±

   f. It is only in the face of loss of responsivity (i.e., episodes are now breaking through a treatment that had been initially effective) that a period of time off drug can be considered as a therapeutic strategy (with the intent to restart the same drug later). ±

   g. If the illness is continuing to remain in remission on a given treatment regime, then having a period of time off may be the last thing that one would want to do. ++

5. Negative consequences of stopping an effective treatment could include:

   a. Relapse and its secondary consequences. ++

   b. Hospitalization. +

   c. Much time required to become stabilized. +

   d. The remote possibility (perhaps about 10%) that the same (previously effective) treatment will no longer be as effective. +

   e. It may not again be effective at all. ±

TAKE-HOME MESSAGE

Gabapentin is generally well tolerated and may help some primary or comorbid symptoms of bipolar illness when used as an add-on to previously ineffective regimens. Since tolerance can occur to almost any prophylactic approach, maintenance of full-dose treatment (in the absence of side effects) appears a conservative course of action rather than lowering doses and risking earlier tolerance development.

29

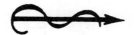

Prophylactic Response to Topiramate With Valproate in an Ultrarapid Cycler

CASE HISTORY

Throughout 1997, 1998, and the first half of 1999, this patient showed ultrarapid cycling between mild to moderate hypomania and moderate to severe depression. This cycling occurred despite treatment with doses as high as 4,000 mg/day of valproate, 1,000 mg/day of carbamazepine, 125 mg of lamotrigine, and 3,600 mg of gabapentin. Treatment with topiramate (Topamax) was initiated in early 1998 with the dose slowly titrated from 25 mg/day to 300 mg/day in the first several months and to 400 mg/day after about 1 year, which was associated with 4 months of euthymia.

Therapy with topiramate had been considered in an attempt both to halt the weight gain associated with the previously ineffective regimen and to find a more successful mood-stabilizing regimen. When the dose reached 330 mg/day, both the hypomanias and the depressions became shorter, less frequent, and usually reached only mild levels of severity (Figure 29.1). With only several weeks' exception, almost all of these 2 years on topiramate (1999 through 2001) were rated euthymic.

Although various medications other than topiramate were briefly used, and treatment with 1 mg of risperidone was initiated in mid-1999, these did not appear primarily responsible for the major clinical improvement (that had also

been observed prior to these adjunctive treatments). Similarly, valproate, either alone or in combination with three other anticonvulsants—carbamazepine, lamotrigine, and gabapentin—did not appear critical to the efficacy of this regimen, because little improvement was observed even with doses of valproate as high as 5,000–7,000 mg/day. An important contribution of valproate to the improvement, of course, could only be definitively demonstrated in this patient by a clinical trial of its discontinuation.

BACKGROUND LITERATURE

Clinical Use of Topiramate

A number of case series in the literature have reported clinical improvement in mania and rapid cycling when topiramate has been added openly to other previously ineffective regimens, similar to that reported in this patient (Calabrese, Keck, McElroy, & Shelton, 2001; Carpenter, Leon, Yasmin, & Price, 2002; Chengappa et al., 1999; Ghaemi, Manwani, Katzow, Ko, & Goodwin, 2001; Grunze et al., 2001; Marcotte, 1998; McElroy et al., 2000; McIntyre et al., 2002; Vieta, Torrent, et al., 2002). Vieta and colleagues reviewed 10 studies in 689 bipolar patients and found the average response rate to be 66% in open adjunctive treatment. Some

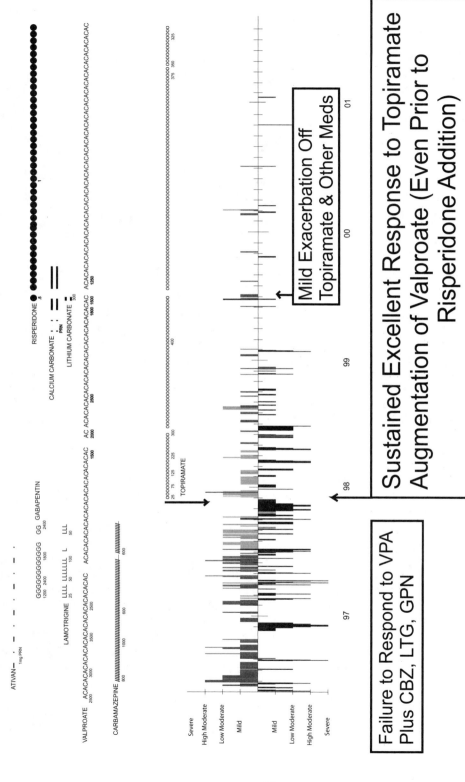

Figure 29.1 Prophylactic response to topiramate. After failing to respond to four anticonvulsants in various combinations and with other agents, the addition of topiramate to previously ineffective valproate was associated with dramatic improvement for this patient. VPA, valproate; CBZ, carbamazepine; LTG, lamotrigine; GPN, gabapentin.

of these studies included rapid- and ultrarapid-cycling patients, as illustrated here.

In the study of McElroy et al. (2000), the prophylactic effects of topiramate in mania and cycling appeared more robust than the degree of clinical improvement achieved when topiramate was used acutely for treatment of a breakthrough depressive episode. However, as in the current case, when an antimanic and anticycling response did occur, there also appeared to be concomitant improvement in the depressive phases.

Yet topiramate is not an effective acute antimanic drug in monotherapy in adults. Four large multicenter studies of topiramate monotherapy versus placebo in acute mania failed to show efficacy (Kushner, Khan, Lane, & Olson, 2006). At the same time, the active comparator drug lithium used in two studies did show efficacy. The lithium response data indicate that these are not flawed studies, but represent a clear failure of topiramate to show acute efficacy (at least in monotherapy). However, one study (DelBello et al., 2005) in adolescents with acute mania (stopped early when the other four adult studies failed to show topiramate's effectiveness) did reveal a significant benefit over placebo in these adolescents. This leaves the issue of efficacy in adolescents unresolved. Bahk et al. (2005) found that topiramate (average peak dose 276 mg/day) was as effective as valproate (average peak dose 912 mg/day) when added to risperidone (about 3.5 mg/day). Importantly, patients with valproate added for 6 weeks gained 2.5 kg (about 5.5 lb), while they lost weight (about 0.25 kg) with added topiramate.

McIntyre and colleagues (2002) compared adjunctive use of topiramate and bupropion for patients with bipolar depression breaking through ongoing mood stabilizer treatment. In a randomized but open comparison, both drugs were effective in about 56% of the patients, and both were associated with some degree of weight loss, although this was greater with topiramate than bupropion. This study contrasts, to some extent, with the results of McElroy and associates (2000), and the delineation of acute antidepressant effects and efficacy in prophylaxis awaits further controlled clinical trials.

Effects on PTSD, Primary Alcoholism, Cocaine Abuse, and Bulimia

Berlant (2001; Berlant & Van Kammen, 2002) reported considerable success in the open-label use of topiramate in PTSD, and there are mechanistic reasons why this might have been expected, as discussed in the following paragraphs. Moreover, in patients with primary alcoholism, Johnson and colleagues (2003; 2007) found topiramate robustly more effective than placebo on most clinical and laboratory measures of alcohol abstinence as well as a self-rated measure of craving for alcohol. In addition, Kampman et al. (2004) found topiramate more effective than placebo in cocaine abuse.

These perspectives suggest that topiramate may continue to have an important role in the clinical therapeutics of bipolar illness and its comorbidities, including bulimia (Knable, 2001; McElroy et al., 2003), overweight (Appolinario, Fontenelle, Papelbaum, Bueno, & Coutinho, 2002; Carpenter et al., 2002), alcohol and drug (cocaine) abuse, and PTSD, even though it does not have primary antimanic effects in monotherapy.

Mechanisms of Action

The mechanisms of action of topiramate (Perucca, 1997; Post, Chalecka-Franaszek, et al., 2002; Suppes, 2002; White, 1999) extend beyond those of other anticonvulsants, and its multiple targets could account for many of its therapeutic and side effects.

Topiramate is a blocker of sodium influx into the presynaptic terminal (like many other anticonvulsants), and thus decreases release of excitatory amino acids such as glutamate. However, topiramate is uniquely a direct blocker of two subtypes of the glutamate receptor, that is, of the AMPA and kainate subtype, but not of the N-methyl-D-aspartate (NMDA) receptor. This is of considerable interest because NMDA receptors are required for the induction of long-term learning and memory as revealed in the model of long-term potentiation in hippocampal slices, whereas the maintenance or expression of long-term potentiation is dependent on AMPA receptors. This action of topiramate in blocking AMPA receptors could account for cognitive and word-finding difficulties seen in a small percentage of patients treated with topiramate (Thompson, Baxendale, Duncan, & Sander, 2000). At the same time, it could account for its unique spectrum of clinical actions in PTSD and other disorders with a prominent conditioned component. It has been postulated that the heightened memories of PTSD and their autonomous replay (flashbacks) could also involve enhancement of AMPA receptor activity, which would theoretically be ameliorated with topiramate. Kainate receptors are prominent in the amygdala and are likely involved in normal and pathological processes of emotional memory, as well as in neurotoxicity (Li, Chen, Xing, Wei, & Rogawski, 2001). Some data indicate decreased glial numbers in the amygdala as well as in the prefrontal cortex in bipolar illness. Topiramate blockage of AMPA-kainate receptors could thus be important to several of its psychiatric and anticonvulsant effects.

Topiramate also increases brain gamma-aminobutyric acid (GABA) as measured in humans with magnetic resonance spectroscopy (Kuzniecky et al., 1998), apparently via an indirect effect, and not one acting on GABA receptors per se. This could account for some antianxiety and putative antidepressant effects.

Topiramate also inhibits carbonic anhydrase, like acetazolamide and zonisamide, and is thus associated with a 1–2% incidence of renal calculi (kidney stones). These calculi contain calcium and are readily subject to destruction with sonication (i.e., lithotripsy), which can be rapidly performed in emergency rooms. Therefore, one would not have to tolerate the extreme pain of kidney stones until they were passed naturally. This action also leads to a considerable incidence of paresthesias (tingling or other unusual sensations), mostly in the extremities.

Other Effects and Side Effects

Topiramate is metabolized by liver enzymes (the 3A4 type) and can affect the blood levels of other compounds. Most important, if one is on topiramate and taking oral contraceptives containing an estrogenic component, topiramate enhances estrogen metabolism (breakdown), and a higher estrogen dosage form should be used to prevent unwanted pregnancies.

Topiramate can cause acute glaucoma in the very small subgroup of those in the population predisposed to narrow-angle glaucoma, and anyone developing eye pain or poor vision on the drug should immediately contact their physician.

Weight Loss

Another prominent side effect of topiramate, which is often considered a positive asset, is weight loss. This side effect was initially observed in the trials of topiramate in epileptic patients and has subsequently been consistently replicated in studies in bipolar patients as well. The mechanism of the weight-reduction effect is unknown but appears to involve both a decrease in appetite and a change in the metabolic set point. It is noteworthy that another direct antiglutamatergic drug such as felbamate also includes weight loss as a potential positive side effect; however, the weight loss effects of zonisamide (see Chapter 30) would not be explained by this mechanism.

Weight loss on topiramate often averages 10 to 15 lb at 6 months and is prominent in about one third of patients. As opposed to many other weight-loss regimens, the chronic administration of topiramate does not appear to be associated with breakthrough weight gain or tolerance to the weight loss effects during continued treatment with the drug. The weight loss effect does stop when the drug is discontinued, however.

McElroy, Frye, and associates (2007) compared the weight loss effects of topiramate to those of sibutramine, an FDA-approved drug for weight loss, in a randomized open comparison. Parallel degrees of weight loss were seen on both agents (about 0.33 lb/week). However, patients appeared to drop out early (for side effects) on topiramate, and late on sibutramine (for mood instability).

Preliminary evidence also suggests that topiramate could have direct salutary effects on blood glucose, triglycerides, and cholesterol, questionably independently of its degree of weight reduction (Chengappa, Levine, Rathore, Parepally, & Atzert, 2001). As such, it may have considerable utility in reducing both the weight gain associated with a variety of the psychotropic drugs widely used in the treatment of bipolar illness (see Table 45.1) and (theoretically) the proclivity of some patients treated with atypical antipsychotics to develop adult-onset diabetes and related weight-associated metabolic alterations.

PRINCIPLES OF THE CASE	STRENGTH OF EVIDENCE
1. This patient is illustrative of the small group of patients with bipolar illness who are not responsive to a variety of anticonvulsants even when used in complex combination therapy; anticonvulsants ineffective in this patient included valproate, carbamazepine, lamotrigine, and gabapentin.	++
2. Even though topiramate shares the ability to block sodium influx and thus the release of glutamate (as do valproate, lamotrigine, and carbamazepine), it is apparent that other aspects of its chemical profile would likely be involved in the clinical response in this patient.	++
3. The addition of topiramate to valproate appeared crucial to this patient's clinical improvement in her previously treatment-resistant ultrarapid cycling pattern, although this could not be definitively ascertained unless an off-drug exacerbation was observed upon tapering of topiramate.	+
4. As the patient had experienced many years of incapacitating severe and rapidly recurring mood	

fluctuations, acquiring such confirmation of responsivity would not at this time appear in the patient's best clinical interest, and she chose to accept this beneficial result as a likely topiramate response when added to valproate and later augmented by risperidone.   +

a. To some extent, the same principle could apply (as in no. 3, above) for maintaining the excellent response to the combination treatment with valproate (also continued without a definitive off-drug trial), but with an additional caveat: Valproate can be associated with a substantial degree of weight gain, and excess weight persisted in this individual despite reduction of the valproate dose from the 5,000–7,000 mg/day range to a 2,000–2,500 mg/day range.   +

b. This might be an area in which careful discussion of the risk-to-benefit ratio of a trial of valproate taper between the physician and patient is warranted.   +++

c. Although valproate may be important to the patient's mood stabilization, the ultimate choice to test this (and likely obtain further weight reduction, but risk illness reemergence) is made on the basis of physician and patient discussion and discretion.   ++

5. The possibility that risperidone (1 mg/day) is necessary to her clinical response (when added to topiramate and valproate) is likewise unknown, but could also play a role in either adding to valproate-associated weight gain or to the possibility that topiramate (plus

risperidone) would have the ability to maintain an excellent prophylactic response even if valproate were discontinued.   ±

   a. The decision of when to leave well enough alone is part of the art of clinical medicine, and it can diverge radically from the academic science of clinical medicine.   ++

   b. We do not advocate taking unproven medications, but when a medication regimen is working for a patient, staying the course and staying *on* course may sometimes be the best strategy.   +

   c. Watch out for people who say, "Why are you taking all these medications? You are doing so well, you probably don't need them anymore." They may have good intentions, but they may also be grossly misinformed.   ++

   d. Information derived from your own mood chart and individual experience is much more reliable than generalities from the literature.   ++

6. After the several-day depression of low moderate severity in November 2000, this patient began to take gingko biloba. The utility of this compound for enhancing memory or augmenting psychotropic response to other agents is not known. Removal of this agent to assess its role in this patient might be considered because there is little reason to assume that this supplement is a primary factor in her response.   ±

7. The differences among suggested action principles (4), (5), and (6) above are largely based on whether the agent has proven effi-cacy in others or not. In (4) and (5), each drug (risperidone and valproate) has proven efficacy in others with bipolar illness based on studies in the literature; this is not the case for gingko biloba.   ±

8. This case clearly illustrates that lack of response to even many different anticonvulsants (with slightly to very different mechanisms of action) does not preclude response to another agent with a different mechanism of action, such as topiramate.   ++

9. The apparent effectiveness of adjunctive topiramate in this patient parallels that reported in about 60% of patients in open case series and randomized trials of topiramate added to other previously ineffective treatments.   ++

10. Topiramate may be usefully considered in situations in which patients:

   a. Are at high risk for weight gain with other psychotropic agents   +++

   b. Have already gained weight on other agents   ++

   c. Have concomitant diabetes mellitus or other elevated blood lipid cardiovascular risk factors   +

   d. Have comorbid PTSD   +

   e. Have a comorbid alcohol abuse disorder (naltrexone may also be considered)   ++

   f. Have bipolar illness comorbid with bulimia   ++

   g. Have comorbid cocaine abuse   ++

   h. Have comorbid migraines   ++

11. Only anecdotal reports exist about topiramate's potential utility in childhood, and there is one positive small (but double-blind, placebo-controlled) study of topi-

ramate in adolescent bipolar illness.

   a. However, because of its relative safety, further systematic exploration of the drug's potential utility in these younger populations should be further pursued.   ±

   b. Especially if there are comorbidities (see no. 10 above) adding further rationale.   ++

   c. Individual clinical trials with this agent in these conditions may be rewarding and beneficial, even though none of these are FDA-approved indications at this time.   ++

12. Although this patient was treated with 300–400 mg/day doses of topiramate, more typical doses usually range around 200 mg/day.   ++

13. It is wise to start at one 25-mg pill per day and increase slowly about 25 mg every 5 days to 1 week to avoid cognitive dysfunction on this drug.   +

14. Topiramate can cause kidney stones and paresthesia (unusual feelings in the limbs) and, rarely, narrow-angle glaucoma.   ++

15. Those patients on birth control pills should take the formulations with higher doses of estrogen, because topiramate can decrease estrogen blood levels.   ++

16. Topiramate may have utility in many different aspects of bipolar disorder even though it clearly is not an effective acute antimanic agent in monotherapy in adults.   +

TAKE-HOME MESSAGE

Even with many years of highly treatment-resistant ultrarapid cycling of moderate to severe hypomania and depression, a substantial remission in symptomatology can still be achieved with the addition of a novel agent, in this case an anticonvulsant compound such as topiramate.

30

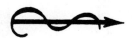

Zonisamide: A Positive
Side Effect of Weight Loss

CASE HISTORY

This patient had a long history of bipolar illness culminating in a pattern of ultrarapid cycling. Despite treatment with a number of psychotropic agents, the patient continued to have a pattern of continuous cycling between brief depressions of moderate to incapacitating severity and brief hypomanias. This continued despite treatment with 2,000 mg of divalproex sodium, 30 mg of tranylcypromine, 4 mg of risperidone, 100 μg of T_4, 300 mg of quetiapine, and 300–400 mg of topiramate. Percocet was needed approximately half the days per month for arm and shoulder pain. Upon the addition of zonisamide beginning at 100 mg/day and titrated up to 400 mg after several weeks, the patient's hypomanic episodes were attenuated in severity, frequency, and duration (Figure 30.1). Her depression entered the low moderate range rather than high moderate severity prior to beginning zonisamide.

The patient thus appeared to have a partial overall response with a good antimanic but weak antidepressant response to adjunctive treatment with zonisamide. However, even this degree of response remains uncertain because the MAOI tranylcypromine had been discontinued about 1 month early, and this could have helped in the achievement of cycle deceleration.

BACKGROUND LITERATURE

Zonisamide is a drug approved in Japan for more than a decade and approved in the United States for the treatment of seizure disorders only in the last several years. It has a number of properties that make it particularly interesting for a clinical trial in treatment-refractory affective disorders. In addition to its effects shared by several other anticonvulsants, including blockade of sodium channels, indirect enhancement of the GABA-benzodiazepine receptor complex, and reduction in T-type calcium channels (Kito, Maehara, & Watanabe, 1996; Schachter, 2000), it has a variety of other actions that make it particularly interesting in the affective disorders.

It facilitates both dopaminergic and serotonergic neurotransmitter turnover utilization at low doses (Okada et al., 1995, 1999), suggesting that it might possess antidepressant properties in parallel with other compounds with dopaminergic and serotonergic effects, such as bupropion and serotonin-selective antidepressants, respectively. Its ability to inhibit dopaminergic and serotonergic turnover at higher doses could be pertinent to its putative antimanic effects.

In addition, zonisamide increases GABA release in the hippocampus and blocks potassium-invoked glutamate-mediated synaptic effects (Mi-

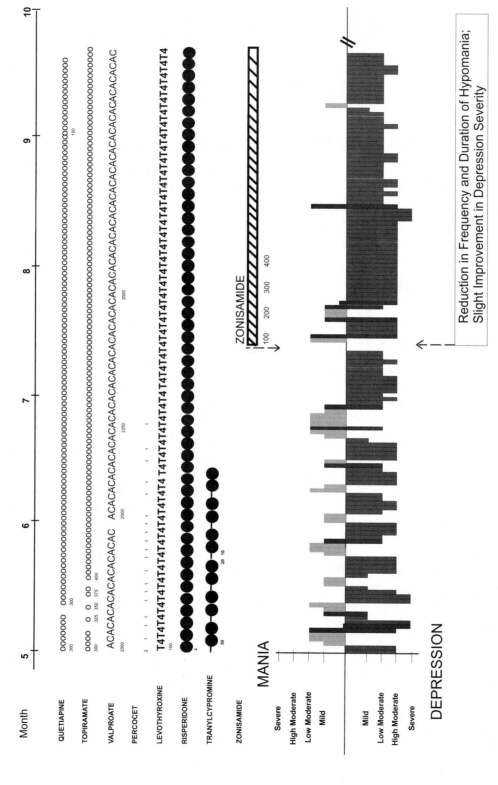

Figure 30.1 Possible antimanic effects of zonisamide in an ultrarapid cycler. This life chart shows ultrarapid cycling despite unusual treatment with two atypicals (quetiapine and risperidone) and two anticonvulsants (topiramate and valproate), as well as the MAOI tranylcypromine and T₄. There was a possible antimanic and anticycling effect of zonisamide, but an effect of tranylcypromine discontinuation is also possible.

maki, Suzuki, Tagawa, Karasawa, & Yabuuchi, 1990; Okada et al., 1998), both of which have been associated with possible antidepressant effects. It is also a weak inhibitor of carbonic anhydrase, but it is only 1% as active as acetazolamide, an anticonvulsant that is rarely used for seizures but is widely used for altitude sickness, that is, preventing pulmonary edema on mountains over 20,000 feet high. This carbonic anhydrase inhibitor component increases the risk of having kidney stones in a very small percentage of patients (about 1%) and, more frequently, the experience of unusual sensations in the limbs (paresthesias).

In addition to these effects, zonisamide is an interesting candidate for the ability to exert some degree of neuroprotection, although this is not well delineated in the literature. Many of its properties consistent with such an action include its action as a free radical scavenger; a hydroxy radical scavenger; an inhibitor of nitric oxide synthase; an inhibitor of lipid peroxidation (i.e., antioxidant effects); a protector against global hypoxia; and an inhibitor of oxidative DNA damage (Leppik, 2002; MacDonald, 2002). These findings are not only of interest for possible protective effects in a variety of neurological illnesses, but given the evidence for neuronal and glial dysfunction in bipolar illness, as reviewed in Chapter 10, some of these properties could be relevant to clinical effects and protecting the brain in the affective disorders.

Studies are just beginning to be conducted in the United States regarding zonisamide's potential role in bipolar illness. Researchers await a series of controlled investigations. However, in Japan, an open-label study was conducted in 24 patients (15 bipolar in the manic state, 6 schizoaffective manic, and 3 with schizophrenic excitement). Of the entire group, 71% and 80% of the bipolar group displayed moderate to marked global improvement using doses ranging from 100 to 600 mg/day with a study duration of 4 to 5 weeks (Kanba et al., 1994).

McElroy et al. (2005) completed an open study of zonisamide added to previously ineffective drugs in 62 bipolar patients. Rapid onset (in the first week) of antimanic effects was ob-

served in 56% of 34 patients given the drug for mania or cycling. Slower onset (improvement seen especially after Week 3) antidepressant effects were seen in 9 of 22 (41%) acutely depressed patients. Parallel incidence and course of antidepressant effects were seen in the patients treated for (dysphoric) mania and cycling. Manic/cycling (34), depressed (22), and euthymic (6) patients (given zonisamide for weight loss) all lost weight in a parallel fashion ($p < .001$ for whole group and averaging about 0.33 lb/week). Ketter et al. (personal communication, 2006) also showed substantial degrees of weight loss in their overweight bipolar patients.

Baldassano, Nassir, Chang, Lyman, and Lipari (2004) saw positive effects of zonisamide on bipolar depression in her cohort of patients. Anand et al. (2005) found very substantial antidepressant effects of zonisamide in treatment-resistant bipolar depressed patients. The best responders who were on monotherapy had not failed multiple previous trials and were not on multiple drugs in combination.

In epilepsy, zonisamide has been given to 750,000 patients, with 1.9 million patient years of experience. Most of the adverse events were mild to moderate, and 88% of zonisamide patients completed the clinical trials. Most frequent adverse events in 269 zonisamide patients versus 230 on placebo were somnolence (17% versus 7%), dizziness (13% versus 7%), anorexia (13% versus 6%), headache (10% versus 8%), nausea (9% versus 6%), and agitation-irritability (9% versus 4%). The risk of kidney stones increases with doses above 600 mg, and there was a 1.2% incidence of symptomatic kidney stones in all clinical trials (Chadwick & Marson, 2002).

Zonisamide is structurally related to sulfa drugs, and those with sulfa allergies are not supposed to be exposed to the drug. However, in a meeting of epilepsy experts in 2003, none of the experts had seen or ever heard of such a case, and the recommendation appears to be based solely on theoretical grounds.

While 49 cases of serious skin reactions requiring emergency medical attention were reported in postmarketing in Japan, with the estimated incidence being 46 cases per million patients exposed, no cases were reported in the U.S. and European development programs.

Two cases of aplastic anemia and one case of agranulocytosis were also reported in Japan. This incidence rate is very close to the background incidence rate for these life-threatening hematological illnesses, which are each estimated to occur in 1 in 1 million individuals in the general population. Two cases of agranulocytosis were reported during the U.S., European, and Japanese development experience.

Decreased sweating (oligohydrosis) and accompanying increased temperature (hyperthermia) have been reported with zonisamide use, with 13 cases noted in Japan among young patients ranging from 1.6 to 17 years of age. This may be a cultural vulnerability because Japanese individuals are thought to have a decreased number of sweat glands compared with North Americans. As is evident from the profile of 13% of epileptics experiencing anorexia, zonisamide is usually associated with some weight loss, which may be a positive side effect for some individuals, as we have seen (Leverich et al., 2005; McElroy et al., 2005). In our study of 62 bipolar patients, none developed kidney stones or overheating from decreased sweating.

PRINCIPLES OF THE CASE	STRENGTH OF EVIDENCE
1. This patient represents a number of other individuals who are highly treatment resistant, as he continued to cycle despite treatment with two putative mood-stabilizing anticonvulsants (valproate and topiramate), two atypical antipsychotics (risperidone and quetiapine), T_4 augmentation, and antidepressant treatment with an MAOI (tranylcypromine).	++
2. The overall response to zonisamide in this patient must be considered equivocal because of the simultaneous taper of the	
MAOI tranylcypromine, which could have contributed to the pattern of ultrarapid cycling.	±
3. In order to attempt to achieve a more complete response in a patient such as this, one might consider:	
a. A reexposure to lithium augmentation, even if it had not been effective previously.	++
b. A trial of lamotrigine, for its antidepressant properties.	+++
c. Antidepressant augmentation strategies including the dopamine-active bupropion or the dopamine D_2, D_3 agonist used in Parkinson's disease (pramipexole).	++
d. Revision of the atypicals to include trials of ziprasidone or aripiprazole	++
e. T_3 augmentation of T_4	+
f. Augmentation with 1–2 mg of folic acid (Coppen, Chaudhry, & Swade, 1986)	++
g. Adjunctive light therapy	+
h. Omega-3 fatty acids (as discussed in Chapter 60).	+
i. Discontinuing the T_3 and slowly increasing the dose of T_4 to supraphysiological ranges (i.e., 400–500 μg/day) in order to push the patient to the edge of mild hyperthyroidism as described by Whybrow (1994) and Bauer, Berghofer, and associates (2002) in Chapter 62	+
4. Open studies of zonisamide in bipolar illness suggest rapid onset, antimanic effects, and weaker, slower onset antidepressant effects that deserve further study.	+
5. Zonisamide has a distinct potential for the positive side effect	

of weight loss for those wishing for either added mood stabilization or assistance with weight loss, or both.   ++

6. Its long half-life in blood (63 hours) makes it convenient for once-daily dosing at night.   +++

7. It is metabolized by liver enzymes 3A4 such that enzyme inducers such as carbamazepine will decrease the half-life to 28 hours and lower zonisamide blood levels.   +++

TAKE-HOME MESSAGE

The promising antimanic and weaker antidepressant effects of the anticonvulsant zonisamide in treatment-refractory bipolar illness remain to be demonstrated and confirmed in controlled clinical trials. In the meantime, its substantial weight loss effects make zonisamide a potential alternative for those patients who do not respond to or tolerate topiramate, wishing for weight loss in the context of greater mood stability.

31

Levetiracetam: Mysterious Mechanism of Action and Psychotropic Profile

CASE HISTORY

This patient's major mood symptomatology had resolved upon treatment with valproate, olanzapine, and bupropion, but she remained persistently mildly depressed, anxious, and insomniac. The addition of levetiracetam was associated with a full remission for the first time in several years (Figure 31.1).

This potential antidepressant response following the addition of levetiracetam could be attributable to either drug response or the natural course of illness. In other mildly or moderately depressed individuals we also saw positive responses, but none of our severely depressed patients showed a good response to levetiracetam (Post, Altshuler, et al., 2005). Similarly, the potential antidepressant response following the addition of levetiracetam (in Figure 31.1) could be attributable to either variation in either the drug regimen or course of illness.

BACKGROUND LITERATURE

Levetiracetam is an anticonvulsant approved for adjunctive therapy for the treatment of refractory seizure disorders, particularly complex partial seizures or what was formerly known as temporal lobe or psychomotor epilepsy. Its anticonvulsant profile has a number of aspects that make it unique among this class of drugs.

Almost all of the other anticonvulsants are effective in the two major seizure models used to assess efficacy of anticonvulsants, that is, maximal electroshock and pentylene tetrazole (Metrazol) seizures for grand mal and petit mal (absence) epilepsy, respectively. Levetiracetam is effective in neither of these models (Klitgaard, Matagne, Gobert, & Wulfert, 1998).

Moreover, levetiracetam has no direct receptor effects on any of the possible neurotransmitter and receptor systems that are thought to be involved in the seizure disorders. Yet it does have its own specific binding site in the brain, but the endogenous ligand for this site and its actions have not yet been identified (Klitgaard, 2001).

In contrast to levetiracetam's lack of efficacy in the typical seizure models, it is effective in preventing both the development and fully manifest seizures of the amygdala-kindling model (Loscher & Honack, 1993; Loscher, Honack, & Rundfeldt, 1998). As noted earlier in this book, many drugs such as carbamazepine and lamotrigine, although they are highly effective anticonvulsants for completed kindled seizures, are not effective in preventing kindling development. The ability to prevent both the development and completed phases of amygdala-kindled seizures is a property of levetiracetam shared with valproate, diazepam, and phenobarbital, but few other drugs.

Recently, several new hints about levetiracet-

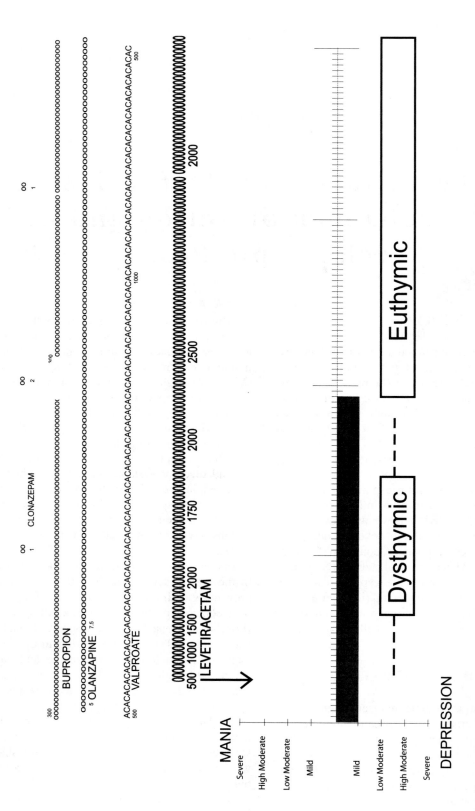

Figure 31.1 Possible response to levetiracetam augmentation for mild depression. Mild depression that persisted during treatment with bupropion (300 mg/day), valproate (500 mg/day), and olanzapine (7.5 mg/day) remitted following the addition of levetiracetam in a slow titration to 2,000 mg/day.

256

am's possible mechanism of action have been elucidated. It appears that it does not exert direct actions at the benzodiazepine-GABA receptor complex, which modulates chloride influx and provides the major mechanism of inhibition of neuronal firing in the central nervous system. Rather, it has an indirect effect at this site and it blocks negative modulators of this site (Rigo et al., 2002). There is a zinc binding site and a beta-carboline binding site, both of which, when occupied, make the benzodiazepine-GABA receptor less effective (Figure 31.2). Similar effects occur for glycine gated currents.

Levetiracetam, in blocking zinc and beta-carboline inhibitory modulation, thus makes the chloride channel more effective. Whether this particular mechanism explains its unique anticonvulsant properties remains to be demonstrated, but it could account for levetiracetam's generally benign side effects profile, because no transmitter or receptor system is completely blocked directly. Thus, normal functioning would proceed, but only in instances of abnormal excitation, such as an epileptic seizure, would levetiracetam's action become important.

Lynch et al. (2004) reported that levetiracetam binds to a synaptic vesicle protein, SV2A, that is critical to calcium-mediated release of transmitters in synaptic vesicles (Figure 31.2; presynaptic). SV2A interacts with synaptotagmin, which is thought to be the key calcium sensor regulating vesicle release of transmitters. Levetiracetam also partially inhibits N-type voltage-gated Ca^{++} channels, which modulate transmitter release.

One other suggestion has emerged about the potential efficacy of levetiracetam pertinent to psychiatry. In an animal model of mania, wherein animals become hyperactive following treatment with meprobamate (Librium) in combination with a psychomotor stimulant, levetiracetam and valproate were both active in decreasing activity (Lamberty, Margineanu, & Klitgaard, 2001), but the two drugs in combination are particularly effective in normalizing this motor hyperactivity. Whether or not levetiracetam will emerge as an effective agent in any phase of affective illness remains to be delineated (Post, Altshuler, et al., 2005), but, based on the results

of this preclinical model, one would also want to assess the efficacy of this drug eventually in combination with valproate.

Prominent side effects of the drug include sedation and dizziness; minor degrees of weight loss were associated with its use in patients with seizure but not affective disorders. A nonsignificant increase in irritability, depression, and psychosis (the latter about 1%) has also been reported during add-on therapy of patients with epilepsy (Cramer, De Rue, Devinsky, Edrich, & Trimble, 2003).

Several isolated case reports have suggested possible antimanic or antidepressant efficacy in several instances (Braunig & Kruger, 2003; Goldberg & Burdick, 2002; Soria & Remedi, 2002), but long-term controlled studies have yet to be conducted. Grunze, Langosch, Born, Schaub, and Walden (2003) provided suggestive evidence of the utility of levetiracetam in acute mania when he studied it as an on-off-on adjunct to haloperidol. Patients improved on, worsened slightly off, and improved again on levetiracetam.

In our own series of 34 bipolar patients exposed to levetiracetam, several patients appeared to have a good acute antimanic and long-term response to the drug, but many patients dropped out early because of sedative side effects, lack of efficacy, or illness reemergence after an initial apparent acute response (Post, Altshuler, et al., 2005). The drug is often started at a dose of 250 to 500 mg at night and increased to approximately 2,000 mg slowly, in order to avoid sedative side effects.

As this drug so far appears to have few serious or life-threatening side effects and possesses a mechanism of action different from most other anticonvulsant and psychotropic agents, one looks forward to further elucidation of its possible utility in mood and other neuropsychiatric disorders. In patients with epilepsy, Trimble (2000) reported that levetiracetam had fewer adverse effects on mood than topiramate. He also found that levetiracetam (or topiramate) cotreatment with lamotrigine further reduced behavioral side effects. However, Zhang, Xing, Russell, Obeng, and Post (2003) found that in amygdala-kindled animals, levetiracetam tolerance crossed to car-

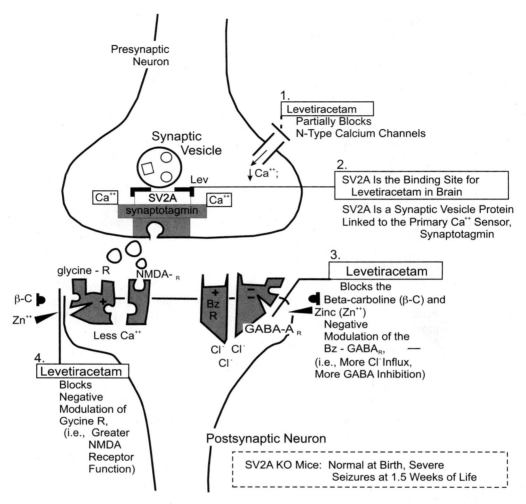

Figure 31.2 Levetiracetam decreases Ca^{++}-mediated transmitter release via SV2A binding site and indirectly enhances $GABA_R$ and decreases $glycine_R$ function. Presynaptically, levetiracetam blocks N-type calcium channels and the SV2A site on synaptotagmin, both of which affect transmitter release. In addition, levetiracetam indirectly enhances GABAergic inhibition by blocking the negative modulatory effects of zinc and beta-carboline at this chloride influx channel.

bamazepine, but, interestingly, animals that were tolerant to carbamazepine still showed anticonvulsant responses to levetiracetam (i.e., unidirectional cross-tolerance).

In the kindling model in rats, there is evidence that tolerance to levetiracetam arises rather rapidly, but, as one might expect based on their differences in mechanism of action, there is not cross-tolerance between this drug and valproate (Krupp, Heynen, Li, Post, &

Weiss, 2000). One analysis of seizure response has suggested that a subgroup of patients with epilepsy may also show the rapid onset of tolerance to levetiracetam's anticonvulsant effects, although this remains to be further evaluated (Ben Menachem & Gilland, 2003).

However, another study reported an extremely high success rate when levetiracetam was administered to patients who had an unsuccessful response to epilepsy surgery, with a large percentage of these patients achieving complete remission on the drug (Motamedi et al., 2003). In that series, three patients showed the new onset of psychosis after 4 to 9 months of treatment with this drug, however. Whether this represents an interaction of the drug's properties with the effects of epilepsy surgery or a proneness to inducing psychosis in patients with epilepsy is not known. Another anticonvulsant, ethosuximide, is widely recognized as inducing psychosis in patients with epilepsy in a process called forced normalization, wherein seizures may be improved and the EEG regularized, but behavior becomes bizarre (Landolt, 1953; Yamamoto, Pipo, Akaboshi, & Narai, 2001). It is not known whether the levetiracetam-related psychosis is a similar manifestation of forced normalization or whether it may or may not be pertinent to patients with psychiatric illness.

	STRENGTH OF
PRINCIPLES OF THE CASE	**EVIDENCE**

1. Levetiracetam is an anticonvulsant with a unique mechanistic profile because it is not effective in the traditional animal seizure models that are positive for the existing anticonvulsants (i.e., metrazol for absence and maximum electroconvulsive seizures for major motor seizures). +++

2. Levetiracetam is effective in preventing the initial development of amygdala-kindled seizures as well as in inhibiting fully manifest seizures as well. +++

3. Although tolerance rapidly develops to levetiracetam's anticonvulsant effects on amygdala-kindled seizures, whether this would become a problem with the drug in the clinical treatment of seizure disorders remains to be further assessed. +

4. The patients illustrated in the two case reports are examples of a highly ambiguous response to this agent because dramatic improvement did not occur, nor was there an attempt to confirm evidence of efficacy based on a period off drug. ±

5. Since the drug has a long half-life and is moderately sedating, it should be used in a single nighttime dose to take advantage of its positive ability to enhance sleep. ++

6. One study in normal volunteers suggests that the drug increases rapid eye movement sleep phases that are associated with dreaming (Bell et al., 2002), which is an unusual property not shared by most other psychotropic drugs. ++

7. Levetiracetam was weight neutral in our open-label add-on case series. +

8. Neither consistent antimanic nor antidepressant effects of levetiracetam have been observed in our initial case series (Post, Altschuler, et al., 2005). ++

9. Further investigation of the effects of levetiracetam on mood is warranted in light of other, more positive reports in the literature. +

10. Levetiracetam indirectly enhances the main inhibitory neurotransmitter system in the brain (the benzodiazepine and GABA receptor-chloride ionophore complex). It also binds to the SV2A synaptic vesicle protein, which modulates presynaptic neurotransmitter release. +++

TAKE-HOME MESSAGE

Levetiracetam is an anticonvulsant with a novel mechanism of action and a generally benign side effects profile, but its utility in the affective disorders remains to be further examined in exploratory case series and then, if positive, verified in controlled clinical trials.

Part VI

CALCIUM CHANNEL

BLOCKERS

32

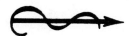

Unequivocal Response to Nimodipine: Cross-Responsivity to Isradipine, but Not to Verapamil

CASE HISTORY

The patient is a 42-year-old married woman with a 20-year history of mood dysregulation characterized by moderate to severe depression and anxiety with comorbid panic attacks. She was diagnosed as bipolar type II because she had never experienced a full-blown manic episode (Figure 32.1). A detailed retrospective life chart was constructed. In the year prior to her admission she exhibited persistent depressive symptoms, but the life chart revealed previous patterns of rapid cycling and refractoriness to imipramine, doxepin, alprazolam, fluoxetine, lithium, carbamazepine, trazodone, and phenelzine. The induction or remission in rapid cycling could not be clearly correlated with initiation or discontinuation of these prior treatments, including fluoxetine (see Figure 32.1).

As can be seen in Figures 32.2 and 32.3, daily prospective life chart (NIMH-LCM) ratings yielded clear evidence that active nimodipine was superior to nonnimodipine trials (two placebo phases and one verapamil phase) in its ability to maximize the number of days the patient was euthymic. The percentage of days euthymic (Figure 32.3) during verapamil therapy (28%) was roughly comparable to that of the two placebo phases (42% and 30%), and substantially below the average of 93% observed on stable doses of nimodipine. The observations

suggest that although the patient responded to nimodipine, this response was not generalized to another class of L-type calcium channel blocker, the phenylalkylamine verapamil, at the highest doses tolerated.

There were no days rated manic in the first placebo period nor in the three nimodipine periods. However, during the second placebo period, 66% of the ill days were characterized by mania; during the blind verapamil phase, 24% of ill days remained characterized by mania. A chi-square test revealed that the patient had a statistically significantly greater number of days euthymic during nimodipine treatment (all phases combined) than during nonnimodipine phases (all phases combined), $\chi^2 (1) = 143.02$, $p < .00001$ (McDermut et al., 1985).

This visual inspection and statistical analysis of prospective daily life chart ratings of percentage of days euthymic and of mean Hamilton depression and Young mania ratings clearly indicate the efficacy of nimodipine in this patient (Figure 32.3).

BACKGROUND LITERATURE

The results of this single-case off-on-off-on replication design study yield both clinical and theoretical perspectives. First, the findings suggest that this patient was a selective responder to only

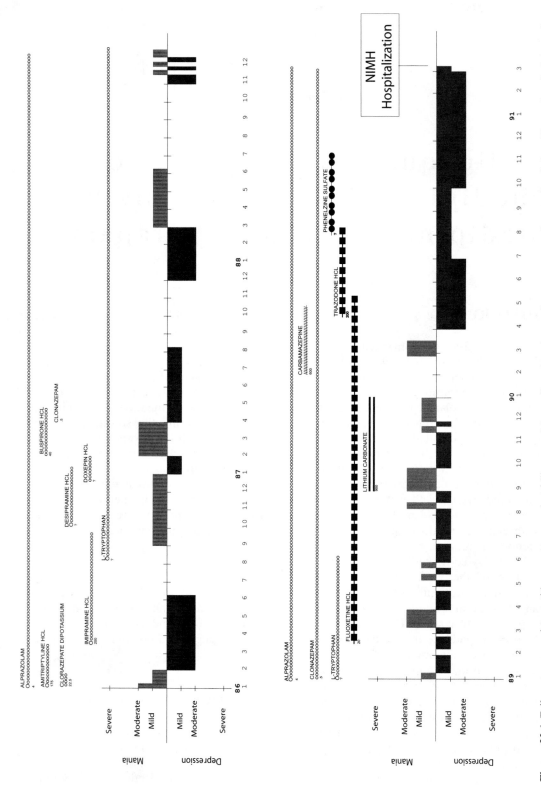

Figure 32.1 Failure to respond to antidepressants, mood stabilizers, and benzodiazepines in a subsequent responder to nimodipine. The patient had a continuous ultrarapid cycling pattern of bipolar type II affective disorder by history. Her past cycling pattern was ultrarapid, but 2.5 years before admission to NIMH, this patient developed a persistent depression of moderate to severe intensity.

264

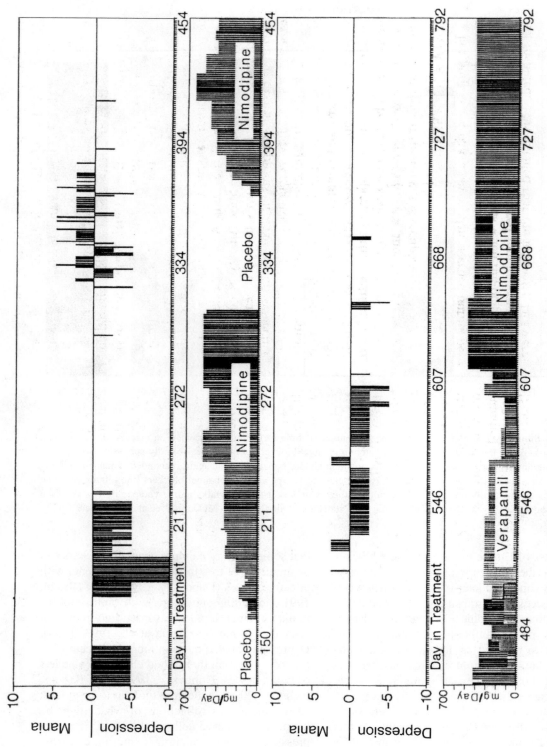

Figure 32.2 Consistent improvement in depression and cycling on nimodipine trials I, II, and III; effect not matched by verapamil. An essentially complete response to nimodipine was documented by nurses' blind functional impairment ratings in a B–A–B–A design, wherein B was placebo and A was active nimodipine. Similar to some other patients with histories of anxiety, this patient developed transient episodes of nocturnal panic during upward dose titration (between 180 and 330 mg/day); anxiety symptoms subsequently decreased at higher doses that were associated with improvement in affective symptoms. Upon nimodipine discontinuation (with placebo substitution), her pattern of ultrarapid mood fluctuation returned, which again responded to an active nimodipine (420 mg/day) maintenance dose. Her symptoms re-emerged during blind verapamil substitution and then again cleared a third time upon blind reintroduction of nimodipine treatment.

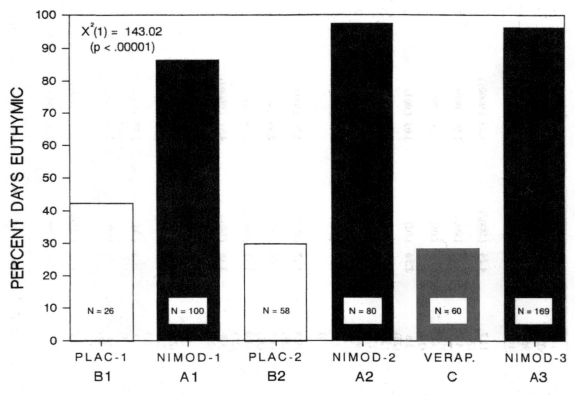

Figure 32.3 Summary of Figure 32.2 showing percentage of time well (euthymic) when on placebo or nimodipine (or verapamil). When the widely used L-type calcium channel blocker verapamil was blindly substituted (in a dose up to 320 mg/day), improvement in mood was not maintained, but the patient again responded when nimodipine was blindly reinstituted for the third time. Thus, one class of L-type calcium channel blockers (the dihydropyridine nimodipine) was repeatedly effective while another (the commonly used phenylalkylamine verapamil) was not. N = number of days in a given phase. (The within trial statistics as described in McDermot et al., 1985 were highly significant.)

one subclass of L-type calcium channel blocker medication (the dihydropyridine type). This view was further supported later in her treatment when she was successfully transitioned to another dihydropyridine, isradipine (21 mg/day), also in the context of the double-blind trial. However, her failure to respond as adequately to the diphenylalkylamine calcium channel blocker verapamil on most measures (Figure 32.2, Table 32.1) indicate either (a) a poor ability to tolerate what might otherwise have been therapeutic doses of this drug, or (b) unresponsivity to this different calcium channel blocker because of its difference in site and mechanism of action compared with the dihydropyridines.

The findings also support the growing belief

that some types of calcium channel blockers can be an effective treatment for some patients with affective illness (Dubovsky, 1993, 1995; Hoschl, 1991), including subgroups with rapid- and ultradian-cycling bipolar disorder and recurrent brief depression (Pazzaglia et al., 1993, 1998). Depressed patients have an increased accumulation of calcium in their blood elements (platelets or lymphocytes; Dubovsky, 1995; Post, Pazzaglia, et al., 2000), which are thought to be at least partial models or reflections of what might be happening in nerve cells in the brain. If in depression too much calcium is entering cells (associated with overactive cell firing), it could provide the rationale for treatment with drugs that block calcium entry.

Table 32.1 *Half Lives, Dosages, and Effectiveness of L-Type Calcium Channel Inhibitors in Mood Disorders*

	Phenylalkylamine (On outside of Ca^{++} Channel)	Dihydropyridines (Inside Membrane and Ca^{++} Channel)		
	Verapamil (Calan, Isoptin)	Nimodipine (Nimotop)	Isradipine (DynaCirc)	Amlodipine (Norvasc)
Half life	Short (5–12 hours)	Short (1–2 hours)	Short (8 hours)	Long (30–50 hours)
Starting dose	30 m.g. T.I.D.	30 mg T.I.D.	2.5 mg B.I.D.	5 mg H.S.
Peak daily dosage	480 mg	240–480 mg	15 mg	10–15 mg
Antimanic	++	++	(++)	( )*
Antidepressant	±	+	(+)	( )*
Antiultradian	±	++	(++)	( )*
Anticocaine (Dopamine)	–	++	++	( )*

Note. Strength of evidence: ++ = very strong; + = strong; ± = equivocal; – = none; * = no systematic studies; only case reports and clinical observation; ( ) few patients studied.

We can only conjecture how some of the idiosyncrasies of this case (e.g., marked co-occurrence of anxiety symptoms as well as lithium and other antidepressant refractoriness) may have influenced or selected for the finding of robust clinical effectiveness of nimodipine in this patient. Larger clinical trials using other designs are now required to document the extent of the efficacy of nimodipine in different patient subtypes and to help identify possible clinical and biological markers of who will most likely respond.

PRINCIPLES OF THE CASE

STRENGTH OF EVIDENCE

1. The failure to respond to the mood stabilizers (lithium and carbamazepine), the tricyclic antidepressants (imipramine and doxepin), other antidepressants and anxiolytics (trazodone and alprazolam), the MAOI (phenelzine), and the SSRI (fluoxetine) does not preclude a positive response to the L-type calcium channel blocker nimodipine (see also Chapter 66).   +

2. Improvement occurred on nimodipine in both manic and depressive phases in this bipolar II patient who also had prominent anxiety and agoraphobia.   +

3. Anxiety symptoms (and the new onset of nighttime panic attacks) were initially worse at lower doses (180–380 mg/day) prior to a positive therapeutic effect on anxiety at higher doses (400 mg/day) and more chronic treatment.   +

4. As this patient's history reveals, single-case designs and statistics can confirm response to a given drug in a given individual (McDermut et al., 1995).

   a. "Once a true process or effect has been established as having occurred in one person, it can reasonably be assumed, or inferred, that there will be other persons as well in which the process or effect will occur" (Chassan, 1992, p. 177).   +++

b. Further studies remain to be performed to assess the percentage of response in different subtypes of affectively ill patients in the general population. +

c. This patient's refractory depression (extensive nonresponse to conventional drugs) responded to nimodipine. ++

d. Other patients with ultra-ultrarapid (ultradian) cycling are among those who also responded (see Chapter 33). +++

5. All calcium channel blockers may not be equivalent. +++

   a. Response generalized from nimodipine to another dihydropyridine L-type calcium channel blocker, isradipine, but not to the phenylalkylamine L-type blocker verapamil. +

   b. The dihydropyridines, compared with verapamil, also show differences in the site of action within the L-type calcium channel pore; blockade of cocaine hyperactivity affecting dopamine levels in reward areas of brain (nucleus accumbens); and in animal models of depression. +++

6. The calcium channel blockers may also be a substitute for lithium in some patients who cannot tolerate lithium because of side effects. +

   a. Dubovsky feels that lithium responders are particularly likely to respond to verapamil (and by inference also to the dihydropyridines nimodipine, isradipine, or amlodipine). ±

   b. Dubovsky reports that verapamil and related drugs could also substitute for lithium in pregnancy, as no syndrome or congenital malformation has yet been linked to its use. ±

   c. Whether the diphenylkyamine calcium channel blockers are as effective as lithium and truly safer in pregnancy remains to be more directly assessed (see Wisner et al., 2002). ±

7. While patients with concurrent (comorbid) mood and anxiety symptoms may be more difficult to treat than those without, even those with a highly recurrent and treatment-refractory course can essentially be brought to full remission with appropriate and sometimes unusual classes of medications. +

8. If a patient like this individual had only a partial or therapeutically inadequate response, one could consider augmenting nimodipine or isradipine with one of the following:

   a. Mood stabilizers

      i. Lithium for cyclic breakthrough (Manna et al., 1991) +

      ii. Carbamazepine (see Pazzaglia et al., 1993; and Chapter 33) +

      iii. Valproate (remains virtually untested) (±)

   b. Atypical antipsychotics (such as quetiapine) ++

   c. antidepressants or anxiolytics (±)

9. Nimodipine consistently increases somatostatin in the spinal fluid of affectively ill patients (see Chapter 9). ++

10. This could account for further preliminary evidence of its small positive effects in:

   a. Alzheimer's disease (which has low brain somatostatin) +++

   b. Memory and cognition in depression (in which CSF somatostatin is transiently low) ++

   c. Better antidepressant response to nimodipine in those with low CSF somatostatin at baseline (Frye, Pazzaglia, et al., 2003) +

11. A pattern of frontal hypometabolism on positron emission tomography (Ketter, Kimbrell, et al., 1999) is more often associated with a response to nimodipine, while a pattern of hypermetabolism, particularly in the left insula, is associated with response to carbamazepine. ++

TAKE-HOME MESSAGE

The calcium channel blockers may provide an alternative to lithium in refractory depression and ultrarapid cycling. Of the several classes of L-type calcium channel blockers, the dihydropyridines may be more effective than some of the others.

33

Ultra-Ultrarapid (Ultradian) Cycling Responding to the Combination of a Calcium Channel Antagonist and Carbamazepine

CASE HISTORY

This woman's prior course of illness is discussed in detail in Chapter 36. She was treated without much success with a series of antidepressant and mood-stabilizing drugs including imipramine, doxepin, alprazolam, fluoxetine, lithium, carbamazepine, trazodone, and phenelzine. During fluoxetine administration, the patient showed a marked increase in cycle frequency that was minimally responsive to carbamazepine alone. Other agents did not markedly affect her cycle frequency. The patient became disabled and dysfunctional because of these rapid mood oscillations and was rarely able to work at her usual professional activities as a teacher and artist.

During her admission to the NIMH, she was initially studied on placebo and was observed prospectively to demonstrate the ultradian cycling frequencies (Kramlinger & Post, 1996) that she had previously described. Very often she would wake up in a very low mood but suddenly become activated, energized, and highly talkative. After several hours, she would suddenly shift down into a severe, retarded depression with impaired concentration and cognition, decreased speed of thoughts, and feelings of hopelessness and suicidality. After a period of

minutes to hours, her mood would again shift to an activated hypomanic phase that could be either euphoric or dysphoric (with pressure, anxiety, and discomfort) in its quality. Two additional shifts like this within a single day were characteristic, with the patient often showing five or more switches per day in the absence of apparent triggers (Figure 33.1). We observed that her retrospectively described extreme mood fluctuations occurring multiple times within a 24-hour period were clearly able to be rated by herself and by the nursing staff, especially when ratings every 2 hours (while awake) were used.

When active medication with nimodipine, an L-type calcium channel blocker, was blindly substituted for placebo, the severity and frequency of these mood fluctuations was attenuated (Figures 33.1 and 33.2). The hypomanic phases responded slightly more than the depressed phases, but significant improvement was observed in both. The question was raised as to whether this was a spontaneous remission due to an increased duration of time hospitalized on an active research and treatment ward. To determine whether this was the case, placebo was again substituted in a blind fashion. As is evident from Figure 33.2, increased severity of manic and depressive episodes was again observed, and, after reinstitution of active nimo-

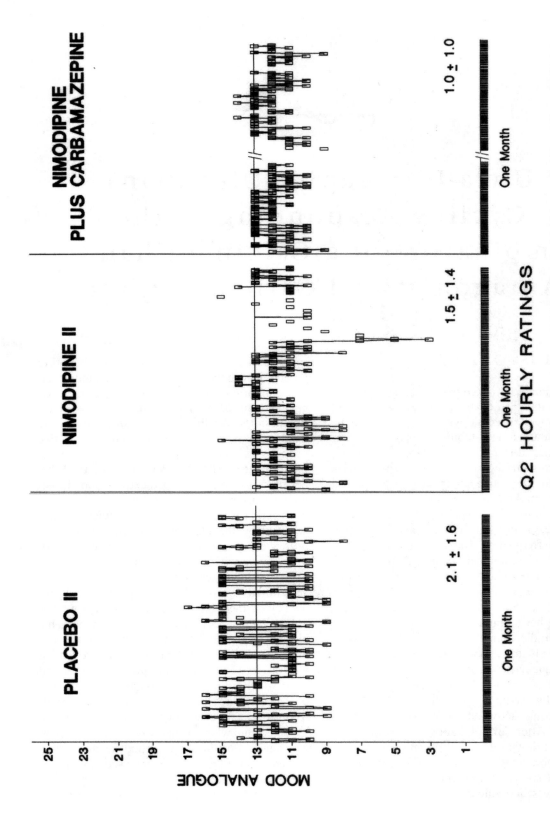

Figure 33.1 Nimodipine plus carbamazepine attenuated the amplitude of ultradian cycling in a bipolar II female. Multiple mood shifts within a single day were recorded by staff and the patient using 2-hourly rating. Only the first month of several of the treatment phases is illustrated here. The mean deviations from a stable baseline (13) in the right lower corner are for the entire duration of the second placebo trial and nimodipine trial (illustrated in Figure 31.2), and were significantly decreased in amplitude on both nimodipine and its combination with carbamazepine.

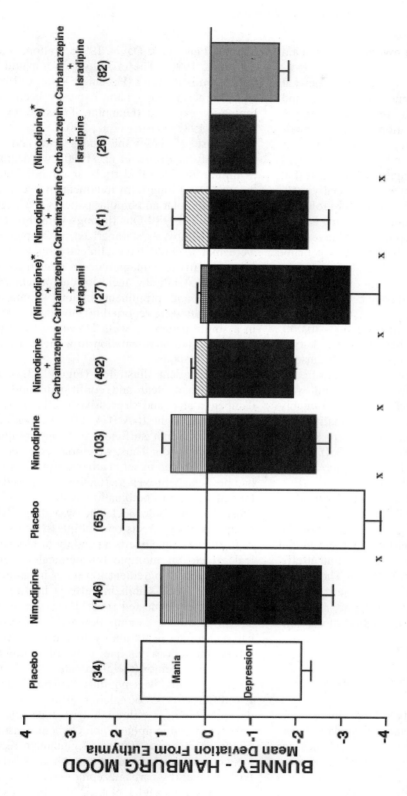

Figure 33.2 Efficacy of dihydropyridine L-type calcium channel blockers in a bipolar II female: nurse ratings. This is the same patient (Chapter 36) who showed a pattern of general increases in severity of illness over time, after a relatively prolonged phase of moderate illness. Her illness showed a distinct jump in cycle frequency to marked oscillations in mood within a single day. The amplitude and frequency of these oscillations diminished with blind nimodipine treatment, increased again on placebo, and reresponded to active nimodipine, confirming the partial efficacy of this calcium channel blocker. However, the patient's response was inadequate, and carbamazepine was added to the regimen on a blind basis. This addition resulted in further amelioration of the frequency and amplitude of mood shifts within a day. When verapamil was substituted for nimodipine, this patient's excellent response was not maintained. However, she did respond to nimodipine a third time and was switched to another dihydropyridine (isradipine) with a continued good response. *Nimodipine slowly tapered to zero. X = p < .05.

273

dipine, clear clinical improvement was again achieved.

However, the patient remained somewhat symptomatic on nimodipine monotherapy and continued to be functionally impaired due to her episodic depressive fluctuations of mild to moderate proportion. Therefore, carbamazepine was added on a blind basis, and this addition was associated with further improvement, such that the patient was now no longer functionally incapacitated and was able to begin a return to work. This improvement was maintained during a combined inpatient-outpatient phase, and there were only periodic mild exacerbations during many stressful situations with which she was confronted.

Since nimodipine would have been extraordinarily expensive, with a year's supply at her current treatment dose costing $25,000–30,000, it was decided to switch her to another L-type calcium channel blocker, verapamil. Because of its availability for a variety of indications in cardiology, generic preparations of verapamil were available, and it was therefore more reasonably priced. Verapamil, however, at maximally tolerated doses was insufficient to prevent her depressive mood oscillations (Figure 33.2). It was discontinued on a blind basis, and the patient was transitioned to nimodipine.

The patient again had a sustained period of improvement and was finally able to be transitioned to another dihydropyridine-type calcium channel blocker (isradipine) without substantial problems of side effects or loss of clinical efficacy (Pazzaglia et al., 1993, 1998). The patient continued working and, at last report several years following her NIMH discharge, remained essentially well on the combination of carbamazepine and isradipine.

BACKGROUND LITERATURE

Considerable evidence shows the clinical efficacy of L-type calcium channel blockers in the treatment of acute mania. However, most of these studies involve the use of the nondihydropyridine L-type calcium channel blocker verapamil (Dubovsky, 1995; Hoschl, 1991; Janicak,

Sharma, Pandey, & Davis, 1998; Walton, Berk, & Brook, 1996). The efficacy of verapamil in depression is doubtful (Hoschl & Kozeny, 1989) and long-term prophylaxis has only been preliminarily explored (Giannini, Taraszewski, & Loiselle, 1987; Wisner et al., 2002).

Because of these ambiguous data and the open study of Brunet et al. (1990), we decided to initiate double-blind trials of nimodipine in the acute and long-term treatment of cyclic refractory unipolar and bipolar patients (Pazzaglia et al., 1993, 1998). Our findings with this drug in monotherapy, as summarized in Chapter 32, were that it could have clinically relevant effects of sufficient magnitude to remain as the sole mood-stabilizing agent for one patient with bipolar II and prominent anxiety symptoms. Good results were reported by Goodnick (1995) in a single patient as well. However, most patients required augmentation to achieve a more complete response.

In the patient illustrated (Figure 33.2), nimodipine had clear and confirmed ability to dampen manic and depressive oscillations, as documented in the B-A-B-A (off-on-off-on) design, but was not sufficient to bring complete clinical remission. Thus, we employed a second mood-stabilizing agent, carbamazepine, which had previously proven ineffective when used either alone or in combination with lithium. As illustrated in Table 33.1, the two drugs have complementary effects on multiple systems.

Carbamazepine exerts a panoply of biochemical effects on multiple biochemical systems, and the crucial ingredient for either its anticonvulsant or mood-stabilizing effects has not yet been clearly delineated (Post, Pazzaglia, et al., 2000). However, among the many effects of carbamazepine is its ability to inhibit calcium influx through a unique type of excitatory amino acid receptor (the glutamate NMDA-type receptor). Thus, it is possible that blockade of two different types of calcium influx—voltage-dependent increases through the L-type calcium channel (by nimodipine; Pani, Carboni, Kusmin, *Gessa, & Rossetti*, 1990) and glutamate receptor-mediated calcium influx through the NMDA-type channel (by carbamazepine)—could be additive (Post, Pazzaglia, et al., 2000). Perhaps the

Table 33.1 *Complementary Effects of the Anticonvulsant Carbamazepine and the Dihydropyridine Calcium Channel Blocker Nimodipine**

Findings	Carbamazepine	Nimodipine
Blockade of Ca^{++} influx	Via ligand-gated NMDA receptor	Via voltage-gated L-type Ca^{++} channel
Ca^{++} channel blockade	Weak	Strong
Anticonvulsant	Potent	Weak (not used clinically)
Somatostatin in CSF	Decreased	Increased[a]
Memory	Unchanged	Enhanced
Dopamine	Turnover reduced[b]	Cocaine-induced dopamine overflow decreased
Cocaine hyperactivity	Little effect	Inhibition
Left insula metabolism on PET scan correlates with antidepressant response	Hypermetabolism and response $r = 0.516$ (*df* 22, *p* < .02)	Hypometabolism and response $r = -0.519$ (*df* 16, *p* < .005)

[a]Better response to nimodipine in those with low CSF somatostatin at baseline.
[b]Better response to carbamazepine in those with low versus high baseline CSF homovanillic acid, the major metabolite of dopamine.
*Table 18.1 is reproduced here to make the point that two drugs with very different mechanisms of action may not only show differential responsivity within individuals, but in combination may provide additive effects on inhibiting calcium influx and on clinical response as seen here.

two together might provide sufficient calcium-buffering capacity to attenuate cellular hyperresponsivity (Dubovsky, Murphy, Christiano, & Lee, 1992) that could underlie the excitatory and inhibitory overexcursions (Figure 33.1) that are thought to be involved in the affective disorders.

Although this theory has not been definitively established, there is evidence from peripheral blood cells that intracellular calcium levels are significantly increased, both at baseline and following stimulation with a variety of agents including thrombin, serotonin, and thapsigargin. Calcium levels are elevated in platelets, lymphocytes, red cells, and other white cells of patients with affective disorders and, in particular, bipolar illness (Dubovsky, Lee, Christiano, & Murphy, 1991; Post, Pazzaglia, et al., 2000). To the extent that this proclivity for increasing cellular accumulation of calcium in blood elements in the periphery is reflected by similar accumulations of calcium in neuronal elements in the brain (Pani et al., 1990), the combined drug approach of nimodipine plus carbamazepine hypothetically might be sufficient

to block these observed increases in calcium and their associated mood swings in patients with bipolar illness.

Of course, it is entirely possible that other aspects of carbamazepine's actions (Ketter, Kimbrell, et al., 1999) contribute the needed extra ingredient to the L-type calcium channel blockade provided by nimodipine; this remains to be more definitively tested by augmenting with other drugs with other mechanisms of action. Because this patient was markedly improved for the first time in many years, we and she did not feel that it was in her best interest to explore this issue further by substituting carbamazepine for other drugs with other effects on calcium, that is, valproate or lithium. A more direct test of this hypothesis of carbamazepine's beneficial adjunctive effects would be to use another type of weak NMDA receptor antagonist to see if it would match carbamazepine's therapeutic effects.

There is evidence from the study of Manna (1991) that nimodipine in combination with lithium exerts greater therapeutic effects in long-term prophylaxis than treatment with either agent alone. In this regard it is of some interest that lithium is also thought to exert direct and indirect effects on calcium-related systems, both through weak blockade of calcium influx through the NMDA receptors and through effects on a variety of second-messenger systems such as adenylate cyclase and phosphoinositol turnover (Post, Weiss, et al., 2000). Nimodipine increases a peptide in CSF, somatostatin, that is low during periods of active depression and is consistently low in Alzheimer's disease (Pazzaglia et al., 1995). Increased somatostatin function in the brain could contribute to nimodipine's actions and account for the preliminary evidence of nimodipine's efficacy in the treatment of depression, especially that associated with low somatostatin levels in the spinal fluid (Frye, Pazzaglia, et al., 2003) and Alzheimer's disease.

For clinical purposes, the exact mechanisms of action by which nimodipine and carbamazepine combine to exert better therapeutic actions than either drug alone is not the crucial question. Rather, as in other branches of medicine, targeting a dysfunctional system with several different types of drugs may be more effective than relying on a single drug at high doses that may also increase side effects. For congestive heart failure, for example, patients are often treated with digitalis to stimulate the heart, diuretics to decrease fluid load, and antihypertensives to reduce vascular resistance. Similarly, effective treatment of tuberculosis requires a combination of three or even four different types of antibiotics with different mechanisms of action.

This patient's pattern of cycling within a day was reported by almost 20% of outpatients in the Bipolar Collaborative Network. It can clearly occur in patients without borderline personality disorder (as in this patient), even though chaotic mood lability can often occur in patients with that diagnosis as well. However, in those patients: (1) the mood lability is often triggered by the external environment; 2) sustained periods of good functioning do not typically occur; and (3) the presence of polysubstance abuse and poor interpersonal relationships differentiates their ultradian cycling from that observed here and in classical bipolar disorder.

PRINCIPLES OF THE CASE

STRENGTH OF EVIDENCE

1. Patients with classic manic-depressive illness can present with extreme ultradian cycling frequencies. These may be difficult to treat with conventional and monotherapy approaches.   ++

2. Calcium channel blockers of the dihydropyridine class (but not necessarily those of the phenylalkylamine class, such as verapamil) may be effective in this disorder.   ++

3. If response to an L-type calcium channel blocker is not complete, a patient may show further improvement with the addition of another mood stabilizer, such as carbamazepine or lithium. This may or may not depend on dual approaches to inhibiting calcium influx.   +

4. Whether antidepressants and the SSRIs, as observed in this case, predispose to the induction of ultradian cycling remains to be delineated (Chapter 36).   +

5. Even the most rapidly cycling patterns of affective dysregulation may ultimately be brought under control by appropriate therapeutic approaches. These may often require complex polypharmaceutical treatment regimens, however.   ++

6. Use of moderate doses of two drugs in combination could even have a lower side effects burden than very high or maximum therapeutic doses employed in monotherapy.   +

7. It is possible that shifts to ultra-ultrarapid (ultradian) cycling frequencies involve intracellular calcium dysregulation and calcium waves and oscillations that (via emergent properties and principles

illustrated in chaos mathematics theories) become manifest at the level of behavioral dysregulation. As such, approaches to calcium channel blockade and its augmentation with other agents may be effective in this particular stage of illness.   (+)

8. Nimodipine increases somatostatin, a peptide low in the CSF of Alzheimer's patients (permanently due to loss of neurons) and of depressed patients (transiently during depressive phases only). This could also account for the preliminary evidence of nimodipine's efficacy in depression and Alzheimer's.   +

9. Those depressed patients with the lowest CSF somatostatin levels at baseline responded best to nimodipine.   ++

TAKE-HOME MESSAGE

Classical bipolar illness can present with extreme cycle frequencies, that is, multiple switches within a day. Even very transient hypomanic switching episodes can be extremely unpleasant and dysphoric and impair patients' functional capacity. These episodes, and the accompanying depressive bursts, may respond to a calcium channel blocker. A combination of this and another mood-stabilizing agent (such as carbamazepine or lithium) may be more effective than a single agent.

Part VII

ANTIDEPRESSANTS

TCAs, MAOIs, and SSRIs

34

Antidepressant-Associated Mania in a Bipolar I Patient With a Major Depressive Episode Breaking Through Lithium Prophylaxis

CASE HISTORY

This middle-aged gentleman experienced two severe spontaneous manic episodes, each requiring hospitalization because of their severity, with impaired judgment and full-blown psychosis. The first episode, in 1985, responded well to treatment with lithium, and a phenothiazine, chlorpromazine. The next episode responded in a similar fashion, and lithium prophylaxis was initiated and maintained.

Despite this, a severe depression began in 1987. This depression was initially treated with adjunctive use of the tricyclic antidepressant (TCA) nortriptyline (Pamelor) which is largely noradrenergic in its mechanism of action. The patient rapidly escalated into a full-blown mania, at which time nortriptyline was discontinued and chlorpromazine was readministered. This resulted in rapid resolution of the mania and a return to a depression of moderate severity (Figure 34.1).

Because the patient remained substantially impaired, a new trial with trazodone (Desyrel) was initiated, which again resulted in a rapid switch (Figure 34.1). In 1988 the patient was admitted to the NIMH for participation in double-blind clinical trials with carbamazepine and other potential alternatives to lithium, which had proved inadequate as a mood stabilizer. This was evident because: (1) a depression of severe proportions broke through lithium prophylaxis; and (2) lithium was not sufficient to prevent switches on two occasions into full-blown mania with antidepressants with different mechanisms of action.

The two episodes of antidepressant-related mania were thought to be likely antidepressant induced and not related to the spontaneous course of the patient's illness on the basis of a number of factors:

1. They occurred in the context of an ongoing depression of moderate to severe proportions.

2. They occurred within an acute time frame of drug initiation.

3. Drug termination was associated with their rapid cessation.

4. The phenomenon of onset and offset was replicated on two separate occasions with two differentially acting antidepressants.

However, these episodes are considered only likely antidepressant related, based on the possi-

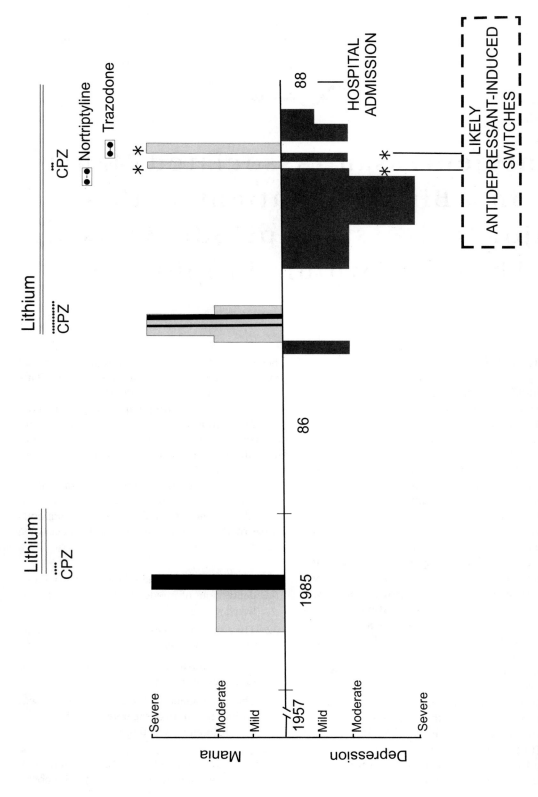

Figure 34.1 Antidepressant-associated mania in a bipolar I male. Following two spontaneous full-blown manic episodes requiring hospitalization in 1985 and 1987, the patient entered a severe depression. Upon two separate occasions with two differently acting antidepressants, the drugs were associated with switches into mania despite concurrent treatment with lithium. CPZ, chloropromazine (Thorazine).

bility that a third manic episode may have been expected in approximately this time frame after an interval of approximately 1.5 years between the first and second episode, and approximately 1 year between these second and third antidepressant-related episodes.

BACKGROUND LITERATURE

This patient was treated with the standard of care in the community in 1987 and 1988, as well as what is generally considered the recommended treatment approach to bipolar depression currently, that is, the addition of a unimodal antidepressant to a mood stabilizer (lithium) in the face of a breakthrough depressive episode (Grunze et al., 2002). However, instead of treatment with the traditional first-generation TCA (nortriptyline) and tetracyclic antidepressant (trazodone), one would now recommend a second-generation antidepressant, such as the selective serotonin reuptake inhibitors (SSRIs), bupropion, or venlafaxine. Even among the first-generation TCAs, the secondary amines nortriptyline and desipramine (which act predominately on norepinephrine) are better tolerated than their older tertiary amine close relatives, that is, amitriptyline and imipramine, respectively (Table 34.1).

In bipolar I patients, switch rates on the first-generation antidepressants have been estimated to occur in the range of 25% to 50% in most studies, with cotreatment with lithium or another mood stabilizer reducing the incidence to approximately 25%, which is the assumed spontaneous base rate that one would expect to see with placebo (Rouillon, Lejoyeux, & Filteau, 1992). However, in this patient, one would not have expected these manic breakthroughs within this time frame (without the administration of the unimodal antidepressants).

More recent data suggest that with second-generation antidepressants the switch rate is more in the range of 5% to 15% acutely when these drugs are used as augmentation of a mood stabilizer (Gijsman, Geddes, Rendell, Nolen, & Goodwin, 2004; Nemeroff et al., 2001; Post, Altshuler, et al., 2001; Post, Leverich, Nolen, et al., 2003; Sachs et al., 2007). Young et al. (2000)

performed a randomized comparison of the addition of a second mood stabilizer (either lithium or valproate) to the existing mood stabilizer, or the addition of the SSRI paroxetine (Paxil), and found that although the acute switch rates did not differ, paroxetine was better tolerated than the addition of the second mood stabilizer. That study, along with a wide range of clinical experience, provided the rationale for the earlier general recommendations for adjunctive use of second-generation antidepressants as a first-line treatment approach to a depression breaking through a mood stabilizer in a non-rapid cycling bipolar depressed patient (Figure 34.2). However, Nemeroff et al. (2001) found paroxetine no more effective than placebo except when lithium levels were low. Now, the latest study from the STEP-BD network indicates that neither paroxetine nor bupropion were more effective than placebo as adjunctive treatment to mood stabilizers for bipolar depression (Sachs et al., 2007).

Sachs and colleagues (Guille, Shriver, Demopulos, & Sachs, 1999; Sachs et al., 1994) further suggested that the switch rate on the older tricyclic antidepressants is higher than that with the second-generation agents such as bupropion. During long-term follow-up, Sachs found a switch rate of 13.3% on bupropion and 37.5% on desipramine. Desipramine, like nortriptyline, is a highly noradrenergic drug (by blocking the reuptake of norepinephrine rather selectively compared with serotonin reuptake). Some have questioned whether it is the noradrenergic properties of desipramine that make it particularly prone to cause switches.

This case example indirectly makes the argument that it is not likely to be only the norepinephrine property of an antidepressant (such as desipramine or nortriptyline), because a completely different agent acting largely on the serotonergic system appeared to be associated with the same switch liability. Trazodone is: (1) a weak reuptake blocker of serotonin, (2) an agonist at 5-HT_{1A} receptors, and (3) a blocker of 5-HT_2 receptors, the last of which is the reason that trazodone is a good treatment for the insomnia of depression. Blockade of the 5-HT_2 receptor has been associated with increases in

Table 34.1 *Adverse Effects of Antidepressant Treatments Used in Bipolar Disorder Patients*

Antidepressants (Dose in mg/day)	Manic Switch	Sedation	Hypotension	Anticholinergic	NE/5-HT	Weight	Sexual Dysfunction	Lethality in Overdose	Other/Comments
Bupropion (75–450)	+	±	0	+	+/0	0, ↓	±	Low	Seizures at high dosages; ↑ dopamine in caudate and nucleus accumbens
SSRIs	+	±	0	0	0/+++	↓, ↑	++	Low	Insomnia, headache
SNRI:[a]									
Venlafaxine (37.5–250)	+++	+	—	±	+++/+++	↓, ↑	++	(Low)	↑ Blood pressure by several mmHg
Trazodone (50–600)	++?	+++	+++	0	0/++	↑↑	++	Low	Priapism risk
Nefazodone (100–600)	++?	++	0	0	0/+++	?	0	?	Increase in slow-wave sleep; liver toxicity
Mirtazapine (15–45)	++?	+++	—	—	++/+++	↑↑	0	?	α_2 blocker; increases NE and 5-HT release
MAOIs[b]	++?	+	+++	0	++/++	↑	++	High?	Off SSRIs by 1 month, diet to avoid tyramine, avoid opiates
RIMAs									
Moclobemide[c] (150–1,600)	+?	+	+	0	++/++	(↑)?	?	?	Not need diet? Less effective than MAOIs
Desipramine (75–300)	+++	+	+++	+	+++/0	↓,0	+	High	Switch rate higher than buproprion
Nortriptyline (50–150)	++	++	++	++	+++/+	↑	+	High	Possible invert U-type blood concentration clinical response
Lithium (600–1,500)	0	±	0	0	±	↑	0	Moderate	Especially for augmentation; may require thyroid supplementation
Lamotrigine	0	0	0	0	?	0	0	Low	Rash
ECT (6–12 treatments)	+	+	—	++ (atropine)	++/++	0	0	N/A	Anesthesia; seizure, memory loss

Note. NE, noradrenergic; SNRI, serotonin and noradrenaline reuptake inhibitor; RIMA, reversible inhibitor of monoamine oxidase type A; SSRI, selective serotonin reuptake inhibitor. Ratings: 0, none; ±, equivocal; +, minimal; ++, moderate; +++, marked or frequent; ↑, increase; ↓, decrease; −, no change or not present; ?, questionable or equivocal data. N/A, not applicable.

a. Duloxetine (Cymbalta) is also an SNRI.

b. Selegeline is a reversible inhibitor of MAO type B; its patch preparation has less need for the MAOI diet.

c. Not available in the United States, but is in Canada.

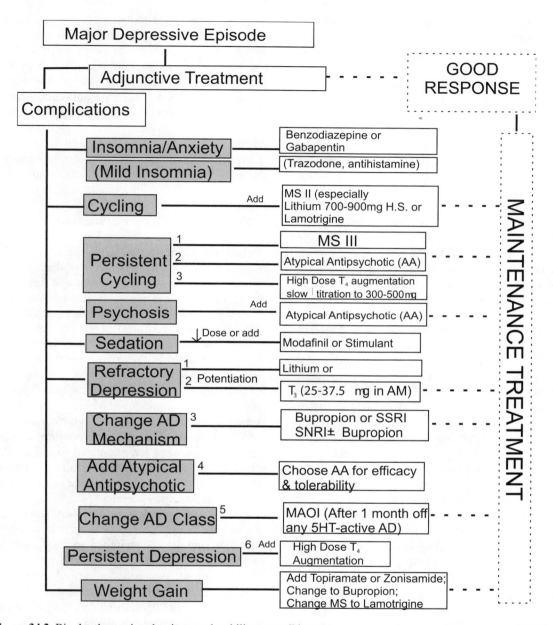

Figure 34.2 Bipolar depression despite mood stabilizer: possible treatment approaches to symptom targets. With the older traditional strategy of adding an antidepressant to a mood stabilizer in a non-rapidly cycling bipolar depressed patient, residual symptoms are still likely to be present. This figure suggests possible adjunctive appropriate approaches, depending on the type of symptoms that remain. Treating depression to complete remission is important for both enhanced functioning and prevention of subsequent depressive relapses. AD, antidepressant; MS, mood stabilizer; AA, antipsychotic.

slow-wave sleep, the deep form of sleep, and this has been documented with EEG studies (Idzikowski, Mills, & Glennard, 1986).

If one assumes that this patient was particularly vulnerable to switching into mania with the addition of any unimodal antidepressant (including second-generation antidepressants), what then might be the most appropriate treatment algorithm? Prior to the late 1990s and the availability of lamotrigine, one would have recommended the augmentation of lithium with a second mood stabilizer such as carbamazepine or valproate in an attempt to better prevent depressive recurrences and augment the antimanic effects of lithium (which in this case was not effective enough to prevent the antidepressant-induced switches into mania). If another depression still occurred, many physicians would then recommend the addition of an antidepressant (such as bupropion) to the two mood stabilizers for the acute treatment of depression, and then withdrawal of the antidepressant as soon as possible.

These current standards of care and recommendations are being reevaluated from a variety of perspectives. With the breakthrough depression in 1987 (as seen in Figure 34.1), many clinicians (Keck et al., 2004) would now recommend the adjunctive use of lamotrigine, given its evidence of both acute (Calabrese et al., 1999) and prophylactic antidepressant efficacy (Bowden et al., 2003; Calabrese, Bowden, et al., 2003). In a combination of two studies comparing the prophylactic efficacy of lithium, lamotrigine, and placebo, lithium was found to be superior to lamotrigine in the prevention of manic episodes, but lamotrigine was superior to lithium in the prevention of depressive episodes. Lamotrigine was FDA approved in the summer of 2003 for prevention of episodes of bipolar I illness (i.e., a depressed, mixed, or manic episode).

A patient such as this one might optimally have the best of both worlds with the use of lithium for the prophylaxis of bipolar I mania and lamotrigine for prevention of bipolar I depression (such as the depression that occurred during lithium prophylaxis in 1987). In the acute and long-term studies noted above, there

was no excess of lamotrigine-induced switching, as might be expected from an otherwise unimodal antidepressant. If one did not wish to use lamotrigine, augmentation with carbamazepine or valproate would also have merit prior to the use of a second-generation antidepressant if a breakthrough depression did occur. One could also consider an atypical (such as quetiapine) in an individual who was prone to switching, because quetiapine has both substantial antidepressant (Calabrese, Keck, et al., 2005) and antimanic effects. Other options are schematized in Figure 34.2.

Switch rates with three of the second-generation antidepressants—bupropion, sertraline, and venlafaxine—were assessed in patients in the Stanley Foundation Bipolar Network during acute clinical interventions for depression breaking through one or more mood stabilizers. Post, Altshuler, et al. (2001) reported switch rates on the first 64 patients given 95 acute antidepressant trials. In an extension of that study in 126 patients and 175 trials, the acute switch rate in the first 10 weeks on these drugs as a group was 9.1% into a hypomania (lasting at least 7 days) and another 9.1% incidence of hypomania (with some dysfunction) or a full-blown mania (Post, Leverich, et al., 2003). Nonresponders to one antidepressant were rerandomized to one of the others on a double-blind basis, and antidepressant responders were offered a year of continuation treatment ($N = 73$ trials).

During the intended year of antidepressant continuation, another 16.4% switched into hypomania, and 19.2% switched into hypomania (with some dysfunction) or full-blown mania. Whether these switch rates would have exceeded that of the expected course of illness cannot be inferred from these data because there was no placebo control in this study.

In the completed study, now unblinded, venlafaxine was more likely to be associated with switches into hypomania or mania than was bupropion or the SSRI sertraline (Leverich et al., 2006; Post, Altshuler, et al., 2006). Since venlafaxine acts on both norepinephrine and 5-HT, and sertraline only on 5-HT, the norepinephrine effects of venlafaxine may account for its higher switch rate than bupropion or a traditional SSRI. Rapid-cycling patients appeared to be at an increased risk of switching on venlafaxine.

Newer data from two studies of Altshuler and colleagues (2001, 2003) also indicate that if one remains well for at least 2 months on antidepressant augmentation of mood stabilizer treatment, the risk of relapsing into another depression is reduced if one remains on the antidepressant, compared with its discontinuation. Moreover, if the antidepressant is continued in this initial small subgroup of good responders, there is no increased incidence of switching into mania over the following year. Therefore, these data suggest that the older policy of removing antidepressants as soon as possible in those with bipolar depression (in order to avoid a potential switch into mania) may need to be reevaluated and reconsidered for the small subgroup (about 15%) who are placed on an antidepressant and respond well for 2 months without a switch into mania.

PRINCIPLES OF THE CASE	STRENGTH OF EVIDENCE
1. The unimodal antidepressants carry a risk of switching patients out of depression directly into hypomania or full-blown mania, as seen in this patient.	++
2. The switch into mania might occur independently of mechanism of action of the antidepressant, since either the noradrenergic (nortriptyline) or serotonergic (trazodone) drug carried this liability.	+
3. Lithium prophylaxis is likely to reduce the proclivity to manic switch, but, as seen here, does not appear capable of preventing it in all patients.	++
4. Adjunctive lamotrigine may be considered as an alternative to a unimodal antidepressant for breakthrough depression, as some studies report substantial acute antidepressant efficacy as well as efficacy in long-term prophylaxis without an increased risk of switching into mania.	++
5. If lamotrigine is used in this regard, one needs to proceed extremely slowly, for example, one 25-mg pill per day for the first 2 weeks, and then two pills for the next 2 weeks, and no greater increase than 25 mg per week thereafter, in order to avoid a severe, potentially life-threatening rash.	++
6. The incidence of this rash is not high with this slow titration of dose and is estimated to be 1 in 5,000 adults and 1 in 2,500 children.	++
7. When assessing the risk-to-benefit ratio of the addition of lamotrigine compared with other agents, one should be aware that the risk of hospitalization for aspirin-induced bleeding is thought to be in the same range or higher than that of a lamotrigine-induced severe rash.	++
8. One should avoid early use of first-generation tricyclic and tetracyclic antidepressants, because they appear to carry a greater switch liability than the newer antidepressants.	+
9. First-generation antidepressants compared with second-generation antidepressants also have more problematic side effects and are more toxic in overdose.	+++

10. Bipolar I and bipolar II depres-

sion can be incapacitating and should be treated with adjunctive mood stabilizers, atypical antipsychotics, or, in some instances, antidepressants (with an eye to balancing the various risk-to-benefit ratios).   ++

11. If the patient has rapid or recurrent cycling depressions, we would advocate the adjunctive use of a second or third mood stabilizer or an atypical antipsychotic over adding a unimodal antidepressant.   +

12. If the patient had a single sustained depressive episode, as in this individual, one might consider augmentation with the following:

    a. A mood stabilizer such as lamotrigine   +

    b. An atypical antipsychotic   +++

    c. Another mood-stabilizing anticonvulsant such as carbamazepine, oxcarbazepine, or valproate.   ±

    d. A second-generation antidepressant   +

TAKE-HOME MESSAGE

One should avoid the initial use of first-generation antidepressants (TCAs) in the treatment of breakthrough bipolar depression (even as adjunctive treatment to a mood stabilizer), because these agents appear to carry a greater switch liability, a more problematic side effects profile, and are more dangerous in overdose than the second-generation antidepressants (bupropion and SSRIs) or other treatment options.

35

Rapid Cycling Associated With Antidepressants and Loss of Responsiveness to ECT: A Sample Consultation About Alternative Treatment Approaches

CASE HISTORY

This patient was a middle-aged married female with a history of mild depression or dysthymia from 1956 to 1958, followed by a period of mania and more severe depressions with three serious suicide attempts in 1962, 1965, and 1968. Persistent continuous cycling occurred despite psychotherapy and acute interventions with antipsychotics and antidepressants. In 1975 she reentered therapy and was treated with lithium in conjunction with a variety of antidepressants. These antidepressants included the tricyclics imipramine and amitriptyline, the monoamine oxidase inhibitors isocarboxazid and phenelzine, and the atypical antidepressants amoxapine and trazodone. Despite concurrent treatment with lithium, these antidepressants appeared to be associated with a more rapid pattern of cycling than experienced at any time previously (Figure 35.1, middle line).

One might have assumed that this was a natural evolution in her course of illness, except for the fact that during her NIMH admission, when she was initially treated with placebo and then carbamazepine and lithium, the depressions returned to the longer durations that were characteristic of 1959 and 1970. She also experienced a well interval of several months between episodes. When she was again cotreated with tranylcypromine, it was associated with a reinduction of her more rapid cycling pattern in 1985 (Figure 35.2).

The first ECT treatment was dramatically effective in ending her severe depression. Several more ECT treatments were combined to treat her ensuing hypomania. The patient was discharged with the recommendation of pursuing ECT prophylaxis. This prophylaxis was initiated approximately once per week when she returned to New York City but was not successful in preventing the onset of a full depression. The patient again required hospitalization in New York and had a new course of eight ECT treatments. However, upon failing to show substantial improvement, the patient was started on another antidepressant (nomifensine) with a novel mechanism of action targeted to the dopamine reuptake system (this drug was subsequently removed from the market). Her depression remained severe and she succumbed to bipolar depressive illness, committing suicide. She returned to the

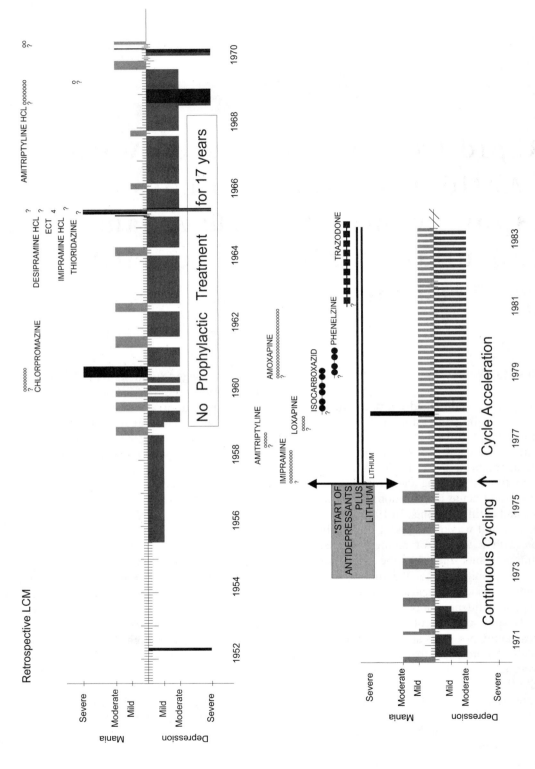

Figure 35.1 Antidepressant-related cycle acceleration despite concurrent lithium treatment. The patient showed a slow, relatively stable cycle frequency on no medications, but in 1975, with the onset of more continuous antidepressant medication (in concert with lithium prophylaxis), the patient showed a much more rapid cycling pattern. This slowed again during her NIMH admission (see Figure 35.2) when she was treated with lithium and carbamazepine with only a partial response. The patient had a good acute response to ECT at the NIMH, but then failed to rerespond to ECT.

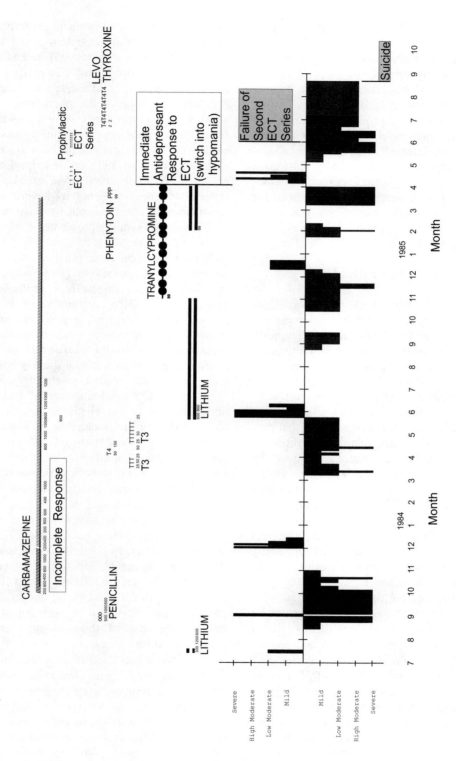

Figure 35.2 Partial response to carbamazepine (several months well between less severe depressive episodes), but failure of adjunctive lithium and MAOI or prophylactic ECT.

most lethal of the three ways she had previously tried to kill herself.

This patient was a warm, loving, caring person who heroically struggled with her recurrent bipolar disorder that occurred almost continuously over the course of her lifetime. During her depressions she was profoundly anergic and showed prominent psychomotor slowing, yet was anxious and internally agitated. The moderate manias observed at the NIMH showed a classical picture of euphoric hypomania characterized by increased energy, decreased need for sleep, increased social interactions, and intrusiveness and overexuberance.

BACKGROUND LITERATURE

Kukopoulos et al. (1980) highlighted a substantial case series suggesting that antidepressants could be associated with an increased rapidity of cycling or a conversion to a more continuous cyclic pattern in a subgroup of patients. One group that was particularly likely to show cycle acceleration was characterized by the patient illustrated, that is, the continuous cycling pattern without a well interval. It also appears that rapidly cycling patients are particularly prone to this issue of cycle acceleration, as noted by Wehr, Sack, Rosenthal, and Cowdry (1988), where systematic treatment with antidepressants and their withdrawal led to increased rapidity of cycling (on an antidepressant) and slower cycling in the off-antidepressant period. In several of his patients this was documented repeatedly in an on (drug)-off (placebo)-on design, clearly confirming the phenomenon.

In our retrospective case series of patients referred and admitted to the NIMH (Altshuler et al., 1995), we found evidence of this type of convincing cycle acceleration on antidepressants and a slowing during their discontinuation in only a small subgroup of 9 out of 35 patients (26%). Thus, the phenomenon is not a regular occurrence associated with antidepressant treatment (Kupfer, Carpenter, & Frank, 1988) but does appear to be a robust phenomenon in some individuals such as this patient. In these instances, as in her case, lithium and other mood stabilizers are not always sufficient to hold back this increased rapidity of cycling.

When Altshuler et al. (1995) looked for predictors of who might show this pattern of antidepressant-induced cycle acceleration, they found a higher incidence of the phenomenon in patients who had previously shown a switch into mania during treatment with antidepressants, as evidenced by this patient in 1964 on desipramine and again in 1970 on amitriptyline. Stoll et al. (1994) observed that antidepressant-related switches were not as severe as those spontaneously observed, but we have seen full-blown manias on antidepressants on many occasions (see Figure 34.1).

How might one conceptualize this process? In previous chapters, we have discussed the possibility that cycling in bipolar illness could relate to the relative predominance of factors associated with depression that are part of its primary pathophysiology (such as increased secretion of corticotropin-releasing factor and attendant hypercortisolemia), whereas periods of euthymia or hypomania might be associated with the relative predominance of endogenous antidepressant factors (such as increased thyrotropin-releasing hormone; Post & Weiss, 1992, 1996). To the extent that medications exerting potent exogenous antidepressant effects add together with the endogenous antidepressant ones (i.e., the body's own natural adaptive process) normally associated with the swing out of a depression, the two might combine to shorten the period of depression, as occurred in 1975 in this patient. However, in some instances, such as in the patient illustrated, this period of euthymia or hypomania may be relatively short lived and associated with the rapid swing into the next depressive episode, which is again of shortened duration because of the antidepressant treatment, and so on.

The crucial mechanisms involved in antidepressant-induced cycle acceleration are not known, but would appear to be an element common to many different antidepressants. Others have postulated that it is the noradrenergic components of the drug, such as desmethylimipramine, that are associated with the switch process, since those with higher levels of the norepinephrine metabolite 3-methoxy-4-hydroxy-phenylglycol in the urine appear to switch faster upon antidepressant treatment (Zis, Cowdry, Wehr, Muscettola, & Goodwin, 1979).

A potential test of this hypothesis would be to examine the switch and cycle acceleration rates on the SSRIs versus the selective norepinephrine reuptake inhibitor (SNRI) venlafaxine. This latter drug inhibits the reuptake of both norepinephrine and serotonin, and to the extent that noradrenergic mechanisms were involved in the switch process, one would postulate that there would be a higher incidence of switch and cycle acceleration on venlafaxine compared with the pure serotonin-selectives such as fluoxetine, paroxetine, sertraline, and fluvoxamine. Recent data of Vieta, Martinez-Aran, et al. (2002), Leverich, Altshuler, et al. (2006), and Post, Altshuler, et al. (2006) suggest that this is the case and that venlafaxine has a higher switch rate than the SSRIs (paroxetine or sertraline) or bupropion.

HYPOTHETICAL PSYCHOPHARMACOTHERAPEUTIC CONSULTATION IN 2007

Should a patient such as this arrive in one's office or in the hospital, a great many more options would be available in 2007 compared with the available treatments in 1985. Although a number of principles and practicalities dealing with complex combination treatment are spelled out in other chapters in this book, it may be useful for the clinician and patient to see what a more current consultation focused on this patient and her case history might have looked like.

Dear Treating Physician:

Thank you very much for the opportunity to see this patient in consultation. She has had an almost 30-year history of continuous cycling bipolar I illness, with three serious suicide attempts during periods of profound depression. Treatment initiated in 1975 with lithium plus a variety of antidepressants was associated with a lesser severity of mania and depression, but with markedly increased cycle acceleration and an overall Clinical Global Impression score of 3 (only minimally improved; grade C).

During an extended hospitalization on a clinical research unit, she experienced more time euthymic than at any previous time in her recent memory, but her illness was still punctuated with moderate to severe depressions and hypomanias despite carbamazepine monotherapy and its augmentation with lithium and tranylcypromine. She had a dramatic response to the first ECT treatment, and several other ECTs were continued in order to moderate her hypomania. She was discharged euthymic and on intended prophylactic ECT, but her mood plummeted and she subsequently failed to respond to a course of bilateral ECT. An attempt to treat her with a novel dopamine reuptake-blocking antidepressant (nomifensine, which is no longer on the market) did not yield impressive clinical effects.

Given this history of inadequate treatment response, I would suggest consideration of the following:

A. Employ a general strategy of increasing the numbers of mood stabilizers in hopes that they convey sufficient anticycling and antidepressant effects to avoid the use of antidepressants.

1. In the first phase of treatment I would reinitiate treatment with lithium because this drug, in conjunction with antidepressants, appeared to prevent the occurrence of her most severe depressions, and for more than 8 years on the drug she made no further suicide attempts. Moreover, as similar bipolar depressed patients have a variety of physiological and biochemical evidence of frontal lobe hypofunction and limbic dysfunction based on both neural and glial deficits, I would reinitiate lithium treatment even in light of its previous inadequate efficacy in this patient because of its newly recognized neurotrophic and neuroprotective effects on both neurons and glia. Lithium increases brain-derived neurotrophic factor (BDNF) and the anti-cell-death (apoptosis) factor Bcl-2, inhibits cell death factors such as Bax and p53 (in cell culture), increases neurogenesis in vivo, and in patients increases markers of neuronal integrity, such as N-acetyl-aspartate as measured on magnetic resonance spectroscopy, and increases brain grey matter volume as measured on magnetic resonance imaging.

2. Almost coincidentally with this approach, I would initiate low-dose lamotrigine treatment (25 mg/day for 2 weeks) with a very slow titration (in hopes of avoiding a severe rash) toward efficacy or a target dose of about 200 mg/day in light of new data on its useful antidepressant preventive effects (exceeding those of lithium and placebo).

3. I would add 1 mg/day of folate for a variety

of rationales, but particularly in light of data on folate's ability to enhance lithium prophylaxis and facilitate antidepressant effects (Coppen et al., 1986; 2000).

4. I would also add 25 μg of T₃ in the A.M. (and increase this to 37.5 μg in the absence of clinical efficacy or side effects) for antidepressant acceleration and potentiation.

B. If the above regimen is insufficient, I would suggest consideration of adding an atypical antipsychotic to the regimen in light of their recent evidence of antimanic and, in some instances, antidepressant efficacy as well. Depending on your and the patient's preference, I would suggest proceeding with either B1 or B2.

1. Consider adding quetiapine h.s. (at night). Calabrese and associates (2006) presented striking antidepressant data on quetiapine (300 or 600 mg/day) compared with placebo. Mood, anxiety, and sleep were all highly significantly improved versus placebo from Week 1 onward. If response is not complete, one might consider ziprasidone in the A.M. (since it is somewhat activating for some individuals).

2. Initiating treatment with very low dose aripiprazole (2.5–5 mg/day to avoid akathisia and activation) could also be considered or used in place of B1 if that was tried but not tolerated. A series of studies have shown that aripiprazole has acute and preventive antimanic effects, and its partial agonist effects at dopamine D₁, D₂, D₃, and serotonin 5HT₁ₐ receptors, as well as full antagonism of 5-HT₂ receptors, suggest a variety of mechanisms that could also convey antidepressant effects, as now seen in unipolar depression. McElroy, Suppes, et al. (2007) have seen good antidepressant effects in open add-on studies. Nickel et al. (2006) also reported marked antianxiety and antidepressant effects compared to placebo in patients with borderline personality disorder.

C. If the above regimen were insufficient, I would suggest considering adding valproate (all h.s. with 250 mg and increasing the dose until efficacy, side effects, or a target dose of about 1,500 mg is achieved). Prior to or coincident with the initiation of valproate, I suggest lowering the dose of lamotrigine by one half in light of valproate's ability to double the blood levels of lamotrigine and accordingly increase the risk of a lamotrigine-related severe rash.

D. Should severe depressions continue to break through the above regimens, I would suggest that the patient consider augmenting these approaches with a single night of sleep deprivation to help terminate the depressive episode earlier than otherwise expected. The sleep deprivation can be followed by a circadian phase advance such that hours of sleep are initiated on the sleep depriva-

tion day at 5 P.M. to 1 A.M. (awakening with an alarm clock), 6 P.M. to 2 A.M. the next day, 7 P.M. to 3 A.M. the next, and so on, until the patient's normal sleep-wake cycle is achieved. This has been reported to help hold the sleep deprivation-induced mood improvement in some patients, along with concurrent treatment with lithium.

1. If B and C were insufficient to stabilize mood and prevent depressive recurrences, I would suggest considering initiating treatment with: a) the addition of the dopamine active agent bupropion; if this is only partially effective, one might also consider b) the dual serotonin and norepinephrine reuptake inhibitor venlafaxine despite its increased propensity for manic switching. This would enhance all three neurotransmitter amine systems (DA, NE, 5-HT) in an attempt to exert maximum antidepressant effects (similar to those achieved by monoamine oxidase inhibitors, which act on all three neurotransmitter amine systems via a different mechanism). Hopefully, the several different types of mood stabilizers and atypical antipsychotics would be sufficient to avoid cycle acceleration on this combination.

2. Supplemental rTMS could also be considered if available.

3. One might also consider h.s. doses of gabapentin or clonazepam should the patient continue to experience periods of breakthrough anxiety or insomnia.

E. If cycling persists, one might discontinue T3, and consider high dose T4 (in the range of 200 to 400 ug/day arrived at extremely slowly) as suggested Bauer and Whybrow (1990) and Bauer et al. (2001; 2005).

F. If the above regimens are insufficient, I would suggest considering vagus nerve stimulation (VNS) device implantation according to the studies of Rush, George, Marangell, and colleagues.

G. If VNS were not available, one might reconsider a new trial of high-intensity, ultrabrief pulse right unilateral ECT in conjunction with clozapine pharmacoprophylaxis in an attempt to provide both an alternative mode of mood stabilization and a mechanism for lowering the ECT seizure threshold, which tends to increase with each ECT treatment and make it progressively more difficult to induce the next seizure. Should the patient have untoward degrees of weight gain during clozapine continuation treatment, one might also consider augmenting it with topiramate or zonisamide in order to (1) facilitate weight loss; (2) prevent clozapine-related seizures that are common on high doses; and (3) potentially also provide augmenting effects for mood stabilization.

H. I would encourage the patient to continue nightly charting of mood in order to help optimize and tailor what might become a very complex pharmacological regimen and to monitor and minimize side effects.

I. I would also suggest engaging the patient in either cognitive behavior therapy or existential psychotherapy focused on making maximum use of her euthymic intervals (if she is not eventually able to achieve and sustain a full remission).

My very best wishes for the rapid and sustained mood improvement in this wonderful individual who has struggled heroically with her treatment-refractory bipolar illness. Despite this long and difficult history, I am confident that further improvement will be achieved with some of the therapeutic approaches recommended here or others that you and she consider as alternatives.

Sincerely,
RMP, MD

P.S. (to the treating physician)

I have provided the patient with a chart that outlines some of the potential mechanisms of action of the treatments recommended and have given her several personal calendars containing a compact form of the NIMH-LCM so that she can conveniently proceed with nightly mood charting along with sleep, medications, and side effects. She has a copy of these written recommendations, and I have also given her an extra one for her psychotherapist. The patient's husband has been wonderfully supportive throughout, and periodic meetings that include him may also be of further assistance.

PRINCIPLES OF THE CASE

STRENGTH OF EVIDENCE

1. Antidepressants may precipitate switches into mania in vulnerable individuals. ++

2. Antidepressants may be associated with cycle acceleration. If the cycling again slows when the drug is removed, a causal link is likely. +++

3. Lithium and other mood stabilizers in monotherapy are not always sufficient to hold back switches or cycle acceleration. ++

4. Several mood stabilizers in combination may help prevent

this process, but this remains to be directly tested. +

5. ECT can be associated with a postdepression-related hypomania and loss of antidepressant increases as a function of the number of weeks following the end of a series. ++

6. The evidence for prophylactic effects of ECT in bipolar illness is based only on very small, uncontrolled case series, and remains to be systematically demonstrated. ±

7. In unipolar depression, the efficacy of prophylactic ECT did not exceed that of lithium plus nortriptyline. ++

8. Tolerance can develop even to the effects of ECT, as suggested by the failure to respond to a new series in this patient and others. +

9. This patient who died in 1985 might have responded to one of the many new approaches outlined in subsequent chapters, including lamotrigine, atypical antipsychotics, nimodipine, valproate, or hypermetabolic doses of T_4, in combination with antidepressants and as described in detail in the hypothetical consultation noted above. +

TAKE-HOME MESSAGE

Antidepressants, even when added to a mood stabilizer, are sometimes associated with cycle acceleration. Whereas 20 years ago there were few treatment options for the lithium- and antidepressant-nonresponsive patient, a wealth of alternative possibilities now exist and should be systematically explored.

36

A Potential Liability of Unimodal Antidepressants in Bipolar Depression: Cycle Acceleration and Conversion to Ultradian Cycling

CASE HISTORY

Previous chapters discussed antidepressants and how they can be associated with a switch into acute mania (Chapter 34), and cycle acceleration and continuous cycling (Chapter 35). This patient illustrates the coincident occurrence of fluoxetine treatment and an extremely fast pattern of multiple switches in a single day (i.e., ultradian cycling). This patient had a clear bipolar II history, although most of the episodes were only mild to moderate and were graphed with dotted lines to indicate that the exact temporal placement of the episode could not be verified by outside records (Figure 36.1). These periods of more mild to moderate depression alternated with distinct periods of hypomania that were usually not dysfunctional.

The patient did have distinct major depressions around age 13 and again around age 28 (in 1971), around age 35 (in 1977), and around age 42 (in 1985). However, upon treatment with alprazolam in 1979, a major manic episode was induced.

Alprazolam is a short-acting triazolo-1, 4-benzodiazepine analog that is thought to have more prominent antidepressant effects than other high-potency benzodiazepines such as clonaze-

pam and lorazepam. Just prior to this alprazolam-related switch into mania, the patient experienced some ultrarapid cycling (not illustrated) prior to entering the more sustained depression in 1978. She also reported periods of ultradian cycling in 1964 and in 1969 between mild depression and mild mania. These spontaneous occurrences raised the question as to whether the persistent pattern of ultradian cycling observed upon fluoxetine administration was directly drug related or merely a coincidental course-of-illness phenomenon. However, the prior treatment with the weaker antidepressant trazodone for insomnia and mild depression did not appear associated with such a transition in the course of illness.

Treatment with fluoxetine did appear, at least temporally, closely linked to the transition to ultradian cycling (Figure 36.1). The derivation of the word *ultradian* is *ultra* (or *very much*) and -*dian* (or *within a day*), and this patient experienced an average of three to five distinct mood shifts within a day. These shifts typically ranged from tearful, immobilizing depression to either euphoric (pleasant) or dysphoric (unpleasant) hypomania.

As indicated in Chapter 33, this new phase of illness completely incapacitated the patient.

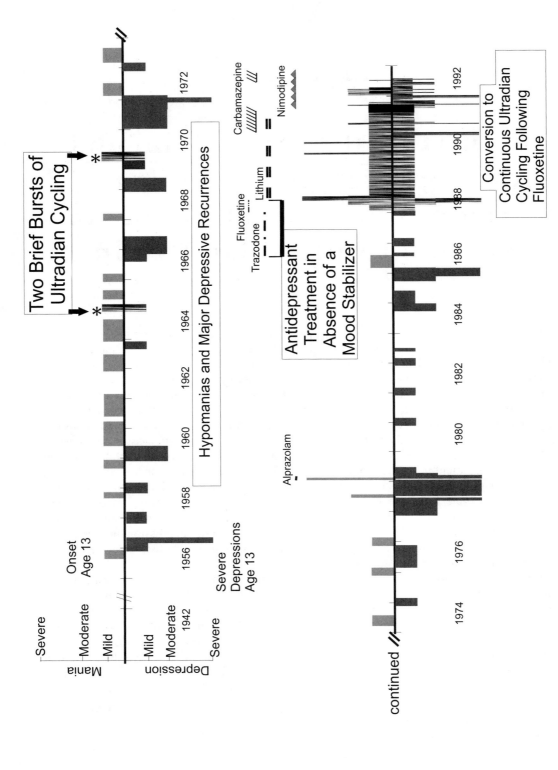

Figure 36.1 Initiation of sustained ultradian cycling during unopposed antidepressant treatment in a bipolar II female. This figure shows the initial course of illness of the patient discussed in Chapter 33 on response to L-type calcium channel blockers. Here we highlight the impact of using antidepressants, in the absence of a mood stabilizer, in the potential destabilization of the patient's illness in late 1987 following treatment with fluoxetine (Prozac). The patient began ultra-ultra rapid (ultradian) cycling. However, two brief bursts of ultradian cycling occurred in 1964 and 1969 in the absence of antidepressant treatment.

Her mood switched dramatically multiple times within a day from despondency and inability to function to a hyperactive state with a flight of ideas and an inability to follow through effectively in work or social situations. As noted above, the quality of the hypomanias could differ considerably, ranging from euphoric (subjectively seen by the patient as quite positive) or dysphoric with much anxiety, irritability, and an uncomfortable sense of pressure and being driven (subjectively viewed by the patient as very uncomfortable). With the transition to this phase of ultradian cycling, she was unable to work in her profession as a teacher and in her avocation as an artist.

BACKGROUND LITERATURE

This patient illustrates one of the most feared scenarios in the use of unimodal antidepressants in bipolar I or bipolar II depressed patients without the coverage of a concomitant mood stabilizer. Not only is there a potential risk of induction of mania (as illustrated in Chapter 34) and rapid continuous cycling (Chapter 35), but in this case, continuous, chaotic, and immobilizing ultradian cycling. This single case example is inconsistent with observations of Amsterdam and associates (1998; Amsterdam & Garcia-Espana, 2000) suggesting that the use of fluoxetine or venlafaxine alone in two studies of a mixed population of depressed patients (including some bipolar II patients but without a prior rapid cycling course) was not associated with manic inductions or rapid cycling. How often one can safely use such antidepressants without coverage by mood stabilizers is not known, but such an approach is generally considered inadequate treatment because of the risks of ultradian cycling (illustrated here) or of manic switching and cycle acceleration illustrated in the two previous chapters.

Kukopulos et al. (1980) discussed his patient series in which a substantial group of patients did convert to continuous cycling upon administration of antidepressants. In his experience, such prior antidepressant treatment and continuous cycling also rendered patients less likely to

respond to mood stabilizers thereafter. This patient would conform to that subgroup because she was subsequently an inadequate lithium responder, even though fluoxetine had been discontinued.

In contrast to the findings in the series of Kukopulos et al. (1980) and the last several chapters, the NIMH Collaborative Group found that use of adjunctive antidepressants (i.e., when added to a mood stabilizer) was no more likely to be associated with switches or cycle acceleration than their absence (Coryell et al., 2003). While the controversy continues, what is clearly agreed upon now and in the guidelines for treatment of patients with bipolar depression is that antidepressants, if they are used, should be given with concomitant mood stabilizer treatment. Whether the use of mood stabilizers would have prevented the malignant progression to ultradian cycling in this individual can only be speculated. It is also of interest that this patient had the initiation of this phase of cycling in the perimenopausal period.

However, we have seen ultradian cycling in men and women of all ages. Almost 20% of the outpatients in the Stanley Foundation Bipolar Network (SFBN, now called the Bipolar Collaborative Network, BCN) reported ultradian cycling, and this was subsequently confirmed in prospective clinical observations and clinician ratings on the LCM in the majority of these patients despite naturalistic treatment (Post, Denicoff, et al., 2003). In this patient, ultradian cycling occurred during treatment with fluoxetine, but it persisted after fluoxetine discontinuation and the institution of lithium prophylaxis. Causal relationships thus cannot be inferred from this case. However, this patient raises the question of whether such an illness transition, once triggered, may no longer require the inducing agent. This process may be thought of as similar to the triggering of episodes of postpartum depression or mania as the first episode of bipolar illness when, in the absence of further endocrine triggers, the illness continues to recur spontaneously.

Thus, while controversy continues about the role of antidepressants even as adjunctive treatment to mood stabilizers (Post Altshuler, et al.,

2006), this patient illustrates the potential hazards of proceeding with treatment with antidepressants alone. The persistence of the fluoxetine-related ultradian cycling in this patient also contrasts with observations that antidepressant-induced cycle acceleration can be attenuated during periods off the drug and then exacerbated again when the antidepressant is reinstituted (Wehr & Goodwin, 1987). In the experience of Wehr and associates (1988), restabilization has usually required the discontinuation of antidepressants. However, in our case example, antidepressant discontinuation was clearly not sufficient, because both lithium alone and lithium in conjunction with carbamazepine were unsuccessful in breaking this pattern of ultradian cycling (Chapter 33).

When we first observed this patient and other patients with ultradian cycling patterns, we thought it was highly unusual and wondered whether it was associated with the presence of a concurrent personality disorder, such as borderline personality disorder, where highly unstable moods are typical. However, this proved not to be the case in the current patient (here and Chapter 33) and in many others whom we carefully assessed (Chapter 2). Ultradian cycling can clearly occur in patients with typical bipolar disorder and no comorbid personality disorder, and it appears to represent a new stage in illness progression based on both the rapidity of the switching and general treatment resistance (Kramlinger & Post, 1996).

In our most recent data, we found that a very substantial group of patients reported such ultradian cycling. Although it is possible that this pattern had previously existed but was simply overlooked, it appears more likely that this pattern was highly unusual some 20 to 30 years ago, but now is becoming relatively common. The reason for this apparent increased incidence of ultradian cycling is not known, but now that it has been identified in one in five patients with bipolar illness, the issue can be more systematically examined.

One can speculate about whether the emergence of ultradian cycling is just another manifestation of the cohort effect. In each birth cohort (decade) since World War I there is: (a) an increased prevalence of unipolar and bipolar affective illness in the population (Gershon, Hamovit, Guroff, & Nurnberger, 1987; Lange & McInnis, 2002; Macedo et al., 1999; Nylander, Engstrom, Chotai, Wahlstrom, & Adolfsson, 1994; Wickramaratne, Weissman, Leaf, & Holford, 1989), and also (b) an earlier age of onset of the illness. Perhaps accompanying these aspects of the cohort effect are (c) more rapid cycling, (d) the emergence of ultradian cycling, (e) greater degrees of treatment resistance, and (f) increased need for complex combination treatment (Frye, Ketter, Leverich, et al., 2000). While (a) and (b) have been clearly documented, it is only clinical impression that supports the other four (c–f) possibilities.

A meta-analysis confirms that first-generation antidepressants are more likely to be associated with a switch into mania or hypomania than the second-generation drugs (Gijsman et al., 2004). This finding, in conjunction with the more problematic side effect profiles of most first-generation drugs and their greater lethality and overdose, should result in the first (and almost exclusive) use of second-generation antidepressants in the treatment of bipolar patients.

Other risk factors for antidepressant-related switching include younger age (Martin et al., 2004, prior substance abuse (Goldberg & Whiteside, 2000), and a history of rapid cycling in the previous year. As noted in the previous chapters, antidepressants with selective or potent effects in blocking norepinehrine reuptake may have an increased switch risk (Vieta, Martinez-Aran, et al., 2002, Leverich et al., 2006; Post, Altshuler, et al., 2006). Patients with mixed depression (depression with racing thoughts and other minor hypomanic symptoms) may also be at higher risk of switching on antidepressants than those with psychomotor slowing (Frye et al. 2006).

PRINCIPLES OF THE CASE	STRENGTH OF EVIDENCE
1. Construction of a retrospective mood chart clearly helps eluci-	

date a bipolar II diagnosis so
that appropriate treatment can
be rendered.   ++

2. This patient was virtually untreated (except with alprazolam in 1979) for 30 years after
her first clear hypomanic
symptoms and first severe major depression at age 13 in
1956.   +

3. As opposed to the other high-
potency anticonvulsant benzodiazepines such as clonazepam
and lorazepam, alprazolam appears to carry an extra liability
of switching patients into ma-
nia.   ++

4. Alprazolam also has a short
half-life and is often associated after 4–5 hours with wear-
ing-off related increases in
anxiety. Thus, alprazolam
should be relatively avoided in
bipolar illness and preference
given to the longer-acting
high-potency benzodiazepines
for this reason and that in (3)
above.   ++

5. This patient represents the occurrence of an all-too-common
long gap in arriving at an appropriate bipolar diagnosis.
She had the onset of a hypomania and major depressive
episode at age 13 (in 1956) associated with clear periods of
hypomania thereafter. Yet her
first treatment with lithium did
not occur until 1988. While
this duration of delay from illness onset to first treatment is
at the extreme end of the continuum, in our outpatients in
the BCN we found this delay
was on the average longest
(16 years) in those with childhood onset prior to age 13 and
still 12 years in those with on-

sets prior to age 19. In contrast, the delay was shortest
(2.5 years) in adults with onset after age 30 (Leverich et
al., 2007).   +++

6. Therefore, much education
and public health effort should
be directed at the earlier treatment of this illness (Post and
Kowatch, 2006).   +++

7. Perhaps early intervention
would have prevented the
seven episodes of major depression prior to 1986 and the
associated suffering.   +

8. Patients with major depression
should be carefully evaluated
for a history of hypomania because 30–40% of presumptive
unipolar depressed patients
will be found to have bipolar
disorder upon closer examination. The easiest screening
question is; "Have you ever
had a period of increased energy and deceased need for
sleep?" This will include those
with a history of dysphoric mania which is particularly prominent in women (Suppes et al.,
2006).   +++

9. The diagnosis of bipolar II depression could readily have
been made in this patient,
even with the most casual history taking. All too often, unfortunately, such patients are
not appropriately diagnosed
and thus are improperly
treated.   ++

10. If a patient checks off more
than seven boxes as positive
on the Mood Disorder Questionnaire (MDQ; Calabrese,
Hirschfeld, et al., 2003;
Hirschfeld, Calabrese, et al.,
2003; Hirschfeld, Holzer, et
al., 2003; Hirschfeld, Wil-

liams, et al., 2000; see Appendix 6), one should further explore the diagnostic criteria, consider getting appropriate consultation on the diagnosis of bipolar illness and obtain appropriate treatment if indicated.   ++

11. Although there is likely a small subgroup of patients with nonrapid-cycling illness who are represented in the experience of Amsterdam (Amsterdam et al., 1998; Amsterdam & Garcia-Espana, 2000) and the initial positive response of the patient illustrated in Chapter 37 to antidepressant monotherapy, it is difficult to predict which patients may show much more deleterious consequences of such treatment, such as induction of mania, rapid cycling, or in this instance, incapacitating ultradian cycling.   ++

12. Once the transition to a pattern of ultradian cycling has occurred, it may take a considerable period of time and the complexity of a combination treatment regime in order to reachieve mood stability.   +

13. This patient failed to respond adequately to lithium monotherapy and lithium in combination with carbamazepine, but showed a consistent partial response to the dihydropyridine L-type calcium channel blocker nimodipine, which

was further augmented by carbamazepine. This combination allowed her to return to active functioning in her usual social and occupational roles (Chapter 33).   +

14. Whether the easier-to-use amlodipine, which is also a dihydropyridine L-type calcium channel blocker, shares the same mood-stabilizing properties as nimodipine remains to be studied.   ±

15. In a survey of more than 85,000 households by Hirschfeld, Holzer, et al. (2003), the vast majority of the patients who had screened positive on the MDQ had not been diagnosed as bipolar in the community. Even more disappointingly, the small minority who did receive a bipolar diagnosis in the community were treated improperly, like this patient, with an antidepressant without a mood stabilizer.   +++

TAKE-HOME MESSAGE

One should take a careful illness history in a patient with presumptive unipolar depression to discover possible symptoms of bipolar II (hypomania lasting greater than 4 days) or bipolar NOS (hypomania lasting less than 4 days) when instituting treatment for depression, because one should avoid the use of unimodal antidepressants without a mood stabilizer in bipolar disorder because of the risks, illustrated here, of marked cycle acceleration.

37

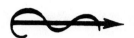

Antidepressant Discontinuation-Induced Refractoriness

CASE HISTORY

This patient was a female in her mid-20s with a history of moderate to severe recurrent unipolar depressions associated with marked psychomotor retardation and brief periods of euphoric or dysphoric hypomania. In 1989, these recurrent depressions of moderate severity were treated with trazodone (150 mg/day), achieving a complete remission for approximately 4 months, after which the patient discontinued treatment (Figure 37.1). She then had several low-level intermittent depressive bursts prior to more rapid cycling and sustained moderate to severe depressions that were again responsive, but at a slower rate, to trazodone (150 mg/day).

After the conventionally prescribed 7 to 9 months of continuation therapy typically recommended for unipolar depression, the patient again discontinued treatment, and in the subsequent year had increasingly rapid recurrences of minor to moderate depression, culminating in 1993 with a more sustained and severe recurrent depressive picture.

However, on this third occasion, the patient failed to respond to trazodone at the previous doses, and also at doses twice as high (300 mg/day) as those that were previously effective. Because of the failure of trazodone, other agents were used including nortriptyline (which appeared to be associated with increased cycle acceleration, which decreased upon discontinuation of this drug on admission), lithium carbon-

ate (which was without effect), and valproate (which was also without effect).

The patient's course at the NIMH (not illustrated) was characterized by repeated episodes of mild to moderate depression that did not respond adequately to carbamazepine, but did respond to the combination of nimodipine and carbamazepine, before the patient began to show breakthrough episodes. These breakthrough episodes responded to the addition of bupropion along with the combination of nimodipine and carbamazepine, which led to a complete remission of symptoms for about 1 month. Upon recurrence of moderate to severe depression, nimodipine and bupropion were discontinued and venlafaxine was added to carbamazepine without effect. Trazodone was explored for the fourth time, this time in combination with carbamazepine and venlafaxine, but was again without effect.

At this point, the patient entered our placebo-controlled comparative trial of lamotrigine, gabapentin, and placebo (Chapters 25 and 26) and showed good partial responses to both agents, but then developed an episode of thyroiditis with first hyperthyroidism and then hypothyroidism during treatment with gabapentin. After resolution of her thyroid problems and in light of the good response to lamotrigine and partial response to gabapentin, the patient was restarted on these agents in a response confirmation mode and then was discharged on the combination of lamotrigine, gabapentin, and a very low dose of

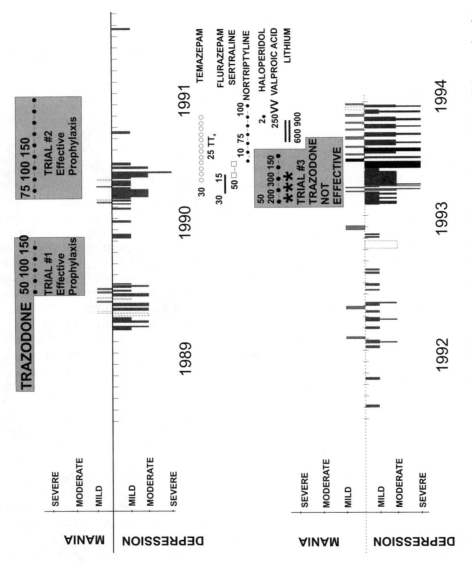

Figure 37.1 Antidepressant discontinuation-induced refractoriness in a bipolar II depressed patient whose recurrent depressions responded rapidly to the first course of antidepressant treatment with trazodone in 1989, a little bit more slowly to the second course of treatment in 1990, but not at all to treatment at the previous doses and at higher doses on the third occasion in 1993. This patient thus appears to be one of a subset of patients in whom repeated discontinuation of effective treatment (such as lithium or here even an antidepressant) results in further breakthrough episodes that are no longer responsive to the originally effective drug. She subsequently responded well to the combination of lamotrigine and gabapentin.

lithium. She continued to do very well for the next 10 years (and has not stopped her medication).

One can only wonder about the potential course of this patient's illness had she remained on the first or second round of treatment with trazodone, which appeared sufficient to maintain a complete remission. Obviously, in retrospect, the suggestion would have been to remain on medications that appear to be highly effective in order to avoid both the likelihood of further episodes and the possibility of failing to rerespond (as seen here).

BACKGROUND LITERATURE

Clinical Considerations About Treatment-Related Discontinuation-Induced Nonresponsiveness

We should emphasize that the initial treatment of this patient represents an exception to standard practice. Patients with bipolar II illness, according to most treatment guidelines, should not be treated with antidepressants without a mood stabilizer. We nonetheless present this patient to emphasize the point that discontinuation of an effective prophylactic medicine in the recurrent affective disorders is not without risk, even when it was just an antidepressant in this instance. This risk includes not only the highly likely recurrence of new episodes, but the less likely possibility of failure to rerespond to the previously effective agent. While the failure to rerespond does not occur in a high percentage of patients, it does in some and should be part of the information provided to patients in their consideration of whether or not they wish to maintain their effective prophylactic regimen for the long term.

The treatment algorithm for reestablishing efficacy in the face of such discontinuation-induced refractoriness to the initial agent is not well established. However, we would suggest a sequential clinical trials approach to this problem, as illustrated in the case of the current patient. After achieving two periods of wellness with this antidepressant, following the second

drug discontinuation, improvement did not occur on a third or fourth occasion. Moreover, the illness appeared to have evolved into a more severe form and did not readily respond to the use of multiple mood stabilizer and antidepressant interventions alone and in combination.

Conventional wisdom, and most formal treatment guidelines for patients with unipolar recurrent illness, state that after two or three prior episodes, one should consider long-term prophylaxis with antidepressants. The second patient's course of illness, depicted in Figure 37.2 showed recurrent major depression emerging from a chronic low-level depression (or dysthymic baseline). Following a year of complete remission, she relapsed upon stopping her MAOI and did not respond to this type of drug again in either 1978 or 1994 and showed a highly treatment-refractory course thereafter. One can only wonder whether this patient would have remained well in the long term if she had decided to continue her first MAOI treatment. In bipolar illness, one might consider the initiation of long-term prophylaxis with a mood stabilizer (rather than an antidepressant) after only the first or second episode according to most clinical and academic guidelines (Post, Speer, & Leverich, 2003).

The first patient (Figure 37.1) began to experience periods of extreme suicidality during her depressive episodes and illustrates the point that inadequately treated bipolar II illness is a potentially fatal medical disorder that should be treated with the same care and respect as other life-threatening medical illnesses. Discontinuation of effective antibiotic prophylaxis can result in irreversible damage to the heart valves in subacute bacterial endocarditis, and discontinuation of effective treatment with digitalis can likewise result in potentially irreversible reemergence of congestive heart failure. Surprisingly, it appears that a moderate percentage of patients with epilepsy are able to discontinue effective treatment without suffering the same high incidence of relapses that seem to occur in the recurrent affective disorders.

Our consistent suggestion remains to treat early episodes vigorously and maintain long-term prophylaxis. The earlier treatment is intro-

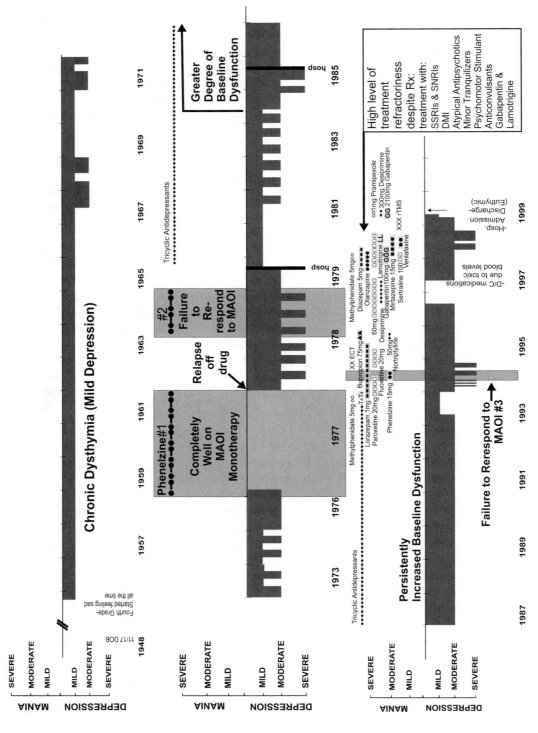

Figure 37.2 Discontinuation-induced refractoriness to an MAOI antidepressant in a patient with unipolar double depression (i.e., recurrent major depressions superimposed on a dysthymic baseline). After a full, complete, and sustained remission for the first time in 19 years on the MAOI phenelzine in 1977, the drug was stopped, the patient relapsed, and then failed to re-respond to phenelzine in 1978 and again in 1995 (bottom line). A partial response to tricyclic antidepressants from 1979 to 1981 resulted in tolerance and a hospitalization in 1985. The depression briefly remitted for about 6 months on high-dose paroxetine (60 mg) plus desipramine in 1997, but relapsed when medications were stopped due to side effects. The patient again failed to respond to a retrial of high-dose paroxetine in combination with multiple adjunctive therapies in 1998–1999. She had a good but partial response to rTMS and was discharged euthymic on desipramine (300 mg/day), which is norepinephrine selective; 1 mg pramipexole, a dopamine agonist; and gabapentin (2,100 mg/day).

308

duced and the longer it is sustained, the better the outcome is likely to be for the patient. Whether maintenance treatment of a sufficient duration will ultimately reveal a lack of need for further treatment has not been documented. To the contrary, we and others have observed that patients who were well for even one to two decades or more still showed relapses upon discontinuing lithium (or other treatments) and, occasionally, these patients demonstrated discontinuation-induced refractoriness (Chapter 13).

As noted in previous chapters (8, 12, 19, 24, and 27), discontinuation of a previously effective treatment during a time when it has lost efficacy due to tolerance may be associated with renewal of responsivity. In contrast, this and other patients (see Chapter 13 on lithium discontinuation-induced refractoriness) suggest that the opposite may occur in patients who were well maintained on a given agent. Not only are recurrences highly likely, but in about 10% of instances, discontinuation of an effective treatment can have consequences much more serious than a single relapse; that is, it may change the illness pattern to a more severe and refractory one. These occurrences reemphasize the importance of recommending long-term maintenance treatment from the earliest point in the illness, not only to prevent the recurrence of a new episode but also hopefully to preserve a good level of treatment responsivity of the illness.

We do not believe this case illustration is a complete anomaly because we have also seen a number of unipolar patients (beyond that illustrated in Figure 37.2) who have the same experience with other antidepressants that were initially highly effective in acute and continuation treatment, but upon repeated discontinuations and subsequent relapses were no longer effective. These observations are not inconsistent with the data of the NIMH collaborative study, wherein approximately 10% of patients with a new episode of depression failed to respond to treatment (Keller & Boland, 1998). One wonders what percentage of these patients were representative of this phenomenon of antidepressant discontinuation-related refractoriness.

Although the mechanisms involved in this effect are not known, we surmise that discontinuation-induced refractoriness is consistent with the general phenomenon of illness sensitization wherein repeated episodes of affective illness engender greater vulnerability to recurrence (Chapter 10). If enough episodes occur, they may no longer respond to previously effective pharmacological interventions.

Episode sensitization has been documented in a Danish study of over 20,000 hospital admissions for unipolar and bipolar disorder (Kessing, Andersen, Mortensen, & Bolwig, 1998). They found that the number of prior hospitalizations was directly related to the incidence and latency to relapse. Mathematical analysis of these data suggest that it was not just a matter of increased severity of illness from the outset in the more recurrent groups, but that the occurrence of episodes themselves contributed to this pattern.

It is also possible that there is an interaction between the changing neurochemistry of the aging process and the neurochemistry of recurrent affective illness, as illustrated in this patient, such that she might have been more responsive in her early and mid-20s and less so thereafter. However, responsivity to antidepressants in general appears to be more age-dependent in the opposite direction, with a considerable body of data suggesting better efficacy in adults than in children and adolescents (Arean & Alvidrez, 2001).

While the discussion has so far focused on the possibility that the occurrence of an additional episode, on its own, may be sufficient to engender changes in the illness that make the illness less responsive than it had been previously, an alternative perspective is that there may also be added vulnerabilities to having an episode while discontinuing antidepressant medication because of the absence of some of the stress-protective effects of the antidepressants.

Mechanistic Considerations: Illness Reappearance Off Medication Could Change Brain Biochemistry and Microstructure

As noted in Chapter 9, the antidepressants as a class increase brain-derived neurotrophic factor (BDNF), which is important not only in early brain development, but also in keeping nerve cells alive in adulthood as well. In addition, BDNF is important for the functioning of normal long-term memory; gene knock-out animals that have only 50% of normal BDNF cannot remember how to navigate a maze that they ordinarily easily could (Linnarsson, Bjorklund, & Ernfors, 1997).

Acute, and particularly chronic, stressors are capable of decreasing BDNF levels substantially in the hippocampus (Smith, Makino, Kvetnansky, & Post, 1995a). Antidepressants exert the opposite effect, and when an animal is on chronic antidepressant treatment during a time of stressor challenge, there is a relative blockade of the BDNF-lowering effects of stress (Nibuya et al., 1995). Similarly, while stress increases neurotrophin-3 (another neurotrophic factor) in the brain stem nucleus that contains neurons with norepinephrine (the locus coeruleus) which modulates arousal and anxiety, antidepressants also counter this change, as well (Smith, Makino, Altemus, et al., 1995).

In addition, stressors decrease the rate of production of new neurons and glia (neurogenesis) (Gould & Tanapat, 1999), which is estimated to involve the generation of about 9,000 new cells in the hippocampus per day in the adult rodent (Cameron & McKay, 2001). Conversely, antidepressants (and lithium) increase neurogenesis and counter some of the effects of stress in decreasing this production of new nerve and glial cell elements (Malberg, Eisch, Nestler, & Duman, 2000). One study suggested that if neurogenesis is blocked (with X-rays), improved animal behavior typically associated with antidepressants fails to occur, at least suggesting the possibility that neurogenesis could be important to some of the effects of antidepressants (Santarelli et al., 2003).

To the extent that antidepressants thus are exerting positive effects on the brain's neuroadaptability and decreasing some of the adverse effects of stressors on neurochemistry, neurotrophic factor induction, and neurogenesis, their discontinuation may remove this series of positive effects. Not only might this make the organism more vulnerable to the effects of stressors, but such stressors may have a deeper impact

on the brain's neurobiology than they would ordinarily if the antidepressant remained in place (Harvey, McEwen, & Stein, 2003). Similarly, an episode of affective illness itself with its associated decreases in BNNF and increases in oxidative stress may have a greater set of adverse consequences for brain neurochemistry during a period off antidepressants as opposed to when they have been continued. Sheline, Gado, and Kraemer (2003) found that unipolar patients not treated with antidepressants very much of the time had age-related decreases in hippocampal volume; hippocampal volume remained normal in those treated with antidepressants more of the time. Thus, with the loss of antidepressant-induced increases in both neurogenesis and neural survival factors (BDNF), the brain may be at increased risk for neural loss.

As in the speculations about one of the possible mechanisms for lithium discontinuation-induced refractoriness, it is likewise possible that in instances of antidepressant discontinuation-induced refractoriness, the new episode of depression occurring off medications is only part of the explanation for the development of the refractoriness. The diverse biological consequences of stressors and episodes may also play a contributing role and reset the central nervous system at a new maladaptive level. This could render a small but particularly vulnerable subgroup of individuals less likely to respond to antidepressants as they had originally.

Whatever the mechanisms involved, the clinical implications are clear. Discontinuation of effective long-term prophylactic treatment not only puts patients at increased risk of relapse compared with their continuation, but the occurrence of each new episode raises the possibility that a more chronic, difficult-to-treat process will also be engendered.

This may be analogous to the process of kindled seizure evolution to the point of spontaneity (Chapter 10). Each stimulation-induced kindled seizure appears behaviorally similar to the previous one, and yet each seizure is participating in the process that is moving the animal closer to the point when vulnerability increases to the extent that seizures occur in the absence of external electrical stimulation. A substantial number of stimulation-induced seizures are required to arrive at this end point of spontaneous seizures, but in any individual animal it cannot readily be determined what precise number of stimulated seizures is actually required to propel them to spontaneity (and the altered response to treatment that accompanies this transition).

From the clinical perspective, one may similarly not be able to discern what number of affective episode recurrences is necessary before a patient becomes less responsive to treatments that were previously effective. It is perhaps not coincidental that in kindled seizure evolution, when animals do progress to spontaneity, their response to drugs also changes. As previously noted, the benzodiazepine anticonvulsants, which are highly effective in the early and middle phases of kindled seizure prevention, are no longer effective against the spontaneous seizures. Conversely, phenytoin, which is not particularly effective in the early phases, becomes an excellent drug for the spontaneous seizure type.

The transition from triggered to spontaneous kindled seizures thus reveals a juncture at which an extra stimulation and seizure finally are enough to produce spontaneous seizures with their new set of drug responsiveness or lack thereof. Perhaps a similar transition is occurring in the small subgroup of patients who have one too many affective episodes and become more treatment resistant.

PRINCIPLES OF THE CASE	STRENGTH OF EVIDENCE
1. Once one stops effective treatment in bipolar illness, relapses are likely.	+++
2. A small percentage of patients (perhaps 10%) do not respond as well following reinstitution of previously successful treatment.	+
3. The number of prior depressive episodes is, in general, a risk factor for vulnerability to the next relapse in both unipolar and bipolar affective illness.	++
4. The number of prior episodes is also related to reduced initial response to lithium (Post, Speer, et al., 2006) or lamotrigine (Obrocea et al., 2002).	++
5. Once the illness has developed past a given point, it may be very difficult to get under control again with the original treatment.	++
6. New approaches may be needed when discontinuation-induced refractoriness is seen.	+
7. The first patient in this chapter eventually had an excellent response to the combination of lamotrigine and gabapentin, further augmented by lithium, but it took several years for this new regimen to be found for her.	+
8. The initially highly antidepressant-responsive unipolar patient illustrated in this chapter struggled for another decade before she restabilized.	+
9. Antidepressants alone (without a mood stabilizer) are not recommended, but the rare bipolar II patient may apparently be sufficiently treated with them for a while;	±
such a trial is now clearly not recommended by expert and consensus guidelines (Keck et al., 2004).	+++
10. Antidepressants as a class increase BDNF in the hippocampus (a structure critically involved in laying down new memories).	+++
11. Stress-induced decreases in BDNF in the hippocampus are inhibited by antidepressants.	+++
12. Antidepressant-induced in-	

creases in neurogenesis and in BDNF may be important for maintaining hippocampal cell number and survival.   ±

13. The second life chart in this chapter illustrates that antidepressant discontinuation-induced refractoriness can also happen on rare occasions (in unipolar depression) with MAOIs or SSRIs. We know a number of other individuals in whom this has happened, and they are extremely regretful that they stopped their effective antidepressant treatment.   ±

14. In unipolar depression, long-term prophylaxis is recommended after three prior major depressions. The first patient had nine prior major depressions superimposed on her dysthymic baseline before her initial good MAOI response (in 1997).   +++

15. If multiple randomized trials in unipolar depression are combined, blindly switching from an effective antidepressant to placebo results in depressive recurrences in about 50% of patients in the first year off antidepressant medications, 75% by the second year, and 85% by the third year. In contrast, staying on the effective antidepressant (blindly)

results in less than 25% of patients experiencing a recurrence in the first year, less than 30% the second year, and less than 40% in the third year. One should note that the drug-placebo difference grows in magnitude over time, that is, the longer one stays on the antidepressant, the relatively more they are protected against relapse compared to no treatment.   +++

16. Davis et al. (1993) calculated that the statistical significance of the likelihood that preventive effects of the antidepressants over placebo were due to chance was infinitesimally small. The probability or p value was $p < 10^{-38}$. Antidepressants do work in the long-term prevention of unipolar depressions, despite the controversies about the magnitude of their acute effects in short-term trials.   +++

TAKE-HOME MESSAGE

In patients with recurrent affective disorders, when an effective prophylactic agent is found and possesses minimal side effects, one should not discontinue that treatment because there is no guarantee that the same degree of responsivity will be achieved upon renewed treatment.

38

Adjunctive Use of a Monoamine Oxidase Inhibitor to Renew Antidepressant Response to Carbamazepine in Bipolar II Depression

CASE HISTORY

This patient is an over-40-year-old married mother (of a toddler) with a 26-year history of bipolar illness. Her first depression occurred at age 14 and she was hospitalized at age 17 for a hypomanic episode that was treated with ECT (not illustrated). Eight weeks of depression was again followed by 8 weeks of hypomania. In 1969 she had a severe depression with a near-lethal suicide attempt with carbon monoxide. She began rapidly cycling following the birth of her first child 1.5 years prior to entering the NIMH (Figure 38.1).

Following the initiation of antidepressant treatment with desipramine, the patient changed from a pattern of isolated, intermittent episodes to more frequent cycling between profound depressions and mild to moderate manias (Figure 38.1). Following discontinuation of this antidepressant and a period of observation off drug at the NIMH, these more rapid cycling patterns were attenuated, but the patient entered a severe persistent depression of psychotic proportions.

Several weeks after beginning carbamazepine on a double-blind basis as active drug was substituted for placebo, the patient's depression began to lift and she achieved a substantially remitted state (Figure 38.1, CBZ I). During the subsequent blind placebo discontinuation at the NIMH, she remained well. When the blind was broken, she wished to be discharged without medications rather than on carbamazepine prophylaxis as recommended by the staff.

Several months later, two mild to moderate depressive episodes occurred and then progressed to a more severe depression that required hospitalization in another institution. TCAs were initially used (not graphed), but these were again without effect (the other institution did not initially believe her NIMH life chart). When carbamazepine treatment was reinitiated, another good response occurred (Figure 38.1, CBZ II). Given this confirmation of her acute responsiveness to carbamazepine, she was given carbamazepine as the focal point of her new prophylactic regimen. On carbamazepine she was essentially well for the next 1.5 years, experiencing only periodic episodes of mild depressive symptoms with little or no associated dysfunction.

However, the depressions began to recur with

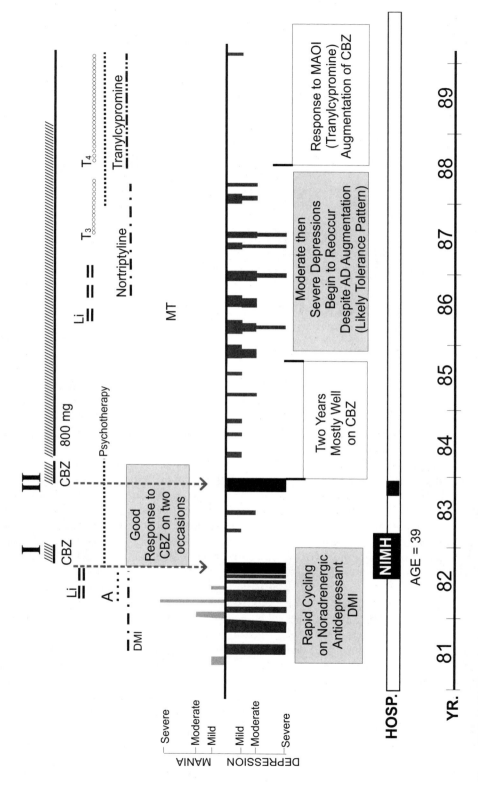

Figure 38.1 Good acute responses to carbamazepine but progressive reemergence of depressive episodes. Severe depressions occurred in 1981 and 1982, which did not remit when carbamazepine was given (CBZ I). When a new severe depression emerged, CBZ II was again given with good effect. However, intermittent depressions of increasing severity and duration emerged despite carbamazepine continuation and adjunctive lithium, nortriptyline, and T₃ as well as psychotherapy. The addition of the MAOI tranylcypromine resulted in a new sustained remission. CBZ, carbamazepine; DMI, desipramine; AD, antidepressant.

314

increasing severity until major depressions of severe proportions broke through carbamazepine prophylaxis in a tolerance-like pattern. Despite a variety of attempts by her outside physicians to maximize carbamazepine dosages and provide adjunctive treatment with antidepressants, T_3 potentiation, benzodiazepines, and psychotherapy, moderate to severe depressions continued to recur.

In the face of this apparent loss of efficacy via a tolerance mechanism, other treatment approaches were considered by her primary physicians in the community. These were not successful until the MAOI tranylcypromine was added to the regimen of carbamazepine, T_4, and psychotherapy, resulting in another period of sustained remission.

BACKGROUND LITERATURE

Antidepressant Efficacy

Although more than 19 controlled studies support the acute antimanic efficacy of carbamazepine, fewer and less rigorously designed studies support the preliminary view that carbamazepine may have acute antidepressant efficacy in a subgroup of refractory depressed patients (Ketter et al., 2004; Post, Denicoff, et al., 1997; Post et al., 1998). In our own double-blind studies at the NIMH, acute antidepressant effects of moderate to marked proportions were seen in approximately 30% of refractory unipolar and bipolar depressed patients (Post, Frye, et al., 1997; Post, Uhde, et al., 1986). While this response rate (in 17 of 57 patients) was not remarkable, it was for our population who were highly treatment resistant. Moreover, upon a second exposure to carbamazepine (also on a blind basis) in 10 of these individuals, a renewed response was confirmed. These double-blind, off (placebo)-on (drug)-off-on data provide strong evidence for the antidepressant effects of carbamazepine in at least a subgroup of refractory affectively ill patients (Post, Speer, et al., 2002).

A double-blind, placebo-controlled parallel group study of Zhang et al. (2007) has also confirmed the acute antidepressant effects of carbamazepine versus placebo in bipolar depression with a response rate of 34.8% for placebo, 63.8% for carbamazepine and 84.8% for carbamazepine plus a combination of 11 Chinese herbs (FEWP; Free and Easy Wander-Plus).

Responders to carbamazepine in our series were among those depressed patients who had an atypical pattern associated with their depression of increased frontal and limbic metabolism (glucose utilization measured by PET), rather than the more usual pattern of hypometabolism of depression (see Chapter 18).

Specifically, many depressed patients have been shown to have decreased metabolic rates (which correlate with decreased neural activity) in their frontal lobes during a depressive episode, and at least nine studies report that this decrement in metabolic function or blood flow correlates with the severity of depression as rated on the Hamilton Depression Rating Scale (Ketter et al., 1996; Ketter et al., 1997). These patients with frontal hypofunction appeared to be among those who responded best to traditional antidepressant modalities, and preliminary data suggest that unipolar depressed responders to venlafaxine or bupropion also have this metabolic pattern (Little et al., 1996). In addition, we have preliminary evidence that antidepressant responders to the calcium channel blocker nimodipine (Chapter 32) and to lamotrigine (Chapter 25) also share this profile of baseline hypometabolism.

In contrast, those with evidence of increased metabolic activity at baseline, particularly in the mediotemporal lobes and insula, are among those who respond best to carbamazepine. We do not believe that patients with mood disorders have a seizure disorder, but only that the anticonvulsant drugs that suppress overexcitability and synchronized neural firing spreading to motor areas of the brain related to seizures can also suppress milder levels of overexcitability in circuits that are pertinent to mood dysregulation.

Mechanisms of Antidepressant Action of Carbamazepine

Carbamazepine acts on a variety of neurotransmitter systems in a way that is dissimilar from many other antidepressants and mood stabilizers (Post et al., 1994; Post, Chalecka-Franaszek, et al., 2002). For example, whereas almost all of the antidepressants upregulate receptors for norepinephrine (NE) in the frontal cortex (beta NE receptors), carbamazepine decreases the number of these receptors. The drug also has an ability to block calcium influx through glutamate receptors, in a fashion that appears somewhat different from many other antidepressants (Hough et al., 1996; Post et al., 1998) (Chapter 9). Moreover, carbamazepine appears to act, at least in part, through peripheral-type benzodiazepine receptors (Weiss, Post, Marangos, & Patel, 1986) as opposed to drugs such as clonazepam and diazepam, which act at the more classical or central-type benzodiazepine receptor. These and many other differences in the biochemical profile of carbamazepine compared with other commonly used antidepressants and minor tranquilizing agents perhaps provide an additional rationale and insight for considering why it may be effective in some patients in whom other antidepressant modalities are not.

Carbamazepine Prophylaxis: Long-Term Efficacy Versus Tolerance

A substantial series of papers have explored the long-term efficacy of carbamazepine in the prevention of both manic and depressive episodes (Post et al., 1996; Post et al., 1997). Although the bulk of these have been open studies, at least 15 have used a randomized, blind, or other similar controlled design. These studies also suggest efficacy of carbamazepine in preventing both manic and depressive episodes in about 50–60% of the patients studied. These preventive effects are usually parallel to those of lithium, although several studies have found superior antimanic efficacy of lithium compared with carbamazepine. Carbamazepine appears to be useful in many patients with potential predictors of lithium nonresponse, that is, those with a negative family history of affective illness in first-degree relatives, patients with more psychotic and dysphoric elements to their mania, those with comorbid substance abuse (alcohol or cocaine), a schizoaffective subtype presenta-

tion, and, to some extent, those with rapid-cycling illness.

In this latter instance, although carbamazepine is often useful alone or in combination with lithium in the treatment of rapid cycling, several studies suggest that the combination of lithium and carbamazepine is substantially better than either drug alone in rapid cyclers. Denicoff, Smith-Jackson, Disney, et al. (1997) and Di Costanzo and Schifano (1991) found that carbamazepine is less effective in rapid cyclers compared with nonrapid cyclers, but when the two drugs are used in combination, an approximately 50% improvement rate is reported.

We have seen tolerance develop after an average of 3 to 4 years of good response to regimens involving carbamazepine in about one third of our treatment-refractory patients (Post, Leverich, et al., 1990; Post, Speer, et al., 2002). Frankenberg et al. (personal communication) also noted loss of effectiveness (presumably some by tolerance) to carbamazepine prophylaxis.

Antidepressant Augmentation of Mood Stabilizers With an MAOI

In a randomized study, Himmelhoch, Thase, Mallinger, and Houck (1991) found the MAOI tranylcypromine had a response rate almost double that of a tricyclic (imipramine) in the treatment of bipolar depression. The MAOIs block the breakdown of presynaptic NE, dopamine, and serotonin, making more of all three available for release. In unipolar depression, MAOIs appear effective in about 50% of tricyclic and SSRI unipolar nonresponders, making them an excellent second- or third-line choice in treatment-refractory depressed patients.

MAOIs are not widely used in the United States because of concerns about side effects, especially a hypertensive crisis. One must go on a diet that excludes substances high in tyramine, because tyramine releases NE. In the absence of functioning monoamine oxidase, that is, because this enzyme for breaking amines down is blocked by the MAOI, ingesting large amounts of tyramine could lead to very high levels of NE and a hypertensive crisis (often indicated by a splitting headache). The new patch preparation with the MAOI selegiline does not require the same dietary cautions at recommended doses, but anecdotal observations suggest higher doses are often required where the drug loses some of its selectivity and dietary precautions again become necessary. It has not been studied in bipolar depression.

Serotonin-potent antidepressants used with an MAOI could also cause a potentially fatal serotonin (5-HT) syndrome and must be avoided. The 5-HT syndrome can induce shakes, high fever, seizures, coma, and even death. The MAOI can cause sleep-wake disturbance, and trazodone is often used to help with insomnia. Episodes of daytime sleepiness may also occur and are more difficult to deal with.

Paradoxically, many patients have problems with low blood pressure on the MAOIs and are especially prone to dizziness and lightheadedness upon standing (i.e., orthostatic hypotension). A high-salt diet, pressure stockings, thyroid augmentation, and fludrocortisone (Florinef) at high daily doses of .6 to .8 mg/day.

PRINCIPLES OF THE CASE — STRENGTH OF EVIDENCE

1. Treatment with TCAs may be associated not only with the induction of mania in some instances (as illustrated in Chapter 34), but also with the occurrence of more severe or more rapid cycling than previously seen in that patient (as in Chapter 36). +

2. The likely relationship of cycle acceleration to antidepressant drug treatment was confirmed by the observations of cycle deceleration (slowing) after discontinuing the antidepressant, as observed during the NIMH placebo phase. ++

3. Antidepressant discontinuation alone (Wehr, 1993) in our experience is typically not sufficient to stop cycling, and a new prophylactic regimen is often required. Other mood stabilizers (lithium, carbamazepine, valproate, nimodipine, and lamotrigine) may be needed. ++

4. Carbamazepine is occasionally dramatically effective in the acute treatment of recurrent unipolar or bipolar depressions. ++

5. Carbamazepine may also be effective in long-term prophylaxis (Chapter 18). ++

6. If this patient carried her mood chart indicating repeated failure to respond to regular antidepressants, she might not have been retreated unsuccessfully with them first when she relapsed following NIMH discharge. A graphic life chart demonstration of prior clear positive or negative drug responsivity may carry more weight with a new treating physician than a casual verbal statement about prior response. ++

7. A subgroup of patients initially responsive to carbamazepine began to experience recurrence and show loss of efficacy via an apparent tolerance mechanism (i.e., the development of progressively more severe, prolonged, or frequent breakthrough episodes). In our series of originally highly treatment-refractory patients, this development of the tolerance type of treatment resistance occurred (in some 30–40%) after an average of 3.8 years of relative wellness on the drug regimen involving carbamazepine. In instances of tolerance development, the treatment algorithm has not yet been clearly specified and the treatment options include:

   a. Increased dosage of initial drug to maximize therapeutic effect. +

   b. Augmentation of the regime with a drug with a new mechanism of action, such as that used in this patient with an MAOI or bupropion (Chapter 39). +

   c. Augmentation with a mood-stabilizing drug with a different mechanism of action (lithium, T_3, or lamotrigine). +

   d. Not using valproate, which has a different mechanism of action than carbamazepine, because there still may be cross-tolerance, based on animal data and clinical vignettes (see Chapters 9 and 10). +

e. Augmentation with a drug active at central-type benzodiazepine receptors such as clonazepam (as opposed to carbamazepine, which is active at different peripheral-type benzodiazepine receptors that control Ca^{++} flux and neurosteroid biosynthesis in mitochondria).   +

f. Consideration of an adjunctive atypical antipsychotic.   ++

g. A period of time off the now ineffective medication, if other approaches fail in the case of the development of loss of efficacy via tolerance (and only in such instances and not when the patient is doing well); a later reexposure to the drug would assess whether there would be a renewal of responsivity, as would be predicted from several case observations (Chapter 19) and an animal model of anticonvulsant tolerance.   ±

8. This patient also helps to support the preliminary view that use of an MAOI with carbamazepine is not contraindicated (Ketter & Post, 1994) although it is stated in the *Physician's Desk Reference (PDR)*. We are not aware of any empirical data suggesting problematic interactions in the literature or from the manufacturers of these drugs. The potential and theoretical reasons for avoiding this combination are also not cogent because carbamazepine is a very weak blocker of NE reuptake, and decreases NE release rather than increasing it.   ++

9. The dietary prohibitions for those on an MAOI center on avoiding foods with high levels of tyramine, which is a potent releaser of NE, and in the absence of functioning MAO to break down excess NE, might cause a rare high blood pressure crisis (see list of foods to avoid on MAOIs in Appendix 7).   ++

10. The *PDR* indicates that the use of stimulants is contraindicated with MAOIs, but in instances of unusual treatment resistance this rule is often violated. Dr. Jan Fawcett suggests that in his experience the only time tolerance does not develop to the antidepressant effects of stimulants is when they are used with an MAOI.   (±)

11. Patients should carry nifedipine or another related pill so that they could take this pill in the event of an impending high blood pressure crisis on an MAOI (i.e., the onset of a splitting headache) on the way to a doctor's office or the emergency room to have their high blood pressure evaluated and treated, often with a blocker of NE alpha 1 receptors (pentolamine).   +++

12. MAOIs may be effective when TCAs and other antidepressants are not, as seen here and reported in the study of Himmelhoch et al. (1991).   +++

13. Whether MAOIs have a lower rate of switching patients into mania than the older TCAs is not clear.   ±

14. One might theoretically be able to mimic some of the unique broad-spectrum amine effects of the MAOIs (on NE, 5-HT, and dopamine) instead by using venlafaxine (for its 5-HT and NE effects) in combination with bupropion (for its dopamine effects). The safety and efficacy of this approach have not been systematically tested, however.   ±

15. The new patch preparation (Ensam) of the reversible inhibitor of MAO type B selegiline requires fewer dietary restrictions, but has not been systematically tested in patients with bipolar depression.   ±

TAKE-HOME MESSAGE

Carbamazepine can work when traditional antidepressants do not, but should tolerance to its prophylactic antidepressant or antimanic effects occur, other approaches need to be considered, occasionally including the adjunctive use of MAOIs.

Bupropion and Venlafaxine

39

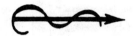

Antidepressant Response to the Carbamazepine-Bupropion Combination, and to Each in Monotherapy

CASE HISTORY

This patient was 34 years old when he was admitted to the NIMH with a 22-year history of increasingly frequent depressive episodes, from an onset at age 13 culminating with a pattern of increasingly severe double depression and a failure to return to a euthymic baseline (as described in Chapter 3). This pattern was further observed and documented during his NIMH hospitalization when, in addition, a pattern of ultradian cycling with frequencies faster than once every 24 hours was manifest.

The manic periods were completely ameliorated during double-blind treatment with carbamazepine, but some depressive symptoms remained, and these were further ameliorated with the blind addition of bupropion. Following discharge from the hospital, the patient discontinued carbamazepine and remained minimally depressed on bupropion for 1.3 years (until March 1991), then restarted carbamazepine monotherapy and achieved a euthymic baseline (Figure 39.1, bottom line).

BACKGROUND LITERATURE

Different Profile of Antidepressant Effects

Bupropion's unusual antidepressant effects (it does not exert potent effects on serotonin reuptake) are thought to be mediated, in part, through increases in dopamine in the brain areas involved in control of motor activity, motivation, and reward (i.e., the caudate or dorsal striatum and nucleus accumbens or ventral striatum; Nomikos, Damsma, Wenkstern, & Fibiger, 1989, 1992). Bupropion can be used in conjunction with any of the three major mood stabilizers and may be less cycle inducing than desipramine, which is selective for the noradrenergic (norepinephrine) system (Guille et al., 1999; Sachs et al., 1994).

In our comparison of the adjunctive antidepressant effects of bupropion, sertraline, and venlafaxine to ongoing mood stabilizer treatment, it appeared that bupropion was the least likely to induce full switches into hypomania or

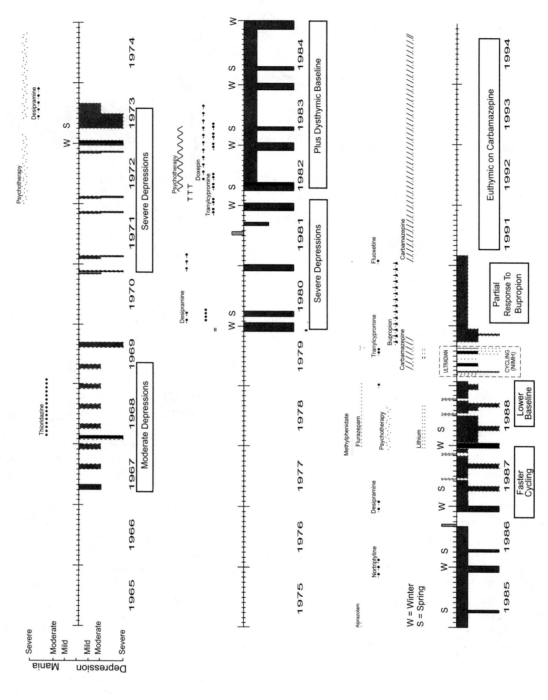

Figure 39.1 Increasing episode severity and baseline dysfunction, with good partial response in 1989 to bupropion and complete response to carbamazepine.

mania (Leverich et al., 2006; Post, Altshuler, et al., 2006). This was also the case for those with a history of rapid cycling, in whom venlafaxine was most prone to induce full switches.

Bupropion is weight neutral or can cause slight weight loss (Anderson et al., 2002). Bupropion is also sold for smoking cessation (Richmond & Zwar, 2003), and rarely causes the sexual dysfunction typical of the SSRIs (Coleman et al., 1999). One of bupropion's prominent side effects—inducing some insomnia—could be beneficial in the treatment of bipolar depression, which often occurs with too much sleep (hypersomnia) as well as other atypical or reverse vegetative features such as increased appetite and weight, compared with the typical anorexia (decreased appetite) and weight loss of unipolar depression.

Potential Predictors of Antidepressant Response to Carbamazepine

The studies supporting carbamazepine's efficacy are reviewed in more detail in Chapters 14–18. In this chapter, we focus on two additional points illustrated by this patient: (1) possible predictors or correlates of antidepressant response to carbamazepine, and (2) pharmacokinetic interactions between carbamazepine and bupropion.

Potential pretreatment predictors of positive response to the acute or long-term antidepressant effects of carbamazepine include patients (1) with a history of recurrent depressions refractory to lithium and conventional antidepressants (Post, Uhde, et al., 1986); (2) with more severe episodic depressive presentations; (3) without a family history of bipolar illness in first-degree relatives; (4) with ultrarapid or ultra-ultrarapid cycling frequencies (such as this patient), although many with this very rapid pattern of mood oscillation require complex combination therapy, and some respond to the dihydropyridine-type calcium channel blockers (Chapters 32 and 33) alone or in combination with carbamazepine; (5) with evidence of the atypical pattern of increased (rather than de-

creased) glucose utilization as measured with positron emission tomography scans (Ketter, Kimbrell, et al., 1999; Chapter 14); and (6) with focal evidence of increased blood flow or metabolism in the structures of the medial temporal lobe, including those of the limbic system (amygdala, hippocampus, and related structures) closely linked to regulation of emotional function.

This last observation is consistent with a view that carbamazepine generally tends to decrease blood flow and metabolism in many areas of the brain, such that those patients with evidence of increased activity in selective structures may be specifically more likely to respond to this agent. In the absence of availability of such a functional brain imaging scan, an empirical trial of carbamazepine in unipolar and bipolar depressed patients nonresponsive to other modalities might be in the patient's interest.

Surprisingly, patients with greater decrements in thyroid hormones, as reflected in blood levels of T_4 or free T_4 (Figure 39.2), have a better response to carbamazepine, not worse, as might have been expected (Roy-Byrne, Joffe, Uhde, & Post, 1984).

Although this observation appears to conflict with the observations that T_3 and T_4 supplementation of many antidepressants can enhance their therapeutic efficacy, the decrement in T_4 might be related to carbamazepine's induction of enzymes that metabolize and break down thyroid hormone. Unlike lithium, carbamazepine does not increase TSH (Liewendahl, Majuri, & Helenius, 1978; Liewendahl, Tikanoja, Helenius, & Majuri, 1985; Strandjord, Aanderud, Myking, & Johannessen, 1981) and is not associated with the same increased incidence of clinical hypothyroidism as lithium.

Many depressed patients are relatively hyperthyroid during their depressive episodes and return toward normal levels with clinical improvement (Bauer & Whybrow, 1986, 1988; Joffe & Sokolov, 1994); therefore, a T_4 reduction could be in the therapeutic direction. When we augment with T_3, T_4 levels decrease by a feedback regulatory process (i.e., higher levels of T_3 are sensed, and this leads to lower TSH levels and less thyroid stimulation). As dis-

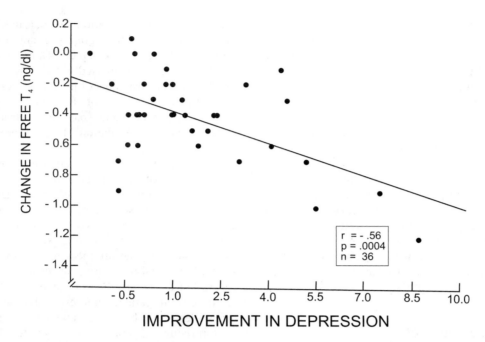

Figure 39.2 Antidepressant effects of carbamazepine: relation to decreases in free T_4. Paradoxically, the greater the drop in T_4 or free T_4 on carbamazepine, the better the antidepressant response.

cussed in more detail elsewhere (Chapter 51), the primary clinical principle when using thyroid supplementation is that it can be considered whether or not there are baseline abnormalities in thyroid indices.

Those patients with higher baseline levels of the dopamine metabolite homovanillic acid respond better to carbamazepine treatment (Post, Rubinow, Uhde, Ballenger, & Linnoila, 1986). Like the other mood stabilizers lithium and valproate, carbamazepine decreases dopamine turnover (Baptista, Weiss, & Post, 1993).

Although these clinical and neurobiological correlates are largely based on limited data from acute antidepressant trials, there is reason to believe that a good acute response may also be associated with a good response in long-term prophylaxis. Although this proposition has not been systematically studied in bipolar illness, most acutely effective antidepressants in unipolar depression, when tested for long-term continuation and prophylaxis, also prove effective.

The guiding principle would appear to be that the full effective dose should be the same one used in prophylaxis (Frank et al., 1990; Kupfer

et al., 1992). There does not appear to be a good correlation of blood levels between carbamazepine and the degree of active antidepressant response (Figure 39.3). There are highly preliminary data more closely linking the CSF levels of the metabolite (carbamazepine 10,11-epoxide) to clinical response, but this remains to be better tested (Post, Uhde, et al., 1983).

Individual side effects thresholds for carbamazepine vary considerably even within the usual therapeutic range (4–12 µg/ml). Doses should be increased slowly and titrated against side effects rather than attempting to target a particular dose or blood level.

As carbamazepine accelerates its own metabolism by inducing liver enzymes (3A4) that break it down into an inactive compound, after 2 to 3 weeks of treatment doses may need to be increased further. This is also likely to be a time during which the drug is better tolerated than in the first few days or weeks.

A number of neurobiological alterations do not appear to be associated with the degree of antidepressant response to carbamazepine. For example, an agitated or retarded presentation

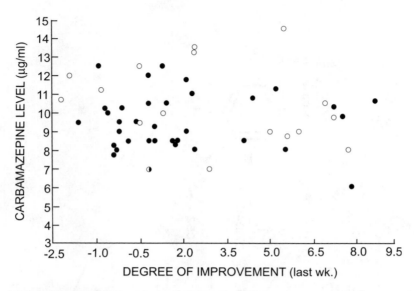

Figure 39.3 Lack of relationship between plasma levels of carbamazepine in the therapeutic range (4 to 12 μg/ml) and individual acute antidepressant response in depression (dark circles) or antimanic response in mania (open circles).

does not, although patients who respond to carbamazepine show normalization of their relatively low motor activity (Joffe, Uhde, Post, & Minichiello, 1987). Since carbamazepine was chosen, in part, because of its ability to quiet limbic hyperexcitability, we thought that an indirect marker of limbic hyperexcitability might be associated with degree of acute antidepressant response. Paradoxically, we found that those patients with more psychosensory symptoms—illusions and sensory distortions typically seen in those with complex partial seizures of the temporal lobe—suggestive of temporal lobe dysfunction are not more likely to respond to lithium, not carbamazepine (Silberman et al., 1985). However, depressed patients with a history of prior problems with alcohol abuse are particularly likely to respond to carbamazepine (Frye, Altshuler, et al., 2003).

There is no evidence of a covert seizure disorder in patients with classical or primary bipolar illness. EEG abnormalities and clinical seizures are not common in those with primary affective disorders, and carbamazepine seems to be just as effective in those without evidence of EEG abnormalities as in those with such evidence (Neppe, 1983). Carbamazepine works rapidly in the treatment of seizure disorders, yet requires some weeks for full therapeutic effect in mania or depression (Post, 1988); thus, it is likely that different mechanisms of action of the drug account for its anticonvulsant versus mood-stabilizing effects. Therefore, while we call carbamazepine an anticonvulsant based on its initial FDA approval status, it is probably not acting directly as an anticonvulsant in its therapeutic effects in the affective disorders.

Carbamazepine lowers cerebrospinal levels of the peptide somatostatin, but this is not related to its degree of clinical response (Rubinow, Post, Gold, Ballenger, & Reichlin, 1985). In contrast, nimodipine increases levels of somatostatin and appears most effective in those with low pretreatment somatostatin levels (Pazzaglia et al., 1995; Chapter 32).

Pharmacokinetic Interactions of the Combination of Carbamazepine and Bupropion

The use of carbamazepine and the antidepressant bupropion in combination is increasingly common because of carbamazepine's mood-stabi-

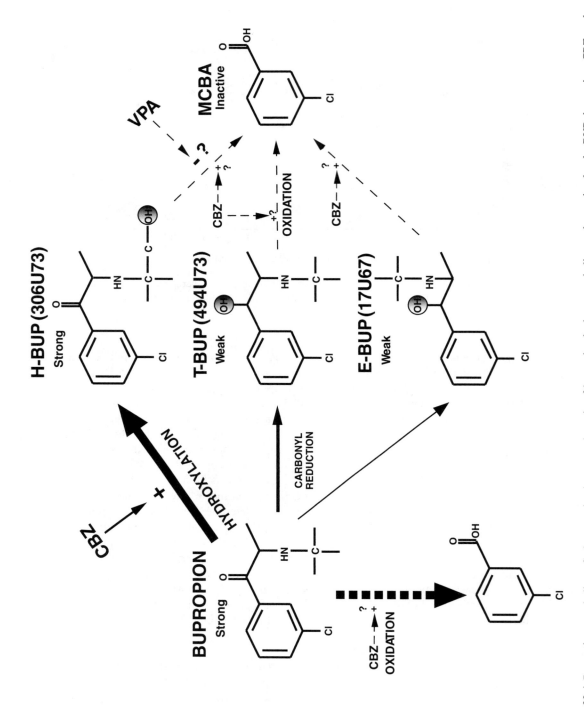

Figure 39.4 Bupropion metabolism. Carbamazepine increases the ratio of bupropion hydroxymetabolites to bupropion levels. BUP, bupropion; CBZ, carbamazepine; VPA, valproate; H-BUP, hydroxy bupropion; T-BUP, theobupropion; E-BUP, Erythrobupropion; MCBA, moncarboxylbupropion.

326

lizing effects and evidence from a variety of studies indicating that bupropion may be different from some of the other traditional antidepressants. Bupropion may possess some mood-stabilizing properties on its own (Haykal & Akiskal, 1990) and causes fewer switches into hypomania or mania than the TCA desipramine during long-term prophylaxis (Guille et al., 1999; Sachs et al., 1994) or the mixed serotonin and norepinephrine blocker venlafaxine (Leverich et al., 2006; Post, Altshuler, et al., 2006). Interactions of carbamazepine and bupropion are thus of considerable interest.

Initial evidence indicates that carbamazepine markedly alters the ratio of bupropion to its hydroxymetabolite (Ketter et al., 1995). Carbamazepine decreases bupropion levels while increasing the hydroxymetabolite substantially (Figure 39.4). Thus, if one is measuring bupropion blood levels during cotreatment with carbamazepine, these levels may appear essentially negligible, but large amounts of active metabolites remain relatively hidden, since conventional assays do not measure these derivatives. Because oxcarbazepine is not a potent enzyme inducer (see Chapter 20), one would not expect this degree of bupropion changes.

When bupropion is used in combination with valproate, this change in the bupropion-to-metabolite ratio does not occur to the same extent (Ketter et al., 1995). If both bupropion and its active hydroxymetabolite convey equal antidepressant therapeutic and side effects profiles, the carbamazepine-induced change in ratio should not be clinically problematic.

However, if increasing levels of the hydroxymetabolite compared with the parent compound are not clinically useful, as one study suggests, then the profile of lower levels of the bupropion metabolite achieved when the drug is used in combination with valproate could be an asset. Further studies are required to determine whether this increased metabolism of bupropion to its active hydroxymetabolite induced by carbamazepine is clinically unimportant or a liability.

Bupropion does not affect carbamazepine levels, in contrast to some other antidepressants such as fluoxetine (Grimsley, Jann, Carter, D'Mello, & D'Souza, 1991; Pearson, 1990), flu-voxamine (Fritze, Unsorg, & Lanczik, 1991), and nefazodone (Ashton & Wolin, 1996; Greene & Barbhaiya, 1997; Chapter 15), which can increase levels of carbamazepine moderately. Other drugs that can increase carbamazepine levels markedly and cause potential toxicity include the calcium channel blockers verapamil and diltiazem (but not nimodipine or nifedipine), the erythromycin-like antibiotics, the anti-tuberculosis drug isoniazid, and acetazolamide.

In contrast, carbamazepine can significantly lower the blood levels of other drugs, including alprazolam, clonazepam, buprenorphine, and lamotrigine (Chapter 15). Most noteworthy is carbamazepine's ability to decrease levels of sex hormones in birth control pills, rendering them ineffective. Higher dosage forms of estrogen must be used to ensure continued effectiveness, or other modes of contraception can be utilized (Ketter & Post, 1994; Ketter et al., 1998, 2004).

Carbamazepine, despite its influence on many other drugs, sometimes helps when other mood stabilizers do not. Bupropion, because of its unique effects on dopamine among the conventional antidepressants, also can have good therapeutic effects and few side effects in the treatment of bipolar depression. Bupropion is an indirect dopamine agonist (via increasing brain levels of dopamine). Several direct dopamine agonists, most recently the D_2, D_3 receptor agonist pramipexole, used in the treatment of Parkinson's disease, have been shown to have antidepressant effects (Goldberg, Burdick, & Endick, 2004; Zarate et al., 2004). These become another option for enhancing dopamine in those unresponsive to or unable to tolerate bupropion.

PRINCIPLES OF THE CASE	STRENGTH OF EVIDENCE
1. Bupropion (with its effects on dopamine) may be effective when other antidepressants with more traditional serotonin or norepinephrine (i.e., nortriptyline and desipramine) ef-	

fects, or the MAOI tranylcy-
promine, are not.   ++

2. Bupropion should be added to
another mood stabilizer such
as lithium, valproate, lamotrigine, or carbamazepine, as seen
here.   ++

3. Bupropion did not induce cycling on carbamazepine, as did
the MAOI tranylcypromine (in
1989).   ++

4. A modicum of data suggest adjunctive bupropion is less
likely to cause switches in hypomania and mania than the
tricyclic antidepressant desipramine or the norepinephrine
plus serotonin reuptake inhibi-
tor venlafaxine.   ++

5. Bupropion has a positive therapeutic profile for bipolar depression in that it is not sedating, is weight neutral, and
usually does not cause sexual
dysfunction, headache, or upset stomach, as the SSRIs
can.   ++

6. Carbamazepine can exert antidepressant effects in monotherapy in some lithium-nonre-
sponsive patients.   +

7. Possible predictors or correlates of carbamazepine antidepressant response are discussed here and in Chapter 17,
and its drug-drug interactions
here and in Chapter 15.   +

8. Even bipolar illness showing a
progressive worsening in
course of illness (as evidenced
by faster cycling, transition
from unipolar to bipolar II,
and acquisition of baseline
dysthymia) can be brought
into remission on appropriate
medication.   ++

9. A clear unipolar course may
convert to a bipolar II or bipolar NOS, even after many de-
pressive episode recurrences.   +

10. Some antidepressants, in the
absence of a mood stabilizer,
may be counterproductive in
the treatment of bipolar depression. In this case bupropion
did not induce cycling, how-
ever.   ±

TAKE-HOME MESSAGE

It may take considerable time and numbers of
revisions of therapeutic regimens to achieve a
good long-term response in unipolar or bipolar
illness with highly recurrent major depressions.

40

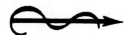

Antidepressant Response to Venlafaxine: Switch Rates, Mechanisms of Action, and Other Augmenting Strategies

CASE HISTORY

This is a 53-year-old patient with a pattern of increasingly persistent depressive recurrences in the context of a single manic episode precipitated during treatment with TCAs and methylphenidate in 1976. As such, he would only be categorized as having substance-induced mania or bipolar NOS according to *DSM-IV*. The patient's last three depressive episodes lasted for successively longer durations of 6.5 months, 14 months, and then 22 months, that is, three times as long as his usual 6-month depressive episode evident in his first four depressive episodes (Figure 40.1). The well intervals between episodes also showed a general pattern of progressive shortening from 6.5- and 10-year intervals between the first, second, and third, to 3 years until the fourth episode (in 1991), and then to 3 months to the fifth episode in 1992, with 1.5 months in between the fifth and sixth episodes in 1993.

In this patient, increased frequency and duration of episodes occurred despite increasingly aggressive psychopharmacology with lithium as the primary treatment and a variety of antidepressant trials, often with thyroid augmentation. Trazodone was used at night for insomnia, and adjunctive trials with alprazolam, lorazepam, and clonazepam were used because of profound anxiety and agitation. A first series of 12 ECT treatments was able to bring the patient out of the episode in 1993, but with the recrudescence of his depression, a second series of bilateral ECT treatments failed to be effective, in a pattern consistent with tolerance development (Chapter 38).

At the NIMH, this patient presented with profound agitation, anxiety, angst, and tearfulness, with an overwhelming sense of hopelessness and despair. The obvious level of extreme psychic pain experienced by this patient made it uncomfortable and difficult for others even to remain in the same room with him for prolonged periods of time. The patient failed to respond to a double-blind trial of the calcium channel blocker nimodipine (Chapters 32 and 33) and was an inadequate responder to rTMS of the brain (Chapter 57). However, he responded dramatically to thyrotropin-releasing hormone (TRH) with an essentially complete, but transient, remission and then reresponded to blind intravenous and intrathecal TRH on multiple occasions (Chapters 61 and 62). This led to an attempt to treat the patient with repeated parenteral TRH administration that was successful

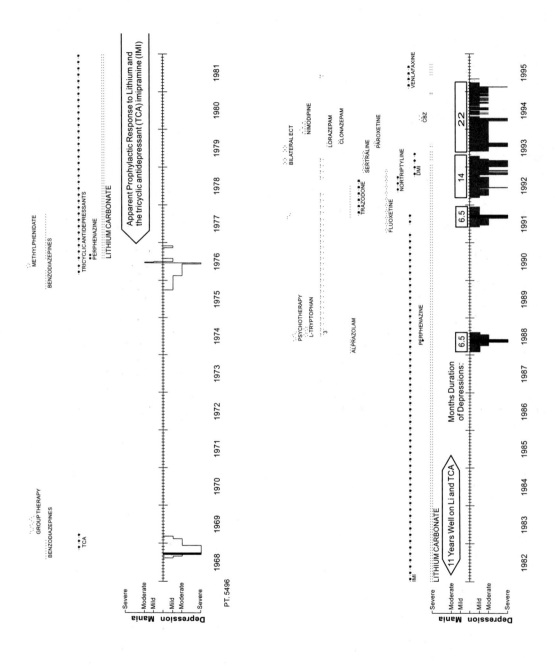

Figure 40.1 Increasing episode duration in a bipolar NOS male. The life chart shows an excellent response to the addition of venlafaxine. The patient's prior history was unusual in that he showed a single brief episode of hypomania when treated with a tricyclic antidepressant and a stimulant in 1976, but this did not recur following subsequent treatments with several SSRIs, or in the current example, with venlafaxine.

for a number of weeks, but he gradually became tolerant to its therapeutic effects.

After experiencing initially severe gastrointestinal side effects (marked diarrhea), the patient responded to the combined noradrenergic-serotonergic reuptake blocker venlafaxine, and the response was further augmented with lithium potentiation, yielding a complete remission in 1995.

His first week of treatment on venlafaxine (37.5 mg/day) was noteworthy in that he suffered marked gastrointestinal distress with severe, multiple daily bouts of watery diarrhea. We suggested that he discontinue treatment with this compound, but he wanted to see if he could acclimate to this side effect, which he did by the second week of treatment. Although most patients have very few side effects on venlafaxine, gastrointestinal side effects occurring in the first weeks of treatment are not uncommon.

However, as in the current patient, side effects are often rapidly attenuated and allow subsequent higher dose escalation, so that patients should be encouraged to try to weather the initial difficulties on this drug if possible. Venlafaxine has a side effect unusual among the psychotropic drugs used for bipolar illness—it can be associated with small degrees of increased blood pressure, such that those patients who have borderline or high blood pressure at baseline should take this into account.

BACKGROUND LITERATURE

Venlafaxine is a dual-action (both serotonin and norepinephrine) reuptake inhibitor (i.e., SNRI; Andrews, Ninan, & Nemeroff, 1997). It is slightly more potent when blocking serotonin reuptake, so that as doses are increased, more adrenergic properties emerge.

The dual action on two transmitter systems is thought to account for venlafaxine's superior efficacy compared to the SSRIs. Recently, several meta-analyses (in unipolar depressed patients) found that venlafaxine compared with SSRIs emerged as a more effective antidepressant in terms of both percentage and magnitude of response (Einarson, Arikiazn, Casciano, &

Doyle, 1999; Entsuah, Huang, & Thase, 2001; Rudolph, 2002; Stahl, Entsuah, & Rudolph, 2002). Thus, it is likely that the noradrenergic actions of venlafaxine, in addition to those on serotonin, account for this superior profile.

These observations are supported by the study of Nelson, Mazure, Bowers, and Jatlow (1991) indicating that the combination of fluoxetine, which is highly serotonin selective, and desipramine, which is highly noradrenergic selective, yielded more substantial antidepressant effects than patients treated with fluoxetine alone. The tricyclic antidepressant clomipramine also has effects on both neurotransmitter systems, and in addition to being the first agent approved for the treatment of obsessive-compulsive disorder because of its potency in blocking serotonin reuptake (Zohar, Insel, Zohar-Kadouch, Hill, & Murphy, 1988), also has noteworthy antianxiety (Gloger, Grunhaus, Birmacher, & Troudart, 1981) and antinociceptive (antipain; Eberhard et al., 1988) effects as well.

The SSRIs are not particularly effective in a variety of pain syndromes, but because of the dual actions of venlafaxine, it appears to be a highly effective adjunct in a variety of acute and chronic pain syndromes (Ninan, 2000; Sayar, Aksu, Ak, & Tosun, 2003). As discussed elsewhere (Chapters 26 and 27), gabapentin is also widely used for its antinociceptive effects, but in this instance they are likely mediated through GABAergic mechanisms and those at a subunit of the L-type calcium channel. The recently approved drug, duloxetine, shares venlafaxine's dual actions on norepinephrine and serotonin reuptake blockade (i.e., an SNRI), is an effective antidepressant in unipolar patients, and also has considerable antipain effects (Brannan et al., 2005; Raskin, Goldstein, Mallinckrodt, & Ferguson, 2003).

As with other antidepressant modalities, the liability of venlafaxine to cause switches into hypomania and mania in patients with bipolar depression remains controversial. One study by Vieta, Martinez-Aran, and associates (2002) reported that venlafaxine was associated with a higher switch rate than the SSRI paroxetine, although, surprisingly, a negligible switch rate was reported in the study of venlafaxine of Am-

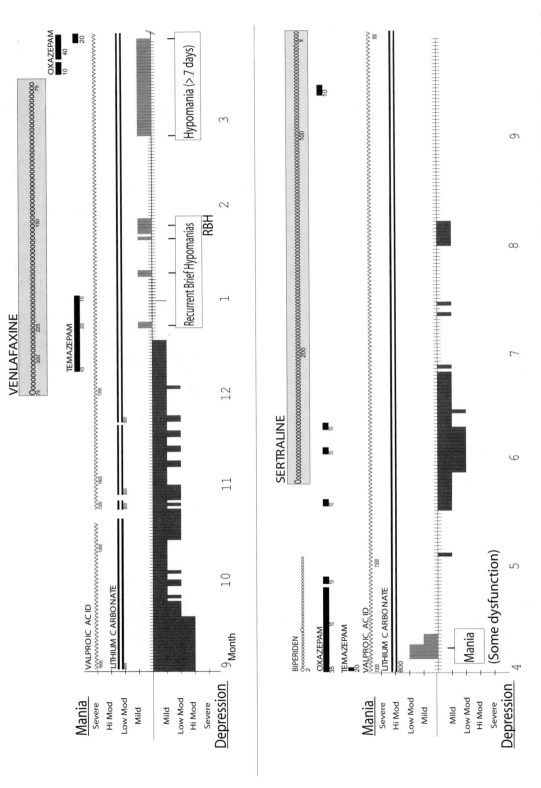

Figure 40.2 Hypomania with venlafaxine but not sertraline augmentation. This patient switched into hypomania and mania after venlafaxine treatment despite the presence of two mood stabilizers. This did not occur with the serotonin selective antidepressant, suggesting that the dual action effect on norepinephrine (as well as serotonin) is implicated in the increased switch rate on venlafaxine.

sterdam (1998) in bipolar II patients who were not even taking a concurrent mood stabilizer. In our Stanley Foundation Network randomized study comparing the efficacy and switch rates of the SSRI sertraline ($N = 62$), the dopamine-active bupropion ($N = 55$), and the SNRI venlafaxine ($N = 67$) as adjunctive treatment in bipolar depression, higher switch rates assessed by most measures were found with venlafaxine compared with bupropion (Leverich et al., 2006; Post, Altshuler, et al., 2006). Three times more manias or full duration hypomanias (>7 days) than brief hypomania was observed with venlafaxine than with bupropion or sertraline (see Figure 40.2).

It is generally thought that those patients with higher initial cycle frequencies are more prone to antidepressant-induced switching and that this could account for some of the discrepancies in switch rates within the literature. Additional concomitants of antidepressant-related switches have been reported, including those with stimulant-related substance abuse problems (Goldberg & Whiteside, 2002), depressed patients who had a contiguous manic episode prior to their depression (Young et al., 2000; and Joffe, personal communication), and those with lower baseline levels of the urinary norepinephrine metabolite 3-methoxy-4-hydroxy-phenylglycol (Zis et al., 1979).

In the study of Sachs and colleagues (Guille et al., 1999), a higher switch rate during continuation therapy was observed with the noradrenergic tricyclic antidepressant desipramine than with the more dopamine-active bupropion. This led to one possible interpretation that the noradrenergic effects of desipramine were responsible for the higher switch rate. If this were the explanation, one would expect (as observed) that venlafaxine (with its added noradrenergic effects) would have higher switch rates than the serotonin-selective antidepressants (or bupropion).

A second possible explanation of Guille et al.'s findings includes the fact that other actions inherent in the profile of the older TCAs (for example, anticholinergic effects of desipramine) could also account for the differences in switch rates. A direct comparison of the older first-generation and newer second-generation antidepressants (Gijsman et al., 2004) supports this proposition. TCAs compared with the second-generation drugs, also have an increased risk of lethal outcomes in overdose as well.

It is interesting that both the first- and second-generation antidepressants with different mechanisms of action all have been reported to increase expression of brain-derived neurotrophic factor (BDNF), which has been implicated in cell survival and in learning and memory. The antidepressants counter effects of stress on BDNF, and this effect remains a major candidate for the common actions of the antidepressant drugs (Chapter 9 and 37).

Lithium reportedly is able to augment the effects of virtually every antidepressant (Bschor et al., 2003). While most of these studies have been in unipolar depressed patients, there is no reason to expect this would not also be true in bipolar depressed patients who do not already have lithium in their treatment regimens. For lithium augmentation, lower doses of lithium (all at night) in the range of 600 to 900 mg/day (achieving blood levels of about 0.75 mEq/L) are often sufficient. Lithium, like the antidepressants, increases BDNF. Antidepressants and lithium also increase (in adult animals) the birth of new neurons (neurogenesis) and new glial cells from the stem cells in the ventricular lining next to the hippocampus (Chapter 9).

PRINCIPLES OF THE CASE	STRENGTH OF EVIDENCE
1. Unlike the SSRIs, venlafaxine inhibits the reuptake of both serotonin and norepinephrine (i.e., an SNRI).	+++
2. This dual action of venlafaxine may account for its greater antidepressant effects in unipolar patients and definitely better antinociceptive profile compared with the SSRIs.	+++
3. Venlafaxine can be associated with minor to clinically relevant increases in blood pres-	

sure, which should be checked in those who are vulnerable (i.e., those with borderline hypertension or actual hypertension at baseline). ++

4. The noradrenergic effects of venlafaxine may also be associated with increased lethality in overdose and the possibility of exacerbating congestive heart failure. +

5. In bipolar patients, venlafaxine also carries a greater liability for causing switches into hypomania or mania compared with bupropion or SSRIs, despite concomitant treatment with at least one mood stabilizer. +++

6. In many individuals, the initial prominent gastrointestinal and other side effects on venlafaxine (in about 10–15% of patients) will be transient and will dissipate completely after the first week or two of treatment. ++

7. Like most other serotonin-potent antidepressants (with the exception of both nefazodone and mirtazapine), venlafaxine can induce the typical range of sexual side effects including slowness to reach orgasm, disinterest and lack of libido, and impotence. +

8. Whether this sexual dysfunction is less frequent with venlafaxine compared with the SSRIs remains to be demonstrated. ±

9. Unproven approaches to antidepressant-related sexual dysfunction include:

    a. Adding bupropion ±

    b. Switching to bupropion or lamotrigine ++

    c. Adding buspirone, which can cause premature ejaculation, and thus counter antidepressant-induced decreases in sexual functioning +

    d. Adding yohimbine, a norepinephrine α_2 receptor antagonist that increases norepinephrine release +

    e. Adding sildenafil, primarily for erectile dysfunction +

10. Venlafaxine is approved for panic and general anxiety disorder, and this patient's overwhelming anxiety and agitation were very well treated in accordance with this general perspective. ++

11. When an SSRI is not effective or tolerated and one is attempting to use another unimodal antidepressant, it would appear prudent to switch to a drug with a different mechanism of action such as an SNRI or bupropion, rather than attempting another trial with a different SSRI, although there is not strong evidence to support this suggestion. +

12. There are reports that switching from one SSRI to another is helpful (in relationship to either side effect tolerability or effectiveness) in some cases, however. +

13. The switch from an SSRI to venlafaxine might be preferable to switching to bupropion where there is extreme anxiety (present case), a comorbid anxiety disorder, or comorbid obsessive-compulsive disorder, because the serotonin system would remain potentiated with the dual actions of venlafaxine. +

14. Principles 11 and 13 would likely also be true for comorbid PTSD symptoms, although this remains to be directly tested. +

15. Those with a prior history of rapid cycling appear particularly prone to switching on venlafaxine. +

16. Switching into mania on one antidepressant does not necessarily mean it will happen again during all other antidepressant trials. +

17. Whether venlafaxine (because of its dual norepinephrine and serotonin mechanisms of action) will have the postulated lower rate of gradual development of loss of efficacy (tolerance phenomenon) than the SSRIs remains to be delineated. ±

18. Lithium augmentation of an incomplete antidepressant response is effective in 40–60% of unipolar patients. +++

19. The dose for lithium augmentation of an antidepressant in unipolar depression is usually thought to be in the range of 900 mg/day (all at night is okay) to achieve blood levels of the 0.75 mEq/L range. +

20. This patient appeared to respond to low lithium doses and levels, however, which were all he could tolerate. +

21. Low doses and blood levels of lithium would likely still begin to produce its neurotropic and protective effects based on animal studies (Chapter 10). ++

22. While venlafaxine has a greater proclivity to induce switches into mania than antidepressants acting on single transmitters, as suggested by two randomized studies, this patient did not switch on venlafaxine as he had initially on a tricyclic antidepressant. +

23. Duloxetine is a dual norepinephrine and serotonin reuptake inhibitor and likely shares venlafaxine's antidepressant and antipain actions. The two drugs would appear to share a roughly similar side effects profile, but perhaps with a lesser magnitude of increased blood pressure on duloxetine compared with venlafaxine. ±

TAKE-HOME MESSAGE

The SNRI venlafaxine can be effective when SSRIs are not, and SNRIs can be considered where there is a prominent comorbid anxiety or pain syndrome. Gastrointestinal side effects, if they occur, will likely dissipate in the first week, so try to hold out. The risk of switching into hypomania or mania is greater with venlafaxine than bupropion or the SSRIs.

Part VIII

BENZODIAZEPINES

41

Adjunctive High-Potency Benzodiazepines for Breakthrough Anxiety and Insomnia of Depression and Mania: Clonazepam and Lorazepam

CASE HISTORY

This patient illustrates a relatively poor response to carbamazepine monotherapy, which was inadequate in preventing a hypomanic episode in 1993 and depressions thereafter, despite treatment with the noradrenergic antidepressant nortriptyline (Figure 41.1). Lithium monotherapy was partially effective from 1994 to 1995, but its augmentation with the combination produced a much more complete response from 1996 onward.

However, periods of mild to moderate depression broke through a number of times each year. These depressions were associated with some degree of insomnia, difficulty in both falling asleep and staying asleep throughout the night, and some increased levels of anxiety. With the addition of lorazepam (0.5 mg each evening), the patient showed improvement in sleep and anxiety and an apparent reduction in time depressed in the latter half of 1999 and early 2000. Again, the response is not unequivocal, because a period between late 1998 and early 1999 had approximately the same degree of improvement prior to the use of lorazepam, suggesting the possibility that this was a course-of-illness-related improvement.

BACKGROUND LITERATURE

Lorazepam, clonazepam, and alprazolam are the high-potency benzodiazepines available in the United States. We call them high potency because they are effective anticonvulsants when administered via the oral route. This contrasts with diazepam, which is a potent clinical anticonvulsant when administered intravenously but is poorly absorbed with intramuscular injections and is ineffective when taken orally as an anticonvulsant. Clonazepam and lorazepam are widely used as adjunctive treatment for insomnia and agitation associated with hypomania, as well as for anxiety and insomnia associated with breakthrough minor depressive episodes, as illustrated in the current patient.

Avoid Alprazolam in Bipolar Illness

Alprazolam is not widely used in the treatment of bipolar illness for several reasons. First, it appears to be somewhat different from the other high-potency benzodiazepines by virtue of its triazolo [4,3-(alpha)] [1,4] ring structure, which apparently helps confer antidepressant proper-

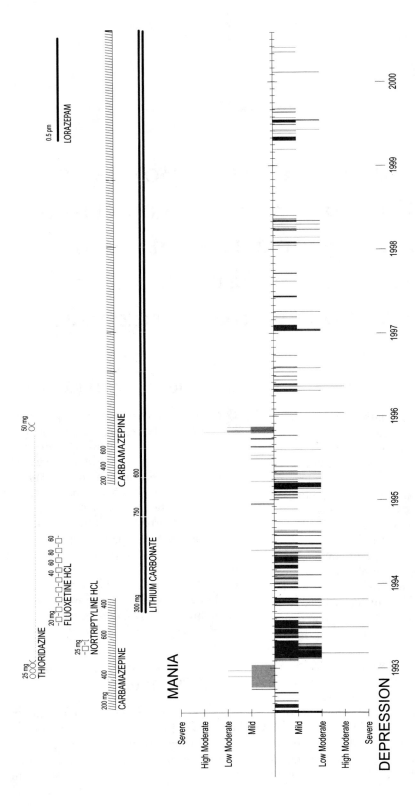

Figure 41.1 Good response to lithium-carbamazepine combination: augmentation with the high-potency benzodiazepine lorazepam for residual depression, anxiety, and insomnia. This patient illustrates a typical use of lorazepam for episodes of anxiety and insomnia associated with mild to moderate depressive recurrences breaking through largely effective treatment with the combination of carbamazepine and lithium. The depressions appeared shorter and less frequent than those seen from 1996 to 1999, prior to treatment with lorazepam.

ties on the drug. However, in association with this added effect beyond benzodiazepine receptor stimulation, there are reports of the induction of mania not only in patients with bipolar illness (see Figure 36.1) but also in those with unipolar illness or anxiety disorders in instances when hypomania had never been previously observed (Pecknold & Fleury, 1986).

Another potential liability of alprazolam is its relatively short half-life of 11 hours and an effective duration of action of only 4–5 hours. With 4–6 hours between drug administrations, the patient may begin to experience increased anxiety from a "mini" alprazolam withdrawal. Likewise, alprazolam may help patients get to sleep, but they may wake up in the latter part of the night or early morning with increased levels of anxiety. The short duration of action often necessitates multiple doses throughout the day and can be associated with increased problems of tolerance, need for drug escalation, and the potential for abuse. A new long-acting preparation may obviate some of these difficulties.

Longer Acting High-Potency Benzodiazepines Are Preferable and Widely Used

A number of controlled or partially controlled studies suggest the utility of lorazepam or clonazepam in the treatment of acute mania (as reviewed in Post & Speer, 2002). Because of a variety of different types of methodological concerns, experts do not consider this group of studies unequivocal in demonstrating the acute antimanic efficacy of these agents. It is for this reason that benzodiazepines are almost always used as an adjunct (i.e., an add-on treatment) in bipolar illness. They are considered a safer and better tolerated alternative to the older (typical) antipsychotics for residual insomnia, anxiety, and agitation breaking through treatment with one or more mood stabilizers.

Sachs, Rosenbaum, and Jones (1990) and Kishimoto et al. (1988) reported that adjunctive clonazepam may be useful in long-term maintenance, although tolerance apparently occurred in a number of the patients studied by Kishimoto et al. In the Stanley Foundation Bipolar

Network (SFBN), benzodiazepines were used in approximately 50% of the first 250 patients followed prospectively for 1 year (Post, Denicoff, et al., 2003).

These drugs were widely used, not only for their action on target symptoms of insomnia and anxiety but also because of their relative safety. Aside from sedative side effects that can be bothersome to some individuals, they are extremely well-tolerated drugs and relatively safe, even in overdose. Clonazepam, like gabapentin (Chapters 26 and 27), is also effective in the treatment of social phobia (Reiter, Pollack, Rosenbaum, & Cohen, 1990), which is a not uncommon comorbidity in patients with bipolar illness.

Among bipolar outpatients in the SFBN, 40% had a lifetime history of an anxiety disorder diagnosis (Suppes et al., 2001). It appears optimal to attempt to treat both the anxiety disorder and bipolar illness on a two-for-one basis with the use of the mood-stabilizing anticonvulsants, such as valproate, carbamazepine, and lamotrigine, but response to these agents is not always complete. Moreover, the presence of prominent anxiety disorder (or a family history of anxiety disorder) is also a predictor of relatively less robust response to lithium.

Thus, in instances of incomplete antianxiety effects of a mood stabilizer regimen or symptoms of an incipient breakthrough or hypomanic depressive episode, or the initial insomnia associated with it, high-potency lorazepam or clonazepam are widely used in clinical practice. Because of their long half-lives, they are less likely than alprazolam to be abused, and many patients who are attempting to withdraw from alprazolam are switched to these agents so that their taper off these longer acting benzodiazepines can proceed more smoothly.

Although the benzodiazepines were extremely widely used for many of the residual symptom areas in bipolar illness, many clinicians are now instead switching to the use of atypical antipsychotics for the same purpose. The rationale for the use of atypicals (in preference to a high-potency benzodiazepine) is that they might provide more primary antimanic or antidepressant effects in addition to their effects on the target symptoms of anxiety, agitation, and insomnia.

The potential better performance of the atypicals in this adjunctive treatment role is based on their FDA approval for the primary (monotherapy) treatment of mania, and in the instance of quetiapine of depression as well, but direct comparisons of the atypical antipsychotics versus the high-potency benzodiazepines for this adjunctive treatment indication have not yet been conducted.

PRINCIPLES OF THE CASE	STRENGTH OF EVIDENCE
1. Some 40% of patients with bipolar illness have an anxiety disorder comorbidity, and sometimes high-potency benzodiazepines are useful in targeting residual anxiety symptomatology or breakthrough agitation and insomnia that occurs with an impending manic or depressive episode.	++
2. While some data support the potential primary antimanic efficacy of the high-potency benzodiazepines, they are virtually never used alone (in monotherapy) in acute or prophylactic treatment of bipolar illness.	++
3. Lorazepam and clonazepam both have a long half-life and relatively low dependence liability.	++
4. One should avoid the use of alprazolam in bipolar patients because of: (1) its short duration of action (half-life), (2) its potential for rebound anxiety and dependence, and (3) increased risk of a switch into mania.	++
5. As noted by Wehr (1989), a night of insomnia is often a precursor to the onset of a manic episode, and attempts to abort this with a high-potency benzodiazepine may help prevent the emergence of a full-blown episode.	+
6. Aside from rare carryover daytime drowsiness or sedation, these drugs are usually very well tolerated, especially with nighttime dosing.	++
7. One should be particularly careful in driving an automobile while taking benzodiazepines, because motor skills pertinent to driving often are impaired on this class of drugs (many times without being recognized by the individual).	++
8. Alcohol and benzodiazepines are a particularly problematic combination, with effects that may be additive or potentiative, and one should avoid this combination, particularly while driving or operating dangerous machinery.	+
9. In those prone to alcohol use, other anticonvulsants such as carbamazepine, valproate, lamotrigine, and gabapentin are usually preferable to the benzodiazepines because of the latters small but real potential for abuse (overuse and progressive need for dose escalation).	+
10. Valproate has been shown to reduce alcohol intake in patients with bipolar illness and alcohol comorbidity, and topiramate has been shown to be highly effective in decreasing intake in patients with primary alcoholism.	++
11. Clonazepam, like gabapentin, is also useful in the treatment of social phobia.	++
12. In many physicians' practices, the very wide adjunctive use of high-potency benzodiazepines is being supplanted by the use of atypical antipsychotics instead because of their presumed greater range of effectiveness.	+
13. The fact that clonazepam and lorazepam are weight neutral, in contrast to some of the atypical antipsychotics, may make them preferable for some patients at risk for weight gain.	+

TAKE-HOME MESSAGE

Bedtime adjunctive use of a high-potency benzodiazepine such as clonazepam or lorazepam may be highly effective in treating anxiety, agitation, and insomnia associated with an imminent manic or depressive episode, and these agents are widely used because of their general tolerability and safety.

42

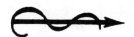

Kindling of Cocaine-Related Panic Attacks: Response to Carbamazepine and Alprazolam

CASE HISTORY

This patient in his mid-20s, without a family history of either affective disorders or panic anxiety disorders, began using cocaine on a regular basis for its euphoria-inducing properties (1978–1981; Figure 42.1). After many months of use, he began to have relatively consistent cocaine-related panic attacks approximately three times a week (January–June 1982). These panic attacks were highly circumscribed and temporally closely linked to taking cocaine, and thus were tolerated relatively well without much associated dysfunction. However, when the panic attacks began to occur spontaneously in July 1982, they were associated with considerable increased generalized anxiety and agoraphobia, because the patient could no longer anticipate when they might or might not occur.

This increasing level of anxiety associated with the now spontaneous panic attacks led him to immediately discontinue all cocaine use. Nonetheless, the panic attacks continued to occur on an intermittent basis and were associated with considerable impairment in his daily life and functioning. He was enrolled in an outpatient study of spontaneous panic attacks, having (supposedly) forgotten that they were initially triggered regularly by cocaine administration. The patient had a moderate response to alprazolam but experienced an occasional breakthrough

panic attack on 3 mg/day of alprazolam and considerable generalized anxiety and agoraphobia. He therefore wished to taper his alprazolam and pursue other therapeutic options.

The initial phase of the alprazolam taper proceeded without difficulty. However, as the dose decreased to the range of approximately 1 mg per day, panic attacks began to reemerge more frequently. This greater difficulty with the last milligram of alprazolam withdrawal is not uncommon and sometimes requires a prolonged period of time to accomplish (i.e., an extremely slow taper). When treatment with carbamazepine was initiated as an alternative to alprazolam, a complete cessation of panic attacks was observed, along with some moderation of his agorophobia. The patient experienced some side effects on carbamazepine and wished to try alternative therapy. Surprisingly, the use of the tricyclic antidepressant imipramine was also associated with a good antipanic response and alleviation of much of his agoraphobia.

BACKGROUND LITERATURE

As alluded to in Chapter 9, there appears to be a sensitization or kindling-like process in the evolution of responses to cocaine (Post, 1977; Post, Weiss, & Pert, 1992; Post, Weiss, Pert, & Uhde, 1987). Animals tested in the same envi-

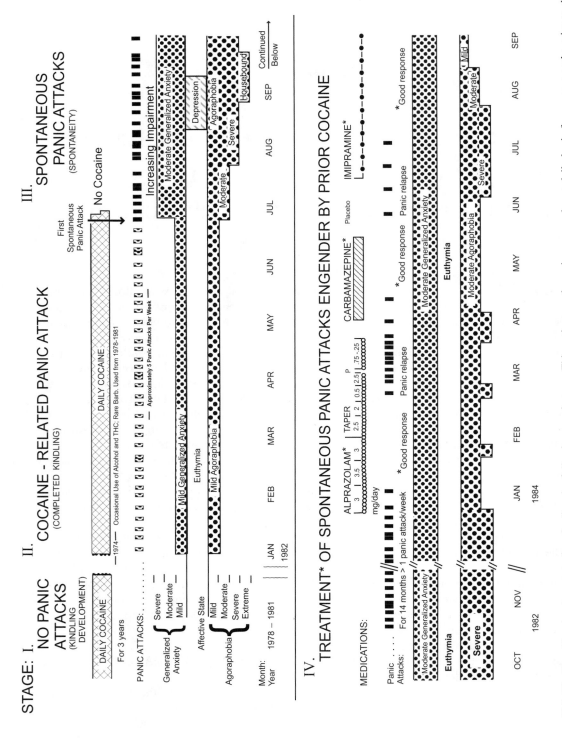

Figure 42.1 Kindling-like development of panic disorder following cocaine use. This patient used cocaine on an almost daily basis for many months prior to the first panic attack and then began to have approximately three to five cocaine-related panic attacks per week (shaded rectangles). In 1982 (at arrow), he had his first spontaneous panic attacks (i.e., in the absence of cocaine administration), and with their continued occurrence despite stopping cocaine use (dark rectangles), he developed more severe generalized anxiety and agoraphobia (top line, right side, and bottom row, left side). His panic attacks subsequently responded in 1984 to the anticonvulsant benzodiazepine, alprazolam, but relapsed on its taper, and then responded to the anticonvulsant carbamazepine, as well as the tricyclic antidepressant imipramine.

ronment become increasingly more hyperactivated by the same dose of cocaine over time, and if one starts with a high enough initial dose, repeated administration of cocaine will eventually be associated with the new onset of full-blown major motor seizures in response to a previously subconvulsant dose of drug (i.e., a pharmacological kindling effect). Following a large number of seizures induced by local anesthetics or electrical stimulation, spontaneous seizures will occur.

Thus, the patient in this case report appears to have followed a kindling-like process, not for seizure evolution, but instead for panic attacks. In other words, he began using cocaine on a regular basis at doses that did not produce panic attacks. Eventually, the threshold was lowered such that panic attacks occurred on an intermittent basis immediately following some, but not all, cocaine administrations. After about 120 such cocaine-induced panic attacks, they then began to occur even in the absence of drug administration. This was clearly documented by the fact that the patient stopped using cocaine altogether and yet continued to manifest panic attacks. These were associated with increasing levels of generalized anxiety and agoraphobia because of their unpredictability.

Following our initial identification of patients such as this, and suggesting that sensitization and kindling-like processes were underlying the evolution of panic attacks, a number of other reports of this phenomenon emerged in the clinical literature (Post, Weiss, et al., 1987). In addition, the number of people whose deaths were related to cocaine use began to become increasingly prominent, not only in emergency room reports, but also in widely publicized deaths of famous Hollywood and sports figures.

In terms of pharmacological kindling in laboratory animals, the seizures induced by the local anesthetics lidocaine and procaine, which are not stimulants like cocaine (because they do not have prominent effects on the release of dopamine and norepinephrine), are well tolerated even for long periods of time and scores of repetitions. In contrast, the seizures associated with cocaine, which is a potent stimulant as well as a local anesthetic, are poorly tolerated, and the laboratory rodent will usually succumb after the first or second cocaine-related seizure. The mechanisms for the increased lethality of cocaine-related as opposed to lidocaine- and procaine-related seizures is not known, but presumably is attributable to cocaine's additional potent effects on increasing levels of synaptic norepinephrine, dopamine, and serotonin by virtue of its reuptake blockade.

The local anesthetic-induced seizure is highly limbic in origin, as revealed by recordings of electrical spiking in the amygdala and related structures of the medial temporal lobe (Eidelberg, Lesse, & Gault, 1963), as well as in directly visualizing this process with 2-deoxyglucose positron emission tomography (PET) scans while animals are experiencing their local anesthetic seizure. The amygdala and hippocampus are strongly activated (Post, Kennedy, et al., 1984). In studies of intravenous procaine in humans, a similar set of structures are involved and activated, although doses well below the seizure threshold are employed (Ketter, Andreason, et al., 1996).

Using 0^{15} blood flow PET scans, we found that in normal volunteers, intravenous procaine infusions increased activity in amygdala, anterior cingulate gyrus, and insula (Ketter, Andreason, et al., 1996). Intriguingly, these were associated with diverse affect changes, ranging from euphoria to anxiety and dysphoria. In addition, some subjects experienced visual illusions or hallucinations, and when this occurred, there was also activation in the occipital (visual) cortex. Volunteers also experienced auditory hallucinations such as buzzing sounds and olfactory illusions including, of all things, smelling tuna fish (Kellner et al., 1987).

All of these findings are of interest in relation to the idea that the limbic system is closely related to emotional regulation and sensory integration of past experiences (LeDoux, 1992), and that its dysregulation may be associated with sensory illusions and hallucinations as well. We note that these experiential phenomena are very similar to those reported by neurosurgeons who have implanted depth electrodes into limbic system structures of patients with refractory epilepsy. Stimulation of these areas produces a wide range of experiential phenomena similar to those evoked by procaine (with the exception of the odor of tuna fish). A sense of anxiety is the most consistent effect elicited (Gloor, Olivier, Quesney, Andermann, & Horowitz, 1982). These observations are also similar to those of Penfield (1955) when stimulating the lateral cortical surfaces of the temporal lobes in neurosurgery patients; these areas of the brain directly overlie the more medial structures of the temporal lobe, such as the amygdala and hippocampus.

Cardiac patients who receive intravenous lidocaine as an antiarrhythmic drug in an intensive care unit situation sometimes spontaneously report the occurrence of doom anxiety, the sense of overwhelming impending threat to one's existence (Saravay, Marie, Steinberg, & Rabiner, 1987). Altogether, these data indicate that the local anesthetics are activating the medial temporal lobe areas of the brain that are associated with the modulation of anxiety, as well as a wide range of affects and affectively laden past experiences.

A critical role for the amygdala has also been elucidated in the conditioning of anxiety to objects in the environment in the work of Davis (1997) as well as LeDoux (1992). They found that if animals are startled by a loud sound, one can condition fear potentiation of this startle response if a light that had been previously associated with the occurrence of a mild electric shock is then paired with the noise startle stimulus. In this fashion, the previously neutral light cues, which now signal an impending aversive experience, potentiate the startle response. Similar conditioned cues could be involved in the cocaine sensitization and kindling responses leading to increasing anxiety and panic.

Recent data suggest that it is quite difficult to decondition or unlearn amygdala-based conditioned responses. Amygdala-based learning is even more impervious to changing cues if parts of the prefrontal cortex are damaged or dysfunctional. The cortex is highly flexible in making new stimulus-response and stimulus-reward conditioned associations, whereas those engendered in the amygdala are very difficult to alter. This is of clinical significance in situations such as depression, PTSD, and cocaine-conditioned anxi-

ety responses, in which there is often decreased neural activity in the prefrontal cortex. This would make it even more difficult than usual for the prefrontal cortex to overrule or inhibit the more primitive and inflexible aspects of conditioned amygdala responsivity.

Davis, Walker, and Myers (2003) have shown that the process of habituation requires active learning and memory itself (requiring unblocked glutamate NMDA receptors) and proceeds best with some degree of emotional arousal. Thus, in attempting to habituate amygdala-based conditioned emotional responses, cocaine-conditioned cues, or PTSD, one must be careful that such attempts are not associated with greater sensitization as opposed to habituation of emotional overresponsivity based on new experience and learning.

Investigators have observed that when experienced users see pictures of cocaine-related cues that elicit craving, there is increased brain activity in limbic areas on PET scans. One can completely subjectively habituate to these cocaine-related cues (i.e., not have the associated craving), but even in the absence of subjective responses, automatic and autonomic conditioned responses in heart rate, blood pressure, and skin conductance still continue. This reveals the extreme difficulties in habituating cocaine-related conditioned cues completely (London, Bonson, Ernst, & Grant, 1999).

This phenomenon perhaps accounts for the fact that patients in rehabilitation can feel that they are completely over their cocaine craving, but when they leave the hospital or return to settings in which they had previously used cocaine, they can relapse in an almost automatic fashion, unaware of the underlying physiological conditioned responses occurring. Case vignettes from Gawin and associates at Yale (personal communication) illustrate this process. Many of their cocaine-addicted patients in the New Haven, Connecticut, area used to take a specific exit from an interstate highway to purchase their cocaine. After these individuals had been through rehabilitation and had been abstinent for a long period of time, they reported that when they intended to drive somewhere else, they unaccountably found themselves automatically driving down the exit ramp they had previously taken to purchase cocaine. This appears to be part of the unconscious or habit memory system, that is, the same mechanism that allows one to automatically drive on the same route to work each day while attention is focused on other tasks such as tuning the radio, talking on the cell phone, and so on. When such a habit is attached to strong emotional cues (via the amygdala), it may be very difficult to unlearn.

From the clinical perspective, these case examples illustrate the importance of desensitizing and habituating cocaine-related cues in their appropriate environment and the difficulty in achieving such a long-term goal. It also, again, indicates the considerable importance of educating patients with affective disorders about not using stimulants recreationally, because one is never sure which people are able to experiment on several occasions and not become addicted, and which will be overwhelmed with eventual compulsive drug use.

Again, cocaine use in the context of bipolar illness is additionally complicated by the phenomenon of cross-sensitization to stress (Sorg & Kalivas, 1991), and it is clear that, in some individuals, stressful experiences can precipitate cocaine craving and relapse. Thus, stress can play a role both in the onset of affective relapses and in those related to stimulant abuse. As noted earlier in Chapter 9, alterations in brain derived neurotrophic factor (BDNF) could underlie this conditioned cross reactivity. If conditioned well enough, affective- and cocaine-related relapses can each also begin to occur in the absence of stressors.

The pharmacology of cocaine-related panic attacks is interesting and appears to be importantly related to anticonvulsant manipulations. Although the patient in this example showed a good antipanic response to the tricyclic antidepressant imipramine, many patients in the literature are resistant to the typical antipanic manipulations if they have had cocaine-related panic attacks and instead require treatment with anticonvulsants. This finding is consistent with the observation that the current patient did have a good response to the high potency benzodiazepine alprazolam as well as the anticonvulsant

carbamazepine, each of which works on a different type of benzodiazepine receptor.

PRINCIPLES OF THE CASE / **STRENGTH OF EVIDENCE**

1. Repeated cocaine administration can be associated with increases in behavioral responsivity (sensitization) rather than the more typically expected decreased responsivity or tolerance that one often sees with opiates. ++

2. As in animals that show increasing amounts of behavioral activity and stereotypy, individual cocaine users may show increasing amounts of activation, dysphoria, and paranoia. ++

3. This sensitization process may be dependent on powerful context-dependent conditioned mechanisms and involve the stimulant (dopamine) properties of cocaine (and amphetamine). +

4. A separate seizure-kindling process can occur with the local anesthetic components of cocaine (also seen with lidocaine and procaine), wherein the repeated administration of the same dose eventually lowers the seizure threshold and seizures begin to occur in response to a previously subconvulsant dose of the drug. +++

5. Local anesthetic seizures, like the electrically kindled variety, if induced enough times, can begin to occur on their own without stimulation (i.e., the stage of spontaneity). ++

6. In this patient, cocaine-related panic attacks seemed to follow a kindling-like process wherein drug administrations that were not associated with panic attacks came to evoke panic (Stage I or

kindling development). Then this association became quite consistent (Stage II or completed kindling) and with enough repetitions of cocaine administration, panic attacks began to occur even in the absence of drug (Stage III or spontaneity). ++

7. When this situation occurs, high-potency anticonvulsant benzodiazepines and other clinically used anticonvulsants such as carbamazepine and valproate may be important therapeutic strategies and are sometimes effective when more traditional antipanic drugs (antidepressants) are not. +

8. It is of interest that cotreatment of an animal with carbamazepine will prevent the development of local anesthetic-related seizures (pharmacological kindling), yet it will not prevent the development of amygdala-kindled seizures based on repeated electrical stimulation, suggesting that different types of kindling have a different neurotransmitter basis. ++

9. Carbamazepine is effective against fully developed amygdala seizures kindled electrically but may not stop local anesthetic seizures once they have fully developed. This finding emphasizes the principle that different stages of kindling evolution may be differentially responsive to drug interventions and that this differs in different types of kindling (i.e., electrical versus pharmacological). ++

10. Although this patient showed a moderate antipanic response to the high-potency benzodiazepine alprazolam, this drug should be relatively avoided in patients with bipolar illness (in favor of clonazepam or lorazepam instead) because alprazolam:

    a. Has a short duration of action ++

    b. After 4 or 5 hours is sometimes associated with increasing amounts of anxiety (a wearing-off effect) and the need for further doses of the drug +

    c. As such, can be more habit-forming and potentially addicting than longer acting high-potency benzodiazepines such as lorazepam and clonazepam +

    d. Can cause switching into mania in both bipolar and nonbipolar individuals ++

11. Some patients have an extremely difficult time withdrawing from alprazolam and, like this patient, have the most difficulty with the last few milligrams of drug. +

12. Many have found that switching from alprazolam to a long-acting, high-potency benzodiazepine (such as clonazepam and lorazepam) makes the benzodiazepine withdrawal process easier. +

13. Carbamazepine cotreatment has also been used with some success in helping patients withdraw from alprazolam. +

14. Chronic carbamazepine administration will induce the metabolism of alprazolam and further reduce blood levels of alprazolam achieved by a given dose of the drug. ++

15. If a patient has one or more cocaine-related panic attacks, or, even more importantly, a single cocaine-related seizure, it would be advisable to stop cocaine use immediately, so that there is no further progression of panic attacks to spontaneity (or seizures that could result in a cardiorespiratory arrest). ++

16. In addition to the above-noted liabilities of cocaine administration, it has also been associated with heart attacks and strokes in young individ-

uals (because of its potent vasoconstricting noradrenergic properties). +

17. If a patient with affective illness develops a cocaine abuse problem, this may present added treatment difficulties, including cross-behavior sensitization to stressors and vice versa. Stressors can reprecipitate cocaine use. ++

18. At the same time, we are fortunate that some of the treatments of bipolar illness can be helpful in the treatment of cocaine-related phenomena. Topiramate and modafinil have been reported to decrease cocaine craving and assist in abstinence in double blind, placebo controlled studies in subjects with primary cocaine abuse. Carbamazepine is effective in those that have an associated mood disorder. +

19. While carbamazepine would theoretically prevent the development of cocaine-related panic attacks and seizures, it might not stop the fully developed ones from occurring. From this case and others in the literature, it appears to prevent the occurrence of late spontaneous panic attacks. +

20. In bipolar patients who have cocaine-related abuse problems, a formal 12-step program and other therapeutic approaches and support groups are highly recommended. +++

21. Cocaine can be an extremely seductive drug because its initial stimulant and euphoric effects (largely dopamine based) appear profound and benign, but with continued use, this pure euphoria becomes harder to achieve (even with dose escalation) and instead is replaced with increasing amounts of anxiety, dysphoria, and paranoia. +++

22. Dose escalation may also engage cocaine's local anesthetic mechanism, contributing to the kindling of panic attacks and seizures. ++

23. The push of hypomania and mania in bipolar disorders to enter new activities, grandiosity, and lack of appreciation of the potential adverse consequences, are ideal mood states for getting into difficulty with cocaine and other drugs of abuse. +++

    a. About 30–40% of patients with bipolar illness do acquire a substance use disorder. +++

    b. Educational and primary preventive programs are particularly indicated for the adolescent or young adult with new-onset bipolar illness. +

    c. One should make a pact (when depressed or euthymic) not to use drugs of abuse when manic, and build in other preventive strategies. ++

TAKE-HOME MESSAGE

Upon repeated administration of the same dose, cocaine's stimulant and behavioral activating effects and its local-anesthetic anxiety and seizure-inducing effects can evolve and increase over time in a kindling-like fashion. Special attention should be given to encouraging bipolar patients to avoid substance abuse in the first place and receiving additional specialized care if they are already experiencing cocaine-related problems.

43

Paradoxical Exacerbation
of Mood Lability by Clonazepam

CASE HISTORY

This patient is a 25-year-old male with a clear history of prolonged mood swings as a teenager and young adult. In the year prior to admission, during a period of treatment with a TCA alone (i.e., TCAs continued when lithium was discontinued), ultrarapid and ultradian cycling began (Figure 43.1). His peer relationships were never well established, perhaps in part because of his early onset mood disorder. The patient met criteria for borderline personality disorder as well as bipolar II.

He failed a number of routine treatments in the community including trials with lithium, benzodiazepines, TCAs, MAOIs, carbamazepine, and antipsychotics. Because of his high levels of anxiety and dysphoria, treatment was continued with clonazepam prior to other NIMH investigational protocols. Mood fluctuations continued unabated, however. They were attenuated during a period off clonazepam, recurred on the drug, and again eased when off clonazepam.

This patient later entered a research study protocol for the calcium channel blocker nimodipine for mood stabilizer nonresponders. His mood fluctuations eventually showed a moderate but unsustained response to nimodipine (Pazzaglia et al., 1993). He showed only a partial response to adjunctive carbamazepine (Chapter 33).

This patient illustrates the potential difficul-ties involved in treating bipolar illness in the setting of a coexistent personality disorder, and the approaches to treatment in these instances are just beginning to be explored. The present case is presented to highlight the unusual exacerbation that can occur with benzodiazepine treatment and reveal the importance of mood charting in order to discern paradoxical or adverse, as well as good, responses to a given treatment.

BACKGROUND LITERATURE

As noted in the previous chapter, there is considerable evidence to support the efficacy of clonazepam and related high-dose benzodiazepines in the acute and long-term treatment of the affective disorders (Chouinard, 1987; Curtin & Schulz, 2004; Edwards, Stephenson, & Flewett, 1991; Pollack, 1993; Sachs, 1990). The high-potency benzodiazepines clonazepam and lorazepam are used in panic-anxiety disorders and social phobia (Beaudry, Fontaine, Chouinard, & Annable, 1985; Charney & Woods, 1989; Reiter et al., 1990; Schweizer et al., 1990; Tesar & Rosenbaum, 1986), as well as being approved for seizure disorders. These drugs, as adjuncts to other primary mood stabilizers, may be particularly helpful in treating the initial insomnia of an imminent manic or depressive episode or the dysphoric component of mania.

Wehr (1989, 1991) has emphasized the impor-

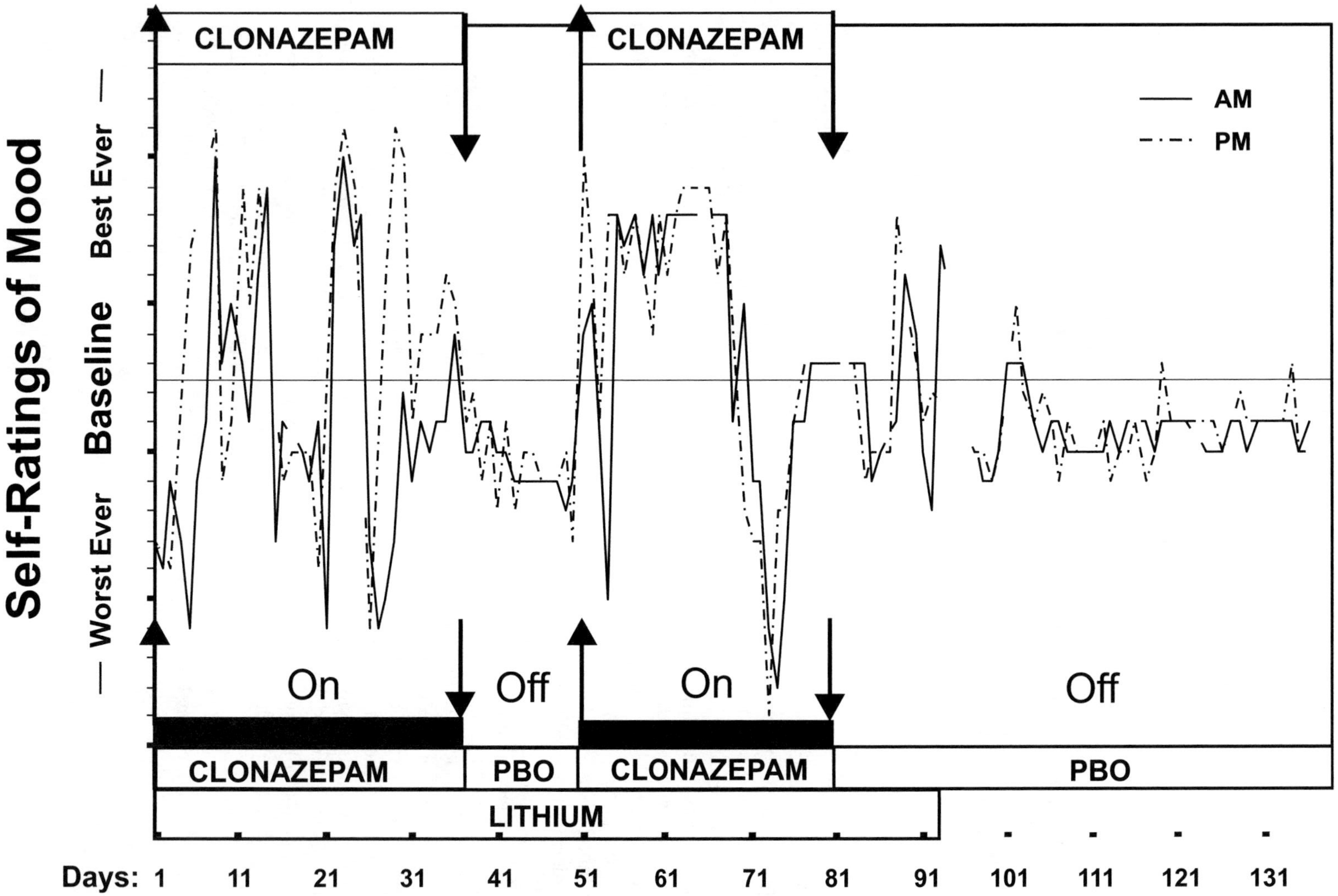

Figure 43.1 Increased mood fluctuations on clonazepam augmentation of lithium: a paradoxical response to a high-potency benzodiazepine. Although clonazepam is a helpful adjunct for a wide range of residual manic, depressive, and anxiety symptoms in bipolar disorder, this patient showed a highly unusual exacerbation of mood lability on the drug, which was confirmed by improvement on placebo substitution, recurrence of the problem on clonazepam a second time, and improvement again off clonazepam. PBO, placebo.

tance of preventing a night of sleep deprivation so as not to precipitate or exacerbate a full-blown manic episode. The nighttime administration of a high-potency, long-acting benzodiazepine such as clonazepam or lorazepam is often a helpful approach in preventing a night of sleeplessness. Kishimoto et al. (1988) has emphasized that clonazepam may be useful in the long-term prophylaxis of recurrent depressive illness of the unipolar or bipolar subtype. Sachs and colleagues (Sachs, 1990; Sachs, Rosenbaum, et al., 1990; Sachs, Weilburg, & Rosenbaum, 1990) also found clonazepam useful in the maintenance treatment of bipolar patients and a suitable replacement for the use of antipsychotic drugs in a substantial percentage of patients.

The report of Aronson, Shukla, and Hirschowitz (1989) suggesting little utility of the high-potency benzodiazepines must be reinterpreted from the perspective that these patients were already shown to be inadequately responsive to antipsychotic drugs (major tranquilizers) from the outset and thus would not be likely to respond to clonazepam (a minor tranquilizer) in any case.

Although the study of Bradwejn, Shriqui, Koszycki, and Meterissian (1990) suggests that lorazepam is more effective than clonazepam in acute mania, considerable data support the utility of clonazepam in a variety of other clinical observations and designs. Moreover, approximately 50% of the 258 patients followed for 1 year in the Stanley Foundation Bipolar Network were treated intermittently with benzodiazepines (Post, Denicoff, et al., 2003).

Thus, the observations in this patient of exacerbation of irritability, lability, dysphoria, and increased amplitude of mood oscillations during treatment with clonazepam and improvement during periods off this medication need to be placed in the perspective that they are highly unusual, perhaps idiosyncratic, reactions. However, the benzodiazepines can cause disinhibitory syndromes in subgroups of patients, particularly in pediatric and elderly patients, as well as in some patients with borderline personality disorder.

This perspective is convergent with the data of Cowdry and Gardner (1988), who observed that the high-potency benzodiazepine alprazolam led to increases in dyscontrol acts in patients with pure borderline personality syndrome (without bipolar illness), in contrast to the substantial therapeutic effects and inhibition of self- and other-related dyscontrol acts during double-blind administration of carbamazepine compared with placebo. Carbamazepine acts through the so-called peripheral-type benzodiazepine (or mitochondrial) receptor (Weiss et al., 1986). The data of Cowdry and Gardner and of this patient suggest that the rare phenomenon of benzodiazepine-induced dyscontrol is mediated through the central-type benzodiazepine receptor at which clonazepam, lorazepam, and alprazolam act.

Patients with borderline personality disorder often have a high incidence of environmental adversities (including a history of abuse) as children, and it may be useful to view them as patients with a complex PTSD syndrome. As such, many of the treatments relevant to PTSD (Chapters 6 and 66) may be useful in patients with bipolar disorder and a comorbid borderline personality disorder.

Patients with bipolar disorder complicated with personality disorder may be at higher risk for an exacerbation of their mood lability with high-potency benzodiazepines and perhaps some antidepressants. Should this occur, other mood-stabilizing approaches should be alternatively considered, including the anticonvulsants carbamazepine, oxcarbazepine, valproate, or lamotrigine, and perhaps topiramate for comorbid alcoholism and PTSD. Reports of Markovitz, Calabrese, Schulz, and Meltzer (1991) suggest that very high doses of the SSRI antidepressants (the equivalent of 60–80 mg of fluoxetine used in conjunction with mood-stabilizing agents) may be required in order to achieve adequate therapeutic effects in bipolar patients with concomitant borderline personality disorder. The same very high doses may also be needed for the treatment of bulimia and obsessive-compulsive disorder, whereas more conventional doses (5–20 mg/day) are usually sufficient for depression and anxiety disorders. In bipolar patients with comorbid borderline personality disorder, the atypical antipsychotics may be particularly useful alternatives to either the benzodiazepines or SSRIs (Fountoulakis, Nimatoudis, Iacovides, & Kaprinis, 2004).

Tolerance and dependence problems are much less prominent with long-acting central-type benzodiazepines such as clonazepam and lorazepam, compared with the short-acting ones such as alprazolam, which can wear off after 4 to 5 hours and is then associated with increases in anxiety. Since alprazolam can also exacerbate or precipitate mania, it should, in general, be avoided in bipolar patients.

Clonazepam or lorazepam substitution for alprazolam may help in the process of benzodiazepine withdrawal. Carbamazepine has been used to help facilitate benzodiazepine withdrawal, although the results are mixed (Schweizer, Rickels, Case, & Greenblatt, 1991). Some of these mixed results might be due to the fact that carbamazepine decreases alprazolam blood levels, perhaps in this fashion inadvertently accelerating the withdrawal process.

PRINCIPLES OF THE CASE	STRENGTH OF EVIDENCE
1. The high-potency (anticonvulsant) benzodiazepines lorazepam and clonazepam may be very useful treatment adjuncts in all phases of bipolar illness.	++
2. These benzodiazepines can help treat the insomnia associated with either depression or mania.	+++
3. They are also effective in the treatment of anxiety and social phobia.	+++
4. Rarely (as seen here), they can cause behavioral dysinhibition in patients with comorbid personality disorder, in children, and in the elderly.	+
5. If benzodiazepine-related exacerbations occur, other mood-stabilizing anticonvulsants or atypical antipsychotics may be more effective.	++
6. Patients can occasionally have unusual (or even paradoxical) reactions to some medications so that a careful monitoring on the life chart of response and side effects is important in clearly delineating and discerning these reactions, and subsequently avoiding them.	++
7. While high-potency benzodiazepines are highly effective acute adjuncts in most anxiety syndromes, they appear less helpful in the chronic phases of PTSD, and other anticonvulsants and the atypical antipsychotics may prove more helpful.	+

TAKE-HOME MESSAGE

Careful documentation of mood ratings can help identify treatments to be avoided, as well as those that are particularly effective in a given patient. Idiosyncratic reactions, even to some of our safest and most widely used treatments, can happen. Individual responsivity and tolerability to a drug (or lack thereof) trumps any general statements about a drug's effectiveness or the percentage of responders reported in the literature.

Part IX

ANTIPSYCHOTICS

Typical Antipsychotics

44

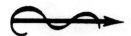

The Role of the Older Typical Antipsychotic Drugs in Bipolar Illness: A Case of Rapid Antimanic Response, but Much Slower Resolution of Psychosis

CASE HISTORY

This patient was a 37-year-old divorced white male who was then unemployed despite a bachelor's degree in anthropology. Over the prior 5 years he had been hospitalized four times for full-blown mania, which had been treated each time with lithium and perphenazine (Figure 44.1). The patient had a history of heavy alcohol use up to 5 years prior to admission and had experimented with marijuana. Eight years prior to admission, he had had a motor vehicle accident in which he apparently lost consciousness for 30 to 40 minutes.

Given this history of full-blown manic episodes despite lithium and a typical antipsychotic, the patient wished to be studied at the NIMH to evaluate the possible antimanic effects of the anticonvulsants carbamazepine and valproate. On the inpatient unit, his mania reached full-blown proportions with a prominent psychotic component (Figure 44.2). His mania and psychosis rapidly improved with the combination of carbamazepine and the typical antipsychotic chlorpromazine, as the atypical antipsychotics described in succeeding chapters were

not available at that time. Chlorpromazine was discontinued and improvement on carbamazepine monotherapy was sustained for about 7 weeks, suggesting response to carbamazepine in average to moderately high doses (1,200–1,600 mg/day). However, these changes were associated with some sedative side effects and occasional dizziness, and response to valproate monotherapy was assessed as an alternative.

Following the taper and discontinuation of carbamazepine, despite therapeutic levels of valproate, a new full-blown manic episode resumed. This new manic episode rapidly responded to carbamazepine treatment, again verifying his responsivity to this anticonvulsant in an on-off-on fashion. However, following the termination of the manic components of the episode, the psychosis persisted despite a variety of treatment interventions, including the reinstitution of first valproate, then lithium, and then the addition of three different typical antipsychotics (Figure 44.2, bottom line). The first was the relatively nonsedating antipsychotic pimozide, then the substitution of the more sedating chlorpromazine for pimozide, and then the high-potency, less sedating trifluperazine for chlorpromazine.

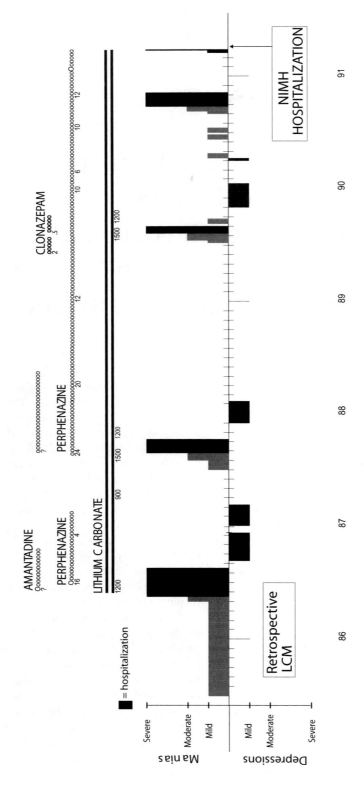

Figure 44.1 Repeated manic hospitalizations despite treatment with lithium and typical antipsychotics. This patient had a manic episode that broke through lithium prophylaxis (1987) and then three more hospitalizations for mania (1989–1991) despite augmentation with a typical antipsychotic, perphenazine.

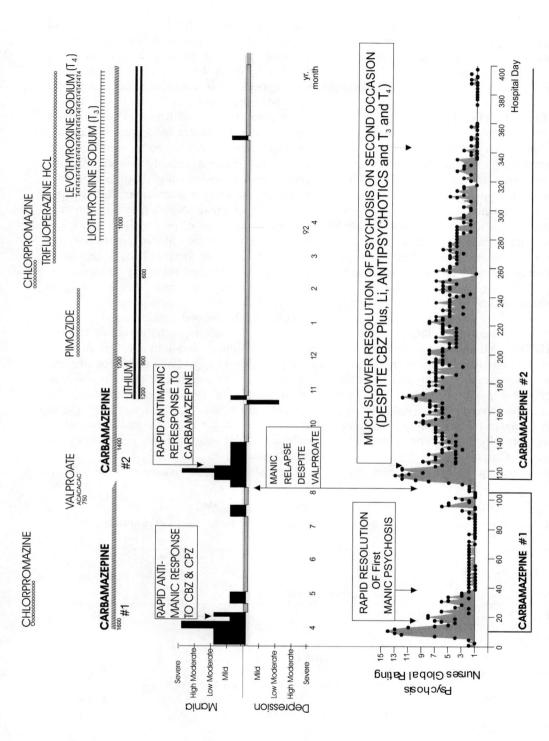

Figure 44.2 Rapid reresponse to carbamazepine, but persistence of psychosis. The patient was admitted to the NIMH with full-blown manic psychosis. Combined treatment with the typical antipsychotic chlorpromazine/thorazine in combination with carbamazepine resulted in a relatively rapid diminution of his mania (top line) and psychosis (bottom line). Valproate was added to see whether it would be sufficient to control his mania, and carbamazepine was tapered. Another full-blown manic psychosis resulted. The reinstitution of carbamazepine monotherapy rapidly improved the patient's manic symptoms (top line), but a persistent high level of psychosis (bottom line) continued for many months despite treatment with multiple medications. Improvement was finally achieved with five medications (top right). CBZ, carbamazepine; CPZ, chlorpromazine; Li, lithium.

It was not until thyroid augmentation with T_3 and then T_4 (instituted to address his persisting depressive symptoms) that the patient's residual psychosis fully disappeared.

BACKGROUND LITERATURE

Prior to the late 1970s and early 1980s, patients with prominent manic recurrences were almost always treated with lithium and periodic augmentation with the typical antipsychotics (neuroleptics) as augmented by benzodiazepines. Those patients, such as this one, with inadequate responsivity often suffered repeated manic recurrences. Carbamazepine and then valproate became recognized as acute antimanic and mood-stabilizing agents that could substitute for, or augment, lithium and neuroleptic treatment regimens.

However, this patient is another example of someone who responds to carbamazepine and not valproate, similar to the patient in Chapter 15, whereas other patients illustrated in other chapters (21 and 22) appear to show the converse pattern of responsivity to valproate but not carbamazepine, again highlighting the issue of individual responsivity among the anticonvulsant compounds (Chapter 16).

We chose to present this patient for an additional reason, however, which is that following a drug taper or discontinuation of an effective treatment (as seen especially with lithium, but occasionally other drugs as well), the resulting manic episode is not always as readily treated as it had been previously. In the studies of Tondo, Baldessarini, Floris, and Rudas (1997), lithium reresponsivity for mania following lithium discontinuation was said to be as good as previously, but patients actually required significantly higher doses of antipsychotics than they had before the lithium discontinuation. This patient would appear to show a parallel phenomenon. While his levels of psychosis were negligible with carbamazepine monotherapy, after his relapse on valproate the psychotic components of the illness remained relatively treatment resistant, even though the manic component again responded as rapidly as previously.

Although the second manic episode was essentially over in 25 days, the psychotic components of his illness persisted for 160 days despite increasingly aggressive treatment attempts with lithium, anticonvulsant mood stabilizers, and a variety of typical antipsychotics. The atypical antipsychotic agents discussed in Chapter 45 were not yet available but would obviously have been a high-priority treatment option for this patient.

This patient is quite unusual in some respects

Table 44.1 *Long-Term Consequences of Using Older (First-Generation) Antipsychotics (Neuroleptics) in Bipolar Illness*

Investigator (N of Bipolars)	Percentage Receiving Neuroleptics	Percentage Tardive Dyskinesia
Yassa et al., 1983 (N = 69)	61% (Current)	41%
Mukherjee et al., 1986 (N = 131)	95% (History) 73% (Maintenance) (avg. 8.7 years)	35%
Waddington and Youssef, 1988 (N = 42)	100% (History) 72% (Current) 300 mg/day CPZ equivalent; avg. 14.6 years	40%
Dinan and Kohen, 1989 (N = 40)	100% (History) (>2 months) 350 mg/day CPZ equivalent; avg. 9.2 years	22.5%
Hunt and Silverstone, 1991 (N = 69)	99% (History) (>3 months) 45% (Maintenance)	19%

Note. From Sernyak and Woods, 1993.

because he is the only individual in whom we have seen an inadequate reresponse to carbamazepine upon its readministration after a period of time off. A failure to reresponse to lithium might occur in some 10–15% of previous lithium responders (Chapter 13), whereas renewed responsivity to carbamazepine is usual and even seen here for manic, if not psychotic, symptoms. However, we think that this case is noteworthy from the more general perspective that the decision to discontinue one's medications after short or extended periods of remission is not uncommon in this illness. As we noted in the chapter on lithium discontinuation-induced refractoriness (Chapter 13), the potential liabilities of this decision are not always readily evident to the patient or family members, or clearly or carefully considered in the risk-to-benefit ratio of the initial decision to stop medication.

The potential liabilities of discontinuing an effective treatment regimen include the following:

1. Symptomatic relapse
2. Full-blown relapse of a manic or depressive episode (illustrated here)
3. An episode requiring hospitalization
4. Further adverse consequences from the above, including loss of job, marital discord, and economic and other losses
5. A much higher risk for a completed suicide (particularly in patients who discontinue lithium)
6. A failure to respond as readily to the same drugs used previously (as illustrated here)
7. A more difficult and persisting psychotic component to the illness, with the requirement for different or more aggressive antipsychotic and other treatment than had previously been needed (as illustrated here)

Episode Sensitization in Psychosis (of Schizophrenia): Increasing Resistance to Typical Antipsychotic Therapy as a Function of Episode Number

The phenomenon of episode sensitization has been most clearly demonstrated in the Hillside

Hospital experience in patients with schizophrenic psychosis (Szymanski et al., 1995). In that study, patients with a first hospitalization for psychosis rapidly responded to their antipsychotic treatment, but when they discontinued their antipsychotic drugs, they suffered relapses requiring rehospitalization. The second round of treatment with antipsychotics required a longer period of time to achieve the same degree of improvement seen the first time. A subgroup of these patients discontinued their antipsychotic drug again and experienced a third episode, which was again more difficult to bring under control than the previous ones. In several instances, patients appeared no longer responsive to their antipsychotic drugs. Thus, an episode sensitization phenomenon may be observed in patients with schizophrenia (Angrist & Schulz, 1990; Sheitman & Lieberman, 1998; Wyatt, 1997) similar to that which we have postulated for manic and depressive episodes in those with bipolar illness (Chapter 10).

Side Effects of the Typical Antipsychotics

The typical antipsychotic agents that block dopamine receptors are effective in the treatment of schizophrenia and bipolar illness (Gerner, Post, & Bunney, 1976), but are associated with a number of adverse side effects, particularly when used in higher doses (Brotman, Fergus, Post, & Leverich, 2000; Cutler & Post, 1982). These adverse effects include acute parkinsonian side effects (stiffness, tremor, rigidity, and slowness in initiating movement); akathisia (restless legs); and dystonic reactions (slow twisting movements), such as opisthotonos (the involuntary contraction of muscles, most noticeably in the neck, causing the head and the back to arch backward) or occulargyric crises (in which the eyes involuntarily move upward behind the eyelids). For these reasons, the typical drugs were often given in conjunction with diphenhydramine hydrochloride or anticholinergic agents such as benztropine.

Despite the improvement in motor side effect profiles these adjunctive treatments achieved,

patients on long-term or intermittent antipsychotics were still at risk for tardive (late onset
of) dyskinesia (involuntary minor motor movements). These involuntary motor movements
typically occur as pill-rolling movements of the
fingers, tongue movements or protrusions, or
lip-smacking movements of the mouth. More
severe tardive dyskinesia can rarely be associated with involuntary contraction of the dia-
phragm and associated difficulty and discomfort
with smooth breathing patterns.

Of bipolar patients exposed to the typical antipsychotics, even on an intermittent basis, 20–
40% may experience the minor forms of tardive
dyskinesia (Hunt & Silverstone, 1991; Table
44.1). This rate exceeds even that seen in patients with schizophrenia, suggesting a relatively increased risk in bipolar illness. This is
one of the reasons that we had previously advised attempting to avoid the use of these older
agents whenever possible in favor of other
mood stabilizers. With the current availability
of atypical antipsychotic agents, we would now
advise their use instead of the typical antipsychotics and in some instances, earlier in the
treatment sequence as adjuncts to another mood
stabilizer for breakthrough manic or depressive
symptomatology, as discussed in the following
chapters.

PRINCIPLES OF THE CASE / **STRENGTH OF EVIDENCE**

1. Some patients are inadequate responders to the older typical antipsychotics (neuroleptics) even when used in combination with lithium (Figure 44.1). ++

2. When lithium and neuroleptics fail, patients may still respond to the anticonvulsants carbamazepine or valproate. ++

3. As in this individual, some patients may respond to carbamazepine and not valproate, although others show the converse pattern. ++

4. This patient's manic symptoms (energy, mood elevation, decreased need for sleep, and hyperactivity) rapidly resolved, but the psychotic components (paranoid delusions and thought disorder) showed a considerable degree of treatment resistance. ++

5. This patient illustrates the difficulties in defining the boundaries of schizoaffective illness (persistent psychosis in absence of an affective episode) in a reliable fashion, even with rigorous formal interviewing techniques and daily ratings of mania, depression, and psychosis. +++

6. The development of a more difficult-to-treat psychotic component of the illness is another risk that is often not considered when patients choose to stop their effective medications. ++

7. The typical antipsychotics are all effective in the treatment of mania; however, the response rate is only about 50%. +++

8. The effectiveness of typical antipsychotics in mania may decrease in those with multiple psychotic episodes. +

9. As opposed to their efficacy in acute mania, there is some evidence that the typicals may increase severity or prolong depressive episodes when used in long-term prophylaxis. +

10. This patient had persisting problems with depression despite two mood stabilizers (lithium and carbamazepine) and a typical antipsychotic un-

til thyroid augmentation was
used.   ±

11. Although the cost of these
older drugs is markedly lower
than the new atypicals (where
generics are generally not
available), use of the atypicals
is preferable (to the typicals)
because of their lower risk of:
(1) acute parkinsonian side effects, (2) tardive dyskinesia,
(3) exacerbation of depression,
and (4) associated decreased
overall tolerability and associated noncompliance.   ++

12. In the past, when patients
were treated acutely with adjunctive antipsychotics, these
drugs were often continued
whether they were needed or
not (Denicoff et al., 2000).   +

13. Of bipolar patients treated
with the older antipsychotics,

even on an intermittent basis,
20–40% develop tardive dyskinesia (involuntary extra minor
movements of the mouth,
tongue, or fingers).   +++

14. Use of intermittent typicals
not only does not prevent the
development of tardive dyskinesia (as previously thought)
but may exacerbate it compared with continuous treatment.   ++

TAKE-HOME MESSAGE

Stopping one's medications and risking having
a new episode of mania or depression is only
one of the liabilities of such a choice; others
include, as illustrated in this patient, a more difficult subsequent treatment course and difficulty
bringing either affective or psychotic symptoms
back to remission.

Atypical Antipsychotics

45

Acute Antimanic Response to Olanzapine in a Patient With a Recurrent Psychotic Depression: Approaches to Weight Gain on Atypical Antipsychotics and Related Drugs

CASE HISTORY

The patient represented in the life chart (Figure 45.1) was a 26-year-old male with a history of recurrent psychotic depressions and full-blown manic episodes. The first manic episode occurred in 1992 at age 20. The second mania in 1995 was associated with tapering of paroxetine during lithium treatment. Lithium had appeared to attenuate the severity of manic and depressive episodes, but even when lithium was combined with valproate and perphenazine, the patient continued to have episodes of moderate severity breaking through prophylaxis. The patient had a brief trial of adjunctive risperidone with lithium and valproate treatment, with only mixed success.

On the inpatient unit the patient suffered from a full-blown manic episode requiring seclusion despite haloperidol treatment. However, he had a good response to the atypical antipsychotic olanzapine only when the dose was increased to 20 mg/day, as noted in Figure 45.2.

This response can still only equivocally be related to olanzapine, because his mania could have ended spontaneously as part of his typical course of recurrent mania punctuated by intervening depression. A subsequent extended period of time well on olanzapine suggested that the response, in retrospect, was likely related to drug treatment, however.

BACKGROUND LITERATURE

Tohen et al. (1999; Tohen, Baker, et al., 2002; Tohen, Chengappa, et al., 2002; Tohen, Goldberg, et al., 2003; Tohen, Ketter, et al., 2003) reported a series of positive studies of olanzapine in acute mania where the rate of response exceeded that of placebo, leading to FDA approval. More recently, olanzapine has been reported to have some efficacy in the treatment of bipolar depression, in which response to olanzapine exceeded that of placebo. More strikingly, however, the combination of olanzapine and fluoxetine yielded markedly significantly greater improvement compared with either olan-

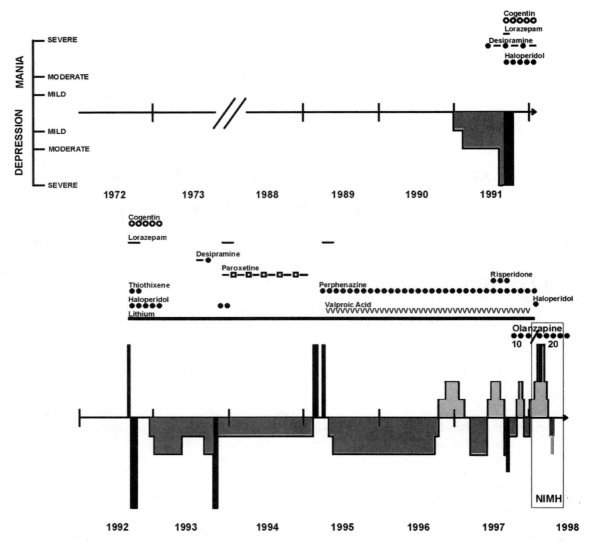

Figure 45.1 Retrospective LCM of repeated manic episodes from 1996 to 1998 despite treatment with lithium, valproate, and the typical antipsychotic perphenazine. Details of prospective course are in Figure 45.2.

zapine or placebo (Shelton et al., 2001; Tohen, Vieta, et al., 2003) leading to FDA approval of the combination for bipolar depression.

Olanzapine is now also approved for long-term prophylaxis. It is also a beneficial adjunct to lithium or valproate (Tohen, Chengappa, et al., 2004). In one study, olanzapine was compared with treatment with valproate and was equally to more effective on all outcome measures (Tohen, Baker, et al., 2002). Most intrigu-

ingly, a study indicated that long-term prophylaxis with olanzapine yielded a better antimanic response than lithium, while there was no difference in depressive breakthroughs (Tohen, Marneros, et al., 2004).

Olanzapine is generally well tolerated with a modicum of sedative side effects and some anticholinergic side effects such as dry mouth, blurred vision, and constipation. More problematic is a moderate to substantial degree of weight

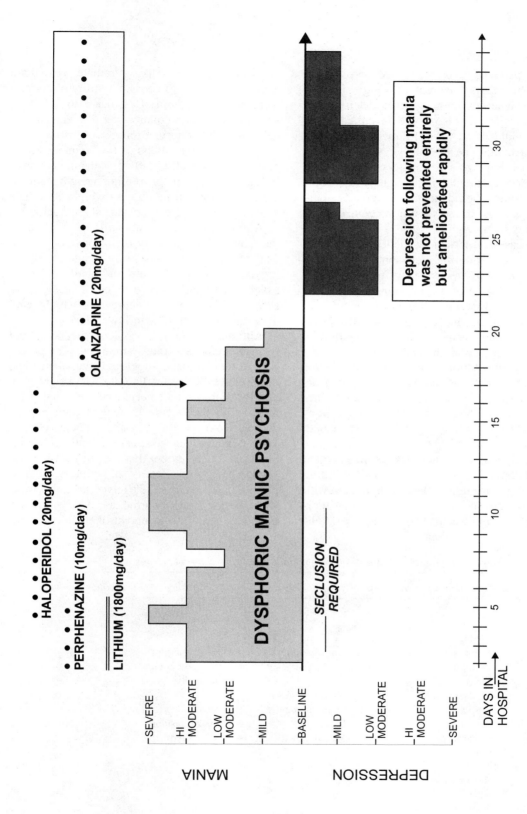

Figure 45.2 Prospective antimanic response to the atypical antipsychotic olanzapine after failing the typical antipsychotic haloperidol.

371

gain in a percentage of patients (McElroy et al., 1998). The relative degrees of weight gain of the atypical antipsychotics are noted in Table 45.1. Olanzapine and clozapine have the highest risk of weight gain (+++), followed by risperidone and quetiapine (++ to +), while ziprasidone and aripiprazole (0) are generally weight neutral, at least in adults. This range of weight gain liabilities should be taken into consideration in patients prone to weight gain or who are already overweight.

Some cases of new-onset diabetes have been reported to occur during olanzapine administration, and this may be secondary to or independent of the degree of weight gain (Buse, 2002; Koller & Doraiswamy, 2002). Clinicians and patients should be alert to this potentially problematic area and ensure the maintenance of adequate exercise, good dietary habits, and certainly, the substitution of noncaloric drinks for those with sugar calories. One study suggests that the risk of diabetes is three times higher with olanzapine than with other antipsychotics or risperidone (Gianfrancesco, Grogg, Mahmoud, Wang, & Nasrallah, 2002).

We and others (Vieta, Sanchez-Moreno, et al., 2004) have had some success in preventing or reversing olanzapine-related weight gain with the concomitant use of the anticonvulsant topiramate. Zonisamide also carries the same likelihood of weight loss as topiramate. Anecdotal evidence suggests the possible utility of cotreatment with a histamine H_2 blocker to help prevent weight gain on olanzapine (Cavazzoni, Tanaka, Roychowdhury, Breier, & Allison, 2003; Pae et al., 2003), although this remains to be more systematically studied. Amantadine may be more helpful in preventing weight gain on olanzapine than in facilitating weight loss once weight gain has already occurred (see below).

Although many patients will show improvement on 5–7.5 mg/day of olanzapine, others appear to require dosages in the range of 20–30 mg/day for optimal acute antimanic and antipsychotic efficacy. These higher doses may be associated with greater degrees of weight gain over one year's time than lower doses.

Although there is some controversy about relative incidence rates among the atypicals, several studies have suggested that olanzapine may possess a greater liability for weight gain and for diabetes (not necessarily associated directly with the degree of weight gain experienced). Both weight gain and diabetes carry a variety of medical risks, as schematized in Figure 45.3. To the extent that weight gain is associated with high levels of cholesterol and plasma lipids such as the triglycerides, they may also increase risk for cardiovascular syndromes, including heart attacks and strokes. In our Stan-

Table 45.1 *Global Assessment of Weight Gain Risk of Psychotropic Drugs*

Lithium and Anticonvulsants		Antidepressants		Atypical Antipsychotics	
Substantial		Mirtazapine	+++	Clozapine	+++
				Olanzapine	+++
Moderate					
Valproate	++	Amitriptyline	++	Risperidone	++
Lithium	++	Imipramine	++	Quetiapine	+±
Mild					
Gabapentin	+	Nortriptyline	+		
Carbamazepine	+	Desipramine	+		
None		SSRI	$0 \rightarrow +$	Ziprasidone	0
Oxcarbazepine	0	Venlafaxine	$0 \rightarrow +$	Aripiprazole	0
Lamotrigine	0				
Mild Loss		Bupropion	−		
Moderate loss					
Zonisamide	−−				
Topiramate	−−				

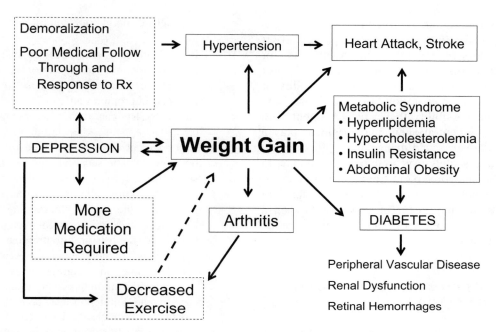

Figure 45.3 Interacting medical consequences of obesity.

ley Foundation Bipolar Network, being overweight was also associated with an increased incidence of hypertension, which itself is also a risk factor for stroke and heart attacks. We also saw an increased incidence of arthritis and other medical problems, with an additional finding of increased severity of depression in those most overweight (McElroy, Frye, et al., 2002). A recent study of olanzepine in childhood and onset mania was highly positive, but many of the side effects were even more prominent than those seen in adults (Tohen et al., 2007)

Approaches to Avoiding Weight Gain

Given these long-term liabilities of weight gain, one needs to be particularly careful in addressing this side effect in choice of drugs for acute, but particularly long-term maintenance treatment of bipolar disorder. One approach that some investigators have used is to aggressively treat patients with an acute manic episode during inpatient hospitalization with, for example,

valproate and olanzapine (both of which can increase weight), but then switch to better-tolerated regimens for long-term prophylaxis (Table 45.1). This could include the weight-neutral anticonvulsants lamotrigine or oxcarbazepine and, if persistent use of antipsychotics is required, the weight-neutral atypicals ziprasidone or aripiprazole.

This approach would appear to have the most utility when the treating physician in the acute phase is the same physician involved in long-term maintenance treatment. Otherwise, there is considerable evidence that once antipsychotic agents are initiated during a hospitalization, other clinicians are slow to withdraw them even in the absence of their demonstrated need. This liability would also likely be the case for the intended conversion to other drugs with more benign side-effect profiles. Although this change may be placed on the long-term treatment agenda, follow through by a different outpatient physician might remain a questionable proposition. There are also some risks involved because response to one set of agents may not directly equate to response to others.

Therefore, an alternative mode is to use better tolerated agents from the start, particularly if there is less severe illness or less pressure for immediate discharge from the hospital after only a few days' treatment. The availability of intramuscular preparations of ziprasidone now raises the possibility that acute treatment with this weight-neutral agent may begin to play a role in the very rapid management of extremely manic and acutely psychotic bipolar patients. In this case, the conversion from intramuscular inpatient medications to orally utilized outpatient medications may occur more smoothly than a transition from one set of atypical antipsychotic agents to another.

Other Approaches to Treatment of Weight Gain

There is a variety of approaches to the prevention or reversal of weight gain that one should consider from the outset of treatment of the bipolar patient:

1. If drugs with weight gain liability are used, patients should be warned of this potential side effect from the outset, and appropriate dietary and exercise regimens should be built into the therapeutic prescription (which is often easier said than done, however).

2. One can choose among the side effects tolerabilities of given classes of agents. Not only are weight-neutral atypical antipsychotics available (ziprasidone and aripiprazole) and weight-neutral antidepressants and anticonvulsants as well, but several anticonvulsants also appear to have beneficial profiles for cutting drug-induced weight gain and enhancing weight loss.

3. Topiramate (Chapter 29) is the best-recognized drug for assisting in weight loss. However, some patients are unable to tolerate its cognitive side effects even at low doses.

4. In these instances, zonisamide (Chapter 30) appears to exert weight loss effects parallel to those of topiramate, and may be an alternative for the bipolar patient who requires both added mood stabilization and weight loss.

5. If antidepressants are to be used, one might give consideration to bupropion instead of an SSRI or mirtazapine because, in some patients, bupropion can cause weight loss and the SSRIs can yield a late rebound increase in appetite after initial periods of slight weight loss. Mirtazapine often has both problematic sedation and weight gain side effects.

6. Another possible alternative to an antidepressant is the use of sibutramine for its FDA-approved indication for weight loss, but not for depression. Sibutramine blocks the reuptake of norepinephrine, serotonin, and dopamine, and originally was studied as a potential antidepressant. It may thus carry some antidepressant potential, but this has not been clearly documented. Moreover, whether this drug, with its theoretical antidepressant profile, would destabilize the illness remains to be ascertained. A preliminary comparison of the weight-loss properties of topiramate and sibutramine reveals equal activity in this domain, but both of these agents were associated with a high dropout rate, topiramate early and sibutramine later for some apparent mood instability (McElroy, Frye, et al., 2007)

7. The antiviral agent amantadine has been reported to significantly attenuate weight gain compared with placebo (Floris, Lejeune, & Deberdt, 2001) but appears less useful for weight loss.

8. Histamine blockers have also been reported to be minimally helpful in attenuating the weight gain with olanzapine or clozapine.

9. One study revealed the norepinephrine reuptake inhibitor reboxetine (not available in the United States) decreased weight gain on olanzapine, although patients still gained considerable amounts of weight during the acute study (but less on the reboxetine versus placebo add-on; Poyurovsky et al., 2003).

10. Psychomotor stimulants are thought to be associated with weight loss, but their effi-

cacy in bipolar illness and ability to sustain this benefit without the development of tolerance has not been clearly established.

11. A novel approach for the future is to use a blocker of the receptor type 1 for endocannabinoids (at which marijuana acts). Rimonabant (20 mg) showed much greater effects than 5 mg or placebo on waist circumference, cholesterol, triglycerides, insulin resistance, and prevalence of the metabolic syndrome (Van Gaal, Rissanen, Scheen, Ziegler, & Rossner, 2005). Concerns about the possibility of increasing depression may limit its usefulness in bipolar disorder.

12. Since weight gain is such a difficult issue to deal with once it has occurred, the best policy appears to be prevention, especially since weight was directly proportional to the number of exposures to previously weight-gain-related psychotropic medications in our outpatient series (McElroy, Frye, et al., 2002). The important point is if there are opportunities to choose among two equally efficacious drugs based on a more benign side effects profile for weight gain, this should at least be factored into the risk-to-benefit ratio for a given approach.

| | STRENGTH OF |
| **PRINCIPLES OF THE CASE** | **EVIDENCE** |

1. Olanzapine was the first atypical antipsychotic specifically FDA approved for use in acute mania, in addition to its original indication for schizophrenia. +++

2. Olanzapine also appears to have a small but significant advantage in acute antidepressant efficacy over placebo when used alone in bipolar depression. ++

3. When olanzapine was used with the serotonin-selective antidepressant fluoxetine, the combination (Symbyax) had very marked antidepressant effects in bipolar depression. +++

4. Olanzapine has a receptor-binding profile that is most similar to clozapine, but olanzapine has a better tolerated side effects profile. ++

5. One problematic side effect of both olanzapine and clozapine is the tendency for weight gain. To prevent weight gain, some have suggested the following:

   a. Topiramate (25–200 mg/day) or zonisamide (100–200 mg/day at night, i.e., h.s.) +

   b. The norepinephrine-reuptake inhibitor reboxetine (Poyurovsky et al., 2003) ++

   c. Amantadine (100 mg once to three times per day (t.i.d.); Floris et al., 2001) +

   d. The H_2 antagonist nizatidine (300 mg twice a day, i.e., b.i.d.; Cavazzoni et al., 2003; Pae et al., 2003) ++

6. In some patients, weight gain can be substantial and can continue to increase with olanzapine use (although the rate of increase moderates after the first 3 to 6 months of treatment). +

7. In association with weight gain, there have been reports of an increased incidence of type II (adult-onset, non-insulin-dependent) diabetes and elevation of cholesterol and lipid profiles. When these occur together and also with increased blood pressure or waist circumfrence, it is called the metabolic syndrome (Table 45.2). ++

8. Patients using olanzapine should be advised to attempt to avoid olanzapine-related weight gain from the outset. ++

Table 45.2 *Diagnosis[a] and Treatment of the Obesity-Related Metabolic Syndrome*

A. Metabolic syndrome (when 3 of 5 criteria are positive)

I. Abdominal obesity	II. ↑Blood sugar	III. ↑ Blood pressure	IV. HDL[b]	V. Tryglycerides
Waist	Fasting B.S. > 100 mg/dL	>130/85 ! mmHg	♀ <50 mg/dL	>150 mg/dL
♀ >35 inches (88 cm)	100–126 mg/dL, impaired;		♂ <40 mg/dL	
♂ >40 inches (102 cm)	> 126 mg/dL, diabetes			

B. Monitoring

Take family history of:
obesity, cardiovascular disease, diabetes
Weight: Buy scale for office
Waist: Buy a tape measure

Blood sugar at:	Blood pressure at:	Fasting Lipids at:
• Baseline	• Baseline	• Baseline
• 3 months	• 3 months	• 3 months
• 1 yearly	• 1 yearly	• every 5 years

C. Clinical symptoms of diabetic ketoacidosis: Note high overlap with lithium toxicity (Li)

a) Polyuria (Li)   d) Nausea/vomiting (Li)   f) Dehydration
b) Polydypsia (Li)   e) Clouded sensorium (Li)   g) Rapid respiration
c) Weight loss (Li)

D. Treatment of Obesity

1. Diet
2. Exercise
3. Behavioral Rx
4. Pharmacotherapy (off label)
   • Topiramate (Topamax)*
   • Zonisamide (Zonegran)*
   • Amantadine (Symmetrel) (300 mg/day)
   • Metformin (Bigwanide, Glucophage) (500 mg tid)
   • Orlistat (Xenical) (120 mg tid) cramps, steatorrhea, ↓vitamins
   • Sibutramine (Meridia) (5–20 mg/day)
   • Nizatine (Axid); H₂ blocker (600 mg/day)

*Drug	Topiramate	Zonisamide
Start	25 mg H.S. or AM	25–100 mg H.S.
Target	50–200 mg/day	100–300 mg H.S.
Max.	300–400 mg	400 mg

a. Diagnosis of Metabolic Syndrome is established when ≥3 risk factors (I–V) are present.
b. HDL = High-density lipoprotein cholesterol.

9. In those who have gained a substantial amount of weight on olanzapine, it would appear prudent to monitor random fasting blood glucose, as well as cholesterol, lipid, and triglyceride levels. A tape measurement of the waist is also recommended. +++

10. Youngsters appear more prone to the side effects of atypical antipsychotics than adults and should also be monitored carefully for the potential liabilities of weight gain and the metabolic syndrome. ++

11. In terms of acute parkinsonian and other extrapyramidal (motor) side effects, olanzapine is clearly better tolerated than the older typical antipsychotics. +++

12. The latest data suggest that olanzapine and the atypicals as a class have the much anticipated lower rate of tardive dyskinesia compared with the older typical antipsychotics, where it was as high as 20–40% in bipolar patients. ++

TAKE-HOME MESSAGE

Olanzapine is an excellent acute and prophylactic antimanic agent and it may also have some acute antidepressant efficacy, but its liability for inducing weight gain should be carefully monitored and in some patients limits long term tolerability and utility.

46

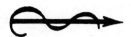

Response to Clozapine in an Olanzapine Nonresponder: Comment on Informed Consent

CASE HISTORY

Prior Clinical Course

The individual depicted in the life chart is a 28-year-old male with a 14-year history of incapacitating psychosis, mania, and depression (Figure 46.1). Prior to his NIMH admission, he had failed to respond adequately to multiple clinical trials of a variety of treatments, and remained substantially impaired by his affective illness. Previous treatment included the mood stabilizers (lithium, valproate, and carbamazepine); the antidepressants (amitriptyline, imipramine, phenelzine, bupropion, fluoxetine, venlafaxine, and nortriptyline); the typical antipsychotics (thiothixine, thioridazine, trifluoperizine, and haloperidol); and the atypical antipsychotics (risperidone and olanzapine).

Upon admission to the NIMH, his depressive episodes were manifested by hypersomnia (increased sleep), anergia (lack of energy), negative ruminations, guilty religious preoccupation, anhedonia (absence of pleasure), and self-deprecatory hallucinations. With an episode switch into a full-blown psychotic mania, his symptoms were characterized by energized grandiose ideas, hyperreligiosity, referential thinking, dysphoria, agitation, and persecutional delusions. His range of past diagnoses (comorbidities) in addition to his bipolar illness was extensive, including alcohol and drug abuse, PTSD, and bulimia nervosa.

Informed Consent and Course During Inpatient Studies and Treatment

Both prior to and throughout his NIMH hospitalization, the patient was made aware of the research context of his hospitalization and repeatedly stated his willingness to undergo double-blind clinical trials with medications that might or might not be of therapeutic value to him. The patient signed a detailed NIMH informed consent statement after a thorough explanation of the potential benefits and risks involved—including the potential for developing a severe, life-threatening rash from one of the compounds (lamotrigine) that he would receive in randomized, blinded fashion. These blinded, randomized protocols would involve an initial phase of medication-free evaluation, if possible; a period of up to 6 weeks on either lamotrigine, gabapentin, or placebo; and the two phases of being crossed over to the other agents. His family was aware of his decision and the risks involved, and supported his entry into the study.

Each week, the patient's willingness to remain in this clinical trial was reassessed by physicians, nurses, and social workers (all of whom

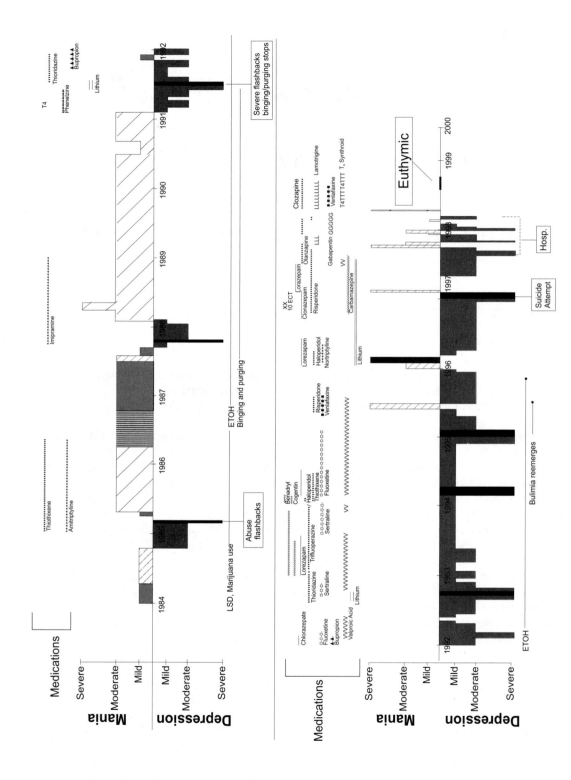

Figure 46.1 Successful mood stabilization with clozapine (plus lamotrigine, venlafaxine, and T_4) following 14 years of incapacitating illness. ETOH, ethanol or alcohol.

were blind to his medication status) during weekly clinical rounds. The patient, because of clinical deterioration, was advanced early from Phase I (which turned out to be placebo) to Phase II, and he remained in Phases II and III for the full 6-week period.

Following completion of all three phases of the study, the patient was offered the option of returning to the previous phase when he had felt best (Phase II), in order to reconfirm response to that medication on a continued blinded basis. The Phase II medication (lamotrigine) at that time was still unknown to both the patient and all staff members, with the exception of the collaborating pharmacist, who was not involved in any of the rating assessments or clinical care decisions. The patient, again, showed a partial, but clinically relevant, degree of improvement in this response confirmation phase.

Treatment Optimization

Because of remaining symptoms, the patient's treatment regimen was supplemented with lorazepam and then topiramate (which were not helpful), before beginning an augmentation trial with olanzapine. Despite the addition of olanzapine to lamotrigine and its supplementation with valproate, the psychotic components of the illness remained severe; thus, the patient was switched to the atypical antipsychotic clozapine with some initial success. However, even with the continued presence of his father on the research unit for support, the patient wanted to return to his hometown and left the NIMH. During a month and a half of further hospitalization at an academic center in the northeast, the dose of clozapine was increased to 300 mg/day, lamotrigine was titrated to 400 mg/day, clonazepam was used for anxiety as needed, venlafaxine was added for residual depression, and T_4 was used for potentiating venlafaxine.

Thus, the combination of (1) an approved agent (clozapine) for schizophrenia (requiring weekly blood monitoring); (2) a then-experimental mood stabilizer (lamotrigine) found to be clearly but only partially helpful in NIMH double-blind clinical trials; (3) thyroid hormone

(T_4); and (4) venlafaxine (approved for use in unipolar depression) were used to achieve, for the first time in many years, an essentially complete clinical remission.

The patient and his father then returned to the NIMH to be further debriefed about the results of his clinical studies. They were both pleased about his research participation and use of information derived from the formal clinical trial about the confirmed partial effectiveness of lamotrigine that was then used in ultimately establishing an effective therapeutic regimen. The clinical staff was amazed with the patient's transformation and could hardly believe he was the same individual who had been so psychotic and incapacitated during most of his inpatient stay.

This case report represents to us an ideal union of (1) acquiring new knowledge from a double-blind, controlled clinical trial series that eventually showed the overall superiority of lamotrigine over gabapentin or placebo, and (2) advancing the patient's individual clinical therapeutics, based partially on information obtained during the formal protocol. The patient and his family, both before and after the blind breaking, appreciated the opportunity to contribute to assessment of the effects of potential new therapies.

Despite being markedly disabled and at times delusional, the patient was able to give explicit verbal and written informed consent about his wish to participate in the controlled (blinded) clinical trials and undergo complex research procedures, including positron emission tomography scans and regional cerebral blood flow with O^{15} water requiring arterial cannulization.

BACKGROUND LITERATURE

Clozapine is the first of a series of atypical antipsychotic agents or major tranquilizers that differ from the first-generation typical antipsychotics in the relative absence of motor side effects. As illustrated in Chapter 10 (Figure 10.11), clozapine retains some of its unique clinical profile because it targets (blocks) dopamine receptors in the mesolimbic (nucleus accumbens, amygdala) and mesocortical (prefrontal cortex) dopamine systems rather than in the dorsal part of the basal ganglia that is primarily involved in motor control. As such, the older antipsychotics are associated with acute parkinsonian side effects (including tremor, rigidity, masked faces, slowness in initiating movement, and dystonic reactions or painful contraction of muscles producing twisted postures). Extrapyramidal side effects occur not because of the loss of dopamine neurons (as in Parkinson's disease) but because of a blockade of dopamine function by inhibiting or antagonizing the dopamine receptor, which is the primary mechanism of action of the antipsychotic drugs.

Another problem with intermittent or chronic use of the typical antipsychotics is the late development of disfiguring involuntary motor movements of the hands, face, and jaw called tardive dyskinesia (see Chapter 44). This occurs in patients with schizophrenia or bipolar illness who are exposed to long-term or intermittent antipsychotic administration, and risk factors appear to be increased age, cumulative dose exposed, and female gender (Brotman et al., 2000).

Patients with bipolar illness are at equal or greater risk of tardive dyskinesia than patients with schizophrenia when exposed to typical antipsychotics. However, with the availability of a whole series of new atypical antipsychotics (Chapters 45–48) that do not possess the same motor side effect liabilities acutely or the late risk of tardive dyskinesia, the role of the atypicals in the sequence of treatments in the overall treatment algorithm of bipolar illness is being reevaluated.

A substantial series of open clinical trials and one randomized study compared with treatment as usual have indicated that clozapine is highly effective for some treatment-refractory rapid-cycling patients with bipolar disorder and also those with dysphoric forms of mania (Calabrese, Kimmel, et al., 1996; Frye, Altshuler, & Bitran, 1996; Frye et al., 1998; Suppes, Erkan, & Carmody, 2004; Suppes, Phillips, & Judd, 1994; Suppes et al., 1992, 1999). Clozapine is unique among the atypicals in that it was available in Europe for many years prior to approval in the United States, because treatment with

clozapine was associated with an approximately 1% incidence of agranulocytosis (absence of white blood cell production), potentially leading to inability to fight infection, overwhelming sepsis, and even death. It was found, however, that close weekly monitoring of the white blood cell count and stopping the drug at the onset of the white count reduction were sufficient to reverse the process and lead to a renormalization of the white cell profile. Thus, mandatory 1-week monitoring schedules were set up, and this novel monitoring program led to FDA approval of the drug in the United States.

In addition to the low but substantial risk of agranulocytosis, clozapine has a series of other noteworthy side effects (Miller, 2000). It is moderately sedating and often associated with weight gain, sometimes of very substantial proportions. Patients also complain of increased saliva accumulation, leading to a wet pillow after a night's sleep. A small group of patients report new onset of panic attacks with the use of this drug.

Perhaps most problematic is the incidence of clozapine-related seizures, particularly in the higher dose ranges. This often necessitates cotreatment with an anticonvulsant. Initially, valproate was widely used for this indication; carbamazepine was avoided because of the possibility of its own hematological side effects. With the availability of other anticonvulsants, particularly those without the liability for weight gain that would add to that of clozapine (such as weight-neutral lamotrigine or weight-reducing topiramate or zonisamide), other drugs are being considered for those requiring high-dose clozapine treatment.

Given this range of potential side effects and the requirement for weekly or biweekly white blood cell count monitoring, clozapine is typically used in bipolar illness only after a variety of other atypicals (with mood stabilizers and other adjunctive treatments) have failed. These are described in the following chapters.

Considerable effort has been expended to understand what makes clozapine different from the typical antipsychotics and possibly more effective than even some of the other atypicals (as illustrated here). It is interesting that olanzapine and clozapine have the most closely overlapping potency profile of blocking a variety of neuro-transmitter receptor systems in the brain, yet clozapine occasionally appears to be superior to olanzapine, as in the current patient.

Moreover, a randomized study in 980 patients with schizophrenia found that clozapine had antisuicide effects superior to those of olanzapine. Although 3% attempted suicide while on olanzapine, and 5% on clozapine, there were fewer hospitalizations and other interventions related to suicidal ideation on clozapine (Meltzer et al., 2003). It remains unresolved which are the crucial elements of clozapine's receptor profile that account for its better spectrum of clinical efficacy than the typical and some atypical antipsychotics.

PRINCIPLES OF THE CASE	STRENGTH OF EVIDENCE
1. Like the patient in Chapter 34, this patient showed switching into mania or hypomania when treated with antidepressants. This included amitriptyline in 1985–1986, imipramine around 1988, bupropion in 1992, venlafaxine in 1995, and nortriptyline in 1996. Some of these switches occurred despite concurrent treatment with antipsychotics or valproate, yet no switch occurred in the latter part of 1992 on the combination of fluoxetine and bupropion, or in 1993–1994 in the face of two further exposures to sertraline and then fluoxetine.	+
2. This pattern is typical of many patients who appear sensitive to switching on antidepressants on some occasions, but not others.	++
3. The patient was found to be a confirmed partial responder to lamotrigine during two separate double-blind trials, but other drugs were required to achieve clinical remission.	++
4. It appeared that clozapine was a crucial element in achieving remission, because other atypicals, such as risperidone and olanzapine, had not previously been adequately effective. Moreover, venlafaxine had been used previously without much success as well. The use of T_4 augmentation may have contributed to the further success of the treatment with this patient, however.	++
5. Thus, it took the combination of four different types of drugs—the atypical antipsychotic (clozapine), the mood-stabilizing anticonvulsant (lamotrigine), the second-generation antidepressant (venlafaxine), and thyroid augmentation (with T_4) to achieve a substantial euthymic interval for the first time in 14 years of otherwise incapacitating illness.	++
6. Complex combination therapy is required for some otherwise highly treatment-resistant patients with bipolar illness.	+++
7. It may take multiple revisions of the regimen to find an effective one, especially since different, equally complex, regimens in the past were not as effective.	++
8. Like many others with bipolar illness, this individual had a past history of substance use, including LSD and marijuana as well as alcohol, which complicate treatment.	++
9. A history of substance abuse and childhood adversity are	

risk factors for eventually developing a rapid-cycling course, but this did not occur until late in his illness.   +++

10. Avoidance of alcohol began in 1996 and brief periods of remission occurred in 1997 and 1998, before his more sustained remission, raising the possibility that avoiding abuse of alcohol helped contribute to the patient achieving mood stabilization.   +

11. Despite being one of the most ill and highly treatment-resistant patients we have seen, this patient was still able to achieve sustained remission. He had previously failed a clinical trial of 10 ECT treatments, and multiple agents in each class of treatments, yielding one of the highest scores on the treatment-refractory index (0–100 maximum; see Appendix 5). Yet he still showed dramatic improvement on the right combination of treatments.   ++

12. This patient had intermittent severe PTSD symptoms and a prior history of binging and purging. These two comorbidities are not uncommon in bipolar disorder and may add to difficulties in treatment.   ++

13. This individual's participation in the clinical trial of lamotrigine helped contribute to the group findings that it was significantly more effective than either gabapentin or placebo (Frye, Ketter, et al., 2000; Obrocea et al., 2002). Yet at the same time it yielded valuable information about his own responsiveness to a (then novel) anticonvulsant.   ++

14. The uncovering of partial responsiveness to lamotrigine in a controlled clinical trial shows the occasional secondary rewards of participating in a new drug study.   +

15. It should be emphasized, however, that an overriding principle in the informed consent process has to be that such research participation may or may not ultimately be directly or indirectly helpful to a given individual.   +++

16. Nonetheless, a positive experience and outcome of being a patient volunteer is not at all uncommon in our experience.   ++

17. Clozapine is superior to olanzapine in reducing suicides and preventing hospitalization for suicide in patients with schizophrenia.   ++

18. Yet given the availability of a range of effective, better tolerated, safer, and more convenient atypical antipsychotics, use of clozapine is generally reserved for those with failure to respond to several other atypical antipsychotics in the class.   +

TAKE-HOME MESSAGE

In some instances, atypical antipsychotic agents may be critical components of the therapeutic strategy in bipolar illness, and sometimes the efficacy of clozapine may exceed that of its close relative olanzapine and other antipsychotics.

47

Atypical Antipsychotics Quetiapine, Risperidone, and Ziprasidone in Bipolar Illness

A UNIQUE PROFILE OF QUETIAPINE?

Rather than present individual patient's responsivity in this chapter, we highlight the general use of quetiapine, risperidone, and ziprasidone for a range of symptom targets in bipolar illness. All three drugs are widely used for adjunctive therapy in the management of acute mania, as typified in Figure 47.1. All existing studies support the general principle that any major tranquilizer (either a typical or atypical antipsychotic) that is approved for the treatment of schizophrenia is also an effective antimanic agent. All of the newer atypicals show about 50% response rates in monotherapy, which is significantly greater than placebo, and all are now FDA approved for acute mania, except clozapine which is likely the most effective. There are isolated case reports that each atypical (with the exception of clozapine) may exacerbate or precipitate mania in rare cases (Frye et al., 1998).

In the Stanley Foundation Bipolar Network series, atypical antipsychotics were often used to address residual depressive symptomatology not responding to more conventional mood stabilizers (such as lithium, carbamazepine, valproate, lamotrigine). In these instances, the ratings of the severity of depression using the Inventory of Depressive Symptomatology (IDS)

were more prominent than the minor degrees of mania (Figure 47.2). Quetiapine was associated with the onset of improvement in IDS depression ratings in the first month and thereafter, which was not seen with the two other agents. These were naturalistic data and did not represent a randomized, controlled clinical trial. They did, however, give a hint that quetiapine might possess some clinically useful antidepressant effects. This has now been documented in the controlled trial of Calabrese, Keck, et al. (2005) and has been replicated (Thase et al., 2007) leading to the first FDA approval of a monotherapy for bipolar depression.

This study by Calabrese et al. and the replication revealed remarkable acute antidepressant effects of both 300 and 600 mg/day of quetiapine versus placebo in acute bipolar depression. Improvement in depression, anxiety, and sleep were prominent in the first week of treatment ($p < .001$). The magnitude of effect was similar to that of the olanzapine-fluoxetine combination and exceeded that of olanzapine in the Tohen, Vieta et al. (2003) studies. Almost identical effects of quetiapine were seen in the second study, supporting antidepressant effects of quetiapine in both bipolar I and bipolar II depression. Two studies of quetiapine in long term prophylaxis are also highly positive in the prevention of both manic and depressive episodes,

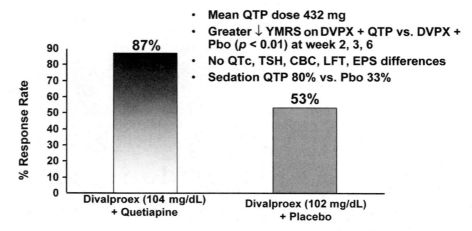

Figure 47.1 Adjunctive quetiapine in adolescent mania. This study from Melissa DelBello and colleagues (2002) at Cincinnati shows the acute antimanic efficacy of quetiapine in adolescents with mania when added to valproate. Their new study (DelBello et al., 2006) also indicates efficacy in monotherapy. QTP, quetiapine; DVPX, divalproex; Pbo, placebo; EPS, extrapyramidal side effects; YMRS, Young Manic Rating Scale; QTc, time interval between Q and T waves on the electrocardiogram; TSH, thyroid stimulating hormone; CBC, complete blood count; LFT, liver function tests.

such this drug will likely be the first drug approved for acute and prophylactic treatment of both phases of manic-depressive illness.

BACKGROUND LITERATURE

Receptor Profiles Versus Efficacy and Side Effects of the Atypical Antipsychotics

The relative affinities of the atypical antipsychotics in comparison with the classic typical antipsychotic haloperidol, with its prominent effects of blocking dopamine 2 (D_2) receptors, are listed in Table 47.1. The atypicals acting on serotonin type 2 (5-HT_2) and other receptor systems are thought to convey potential antidepressant effects and protect, to some extent, against parkinsonian and other extrapyramidal side effects (EPS) along with the inherent anticholinergic effects of these agents. The general profile of side effects, as outlined in Table 47.2, to some extent matches these receptor affinities.

Risperidone, because of its potent D_2-blocking effects, at doses over 6 mg/day may begin to produce parkinsonian and other extrapyramidal

side effects (Simpson & Lindenmayer, 1997). This profile contrasts with most of the other atypical antipsychotics, which have a much wider dose range prior to inducing EPS, and EPS are very rarely produced by clozapine at any dose. In fact, clozapine treatment has been noted not only to acutely decrease one of the more disturbing long-term side effects of the typical antipsychotics, tardive dyskinesia, but also to ameliorate its symptoms in long-term use (Iqbal et al., 2003). It is still unclear whether any of the other atypicals will ameliorate tardive dyskinesia in the same fashion.

In conjunction with this proclivity for inducing EPS at high doses, risperidone is also associated with increases in prolactin because of its relatively unopposed blockade of D_2 receptors. Prolactin elevation is also a consistent effect of all of the older typical antipsychotics, and this elevated production can be associated with menstrual irregularities, sexual dysfunction, and, in some cases, the generation of breast milk from nonpregnant individuals (galactorrhea). As opposed to risperidone, quetiapine and ziprasidone are not associated with increases in prolactin, and aripiprazole even lowers prolactin a little based on its partial agonist properties at the

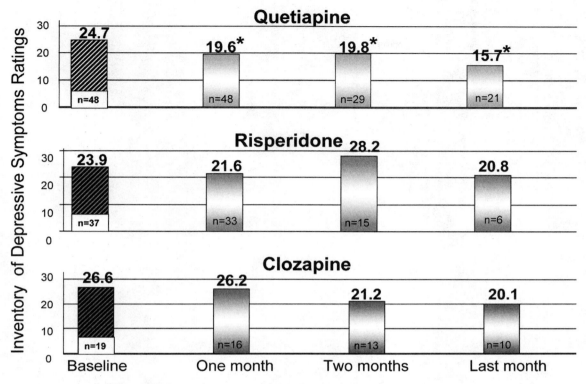

Figure 47.2 Possible antidepressant efficacy of quetiapine: comparison with risperidone and clozapine in an open case series. This figure illustrates the reduction in severity of depression as measured on the Inventory of Depressive Symptomatology (IDS) in Stanley Foundation Bipolar Network patients when quetiapine was added on an open-label basis to previously ineffective pharmacotherapy. Improvement occurred in the first month of ratings and remained significant over the second and third months of follow-up (top row). In contrast, there were no significant decreases in IDS ratings on risperidone (middle row), nor, surprisingly, on clozapine (bottom row).

dopamine receptor (Hamner, 2002; Mullen, Jibson, & Sweitzer, 2001).

As noted previously, risperidone and quetiapine are associated with a moderate liability for weight gain, whereas ziprasidone and aripiprazole are weight neutral. Thus, molindone is the only typical antipsychotic not associated with weight gain, and ziprasidone and aripiprazole are the only atypicals not associated with weight gain (see Chapter 46). Interestingly, these last two antipsychotics are among the least associated with daytime sedation and both are sometimes given in morning doses, whereas the other atypicals are traditionally dosed almost exclusively at night to take therapeutic advantage of their sedative side effects profile in promoting sleep.

An FDA warning accompanies ziprasidone because of its ability to increase the Q-T interval on the electrocardiogram (EKG). The Q-T interval reflects the length of time of cardiac contraction, and widening beyond 500 milliseconds is thought to increase vulnerability to arrhythmias of the type that could be life threatening. However, during postmarketing surveillance, this has not been reported as a problem, and ziprasidone is increasingly being used with minimal amounts of EKG monitoring.

Mechanistically, ziprasidone is also of interest because, in addition to its usual profile as an atypical antipsychotic, it also appears to exert important effects on the blockade of serotonin and norepinephrine reuptake (Tamminga, 2003). These properties are reminiscent of the effects

Table 47.1 *Relative Strength of Receptor Activities Postulated Related to Positive and Negative Effects of Atypical Neuroleptics Relative to Haloperidol*

Receptor	D_1	D_2	5-HT Type 1A	5-HT Type 2	α_1	α_2	Histamine 1	Muscarinergic 1-5
Negative side effects of receptor activity	↓Motor activity ↓Enabling effects on D_2 receptor activity	EPS (relative to 5-HT type 2 receptor); ↑prolactin	—	Weight gain (5-HT type 2C receptor)	Reflex tachycardia, hypotension dizziness	Block blood pressure effects of clonidine; panic attacks	Sedation, drowsiness, weight gain	↓Memory (M_1), blurred vision, sinus tachycardia, dry mouth, constipation, glaucoma ↓EPS; Cognitive Improvement (M_2)
Positive effects of receptor activity	Block stress effects ↑signal to noise ratio	Antipsychotic	Antidepressant Anxiolytic	Antidepressant, ↓EPS (5-HT type 2A receptor) ↑Slow wave sleep (SWS)		Antipanic? Antidepressant?		
Haloperidol (Haldol, butyrophenone)	+++	++++	0	+	+	NA	0	0
Clozapine (Clozaril, dibenzodiazepine)	++	++	+	++	+++	+++	+++	++++
Risperidone (Risperdal, benzisoxazole)	++	++++	+	++++	+++	++	++	0
Olanzapine (Zyprexa, thienobenzodiazepine)	++	+++	0	++++	+++	NA	+++	++++
Quetiapine (Seroquel, dibenzothiazepine)	+	++	↑,↓	+	++++	+	+++	++
Ziprasidone (Geodon)	++	+++	+++	++++	++	NA	+	0
Aripiprazole (Abilify)	↑,↓ +	↑,↓ +++	↑,↓	++++[a]	++	NA	++	0

Note. Ratings: 0, none; +, weak; ++, mild; +++, moderate; ++++, strong; ++++, very strong; NA, not available; ↑,↓, partial agonist; D_1, dopamine type 1; D_2, dopamine type 2; 5-HT, serotonin; EPS, extrapyramidal side effects.
[a] , full antagonist at 5-HT$_{2a}$ receptors.
Modified from Pickar (1995).

Table 47.2 *Clinical Profiles of the Atypical Antipsychotics Relative to Haloperidol*

	Relative Potency, Chlorpromazine Equivalents	Weight Gain Liability	Sedation	Autonomic	Extra-pyramidal Side Effects	Prolactin↑	(Starting Dose)/ Usual Clinical Range (mg/day)	Half-life
Haloperidol (Haldol)	2	+	+	+	+++	+++	(1)/5–20	3 wk
Clozapine (Clozaril)	100	+++	+++	+++	+/–	0	(50)/100–600[c]	8 hr
Risperidone (Risperdol)	1.5	++	++	++	++	++	(1)/4–12[c]	20 hr
Olanzapine (Zyprexa)	4	+++	++	+	+	+	(2.5–5)/10–25	35 hr
Quetiapine (Seroquel)	100	++	++	++	+	0	(25–100)/ 300–900 (limbic selective)	6.9 hr (but single h.s. dose is feasible)
Ziprasidone (Geodon)	50	0	++[a]	++	++	+	(20)/80–200	5 hr
Aripiprazole (Abilify)	15	0	+[b]	0	+	––	(2.5–5)/15–30	72 hr

Note. Ratings: 0, none; ±, equivocal; +, mild; ++, moderate; +++, substantial; –– opposite.
[a]May cause activation; give in morning.
[b]Least sedating, can be given in morning.
[c]Modification from Richelson (1996).
Adapted from Gerlach & Peacock (1995).

of antidepressant compounds, and the relative antidepressant efficacy of ziprasidone requires further exploration. Several cases of ziprasidone-induced hypomania and mania have been reported (Baldassano et al., 2003; Davis & Risch, 2002), as observed on most of the atypicals except clozapine. Ziprasidone may ultimately emerge as useful in depression, as might be predicted on the basis of both its well-tolerated side effects profile and its theoretical mechanistic utility for this phase of the illness via norepinephrine and serotonin.

The receptor profile of quetiapine, with the exception of its lower potency (affinity) in blocking D_2 receptors, only gives some hints as to why it may be a better tolerated antidepressant than several of the other atypicals. Because of this lower affinity, the ability of quetiapine to diffuse on and off the receptor relatively rapidly could also be important to its psychotropic profile, relative lack of EPS, and lack of increase in prolactin (which ordinarily should accom-

pany potent D_2 receptor blockade (Nemeroff, Kinkead, & Goldstein, 2002). Chronic pretreatment with quetiapine blocks the decrease in brain-derived neurotrophic factor induced by stress (Xu et al., 2002; Park et al., 2006), a property shared by all antidepressants (Chapter 9). Moreover, the active metabolite nor quetiapine has now been found to potently inhibit norepinephrine re-uptake process (like many other unimodal antidepressants) and to be a partial agonist at serotonin 5HT-1A effects which increase dopamine release in prefrontal cortex (Goldstein et al., 2007). These effects alone or together could account for quetiapine's apparent superior antidepressant effects compared to other atypical antipsychotics.

Antidepressant Actions

While the antidepressant effects of quetiapine and olanzapine plus fluoxetine are noted above, what is less clear is to what extent these will be representative or a class effect of all atypicals (Ghaemi, Charry, Katzow, & Goodwin, 2000). Some of the old typical antipsychotics could even exacerbate depression (Ahlfors et al., 1981; Denicoff et al., 2000).

The receptor profile of ziprasidone is consistent with its antipsychotic and antimanic effects; in addition, its potent ability to block 5-HT$_2$ receptors as well as increase synaptic norepinephrine and 5-HT levels could be relevant to its potential antidepressant effects. In addition, Kim et al. (2007) reported that ziprasidone prevented the restraint stress induced decrements in hippocampal BDNF, while the typical antipsychotic haloperidol showed the opposite effect and exacerbated the stress effects on BDNF.

As noted, ziprasidone (along with apipirazole) has the advantage over all other atypicals in being weight neutral. Its relative lack of histamine (H$_1$) blocking activity could also account for the fact that it is among the least sedating of the atypicals and can be associated with a sense of mild agitation or activation in some patients, particularly at low starting doses of 20–40 mg. As anecdotal case reports had suggested that this was less likely to happen with higher initial starting doses, these observations have now been directly confirmed in patients with schizophrenia. Vanderburg and associates (2007) compared 40, 80, 120, and 160mg/day (the later two doses achieved by day 3), and found 160mg/day was the most efficacious at 1 week and was equally well tolerated. Whether this would directly extrapolate to patient with affective illness remains to be further studied.

Risperidone was the most widely used atypical antipsychotic agent in the United States until quetiapine recently achieved this status. The efficacy of risperidone has been demonstrated not only in monotherapy for acute mania, but also in trials in which it was added to a previously ineffective mood stabilizer such as lithium or valproate (Bowden, Myers, Grossman, & Xie, 2004; Hirschfeld et al., 2004; Vieta, Brugue, et al., 2004; Yatham, Binder, Kusumakar, & Riccardelli, 2004). Its antidepressant effects have been less well studied (Ostroff & Nelson, 1999) and are more ambiguous.

Vieta et al. (2001) studied 299 patients presenting with bipolar I disorder and 183 with schizoaffective disorder, bipolar type, who were treated with an average dose of 3.9 mg/day of risperidone for 6 months. The mean score on the Hamilton depression rating scale declined in a highly significant fashion, from an initially low baseline rating of 12.8 ± 7.9 to 4.1 ± 4.8 at 6 months. These data suggest good overall antidepressant effects, although one caveat is that this was an open study in patients who were only minimally depressed at baseline. Hillert, Maier, Wetzel, and Benkert (1992) had previously reported a 70% response rate in psychotic depression with risperidone monotherapy, and Dwight, Keck, Stanton, Strakowski, and McElroy (1994) found a 94% response rate in 18 patients with schizoaffective illness of the bipolar depressed type.

General Tolerability and Weight-Gain Side Effects

Risperidone and quetiapine share a moderate liability for weight gain in contrast to the more considerable liability for this side effect with olanzapine and clozapine, and an absence of this side effect for ziprasidone and aripiprazole (Baptista et al., 2004). Despite this side effects profile of some of the atypicals, they are (as a class) better tolerated in bipolar illness than conventional or typical antipsychotics, which have a much higher proclivity for causing acute parkinsonian side effects and other EPS such as akathisia and dystonia, and possibly depression as well. Moreover, long term, even the intermittent, use of the typical antipsychotics is associated with an approximately 20–40% incidence of tardive dyskinesia in patients with bipolar illness, which appears to be in excess of the rate even in patients with schizophrenia (Brotman et al., 2000; Hunt & Silverstone, 1991).

Thus, given the unusual sensitivity of bipolar patients to long-term side effects of the typical antipsychotics, the atypicals should be used whenever possible. Attention to their weight gain liability is also indicated (McElroy et al., 2002). In addition, there are reports of new-onset ype II diabetes in some adolescents and adults treated with the atypicals (Gianfrancesco et al., 2002; Koller & Doraiswamy, 2002; Sernyak, Leslie, Alarcon, Losonczy, & Rosenheck, 2002; but see Regenold, Thapar, Marano, Gavirneni, & Kondapavuluru, 2002; Ryan, Collins, & Thakore, 2003) and the FDA has included a black box warning for all the atypicals. Possible approaches to this problem are discussed in the previous several chapters.

Usual Doses

The typical doses of quetiapine are 25–100 mg h.s. (at night) for effects on insomnia, and substantially higher doses (400–600 mg) are used for antimanic and antipsychotic effects. Doses of 300 and 600 mg/kg h.s. had approximately equal acute antidepressant effects (Calabrese, Keck, et al., 2005), suggesting that 300 mg or below is a target dose. Whether lower doses would also be this effective remains to be ascertained. Calabrese has suggested the utility of a test dose of 25mg of quetiapine on a Friday or Saturday night just in case an individual is extremely sensitive to the sedative effects which can sometimes carryover to the next morning.

The dosing of ziprasidone is slightly more complicated based on its general lack of sedating properties and, in some instances, its ability to produce uncomfortable degrees of activation or agitation at low doses (20–40 mg/day). These effects are reportedly less substantial if one initiates treatment at higher doses such as 80–120 mg/day (Di Lorenzo & Genedani, 2002) or even 40mg on day 1 rapidly titrated to 160mg/day (Vanderburg et al., 2007). Moreover, a preparation of ziprasidone for intramuscular use has recently been developed, and 40-mg injections are highly efficient in helping to stabilize acute manic excitation and may be repeated at 4 to 6 hours as needed (Keck & McElroy, 2004).

The dose of risperidone should be kept under 6 mg/day because higher ones are more likely associated with EPS. 1 to 2 mg may be effective for some affectively ill patients, but still is associated with increases in prolactin. A long-acting or depo form of the drug is available for administration about once over 2 weeks. This may be particularly helpful for the group of patients with euphoric mania and poor insight into the potential adversities of the disorder (i.e., they can have complete denial of illness).

PRINCIPLES OF THE CASE	STRENGTH OF EVIDENCE
1. Like the older typical antipsychotics (neuroleptics), all of the atypical antipsychotics possess acute antimanic efficacy.	+++
2. The older typical antipsychotics have the problem of causing untoward acute motor or extrapyramidal side effects including parkinsonism (motor slowing, rigidity, and tremor), akathisia (restless legs), dystonias (slow twisting movements of muscles), and so on, and often require concomitant medication with anticholinergic drugs to moderate these effects.	+++
3. The atypicals have their own inherent anticholinergic properties via blockade of acetylcholine receptors of the muscarinic type, and thus extra anticholinergics are not needed.	++
4. In addition, the older typical antipsychotics are associated with a moderate incidence of tardive dyskinesia (repetitive and disfiguring movements of tongue, lips, or fingers) in 20–40% of bipolar patients so exposed, even on an intermittent basis.	+++
5. The atypicals have a more benign acute and long-term side-effects profile in terms of EPS, and a relative lack of tardive dyskinesia development in long-term administration.	++
6. The atypicals have a range of tolerability for side effects such as weight gain with olanzapine > clozapine > risperidone > quetiapine > ziprasidone = aripiprazole, the last two being weight neutral.	++
7. Consideration should be given to an individual patient's risk for weight gain (i.e., sedentary lifestyle with no	

exercise) as well as the other drugs being used in the assessment of the risk-to-benefit ratio of using a given atypical.   ++

8. However, in those at high risk for weight gain, many clinicians are switching patients over to better tolerated regimens for long-term prophylaxis once the patient has been acutely stabilized.   +

9. The atypicals also have a range of effects on prolactin, with olanzapine having minimal effects, and risperidone considerable increases, in contrast to clozapine, quetiapine, and ziprasidone, which are prolactin-neutral, and aripiprazole, which actually decreases prolactin based on its partial dopamine agonist effects.   ++

10. The atypicals also are differentially grouped in terms of sedation, with the most sedating drugs being olanzapine, clozapine, and quetiapine. Risperidone and aripiprazole are less sedating drugs, and the least sedating atypical is ziprasidone.   ++

11. The relatively good antidepressant effects among the whole group of the atypical antipsychotics compared with the typicals is likely based on their novel serotonergic mechanisms and anatomical targets of action outside the striatum (motor system).   +

12. Currently, there is strong support and FDA approval for the antidepressant effects of quetiapine (300 mg and 600 mg h.s.) versus placebo in the monotherapy of acute bipolar depression.   +++

13. Significant improvement was seen even by week 1 of quetiapine for depressed mood, anxiety, and sleep.   ++

14. The magnitude of antidepressant effects of quetiapine monotherapy exceeds that of olanzapine and is about equal to the effects of the olanzapine-fluoxetine combination.   ++

15. As quetiapine can be sedating, dosing should be all at night (h.s.).   ++

16. One might start at low (25 mg/day) doses for those highly prone to sedation, and then, as tolerated, rapidly proceed upward as tolerated toward a target of 200–300 mg h.s.   ±

17. Ziprasidone may be associated with uncomfortable degrees of agitation and activation at low doses, but these side effects are reportedly less apparent both with higher initial doses and the intramuscular preparation.   +

18. Quetiapine has also been reported to be effective in augmenting the effects of SSRIs in the treatment of obsessive-compulsive disorder.   +++

19. Extrapolating from above and based on clinical vignettes, quetiapine may be helpful in those with insomnia, agitation, and ruminations associated with both acute depressive and manic episodes and may be an alternative to (and possibly more effective than) the high-potency benzodiazepines that are widely used for the insomnia and agitation of both depressive and manic phases.   ±

20. While aripiprazole and olanzepine are FDA approved for prevention of manic episodes, quetiapine is likely to be the first atypical approved for prevention of both manic and depressive episodes.

TAKE-HOME MESSAGE

The atypical antipsychotics as a class have many advantages over the older typical antipsychotic agents in bipolar illness and, with few exceptions, should be used in place of the typical drugs because of better tolerability (except for weight gain), safety regarding tardive dyskinesia, and antidepressant efficacy (for which quetiapine is now FDA approved).

48

$$\sim\!\rightarrow$$

Aripiprazole: A Dopamine D_1, D_2, D_3, and Serotonin 5-HT$_{1A}$ Receptor Partial Agonist FDA Approved for Acute and Continuation Treatment of Mania

BACKGROUND CLINICAL DATA

Aripiprazole only became available in pharmacies in November 2002 and was not approved for bipolar illness until 2004, and therefore we do not have a good long term life chart case to present. Under Principles of the Case, we present preliminary suggestions about the potential use of this most atypical of the atypical antipsychotic agents.

It is likely that aripiprazole will play an increasing important role in the treatment of bipolar disorder. All of the antipsychotic agents that have been shown to be effective in schizophrenia are also effective in mania. Four placebo-controlled studies in acute mania using aripiprazole were positive (Keck et al., 2003; Keck, Calabrese, et al., 2006; Sachs et al., 2006; Vieta et al., 2005). Two retrospective chart review studies have found aripiprazole to be effective in pediatric bipolar disorder also (Barzman et al., 2004; Biederman et al., 2005). The potential for antidepressant effects (as discussed mechanistically below) is good.

In open studies in refractory depression, Worthington, Kinrys, Wygant, and Pollack (2005)

reported 59% improvement rates with aripiprazole; Barbee, Conrad, and Jamhour (2004) found 47% who improved; Simon and Nemeroff (2005) found that all eight completers of their study achieved remission; and Papakostas et al. (2005) found a 56% response rate when aripiprazole was added to existing antidepressant regimens. A highly positive placebo controlled trial was presented at the APA meeting, 2007 indicating good acute adjunctive antidepressant effects of aripiprazole in unipolar depression (Berman et al., 2007). A second study was equally positive, so it is likely that these data will be submitted to the FDA for approval.

In an open study, McElroy and colleagues (2007) found a substantial rate of effectiveness when aripiprazole was add to previously inadequate treatments of bipolar depression. The moderate dropout rate may have been related to too high a starting dose, often 10 or 15mg/day. In a double blind placebo controlled study, Marcus et al (2007) reported significant antidepressant effects at weeks 6 and 7, but not at end point at week 8. In contrast to the study in unipolar depression where the maximum dose was 20mg/day and the dropout rate low (10%), the study in bipolar depression had a maximum dose of 30mg/day and the dropout rate was high (45%). Thus, aripiprazole may very well be approved for unipolar depression, before further studies are conducted using a slower titration schedule in bipolar depression.

In a double blind study Nickel et al. (2006) reported highly significant effects of aripiprazole compared to placebo for both anxiety and depression associated with borderline personality disorder. Thus, based on mechanistic considerations of the entire class of atypical antipsychotics and the available data on aripiprazole in mania and depression, it is highly likely that this drug with its good tolerability profile will play an increasing important role in the acute and long-term treatment of bipolar illness.

MECHANISMS OF ACTION

Aripiprazole is not a complete blocker or antagonist of the dopamine receptor, as are all of the other typical and atypical antipsychotic agents. Instead, it has minor (20%) agonist or dopamine stimulatory properties on its own, yet it continues to occupy the dopamine receptor in the presence of local, synaptic (endogenous) dopamine that is released from nerve endings. Thus the excess dopamine cannot get to the receptors because aripiprazole is occupying like a partially fitting key in a lock, it only opens the door 20% of the time, but prevents the more effective key (dopamine) from opening the lock. In this fashion aripiprazole provides a functional (80%) blockade while it exerts no more than 20% of receptor activation or agonism (Davies, Sheffler, & Roth, 2004; McGavin & Goa, 2002).

In Parkinson's disease there is a loss of dopa-

mine neurons. With the antipsychotic drugs that are full antagonists, parkinsonian side effects (stiffness, slowness, tremor) can occur because the normal amount of dopamine that is present cannot reach its receptors. In contrast, dopamine agonists stimulate the receptor and help treat Parkinson's disease (Table 48.1).

Full dopamine receptor blockade by the older and some new antipsychotics is also associated with increases in prolactin, since dopamine normally exerts inhibitory control over secretion of this hormone. If dopamine cannot reach the receptor, prolactin increases. Aripiprazole not only does not increase prolactin, but because of its low intrinsic agonist activity, it actually reduces prolactin levels slightly. Thus, it would not cause the side effects sometimes associated with high levels of prolactin, such as menstrual irregularity and, rarely, galactorrhea (the development of milk in the breast tissue when an individual is not pregnant).

Two other properties (summarized in Table 47.1) also raise the possibility of antidepressant effects: (a) aripiprazole is a partial agonist, not only for D_1, D_2, and D_3 receptors but also for 5-HT_{1A} receptors; and (b) it is also a full antagonist at 5-HT_2 receptors. Because 5-HT_{1A} receptors are thought to be involved in the antidepressant effects of compounds such as buspirone, this aspect of aripiprazole's mechanism could also be of theoretical utility in the depressive phase of bipolar illness (Fleischhacker, 2005).

A series of studies have suggested that the 5-HT_{1A} blocker pindolol can accelerate or enhance the antidepressant effects of a variety of unimodal antidepressant agents (Olver, Cryan, Burrows, & Norman, 2000), perhaps by blocking the presynaptic 5-HT_{1A} or autoreceptors that initially inhibit the firing of serotonergic neurons.

Table 48.1 *Full Dopamine Agonists Effective in Depression*

Receptor	Drug	Effective In	Author(s)
D_1	Piribedil (ET 495)	Depression	Shopsin and Gershon, 1978 Post et al., 1978
	Bromocriptine	Depression	Silverstone, 1984
D_2, D_3	Pramipexole	Depression	Goldberg et al., 2004 Zarate et al., 2004

Thus, it is thought that one of the reasons for the delay in the onset of action of the serotonin-selective antidepressants is that they block serotonin reuptake, increase serotonin overflow, and thus initially overactivate these presynaptic or inhibitory autoreceptors. It is proposed that when the 5-HT$_{1A}$ autoreceptors finally become desensitized by chronic antidepressant treatment, serotonergic neural firing can return to normal and antidepressant effects can become maximal.

Pindolol, as a direct antagonist, is thought to speed up antidepressant response because it removes the brake on serotonergic firing at the 5-HT$_{1A}$ autoreceptors from the beginning of antidepressant treatment. To the extent that the partial agonist aripiprazole acts as a functional antagonist at 5-HT$_{1A}$ receptors, it theoretically could also have a pindolol-like effect in acceler-

ating antidepressant responses. This theoretical possibility remains to be directly explored and tested in the clinic, however.

Positive antidepressant effects could also occur via full blockade by aripiprazole of 5-HT$_2$ receptors. This action is thought to be associated with improvement in mood and also increases slow-wave (or deep) sleep, like nefazodone and trazodone, which also block 5-HT$_2$ receptors.

IMPLICATIONS OF PARTIAL AGONISM

Figure 48.1 illustrates how a partial agonist might act like a functional antagonist. On the left side of the figure, direct agonists such as the natural transmitter dopamine itself, or the

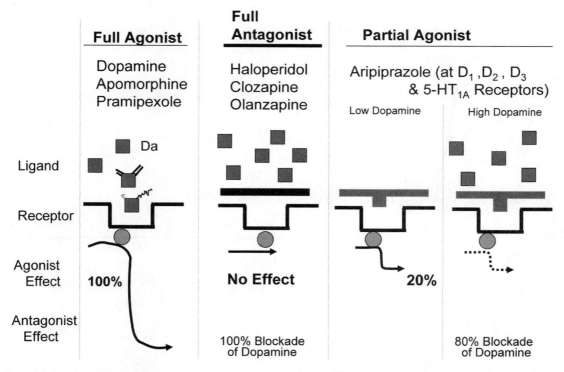

Figure 48.1 Aripiprazole is a partial agonist at dopamine D$_1$, D$_2$, and D$_3$ receptors and at serotonin 5HT$_{1A}$ receptors. Full agonists (left) activate the dopamine receptor and produce full (100%) biochemical and behavioral effects. In contrast, full antagonists (middle) of the dopamine receptor are all antimanic and antipsychotic agents, blocking the receptor and preventing the effects of excess dopamine. A partial agonist (right) stimulates the dopamine receptor a little (like dopamine, but only to 20% of full effect). However, since it occupies the receptor it will also prevent excess dopamine activity (i.e., it produces an 80% functional blockade).

drugs apomorphine and pramipexole are capable of stimulating the dopamine receptor and producing a 100% stimulatory effect. In contrast, the typical and atypical antipsychotic drugs, when they occupy dopamine D_2 receptors prevent dopamine effects (Figure 48.1, middle).

In instances in which dopamine levels are low, aripiprazole acts as a weak or partial agonist, producing a maximum of 20% of full dopamine receptor stimulation. (Figure 48.1, right side) Because it occupies the receptor under conditions of excess dopamine in the brain, that may occur spontaneously or by increased release of dopamine by stimulant drugs such as amphetamine, all of this extra dopamine cannot reach the receptor, resulting in a functional antagonism of the dopamine receptor; only the 20% intrinsic activity of aripiprazole remains (Figure 48.2).

These actions account for aripiprazole's rela-

tively positive side effects profile compared with many other typical and atypical antipsychotic agents. Most of the other antipsychotic agents have dose-related side effects wherein higher doses block more of the dopamine receptors in the brain and produce side effects such as parkinsonian immobility, rigidity, tremor, and many other motor phenomena. In contrast, neither aripiprazole's therapeutic nor side effects appear to be clearly dose related. No matter how high the doses increase, 100% dopamine receptor blockade is never achieved because the 20% intrinsic agonist effect continues to be present (Figure 48.2).

For this reason, 15 mg/day appears to be both an adequate initial and final dose in the treatment of schizophrenia. However, bipolar patients appear to be more sensitive to some side effects. Because of this, it may be useful to start even adult patients at a low or baby dose, 2.5

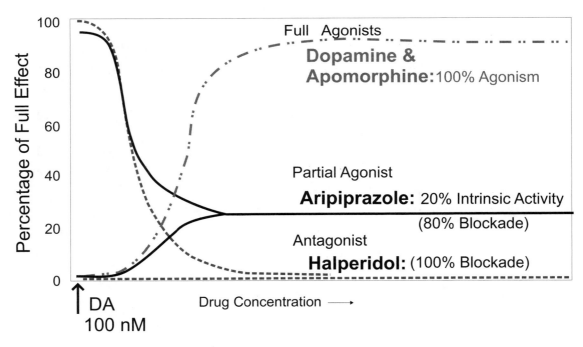

Figure 48.2 Schematic of the receptor-modulating effects of partial agonists. Dopamine or the full agonist apomorphine at high enough concentrations (top, right) produce full effects. In contrast, no matter how high the dose or concentration of aripiprazole, it never exceeds 20% of full dopamine-like effects (middle). If a dose of dopamine is given (arrow left), haloperidol at high enough doses (bottom right) will completely block its effects. However, aripiprazole will still exert its own 20% agonist effects, and its blocking effects will never exceed 80% of full blockade.

mg/day, particularly in an attempt to avoid the uncomfortable side effects of akathisia (restless legs). This low starting dose is a must for children who may experience nausea and vomiting from higher starting doses.

PRINCIPLES OF THE CASE	**STRENGTH OF EVIDENCE**

1. Aripiprazole has a unique mechanism of action because it is not a complete blocker of dopamine D_2 receptors the way all other typical and atypical antipsychotic agents are. +++

2. Instead, aripiprazole acts as a functional antagonist because it occupies the dopamine receptor as a weak agonist (with 20% intrinsic activity) and thus prevents further excess dopamine from reaching the receptor. ++

3. This likely allows for its antimanic effect, and aripiprazole is now FDA approved for acute and continuation treatment for this indication. ++

4. In addition to its partial agonist effects at dopamine D_2 receptors, it is also a partial agonist at D_1, D_3, and serotonin $5\text{-}HT_{1A}$ receptors. This ability to minimally activate or "tickle" multiple dopamine and the $5\text{-}HT_{1A}$ receptors could be relevant to antidepressant and antianxiety effects. Aripiprazole will likely be approved for unipolar depression before it is for bipolar depression. ++

5. Additionally, it is a full blocker of $5\text{-}HT_2$ receptors, an action that is usually associated with increases in deep or slow-wave sleep. +++

6. Because of its inherent partial agonism and consequent functional antagonism, it has a benign and non-dose-related side effects profile (largely similar to that of placebo), with the exception of akathisia. ++

7. Its partial agonist effects allow for mild suppression of prolactin as opposed to marked increases in prolactin with all of the other typical antipsychotics and some of the atypicals. ++

8. A very important side effect property of aripiprazole is that it is weight neutral. This property contrasts with other atypicals, with the sole exception of ziprasidone (which is also weight neutral). ++

9. The drug can cause akathisia (restless legs), apparently more so in patients with bipolar illness than with schizophrenia. +

   a. Therefore, it might be useful to start at very low doses (2.5 mg) and increase slowly to the target range of 10 to 15 mg/day (or higher doses in some patients which have anecdotally been reported to help achieve a more complete remission, i.e., in the range of 30 to 45 mg/day). ±

   b. If one is on another atypical and transitioning to aripiprazole, it might be useful to add aripiprazole to the other agent first. One can then slowly taper the other atypical while increasing aripiprazole. +

10. Children are also prone to akathisia as well as gastrointestinal distress (nausea and vomiting), and starting them at 2.5 mg/day (or every other or third day in the youngest children) is also advisable. +

11. One hopes that aripiprazole's partial agonism at multipe dopamine

receptors will contribute to a good antidepressant profile in patients with bipolar illness, yielding similar positive antidepressant effects of the full dopamine D_2 agonist such as bromocriptine and the D_2 and D_3 agonist pramipexole (Table 48.1).   ±

12. Metabolism or kinetics of aripiprazole:

   a. The half-life ($T_{1/2}$) is about 47 to 68 hours. The $T_{1/2}$ of the active dehydroaripiprazole metabolite is about 94 hours.   +++

   b. Steady-state levels are achieved after 14 days of once-daily administration.   +++

   c. Aripiprazole is metabolized by hepatic enzymes: CYP-2D6 and CYP-3A4.   +++

   d. Slow metabolizers of CYP-2D6 (about 8% of Caucasians) have 60% higher levels of aripiprazole.   ++

   e. Inhibitors of 2D6 (such as fluoxetine and paroxetine) or of 3A4 (such as erythromycin and verapamil) will increase blood levels, and downward dose adjustment of aripiprazole may be considered or needed.   +++

   f. Inducers of 3A4 (such as carbamazepine) will lower blood levels considerably (by half or more), and the dose of aripiprazole can be adjusted upward accordingly.   ++

TAKE-HOME MESSAGE

Aripiprazole's unusual mechanisms of action may account for its excellent side effects profile compared with placebo and should render this drug of considerable utility in the acute and long-term management of bipolar illness.

Part X

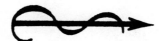

COMPLEX COMBINATION
THERAPY

49

Response to the Combination of Carbamazepine and Valproate in the Absence of Response to Either Drug in Monotherapy and a Comment on Sleep Deprivation

CASE HISTORY

This 57-year-old married professional man with bipolar II disorder had a medical history that was unremarkable, aside from receiving thyroid hormone from ages 16 to 18 for unclear reasons. At age 22 he developed 3-month episodes of mild dysphoria alternating with mild hypomania. At age 49 he had his first major depression (Figure 49.1), which was refractory to 200 mg/day of imipramine plus lithium augmentation. After 8 months of imipramine therapy, he developed a more rapid cycling pattern with depressions and hypomanias that lasted 2 to 6 weeks. This persisted despite adequate outpatient trials of lithium plus imipramine, lithium plus nortriptyline, lithium plus phenelzine, lithium plus carbamazepine, lithium plus carbamazepine and imipramine, carbamazepine plus phenelzine and levothyroxine, and monotherapy with valproate. He was admitted to the 3-West clinical research unit of the NIMH, and after oral and written informed consent, his cyclic mood disorder was evaluated. His depressions were characterized by anhedonia, hypersomnia, psychomotor retardation, passive suicidal ideation, and decreased appetite, energy, memory, and concentration. His hypomanias involved irritability, intrusiveness, racing thoughts, and increased energy, distractability, and verbal productions. Both depressive and hypomanic symptoms, as assessed by nurses' twice-daily ratings and self-ratings, were not affected by adequate and sequential trials of carbamazepine (a 14-week trial of 800 mg/day with plasma levels of 8.2–10.8 μ/ml), carbamazepine plus bupropion, nimodipine alone, and valproate alone (a 23-week trial of 2,125 mg/day with plasma levels of 81–124 μg/ml). In each instance, depressions (Figure 49.2) and hypomanias (not illustrated) of approximately equal severity to those observed on placebo occurred.

Following the lack of response to carbamazepine or valproate monotherapy, it appeared highly unlikely that the patient could have a response to both of these drugs in combination. However, one of our associates (Dr. Terence Ketter) argued that this might occur and encouraged us to perform the combination clinical trial illustrated, despite the qualms of the authors.

There was substantial improvement on the combination of carbamazepine plus valproate

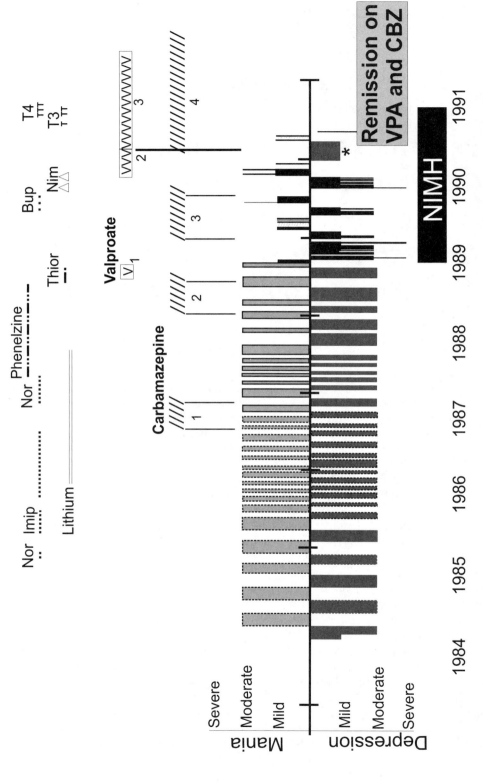

Figure 49.1 Failure to respond to carbamazepine or valproate separately, but a good response to the combination. This patient showed persistent bipolar illness with cycling, which responded to neither carbamazepine (on three occasions in 1987, 1989, and 1990) nor valproate (on two occasions in 1989 and 1990), and yet he had a complete response to combination treatment with both drugs. In 1986 and 1987, he also showed no response to lithium combined with several antidepressants. The apparent decreased severity of depression on valproate monotherapy (*in 1991) was not reflected in his self-ratings, as noted in Figure 49.2.

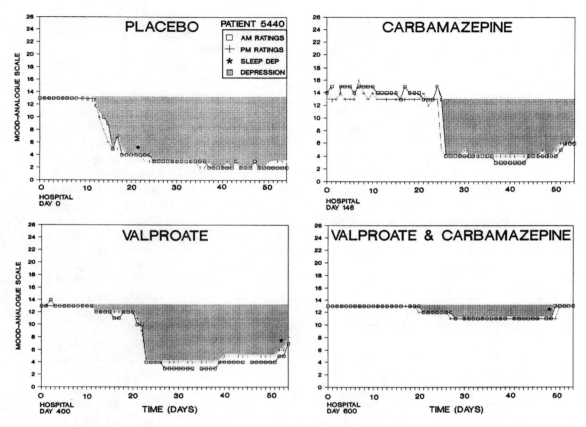

Figure 49.2 Self-rating of depression severity shows the synergistic prophylactic response to the valproate-carbamazepine combination. The first sleep deprivation (*) early in the depressive episode (top left) resulted in no mood improvement, but those near the end of an episode (bottom row) triggered mood improvement.

(carbamazepine 400 mg/day with plasma levels of 6.0–7.1 μg/ml; valproate 2,500 mg/day with plasma levels of 86–111 g/ml). For the first time in 7 years, an expected depression did not occur and the patient remained essentially asymptomatic. In general, he tolerated the combination well. However, he did develop elevated thyroid-stimulating hormone levels (up to 16.9 μg/ml); decreased free T_4 levels (down to 0.8 ng/dl), and symptoms of hypothyroidism (bradycardia and low energy). His thyroid abnormalities were treated initially with T_3 with good results. To assess whether the addition of T_3 contributed to the patient's mood improvement, T_3 was briefly discontinued, and no adverse effects on mood were noted. However, the abnormal thyroid function tests and bradycardia

recurred, so that the T_3 was reinstituted and combined with T_4 to minimize side effects.

BACKGROUND LITERATURE

We have discussed the use of carbamazepine or valproate for rapid or continuously cycling patients in previous chapters. There has been little systematic exploration of these drugs in combination with each other in psychiatry, although the carbamazepine-valproate combination is a more widely studied and utilized approach to patients with treatment-refractory epilepsy (Ketter, Pazzaglia, & Post, 1992). In a number of case series, more complete anticonvulsant responsivity appeared to be associated with the use of these two agents in combination than had been achieved with monotherapy (Froscher, Stoll, & Hoffmann, 1984; Gupta & Jeavons, 1985; Sovner, 1988). What is less clear is whether any of these epilepsy patients were completely nonresponsive to each drug in monotherapy and then showed a good response in combination, as illustrated in bipolar illness in the current individual.

There are a number of medical rationales for the use of these two drugs in combination. They have somewhat different mechanisms of action and side effects profiles (Chapter 9). However, their use in combination is not uncomplicated because they have prominent pharmacokinetic interactions, described later.

Biochemical Rationales for the Combination of Carbamazepine and Valproate

Mechanistically, these two agents both share some actions but differ substantially in others (Post, 1987; Post, Weiss, & Chuang, 1992). Valproate has a variety of effects on gamma-aminobutyric acid (GABA) metabolism, which results in increased brain GABA levels, whereas carbamazepine does not appear to affect GABA levels at clinically relevant doses. Carbamazepine more likely has interactions with $GABA_B$ receptors related to those acted on by the $GABA_B$ agonist baclofen (a drug with antipain and antispasticity effects). Carbamazepine is thought to exert its major actions in seizure disorders by blocking sodium channels and decreasing glutamate release.

It is interesting that valproate also has some efficacy in blocking these sodium channels by a slightly different process. Moreover both drugs (like lithium) appear to be weak inhibitors of calcium influx through the glutamate NMDA receptor. They also can enhance potassium efflux acutely (which stabilizes neuronal membranes) and, like lithium, they both inhibit the inositol transporter and increase $GABA_B$ receptors in the hippocampus upon chronic administration. Clinically, valproate is efficacious in the treatment of petit mal or absence epilepsy by

virtue of its effect on T-type calcium channels. Conversely, carbamazepine can exacerbate absence seizures.

Therefore, these divergences and partial convergences in the mechanistic profile of carbamazepine and valproate could theoretically be helpful in their actions on targets important to therapeutic effects in affective illness. Their side effects profiles are divergent, and even in animal studies there appears to be evidence of an additive anticonvulsant efficacy without additive toxicity. In the animal model of amygdala-kindled seizures, when both drugs are used in combination at marginally effective doses in monotherapy, the combination is able to slow the development of anticonvulsant loss of efficacy or tolerance (Chapter 9).

In the studies of Denicoff, Smith-Jackson, Bryan, and associates (1997), when carbamazepine, which had previously been inadequately effective in a year of monotherapy prophylaxis, was added to the combination of lithium and valproate (which had also been inadequately effective for a year), a number of patients showed clear clinical improvement. These observations, along with the current case illustrated, are at least consistent with the perspective that dual or triple therapy with combinations that contain carbamazepine and valproate may at times be clinically useful.

Drug-Drug Interactions on Blood Levels

The pharmacokinetic interactions between carbamazepine and valproate are somewhat complex, but they can be condensed down to an easy recommendation for action. When the two drugs are used in combination, the doses of carbamazepine should be decreased when compared with usual or previously utilized dosing strategies. The reason for this is that valproate is an inhibitor of the breakdown of the active -10,11-epoxide of the carbamazepine into the inactive dihydroxy compound. As such, because of this inhibition of metabolism to the dihydroxy compound, levels of the -10, 11-epoxide will increase markedly (Brodie, Forrest, &

Rapeport, 1983; Kutt, Solomon, Peterson, Dhar, & Caronna, 1985). Since the epoxide is active in producing anticonvulsant efficacy and contributing to the side effects profile of carbamazepine, such notable increases could contribute to carbamazepine-induced toxicity (Bourgeois, 1988), particularly if one is already near the carbamazepine side effects threshold and valproate is added to the regimen.

It is noteworthy that if one merely measures carbamazepine (and not the epoxide), as is common in many laboratories, the increased levels of the epoxide will not be detected in routine laboratory assays (unless they are specifically requested). We are not suggesting that one needs to assess all of these changes with increased blood level monitoring, but only that the known increase in the epoxide during valproate cotherapy should be compensated for in advance by an overall carbamazepine dose reduction in order to avoid side effects.

An additional factor increasing the amount of carbamazepine with the combination is the fact that valproate displaces carbamazepine from protein binding and thus increases the free fraction of carbamazepine (which is the component that is physiologically active).

On the opposite side, carbamazepine is able to increase the metabolism of valproate, and valproate levels may fall to a minor to major extent with the use of the combination. While this is usually not problematic, it may at times suggest the need for concomitant small increases in the valproate dose.

Risks of the Combination in Pregnancy

If the two drugs are used in combination during pregnancy, there is some potential for additive or potentiative increased risk of spina bifida and other malformations that can occur with either drug alone. The risk of spina bifida is about 0.5% with carbamazepine and 1–2% with valproate. However, the risk of other serious adverse events is 1.0% for lamotrigine, 8.2% for carbamazepine, 10.7% for phenytoin, and 20.3% for valproate, and valproate's effects

were dost dependent (Meador et al., 2006). If at all possible, the combination should be avoided during pregnancy (Lindhout, Hoppener, & Meinardi, 1984), and if this is not possible, high doses of folate supplementation should clearly be utilized along with careful fetal monitoring.

Utility in PTSD

It is also noteworthy that preliminary communications have suggested the potential helpfulness of both carbamazepine and valproate alone in treating components of PTSD (Ford, 1996). Whereas carbamazepine was reported to inhibit the paroxysmal intrusions of nightmares, valproate appeared to improve general sleep characteristics. Although the two drugs have not been studied clinically in combination in a systematic fashion for PTSD, this differential targeting of different clinical components of PTSD with these two differently acting agents at least gives a theoretical rationale for considering such a therapeutic maneuver in the face of an intractable sleep disorder in patients with comorbid PTSD.

Parenthetically, it is noteworthy that we have seen good effects of other anticonvulsants in combination on PTSD symptomatology, such as lamotrigine and gabapentin (Chapter 9).

PRINCIPLES OF THE CASE	STRENGTH OF EVIDENCE
1. The combination of carbamazepine and valproate may be clinically useful even in circumstances when there is little evidence of efficacy of either drug in monotherapy.	+
2. Valproate has a clinically wider anticonvulsant spectrum than carbamazepine (i.e., its efficacy in absence seizures is thought to be attributable to its effects on T-type calcium channels).	+++
3. The factors mediating the wider range of efficacy of valproate in the epilepsies could add further to	

carbamazepine's profile of effects in affective illness. +

4. Since valproate decreases the breakdown of the active -10,11-epoxide metabolite of carbamazepine and displaces carbamazepine itself from protein binding, the dose of carbamazapine should be adjusted downward when the two drugs are used in combination. +++

5. Carbamazapine will reduce valproate blood levels to a minor extent, but this is usually not a major cause for concern. ±

6. Carbamazepine and valproate are one of the few anticonvulsant combinations that appears to increase the therapeutic index (efficacy to side effects ratio) in the treatment of clinical seizure disorders and in animal seizure models. ++

7. However, the two drugs should not be used in combination during pregnancy as there is an increased risk of congenital malformations and developmental delay, particularly related to valproate. ++

8. If either drug alone is used in pregnancy, folate supplementation of 5 to 10 mg/day should be considered. ±

9. If women of childbearing age are using either drug alone, one should consider adding 1 mg/day of folate to the regimen, both as an antidepressant potentiator and to prevent drug-related decreases in folate. Moreover, valproate will increase unwanted levels of homocysteine, and the effect may be countered by folate. +

10. Carbamazepine induces metabolism of the estrogen component of orally active birth control pills, and higher estrogen preparations of oral contraceptives are indicated with this anticonvulsant, as well as when oxcar-

bazepine and topiramate are used. +++

11. In patients with rapid and continuously cycling presentations such as this case, the use of two mood stabilizers in combination may be worth considering prior to the addition of a unimodal antidepressant. +

12. This patient's good clinical response to the combination of carbamazepine and valproate, when each alone was ineffective, adds to the overall rationale of proceeding with augmentation strategies rather than individual sequential clinical trials of monotherapy in patients with highly treatment-resistant affective illness presentations. If the combination did not prove efficacious, one would have saved the time necessary to assess one of the intervening monotherapy trials. +

13. This patient presents a clear example of the ineffectiveness of previous lithium and unimodal antidepressant regimens in some rapid cyclers. The combination of two other mood stabilizers (without a concomitant antidepressant) was effective in substantially ameliorating the severe depressions and intervening hypomanias (i.e., antidepressants are not always needed in the treatment of severe recurrent bipolar depressions. +

14. This patient also showed a lack of response to sleep deprivation at the beginning of an episode, but good responses toward the end of a depressive episode. +

TAKE-HOME MESSAGE

Two mood-stabilizing anticonvulsants with differing mechanisms of action (even when each alone are ineffective) may sometimes yield therapeutic benefit in otherwise treatment-refractory rapidly or continuously cycling patients.

50

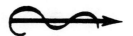

Long-Term Remission Achieved With Complex Combination Therapy (Polypharmacy)

CASE HISTORY

This patient was 35 years old at the onset of her severe depressions in 1984. Antidepressant treatment was associated with the induction of rapid cycling, which was not ameliorated with the addition of lithium carbonate (Figure 50.1). Her depressions were classic and typical of many bipolar patients, consisting of extreme psychomotor slowing, fatigue, anergia, marked social withdrawal, guilt, low self-esteem, and doubt, with complaints of extreme memory loss and indecisiveness. In her most severe depressions, she was unable to choose her clothes, appropriately dress herself, or maintain adequate hygiene. When asked a question, her answers were often so slow in coming that one wondered whether she had forgotten the question or was ever going to answer at all.

Early in her illness, her depressions were marked by increased sleeping; in the later, more agitated variety, she had early morning awakening with many awakenings throughout the night. She felt hopeless, worthless, and profoundly suicidal. She also had mild paranoid ideation during depressive phases.

Her manias consisted of decreased need for sleep, increasing energy, impulsivity, reckless spending, bad check writing, and long-distance calls and trips. She manifested increased social-ization but also increased talkativeness, irritability, and intrusiveness. There was increased physical and mental activity with racing thoughts and increased productivity of writing, hypergraphia, and decreased ability to focus her attention on the tasks at hand; that is, she was usually extremely distractible. She also had an increased appetite with increased carbohydrate craving.

At the time of NIMH admission, during a period on placebo, she again demonstrated these mood phases, although the mania was primarily mild to moderate rather than severe and full blown. The reported cycles of approximately 8 weeks of depression followed by an approximate month of hypomania tapering to a relatively euthymic state was also observed. Antithyroid antibodies and abnormal thyroid indices were consistent with a diagnosis of Hashimoto's thyroiditis, and she was placed on T_4 long-term maintenance treatment. The calcium channel blocker nimodipine did not make a substantial impact on her cycling as it had on several other patients (Chapters 32 and 33), although she had a subjective sense of improvement in alertness, memory, and recall.

Following the addition of valproate to her thyroid supplementation, the patient no longer experienced manias, and depressions appeared to be of lesser severity with the addition of bupropion, but it was not until lithium was added

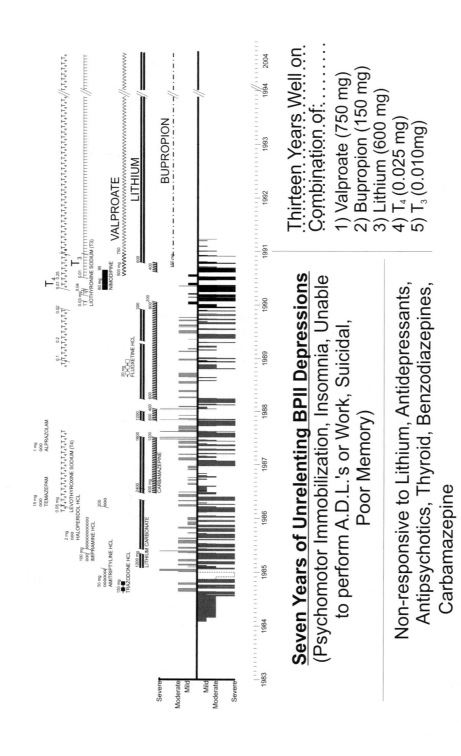

Figure 50.1 Complete and sustained remission with complex combination therapy. Prior to NIMH hospitalization in 1989, this patient had a profound onset of depression in 1984 with rapid cycling following antidepressant treatment that was not moderated by lithium. Lithium alone and with a variety of antidepressants and thyroid treatment failed to substantially ameliorate her illness. Carbamazepine in 1986 and 1988 transiently ameliorated the depressions, but the patient had progressive breakthrough episodes with a loss of efficacy suggestive of tolerance (Chapter 19). At the NIMH she failed to respond adequately to a double-blind trial of nimodipine but following treatment with valproate and T_3 and T_4 augmentation ceased to show hypomanias. With the subsequent addition of bupropion and then lithium, depressive episodes were attenuated in duration and severity. From 1991 to the present she has essentially been euthymic on this regimen.

that the duration and severity of depressive episodes became remarkably attenuated. After discharge from the hospital, the patient continued to report relatively few side effects on this complex combination therapy, and in both her NIMH and subsequent follow-up periods she chose to maintain all of the drugs in this combination for fear that decreasing any one of them could result in the reinstitution of her cycling pattern. This was also the consensus of her physicians at the NIMH and her outpatient physicians.

It should be noted that while each of the drugs in this combination treatment was not proven to be absolutely necessary, many of these drugs had been used alone or in less complicated combination regimens prior to her improvement, suggesting that many, if not all, of the drugs were important to her improvement. The formal academic exercise of discontinuing some of the drugs that might not have been absolutely necessary to the maintenance of her improvement was not considered a reasonable option in light of both the possibility of reactivation of her illness and in the face of a benign side effects profile even on this complex regimen. If the patient had been suffering from a difficult side effects burden, it might have changed the risk-to-benefit ratio in the decision-making process toward considering discontinuation of the likely offending agents, with a very slow taper, however.

This patient had been totally incapacitated by her illness for 7 years despite many different treatments, including antidepressants (trazodone, amitriptyline, imipramine, and fluoxetine), benzodiazepines, antipsychotics, thyroid supplementation, and mood stabilizers (lithium and carbamazepine). However, following discharge from the NIMH on a complex polypharmaceutical regimen of two mood stabilizers, two thyroid hormones, and an antidepressant, she was able to return to work, her family relationships improved remarkably, and she and her husband adopted a child. She was able to maintain her multiple role functions as mother, spouse, and employee in a highly successful and effective fashion. She has had no further episode recurrences for more than 15 years.

BACKGROUND LITERATURE

This patient's ultimate response to a complex polypharmaceutical approach to her treatment-refractory, rapid-cycling bipolar illness reveals many different principles and problems with the formal research literature, which often fails to be directed at ascertaining optimal treatment intervention for bipolar patients after they have not responded to more conventional approaches (Post, 2004b; Post, Speer, et al., 2006). While each of the separate treatments utilized in this patient has some academic backing for use in bipolar illness, there have been few systematic clinical trials of the kinds of complex regimens that are often needed for the highly refractory patient. This is very different from the situation in tuberculosis, congestive heart failure, or cancer chemotherapy, where not only are complex polypharmacy regimens the norm, but in many instances there are specific clinical trials demonstrating that the combination of a given three drugs, or the addition of a fourth drug, is better than a regimen without it. In the absence of this type of formal clinical-trials literature, the patient and clinician are left with isolated case reports and the ability only to synthesize a disparate literature in order to apply agents that are most likely to be effective in combination when monotherapy or more simplified combination therapies are ineffective.

General Principles of Rational Polypharmacy

1. The initial drug use should be based on its general efficacy and side effects profile as well as history (family and personal) of prior responsivity.

2. If the patient cannot achieve clinical response at a reasonable dose and blood level (which cannot be further increased because of side effects), adjunctive therapy might then be pursued with the first drug lowered below its side effects threshold.

3. A patient's dose of a new adjunctive agent

should be slowly increased, titrating against clinical efficacy and side effects burden for the entire regimen.

4. A drug with a new putative mechanism of action can thus be added, and with slow dose titration not add to the overall side effects burden. The new drug may provide enough of this novel mechanism to finally dampen the illness process.

5. Another agent targeting residual symptoms or comorbidities can then be pursued if needed to achieve a more complete response or remission.

While a detailed approach to the mechanisms of action of the drugs used in this and related patients is initially dealt with in Chapter 10, a note on some of the basic clinical and pharmacological principles and rationales may be useful. Since this patient seemed to have acceleration in her cycle frequency with the use of antidepressants, and lithium and carbamazepine alone or in combination were not sufficient to break the cycling themselves (or with the addition of a serotonin-selective antidepressant such as fluoxetine), the direction we took was to use additional possible mood stabilizers. We started with the novel agent nimodipine, a calcium channel blocker with possible antidepressant effects (Chapter 32), and thyroid treatment, which was important to treat her Hashimoto's thyroiditis.

The addition of T_3 to T_4 was felt to be important in light of Cooke, Joffe, and Levitt's (1992) clinical observations that the addition of T_3 to T_4 can be helpful in refractory depression, consistent with the view that T_3 can be of greater effectiveness than T_4 as an adjunct to antidepressant treatment in those with refractory depression (Joffe & Singer, 1990).

These data are also partially convergent with those of Bauer and colleagues (Bauer & Whybrow, 1990; Bauer et al., 2001, 2005; Bauer, Baur, et al., 2002) and others that higher dose thyroid treatment might be efficacious in augmenting other mood stabilizer treatment in refractory and rapid-cycling bipolar patients. Their experience suggests that in some patients even higher doses of thyroid than used here might be effective, although the relative benefit of low-dose (replacement) versus very high-dose (supraphysiological and suppressive) thyroid treatment, with its potential short- and long-term side effects, remains to be systematically explored.

When these mood stabilizers (nimodipine and thyroid, and previously lithium and carbamazepine) proved ineffective, a then-new mood stabilizer (valproate) was added. Nonresponse to one mood stabilizer is not predictive of nonresponse to another. Thus, we were targeting the patient's most prominent symptomatology. Her recurrent hypomanias were less problematic than her completely incapacitating depressions, and these were occurring with a certain rhythmicity and cyclicity, if not absolute periodicity, to suggest the need for additional mood stabilizer treatment.

The patient had a subjective sense of decreased problems with appetite and weight gain when bupropion was added. This clinical vignette deserves further systematic study, although it should be noted that bupropion is one of the few antidepressants that has been associated with weight loss rather than gain, on average (Anderson et al., 2002). Thus, in some instances, the side effects of one drug may help counter rather than exacerbate those of another, and this should be considered in choice of augmenting agents (Post, 2004b; Post, Speer, et al., 2006).

The one prominent side effect that the patient had was tremor, which can be caused by both lithium and valproate alone and additive in combination, but can be minimized with careful dose titration. Bupropion and thyroid treatment can also be associated with a minor exacerbation of tremor. In some instances, tremor can be ameliorated with the addition of a beta blocker, but this has the potential for increasing the risk of depression and would require an additional adjunctive treatment with an unknown impact on the patient's illness process. Bupropion apparently ameliorated some of the depressive symptoms but, in combination with the other agents, was still not sufficient to block the appearance of the next episode.

Return to lithium treatment, which was previously ineffective in combination with other regimens, now appeared to help the patient achieve a complete remission. Lithium, which previously had been only partially effective in ameliorating the intensity of the patient's highs, was now added to attempt to attack the problems of rhythmic recurrence of depression. This combination now appeared remarkably effective, and increasingly so after each putative depressive cycle. Each depressive episode was of lesser duration or severity until finally the patient stopped having depressions altogether.

Putative Mechanism of Action of the Drugs Used in This Regimen

T_3, via its intracellular receptor, is thought to be more transcriptionally active and have differing effects on gene expression compared with T_4, as well as having direct thyroid effects.

Valproate is thought to exert its mood-stabilizing effects in part through enhancing GABAergic systems, the major inhibitory neurotransmitter in the brain. It may, like lithium, also have neurotrophic effects via brain-derived neurotrophic factor (BDNF) and Bcl-2. It also has novel mechanisms such as changing transcription via blockade of histone deacetylase.

Bupropion is thought to be unique among the antidepressants in not being a potent aminergic reuptake blocker, but it nonetheless increases levels of dopamine in the caudate nucleus and nucleus accumbens, the latter of which is thought to modulate mood, motor activity, and reward motivated behavior.

Lithium is thought to act in part by blocking second messenger systems, that is, below neurotranmitter receptors, such as adenylate cyclase, phosphoinositol metabolism, and calcium. It also increases cell survival factors (BDNF and Bcl-2) and decreases cell death factors (BAX and p53), effects that occur at clinically relevant concentrations. Detailed reviews of these drugs and their mechanisms of action can be found in Chapters 9 and 10.

PRINCIPLES OF THE CASE	STRENGTH OF EVIDENCE
1. Complex regimens may be required to bring on a remission in some refractory severe or rapid-cycling bipolar patients.	+++
2. In the absence of formal clinical trial data, systematic sequential clinical adjunctive trials, slowly increasing dose against clinical efficacy and stopping before side effects become prominent, may be most clinically useful.	+
3. In this fashion, adjunctive trials can be assessed for efficacy faster than unsuccessful trials of monotherapy alone in patients in whom rapidity of response is of considerable importance.	++
4. Even 7 years of severe and incapacitating rapid cycling does not preclude complete clinical recovery under an appropriate medication regimen.	++
5. When lithium has been ineffective in the past, it may still be an important augmentation treatment in conjunction with a new basal treatment regimen, as it appears to be a crucial variable in this patient's clinical remission. These data are convergent with other observations suggesting that lithium not only can be an important adjunct for virtually all unimodal antidepressant modalities for unipolar depression, but also may have important long-term antisuicide and other positive effects on medical mortality, even when it is an inadequate treatment on its own for bipolar patients.	++
6. When initial treatment strategies are not effective, one should be increasingly aggressive and innovative in order to attempt to	

bring the patient's illness into remission and sustain recovery.   +

7. A comparison principle is less
    clearly delineated in this patient:
    When the illness is finally brought
    under control, maintenance of the
    regimen that led to clinical im-
    provement might be the most con-
    servative approach (in the absence
    of side effects). In this patient's
    case, her regimen resulted in
    many years of complete clinical re-
    mission.   ++

    a. While it might be argued that
        this could have been achieved
        with perhaps one or even two
        fewer drugs, the potential con-
        sequences of a relapse and
        lack of responsivity made the
        patient and her clinicians and
        physicians hesitant to adopt a
        strategy of drug simplification
        or dose reduction.

    b. Moreover, even the mainte-
        nance of the regimens that
        were acutely effective does
        not guarantee long-term remis-
        sion.

8. Academic medicine and formal
    clinical trials are often far behind
    the innovative clinician in apply-
    ing the most appropriate treat-
    ments for a given individual,
    even when a medicine is not
    FDA approved for this indication
    of bipolar illness. One may have
    to import other treatments from
    endocrinology (thyroid, steroids),
    schizophrenia (atypical antipsy-
    chotics), cardiology (calcium
    channel blockers), neurology (an-
    ticonvulsants and the seizures of
    ECT), and so on to bring this ill-
    ness to remission.   +

9. Systematic life charting of the
    course of illness can help in the
    assessment of the duration and

timing of treatments as well as
the sequencing of the next appropriate treatment.   +++

    a. In this case, the semirhythmic
        and relentless recurrence of ill-
        ness drove certain decisions,
        as well as the careful
        delineation of the past history
        of inadequate response to
        given agents that helped keep
        the development of this com-
        plex polypharmaceutical regi-
        men more rational rather than
        being a random decision-mak-
        ing process.

    b. The art of complicated pharma-
        cotherapeutic management of
        bipolar illness may, in some
        stages of the illness, require
        many different approaches and
        drugs before a fully successful
        clinical result is achieved.

10. While all of the pharmaceutical
    interventions illustrated in Figure
    50.1 in 1990 and 1991 were con-
    ducted on a double-blind basis
    (further suggesting the likelihood
    that this response was not attribut-
    able to placebo effect), similar
    clinical strategies can obviously
    be followed in outpatient clinical
    practice settings with careful
    monitoring of dosages against
    side effect profiles.   ++

11. In this careful fashion, even com-
    plex regimens can be maintained
    in the relative absence of inten-
    sive degrees of blood level moni-
    toring, that is, using the strategy
    of dose titration toward effective-
    ness and the avoidance of side ef-
    fects.   +

12. Conversely, blood level monitor-
    ing may become more important
    in the following cases:

    a. The absence of clinical response (and side effects) in order to see whether adequate blood levels have been achieved in conventional dose ranges. +

b. The presence of unusual or unexpected side effects. ++

c. Concerns about potential toxicity from the newly added drug or its use in combination. ++

d. While none of the drugs illustrated in this patient appears to have prominent pharmacokinetic interactions—that is, they do not affect the blood levels of the other agents to any remarkable degree—this is clearly not always the case and, in particular with the use of carbamazepine, some consideration of its interactions with other agents becomes very important (Chapter 16). ++

13. Whenever possible, a drug should be added in a sequential clinical trial fashion, so that inferences about a given agent's contribution to effectiveness or side effects can best be made. +

14. Although the blind addition of lithium to the other drugs (T_3, T_4, valproate, and bupropion) seemed to be an important step in the amelioration of the patient's illness on this regimen, it is clear that lithium (in combination with previous thyroid and carbamazepine treatment and a variety of antidepressants) was not adequate in the past. This further suggests that many, if not all, of the new elements of the combination treatment were indeed important to her new recovery. The duration of a given individual clinical trial that is necessary to assess effectiveness may be very much a factor

of the patient's prior cycle frequency. ++

a. The faster the episode recurrence, the shorter is the necessary trial.

b. Even in this case of very rapid cycling, waiting on the order of months was required to see whether the next depressive episode was going to be prevented or ameliorated.

15. Taking the appropriate time to evaluate a treatment may also be related to: ++

a. How rapidly one can reach adequate levels.

b. A drug's mechanism of action. This is convergent with an older literature that indicates that at times it may take a cycle or more for lithium to induce its mood-stabilizing effect, and perhaps much longer until it manifests its antisuicide effects to an adequate degree. There is also some evidence with valproate in epilepsy that improvement may continue progressively for some period of time. This also appears to be the case for clozapine in schizophrenia and schizoaffective illness, wherein improvement may continue over 6 months to a year. In vagus nerve stimulation (Chapter 58), improvement can also increase over the course of the first year after implantation.

16. Carbamazepine was not FDA approved for acute mania until 2005. It is not yet approved for long-term prophylaxis. Valproate is also not approved for long-term prophylaxis in bipolar ill-

414   TREATMENT OF BIPOLAR ILLNESS

ness (only for acute mania) and yet was likely a crucial component of this patient's recovery. Prescribing only within the FDA approval framework thus may not represent the best clinical practice, particularly in bipolar disorder. Many different guidelines for treatment of bipolar illness emphasize the importance of using innovative and not yet FDA-approved treatments for patients who do not respond to conventional therapeutics.   +++

a. Lawyers and potentially litigious patients who believe that treating bipolar illness only according to FDA approval or the *PDR* is somehow the only appropriate or ethical approach are indeed sorely misinformed, as this patient (and many others in this volume) most adequately document.

b. The same caveat must also be given for precisely following

or not following any set of published guidelines for treatment of bipolar illness. The expansion, revision, or violation of such guidelines may indeed be very much in the best interests of individual patients, particularly when there is good evidence of the need to pursue novel treatment approaches.

TAKE-HOME MESSAGE

At the time of this case, lithium was the only drug approved by the FDA for the long-term treatment of bipolar illness, but when it is documented repeatedly to be ineffective, it is mandatory that other agents be used. In some instances, in patients such as these with severe and refractory illness, multimodal therapy with several mood stabilizers—lithium, valproate, T_3, and T_4—may be required in addition to antidepressant augmentation with a unimodal antidepressant such as bupropion.

51

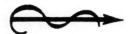

Thyroid Augmentation of Triple Mood Stabilizers Therapy

CASE HISTORY

This is the inpatient record (using blind nurse ratings on the daily Bunney-Hamburg scale) of a 58-year-old single female with a more than 20-year history of almost continuous ultrarapid cycling (four or more episodes per month) of predominantly depressive episodes in her bipolar II illness (Figure 51.1). The pattern continued (Figure 51.2, left side) when she was observed in the medication-free state. This pattern showed some resemblance to that of incapacitating unipolar recurrent brief depression (Angst, Merikangas, Scheidegger, & Wicki, 1990) but also showed brief bursts of hypomania.

The patient had been unsuccessfully treated with antidepressants, including tricyclics and monoamine oxidase inhibitors (MAOIs), in combination with lithium or carbamazepine in the general years prior to her NIMH admission (Figure 51.1). Carbamazepine had initially provided some relief of her depressions, but she developed tolerance to previously adequate doses and could not tolerate increased doses. In the past, valproate had paradoxically induced manias. The patient's depressive episodes began with a loss of physical energy and increased shakiness, followed by fear, sadness, and uncontrollable crying. She was hypersomnic (often unable to get out of bed), unable to perform household tasks, and at times mildly confused. Depressions were also associated with loss of appetite, and previously she had gone up to 18

days without eating. She had made numerous suicide attempts from 1957 to 1984, predominantly with drug overdoses. The patient had multiple hospitalizations for depression and suicide attempts.

The readministration of carbamazepine on a double-blind basis at the NIMH prevented her hypomania but only mildly attenuated the severity of depressive breakthroughs (Figure 51.2). Augmentation with lithium appeared to help considerably, but intermittently the patient became mildly to severely symptomatic. The triple combination therapy with the addition of valproate appeared ineffective, with an apparent prolongation of a depressive episode and a new depressive breakthrough just prior to augmentation with T_3 (50 μg/day; Figure 51.2).

It was not clear whether the initial 2-week period of remission, when T_3 was blindly added, was spontaneous or medication related. This was explored with a brief period of T_3 discontinuation that resulted in the more prominent reemergence of depressions of moderate severity. T_3 was rapidly reinstituted and resulted in several months of virtual remission, confirming her responsiveness to T_3, and the patient was able to be discharged from the hospital.

As an outpatient in private care, she remained stable for several more months, but a MAOI was added to the regimen for a breakthrough depression of moderately severe proportions, and she then maintained her marked improvement for the next 4 months. When the

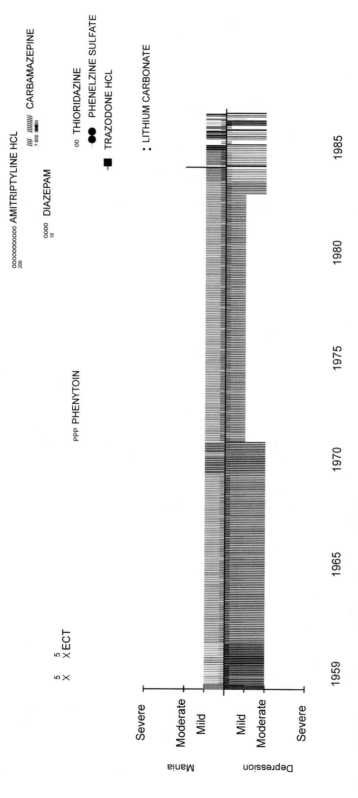

Figure 51.1 Retrospective course: 26-year history of ultradian cycling (bipolar NOS). This patient showed ultrarapid cycling—from mild or moderate depression to hypomania—for much of her adult life and had received minimal treatment.

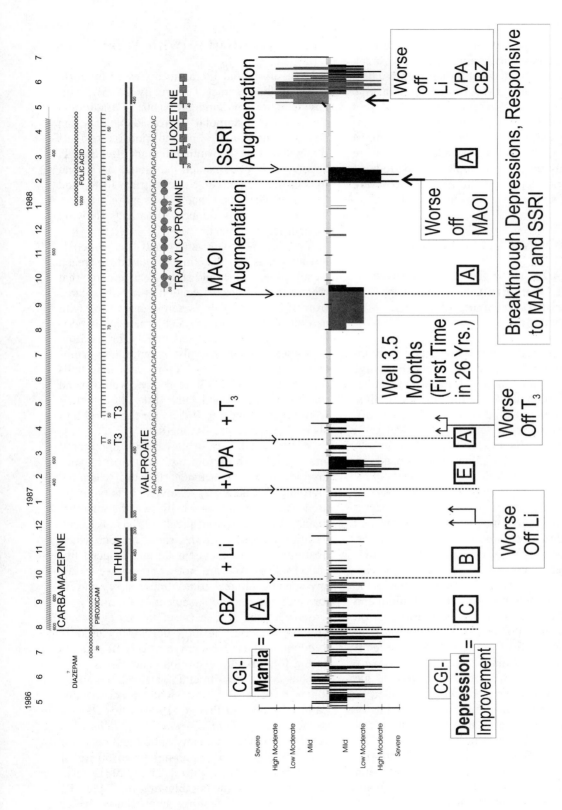

Figure 51.2 Response to triple mood stabilizer therapy (carbamazepine, lithium, and valproate) as augmented by T_3 and later an MAOI or SSRI. This patient with ultrarapid cycling and predominantly depressive recurrences (left side, 1986) failed to respond adequately to trials of: (1) carbamazepine, (2) carbamazepine plus lithium, and (3) valproate, but finally was stabilized using the three mood stabilizers and thyroid augmentation with triiodothyronine, T_3 (50 µg/day). This patient's mania stopped on carbamazepine (A), but there was minimal antidepressant response (C). The addition of lithium further helped her response. Valproate appeared to worsen the duration of depression (E), but T_3 augmentation resulted in remission. CBZ, carbamazepine; Li, lithium; VPA, valproate; CGI, Clinical Global Impressions scale; CGI, improvement scale; A, very much improved; B, much improved; C, minimally improved; D, no change; E, minimally worse.

MAOI was stopped because of side effects, a moderate depression again began to break through her treatment with carbamazepine, lithium, valproate, and thyroid augmentation. She responded when fluoxetine was added, but had a dramatic exacerbation when she transiently stopped all her medications. In contrast to much of the previous 2 decades, which were almost continuously interrupted by periods of recurrent brief depression of moderate to severe proportion, she was well for much of 1987.

BACKGROUND LITERATURE

Lack of Adequate Responsiveness to Triple Combination Therapy With Carbamazepine, Lithium, and Valproate

This inpatient case report represents a substantial group of outpatients inadequately responsive to all three major mood stabilizers used either alone or in combination. In the outpatient clinic work of Denicoff and associates (Denicoff, Smith-Jackson, Bryan, et al., 1997; Denicoff, Smith-Jackson, Disney, et al., 1997) in our group, approximately 37.5% of the patients who initially entered the clinic failed to have a clinically relevant response to any of the 5 years of pharmacoprophylaxis with different mood stabilizers and antidepressants, benzodiazepines, and antipsychotics used as additionally needed. Patients sequentially received a year of blind, randomized treatment with either lithium or carbamazepine, a switch to the other drug in the second year, then a third year of the lithium and carbamazepine combination, the fourth year on valproate (either alone or in combination with lithium), and the fifth year on all three drugs if the patient was still inadequately stabilized.

This patient thus resembled one third of the outpatients in that series because she failed to respond to shorter, but blind, inpatient trials of these 3 mood stabilizers. However, with the addition of T_3 she finally achieved a period of almost complete euthymia, which was briefly interrupted by the reappearance of depression when T_3 was temporarily discontinued but reappeared when T_3 was reinstituted.

Acute Potentiation With T_3 or T_4

A very substantial literature reviewed by Joffe (1998) indicates that T_3 (usually 25–37.5 µg) augmentation of antidepressants in traditional acute trials in unipolar depressed patients can convert some 20–40% of unresponsive patients into responders. The antidepressant effects of T_3 appear better documented than those of T_4, and in one comparative clinical trial Joffe and Singer (1990) found that T_3 was more effective than T_4 in terms of numbers of patients showing clinical improvement.

T_3 has a relatively short half-life, which is advantageous in the time required to reach steady state, and should side effects emerge that require thyroid discontinuation is rapidly cleared from the blood. This is rarely necessary with careful dosing, although a few patients experience palpitations, increased anxiety, or sweating on higher doses. In contrast, should these symptoms emerge with use of T_4, its very long half-life of approximately 5 to 9 days would mean that even after stopping the drug altogether, it would take about 5 to 9 days for the blood levels of T_4 to decrease by one half.

When patients are being carefully monitored and treated with thyroid replacement for hypothyroidism, or replacement therapy when the thyroid gland has been removed, T_4 is typically used because of its longer half-life and a smoother maintenance of thyroid levels. T_4 has also been traditionally used for the same reasons when treating actual or incipient lithium-induced hypothyroidism. We are not aware, however, of any specific clinical trial comparing T_3 and T_4 for such thyroid replacement, particularly in terms of positive effects on mood. However, Tremont and Stern (2000) successfully used T_3 to counter adverse cognitive effects in patients during lithium administration. The closest anyone has come to a direct T_4 versus T_3 comparison is the study of Bunevicius, Kazanavicius, Zalinkevicius, and Prange (1999) who reported in the *New England Journal of Medicine* that in thyroid replaced patients' mood and behavior were better (than on T_4 alone) when 50 µg of the T_4 was replaced with 12.5 µg of T_3 on a blind basis. With the combination of T_3 plus T_4, patients reported feeling significantly better compared with those continued on T_4 alone. Several subsequent attempts to replicate these findings were not successful, and the issue remains unresolved for medical patients on complete thyroid replacement (Saravanan, Simmons, Greenwood, Peters, & Dayan, 2005).

However, isolated case reports by Cooke et al. (1992) also support the view that adding T_3 to T_4 was apparently instrumental in the mood improvement in several affectively ill patients with refractory depression. Thus, this strategy is perhaps worthy of consideration in some bipolar patients with refractory chronic depression or recent depression who have been on long-term T_4 replacement. We used this rationale and strategy in the case report in Chapter 50.

In individuals with treatment-resistant, predominantly bipolar depression (but some unipolars as well), Frye et al. (1997, unpublished data) in our group showed that adding T_3 blindly to existing antidepressant regimens was helpful in 11 of 33 patients (33%) and T_4 was helpful in 8 of 15 instances (53%). Women tended to be nonsignificantly ($p < .10$) more likely to respond than men, for example, 44% versus 10% for T_3, and 70% versus 20% for T_4, respectively.

Supraphysiological Doses of T_4 for Refractory Depression and Cycling

Gjessing (1938) originally reported treating periodic catatonia (in some who were apparently manic-depressive) with higher than normal doses of thyroid extracts (Table 51.1). Stancer and Persad (1982) used this empirical rationale in their case series of patients with refractory bipolar episodes using T_4 doses between 300 and 500 µg as additions to previously inadequately effective treatments. They reported substantial success, although several patients experienced medical complications requiring drug discontinuation. Bauer and Whybrow (1990) reported similar improvement in a case series of patients with rapid-cycling bipolar disorder with high-dose T_4 ranging between 150 and 400 µg/day. Sack and Wehr (personal communication) also reported success with several patients using high-dose T_4 augmentation of previously ineffective regimens but felt that the majority of

their very small group of patients did not tolerate this regimen well.

Michael Bauer, working with colleagues in Germany and then at UCLA, also reported considerable success (greater than 50% response) in both stabilizing mood in refractory cycling patients as well as converting patients with chronic refractory depression to responders with T_4 regimens, usually between 200 and 400 µg/day, achieved with slow upward titration as augmentation to other drugs (Bauer, Baur, et al., 2002; Bauer, Berghofer, et al., 2002; Bauer et al., 2001, 2005). In contrast to several of the previous reports, he indicated that patients tolerated this regimen and had only mild side effects such as tachycardia and sweating.

There has been considerable controversy about the general medical safety of this high-dose T_4 strategy, with many endocrinologists being concerned about an accelerated rate of bone loss (osteoporosis) on this regimen. However, Gold and associates have observed that depression itself seems associated with an increase in bone resorption and low bone density (Cizza, Ravn, Chrousos, & Gold, 2001). Moreover, preliminary examination of patients placed on these supra- physiological thyroid regimens showed no evidence of accelerated demineralization and bone loss in small series studied over a period of about 1 year (Bauer et al., 2004).

Given the several areas of tolerability concern and the fact that one is increasing T_4 levels to approximately 150% of normal free thyroxine index and thus inducing a subclinical state of hyperthyroidism, we have generally reserved this high-dose T_4 treatment as a low priority in the algorithm of sequential approaches to treatment-refractory bipolar illness and thus have rarely had the opportunity to use it. In the several instances that we did, it did not stop the refractory cycling.

Overview

Given the rapid onset of T_3 augmentation and the robust literature on thyroid augmentation in unipolar depression, we are inclined to start thyroid potentiation with T_3. We usually begin with 25 µg in the morning and increase to 37.5 µg if

Table 51.1 *High-Dose L-Thyroxine (T_4) in Affective Illness*

Date	Investigators	N	Diagnosis	Dosage (μg/day)	Responders/ Nonresponders (%)	Comment
1938	Gjessing		Periodic catatonia			Cycle and mood stabilization
1982	Stancer & Persad	7	BP	up to 500	5/7 (71%)	Lack of persistence of Rx effects, however
1990	Bauer & Why-brow	11	Bipolar (RC)	150–400	10/11 (91%) depressed 5/7 (71%) manic	3/4 (75%) relapsed during blind placebo substitution
1994	Baumgartner et al.	6	BP	250–500	6/6 (100%)	No significant side effects (mild perspiration
1997	Afflelou et al.	6	Bipolar (RC)	50–325	4/6 (67%)	
1998	Bauer et al.	17	Depression (12 BP, 5 UP)	500	10/17 (59%)	Chronic, treatment-resistant, one dosage reduction due to tachycardia
1998	Spoov & Lahdelma	22	Depression	200	7/11 (64%) on T_4 vs. 2/11 (18%) on Li	Crossover study
1999	Rudas et al.	7	Depression or dysthymia	150–300	6/7 (86%)	Two patients dropped out early in the study because of side effects at 100 μg/day
2001	Bauer et al.	16	Refractory (schizo) affective disorders	500	15/16 (94%)	Very few adverse side effects reported on two different side effects scales
2002	Bauer, Berghofer, et al.	21	Prophylaxis-resistant affective disorders (13 BP, 4 UP, 4 SA)	up to 500	15/21 (71%)	Long-term prophylactic study (T_4 treatment averaged 51.4 ± 21.7 months) showing significant reduction in recurrences and hospitalizations
2004	Pfeiffer et al.	28	Treatment-resistant depression	350	61%	Serious side effects in 18% of patients
2005	Bauer et al.	10	Depressed women with BP	320	7/10 (70%)	The decrease in relative activity of the left thalamus, left amygdala, left hippocampus, and left ventral striatum was significantly correlated with reduction in depression scores

Note. BP, bipolar; RC, rapid cyclers; UP, unipolar; SA, schizoaffective.

needed. In a patient on minimal to average doses of T_4 augmentation, we would add T_3 (25 μg) to the T_4 in instances of refractory depression. With these more conventional dosage strategies and the combination strategy of T_4 plus T_3 of Bunevicius and colleagues (1999), we rarely use supraphysiological T_4. If the latter strategy is attempted, we would recommend discontinuation of T_3 and very slow dose titration

PRINCIPLES OF THE CASE

STRENGTH OF EVIDENCE

1. A modest percentage of patients fail even triple combination therapy with the three most widely used mood stabilizers (lithium, valproate, and carbamazepine), as evidenced in this patient. (Lamotrigine had not yet been studied when this patient was treated.)   ++

2. The patient apparently responded to T_3 augmentation, relapsed when it was discontinued on a double-blind basis, and reresponded when it was reinstituted. As illustrated, the patient's response to T_3 is not unequivocal as it still might be attributable to the slow onset of response to triple mood stabilizer therapy, with the T_3 relapses being coincidental. In order to definitively establish a role for T_3 in this individual, more systematic clinical trials of thyroid alterations would have had to be explored. These were not pursued in light of the patient's achieving a euthymic state for the first time in many years.   +

3. The patient maintained her general state of euthymia for approximately 9 months (with the

addition of an MAOI) but then, as previously, began to experience some depressive breakthroughs. This patient had developed tolerance to the psychotropic effects of carbamazepine in the past, and eventually did so in spite of its augmentation with lithium, valproate, thyroid, and an MAOI. However, it is our impression that the majority of patients can be stabilized and maintained on such complex regimens without breakthrough episodes, as illustrated in the previous chapter.   +

4. Nonetheless, in many instances of refractory depression or cycling, we believe traditional-dose T_3 augmentation (35–37.5 μg) is often useful and almost never associated with problematic side effects.   +

5. Augmentation of T_4 replacement therapy with T_3 may also be attempted in instances of refractory depression or cycling.   +

6. A nonrandomized study database (Table 51.1) also supports the use of supraphysiological doses of T_4 with very slow titration up to doses ranging between 200 and 400 μg. Our personal preference is to reserve this strategy for late in the treatment algorithm. This could change and move earlier in the sequence if an ongoing randomized study led by Michael Bauer is positive.   +

7. When mood stabilizers are sequentially added and doses slowly titrated toward maximally tolerated doses, most patients (as exemplified by this individual) will have few problematic side effects, even with very complex regimens.   ++

8. While it has not been systematically studied, it is our impression that utilization of combination therapy represents a reasonable approach to slowing or preventing the development of tolerance, which this patient had shown in the past (but then experienced again after discharge).   ++

9. It is also our impression that thyroid augmentation strategies may also be useful in delaying or preventing the development of tolerance, although this too has not been systematically explored in the literature, and the

strength of this observation is weak.   ±

TAKE-HOME MESSAGE

While most of the literature on T_3 (25–37.5 μg) augmentation refers to adding T_3 to unimodal antidepressants for acute episodes of depression, use of thyroid augmentation in treatment-resistant cyclic depressive presentations may also be worthy of consideration relatively early in the treatment algorithm because of its benign side effects profile. Supraphysiological doses of T_4 appear to have a role later in the algorithm, especially if one is faced with a treatment-resistant chronic depression or cycling presentation.

52

Complex Regimen Required to Stabilize a Patient With Antidepressant-Induced Cycling

CASE HISTORY

The patient whose mood and treatment history are depicted in the life chart is a 48-year-old bank executive with no history of depression prior to 1999 (Figure 52.1). Shortly after his wife died at the end of 1999, the patient slipped into an increasingly severe depression culminating in extreme agitation, anxiety, a 60-lb weight loss (on an already thin frame), insomnia, anorexia, and suicidal thoughts. Following a lack of response to several different SSRIs, the atypical antipsychotic risperidone, and mirtazapine, which was also ineffective for both anorexia and insomnia, the patient was referred for ECT.

However, the patient and his family wanted to avoid this procedure if possible and instead elected to participate in an NIMH clinical research protocol involving rTMS for the potential treatment of his depression (Chapter 57).

The patient was randomized to receive high-frequency (20 Hz) rTMS at 110% of motor threshold for 3 weeks (five times per week), which would be followed by a continuation phase of 8 weeks with rTMS. Although the degree of improvement was only from severe to high moderate on the NIMH-LCM (2–01 to 3–01 in Figure 52.1), the patient's Hamilton Rating Scale for Depression scores fell substantially from a very high baseline of 53 to 33 at

the end of 3 weeks of rTMS and to 22 after 8 weeks (i.e., greater than 50% improvement).

With this substantial but clinically insufficient degree of response to rTMS, the patient was started on venlafaxine (a_1) and gabapentin (a_2) for his remaining moderate depression and anxiety, respectively, as augmentation of his lorazepam initially, and then folic acid (c) and T_3 (d). Valproate (b) was added for persisting high levels of anxiety and more severe depressive fluctuations (4–01). Nonetheless, a brief manic switch occurred.

On a dose of 300 mg of venlafaxine and 900 mg/day of gabapentin, the patient's mood switched into a more persistent hypomanic episode (5–01) characterized by increased energy, jocularity, and inappropriate behavior toward other patients and staff, which was only partially responsive to the addition of lithium (e). As the dose of venlafaxine was decreased, this hypomanic episode was followed by another period of moderate to severe depression (6–01), which appeared to improve with increasing doses of venlafaxine and the initiation of lamotrigine (f).

Another rapid mood switch occurred in July 2001 despite a further increased dose of divalproex sodium to 1,750 mg/day. The hypomania persisted for another month despite olanzapine (g). The patient finally entered a period of eu-

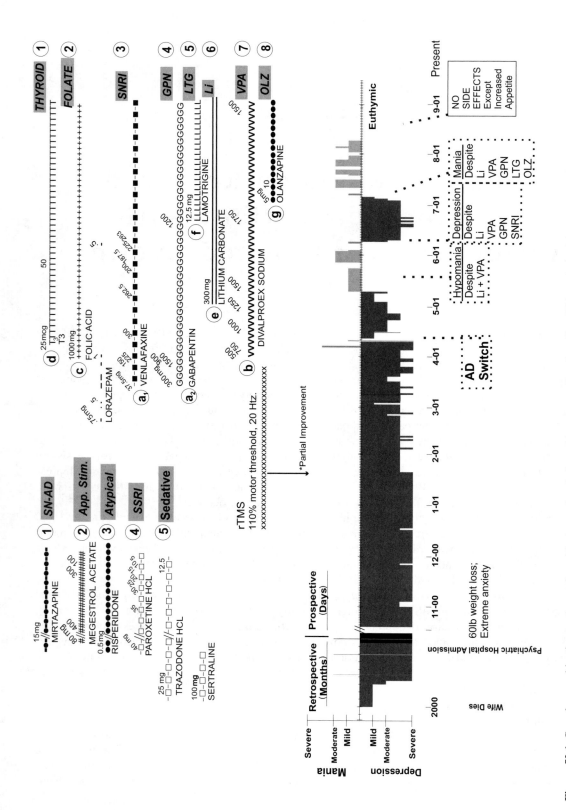

Figure 52.1 Complex combination treatment for achieving euthymia in antidepressant-related cycling. This patient with a severe anxious depression showed a failure to respond to five medications in combination (1 to 5, top, left) and a partial response to rTMS.* The patient began cycling following treatment with venlafaxine despite the presence of several mood stabilizers. Very complex treatment (including 8 medications, top, right) was eventually required to achieve a complete remission.

thymia (no depressive or hypomanic symptoms) in August 2001 and was able to be discharged to his home.

BACKGROUND LITERATURE

This patient's life chart illustrates a number of points of clinical interest. As noted by Kraepelin (1921) and many others over the past century, the first episode of illness often begins with a severe psychosocial stressor, such as the loss or death of others. This patient's profound depression and cachexia (severe weight loss) following his wife's death at the end of 1999 did not respond to five different classes of medication in combination, and he was considered for a trial of ECT based on his rapidly deteriorating physical condition secondary to severe anorexia and weight loss. He and his family elected to have a trial of rTMS prior to the contemplated ECT series. He was only partially responsive to rTMS, in this case administered at 20 Hz at 110% of motor threshold. We had observed previous moderate effects of rTMS at these frequencies utilizing 80% of motor threshold (George et al., 1997) and 100% of motor threshold (Kimbrell et al., 1999) and hoped that by increasing the length of the clinical trial (from 2 to 3 weeks) and the intensity of the rTMS (from 100% to 110% of motor threshold) in a third protocol revision, we would observe more robust and clinically meaningful effects which appears to be the case (Speer, Wassermann, Benson, Herscovitch, & Post, 2006). This parallels the mixed results of some rTMS studies in the scientific literature, but is generally consistent with the observations that higher doses (intensities of stimulation) and longer trials are more effective than others.

Switches Into Hypomania on Antidepressants Despite Multiple Mood Stabilizers

This patient is not representative of the vast majority of patients with unipolar depression who do not switch into mania or hypomania upon treatment with antidepressants. The risk of this occurrence in unipolar patients in acute clinical trials is estimated to be about 1–2%. However, switches from unipolar depression into mania or hypomania can occur at any age, as revealed by data of Angst et al. (2005). It is worth noting that this patient had three prior brief periods of hypomania during antidepressant treatment in 2000 (Figure 52.1, left side), none of which lasted longer than 24 hours. Once engendered, this patient's recurrent, more sustained hypomanias in May and July were not readily responsive to mood stabilizers such as lithium carbonate, divalproex sodium, or lamotrigine. The addition of an atypical antipsychotic (olanzapine) appeared needed to achieve euthymia.

Very Complex Multimodal Treatment Used to Achieve Mood Stabilization

This patient thus represents an unusual situation not only because of his antidepressant-associated recurrent hypomanias (5–01 and 7–01) but also because these and his severe depressive recurrences required extraordinarily complex treatment to achieve mood stabilization. The patient was discharged on a number of different classes of psychotropic drugs, including antidepressants (venlafaxine), mood stabilizers (lithium, valproate), atypical antipsychotics (olanzapine), an anxiolytic (gabapentin), and augmenters (folate and T_3). His recurrent affective disorder would be classified according to *DSM-IV* as bipolar NOS, because his hypomania emerged in association with antidepressant treatment, that is, a substance-induced bipolar illness.

One could readily make the case that following clinical remission, the patient should be weaned from several of the agents noted above. However, in the absence of serious side effects, we and the patient chose to proceed with continuation therapy, especially in light of earlier attempts to reduce doses of the antidepressant venlafaxine in June that appeared to be associated with the reemergence of a severe depression. Our experience at NIMH (Frye, Ketter, Kimbrell, et al., 2000) has been convergent with that of many other groups (Frangou, Raymont, & Bettany, 2002; Kupfer et al., 2002; Levine et al., 2000) who have similarly observed the need for increasingly complex combination therapy for recent patients with both unipolar and bipolar mood disorders in order to achieve substantial improvement or remission.

rTMS Versus ECT

Although our experience and that of a number of other investigative groups with rTMS was not striking until we moved to higher intensities, six essentially randomized studies have openly compared the efficacy of rTMS and ECT.

Grunhaus et al. (2000) reported that rTMS was equal in efficacy to ECT in patients with nonpsychotic depression but was clearly inferior to ECT in those patients with psychotic depression. The parameters used for rTMS were 10 Hz at 90% of motor threshold. ECT in that study was right unilateral and may not have been an adequate comparison because: (1) bilateral ECT is often more clinically effective than unilateral ECT; and (2) only 9.6 ECT treatments were used compared with 20 rTMS treatments. There was an 80% response rate to ECT in the entire group of patients with a range of depressive severities, including those with psychotic depression (16 of 20 patients responded). In contrast, only 9 (45%) of 20 responded to rTMS in this entire cohort of more severely ill patients.

Pridmore, Bruno, Turnier-Shea, Reid, and Rybak (2000) also found that in 32 patients suffering a major depressive episode, an average of 12.2 rTMS treatments (20 Hz at 100% of motor threshold) was about equal to (not significantly different from) an average of 6.2 right unilateral ECT treatments.

Janicak and colleagues (2002) reported that rTMS treatments (10 Hz rTMS at 110% of motor threshold) in 25 patients with either bipolar disorder or major depressive disorder achieved a degree of efficacy not significantly different from that administered with bilateral ECT using bitemporal electrode placements. In this study, there was a nonsignificant trend for rTMS to be less effective than ECT; with a larger number of subjects, this trend might have emerged as statistically significant.

Dannon, Dolberg, Schreiber, and Grunhaus (2002) reported on a study of 3- and 6-month outcomes following a course of ECT or rTMS (10 Hz at 90% of motor threshold), and found no differences in the 6-month relapse rate between the groups.

In 2003, Grunhaus, Schreiber, Dolberg, Polak, and Dannon conducted a randomized controlled trial of ECT versus rTMS (10 Hz at 90% of motor threshold) in 40 patients with severe and resistant nonpsychotic major depression. They found that patients responded as well to either ECT or rTMS. One 6-month, randomized study by McLoughlin et al. (2005) found that bilateral ECT was more effective than rTMS (10 Hz at 110% motor threshold) in 46 patients with major depression but had several methodological confounds and, surprisingly, ECT was not associated with any cognitive side effects.

In two different series, Kimbrell et al. (1999) and Speer et al. (2000, 2006) in our group have found that some patients respond to 1 Hz and not 20 Hz, and vice versa, such that in individual patients the degree of improvement on one frequency was inversely correlated with the degree of improvement on the other.

Thus, it is of interest that five of the six studies comparing rTMS to ECT used the intermediate frequency of 10 Hz (rather than either low [1 Hz] or high [20 Hz] frequencies as in our studies at the NIMH), and excellent results (clinical remissions) were observed in substantial numbers of patients. This raises the prospect that driving neural activity with either low or high rTMS is not optimal and that an intermediate frequency of 10 Hz, much like that which occurs spontaneously in the alpha frequency on the electroencephalogram, might be preferable. However, one study (Pridmore et al., 2000) used 20 Hz at 100% of motor threshold and still saw substantial degrees of improvement. This raises the issue of differences in the degree of treatment resistance in different patient populations and, in particular, what parameters of rTMS may be optimal for a given individual.

In summary, intervening in the affective disorders with rTMS continues to hold promise, and a large multicenter randomized study using the highest parameters to date, 10Hz at 120% of motor threshold was strongly positive and the machine is being considered by the FDA for approval.

Medication Overview

The patient illustrated in Figure 52.1 initially failed to respond to two SSRIs, a risperidone-trazodone augmentation, and then a trial of augmentation with mirtazapine. He ultimately required a combination of eight different agents in five drug classes to achieve remission. Despite this range of drugs, he had a minimal side effects burden and was eager to return home and live independently.

PRINCIPLES OF THE CASE	STRENGTH OF EVIDENCE
1. Antidepressants are associated with mania or hypomania in only 1–2% of unipolar patients, although since half of the episodes of patients with bipolar illness are of the depressive variety, many presumptive unipolars with only one or two depressive episodes will eventually emerge as bipolar; 17% of patients with three prior depressions will prove to be bipolar patients.	+++
2. As originally noted by Kraepelin and others and as seen here, initial episodes of unipolar and bipolar illness often begin after psychosocial stressors such as the death of close relatives, although subsequent episodes appear to require less triggering by stressors.	++
3. This patient had a partial response to high-frequency rTMS that reduced his level of depression, anxiety, social withdrawal, and anorexia from severe to moderate; whether he would have responded more completely to ECT is not known, but he and his family were pleased with the decision to try rTMS and then medications.	+
4. Five of six small studies in the literature suggest equal efficacy of ECT and rTMS in nonpsychotic depression.	+
5. Because this patient's mania developed on antidepressants, he would be diagnosed with substance-induced hypomania and therefore meet the criteria for bipolar NOS, even though he showed a classical pattern of recurrent bipolar II-like illness.	++
6. The patient's hypomanias broke through increasingly aggressive mood stabilizer treatments that included (a) valproate initially, (b) lithium and valproate, and then (c) lithium, valproate, lamotrigine, and olanzapine.	+
7. While many would argue that antidepressants should have been withdrawn in this individual, when dose reductions of venlafaxine were attempted, the severity of recurrent depression appeared to be exacerbated.	+
8. Despite drugs from multiple classes of medication in combination, this patient had a negligible side effects burden, achieved by the sequential additions of agents with a slow upward dose titration.	++
9. The patient's appetite increased and he began to regain weight, but this had not yet become problematic in light of his previous 60-lb weight loss, and whether this would continue to	

increase over his ideal weight
in the future should be carefully
monitored.   +

10. Revisions of drugs associated
with weight gain (such as
switching from olanzapine to
the weight-neutral ziprasidone
or aripiprazole) can be consid-
ered as necessary.   ++

11. In light of the sequential additions to the complex pharmacotherapy regimen, it appeared
that many of the agents were
important to the therapeutic response, although this could not
be definitively ascertained without attempts at regimen simpli-
fication.   +

12. In light of the benign side effects profile, it was recommended that the patient initially
continue on the full treatment
regimen after discharge, and he
and his family agreed with this
suggestion.   +

13. This patient's hypomania included extreme degrees of religious fervor with active proselyt-
izing of the staff, including the
authors; this hyperreligiosity is
not an uncommon symptom of
hypomania or mania.   ++

14. This patient's extreme anorexia
and marked weight loss was endangering his physical health
close to the point at which ECT
would have been indicated as
an emergency medical interven-
tion.   ++

15. At the same time, the patient
and his family were extremely
reluctant to proceed with this
treatment option but were, instead, willing to risk enrolling

in an experimental research protocol. While rTMS was only
marginally effective, the subsequent pharmacotherapy eventually proved effective, but only
after months of aggressive inpa-
tient treatment.   ±

16. Whether a more rapid and positive outcome with the use of
ECT would have been achieved
would still be roughly a 50–50
proposition, because data from
Sackeim and colleagues (1990)
at Columbia suggest that the
roughly 80% response rates for
ECT in non-treatment-refractory
depressed patients decrease to
about 50% in those with a history of strong treatment resis-
tance, as seen in this patient.   ±

17. As suggested in other chapters,
starting over with major revisions to an initial failed complex regimen (as seen in 2000)
may be a useful approach. In
this instance, all of the drugs
that eventually proved effective
were different from those ini-
tially employed in 2000.   ±

TAKE-HOME MESSAGE

This patient with a late-life depression failed to
respond at all to one complex combination treatment involving five drugs (mirtazapine, meges-
trol, risperidone, paroxetine, and trazodone), but
following the induction of antidepressant-related
bipolar II-like cycling, the patient was stabilized
on a regimen involving eight entirely different
drugs (an antidepressant, lithium, three anticonvulsants, and an atypical antipsychotic, along
with folate and thyroid augmentation) whose
carefully titrated doses left him with relatively
few side effects.

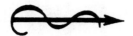

53

Stabilization of Ultrarapid Cycling With Highly Complex Combination Therapy: Rationales

CASE HISTORY

This patient had experienced many years of ultrarapid cycling, as illustrated at the end of 1996 (Figure 53.1), which was unresponsive to standard mood stabilizers and antidepressants, as listed at the end of this section. He underwent a trial of gabapentin that may have only slightly moderated his manias and severity of depression, whereas higher doses may even have exacerbated his manic cycling in the second half of 1997. With the addition of lamotrigine (at 2 on Figure 53.1) there was a reduction in hypomania and in depression from a generally low moderate severity to mostly mild severity. However, with the discontinuation of gabapentin and the taper of lamotrigine, a more severe and sustained depression occurred, despite treatment with a benzodiazepine, an atypical antipsychotic, low doses of lamotrigine, and the addition of 6 g of omega-3 fatty acids in the form of pure eicosapentaenoic acid.

With the persistence of this chronic depression, T$_3$ (at 4) was added with apparent good effect, along with 20 mg and then 30 mg of citalopram (at 5). From December 2000 to April 2001 the patient was substantially improved, but continued to struggle with a mild depressive or dysthymic baseline (Figure 53.1, bottom left). Augmentation with an amphetamine (at 6) was beneficial in helping him to get activated and

motivated in the morning. When donepezil (at 7) was added for his subjective sense of mild cognitive impairment, the patient entered a more sustained euthymic (remitted) phase (see Table 53.1 for a series of approaches to mild cognitive dysfunction in bipolar illness).

His atypical antipsychotic was switched from olanzapine to ziprasidone in September 2001 in an effort to prevent weight gain, yet maintain mood stability. Mood stabilization was thus achieved with the use of seven different classes of medications including the following:

1. A cholinesterase inhibitor (donepezil, 7.5 mg/day)

2. An antidepressant (citalopram, 40 mg/day)

3. An atypical antipsychotic (ziprasidone, 60 mg/day)

4. A high-potency, long-acting benzodiazepine (clonazepam, 0.25 mg h.s.)

5. An anticonvulsant (lamotrigine, 50 mg/day)

6. Augmentation with liothyronine (T$_3$, 37.5 μg/day)

7. An amphetamine (dextroamphetamine, 5 mg in the A.M.)

This remission occurred after the patient had had a 38-year history of bipolar affective illness, with an onset at age 18, and primarily mild to

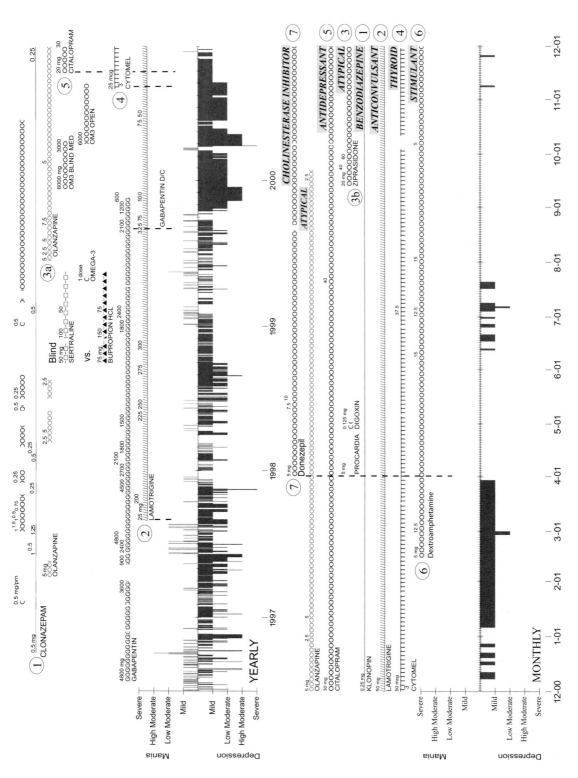

Figure 53.1 Mood stabilization with complex combination therapy: seven medication classes. This patient experienced ultrarapid and ultradian (within a day) mood cycling of high moderate depression severity and hypomania, as well as more extended periods of depression of moderate severity (top right). However, with a variety of medications sequentially added (see circled numbers), this patient became essentially euthymic in the last two thirds of 2001 (bottom line) on a combination of medications from seven different drug classes.

430

Table 53.1 *Approaches to Cognitive Slowing/ Dysfunction in Bipolar Disorder*

		Safety	Efficacy	Utility
1	Folate (1mg ♀, 2mg ♂)	A	+++	A
2	T₃ 25–37.5 μg (independent of baseline values)	A	++	A
3	Modafinil (Provigil)	A	+++	A
4	Optimize symptom remission	B	NR	A
5	Reduce dose of offending agents	B	+++	A
6	Evaluate and treat sleep disorder	A	+++	A–
7	Bupropion	A	+	B+
8	Revise regimen to avoid sedation	B	+++	B+
9	Psychomotor stimulant (amphetamine, methylphenidate)	B	+	B+
10	Memantine (Namanda)	A	(+++)	C+
11	Acetylcholine esterase inhibitor (i.e., donezipil, Aricept)	A–	(+++)	C+

moderate manias, and then many years of mostly moderate to severe depressions, with a progression to rapid and ultrarapid cycling for the 5 years prior to his NIMH admission, despite treatment with lithium, valproate, carbamazepine, desipramine, venlafaxine, bupropion, sertraline, fluoxetine, alprazolam, clonazepam, nefazodone, and T₄.

BACKGROUND LITERATURE

As discussed in Chapter 26, the combination of lamotrigine and gabapentin in this instance was perhaps slightly helpful in moderating depressive severity in 1998, but very substantial morbidity remained. In retrospect, it appears that the taper and discontinuation of gabapentin may have contributed to the appearance of more chronic and severe depression in 1999–2000

(Figure 53.1, top right). With the addition of antidepressants in late 1998 there was an increased amount of cycling and hypomania that appeared to be attenuated following an increase in the dose of olanzapine to 7.5 mg/day. As discussed in Chapter 45, olanzapine has good prophylactic antimanic efficacy, and in one randomized study its effectiveness exceeded that of lithium carbonate. Despite olanzapine's reported antidepressant properties, this patient's depression became more persistent and severe.

Chronic depression was partially attenuated with T₃ augmentation, and further improvement toward an intermittent euthymic baseline was achieved with the SSRI citalopram (Figure 53.1, top right). Dextroamphetamine may have helped with residual morning fatigue and sedation. The cholinesterase inhibitor donepezil has been reported by Jacobson and Comas-Diaz (1999) to help clear cognitive functioning when it has been impaired by a variety of psychotropic compounds, particularly of the antidepressant category. The esterase inhibitor not only appeared to be effective on cognition, but was also associated with the onset of a more sustained euthymic phase. Thus, treatment decisions were made here on the basis of (a) targeting specific symptom presentations, (b) use of novel agents with different mechanisms of action, and (c) those with the most benign side effects profile.

As noted in previous chapters, there has been a trend toward an increasing need for complex combination therapy to bring patients to acute remission following inpatient hospitalizations at the clinical research unit at the NIMH over the past 30 years (Frye, Ketter, Leverich, et al., 2000). Many other investigative groups have noted similar trends.

What are the rationales, then, for use of such complex combination therapies in bipolar illness? We propose the following.

First, the rationale for attempting such heroic measures is evident for this patient with extreme degrees of treatment-refractory bipolar illness inadequately responsive to multiple classes and types of medications within each class for much of the prior 38 years. Thus, the major rationale for the aggressive exploration of combinations is clearly patient need.

A second, indirect rationale is that many other chronic or recurrent medical illnesses similarly require extremely complex medication regimens to bring about remission. These include most cancer chemotherapeutic regimens, resistant tuberculosis, congestive heart failure, AIDS, and rheumatoid arthritis, for which expert clinicians widely and openly advocate combination treatment. Thus, extensive use of multiple medications from different classes is widely practiced throughout many areas of medicine.

A third rationale relates to the previous observations. That is, by using a number of agents with different mechanisms of action, one can often achieve a more effective treatment outcome than with a single targeted approach. Given the number of neurotransmitters that may be altered in bipolar illness (Chapter 10), multiple approaches to these alterations may be required until more specific treatment strategies are found for the illness. However, even when the basic pathophysiology of an illness is known, such as the dopamine deficiency in Parkinson's disease, patients still require multiple and different types of medications to control their illness, particularly in its later phases.

A final rationale is the reduction of side effects. Although this might seem paradoxical, it is apparent that if one judiciously uses doses of drugs that are not only below a patient's side effects threshold but below the side effects threshold of the entire regimen, multiple drugs can often be implemented sequentially without the occurrence of major side effects. This strategy is contrary to pushing individual drugs (when only lithium and typical antipsychotics were available) to and above an individual's side effects threshold. In those instances, patients were sometimes titrated to lithium levels over 1.5 meq/L (often associated with a wide range of side effects) and the use of extraordinarily high doses of antipsychotic agents was widely practiced 20 years ago, despite mounting evidence that they were no more effective than lower dose regimens and were associated with a greater side effects burden.

PRINCIPLES OF THE CASE	STRENGTH OF EVIDENCE
1. Even with many years of severe ultrarapid cycling, remissions can most often be achieved.	++
2. Remission often requires employing a number of different medications and classes of medications.	++
3. Slow titration of the dose of each agent, thus keeping the side effects burden of the entire regimen to a minimum, is the most important treatment principle.	+++
4. When there is some evidence of sequential improvement with additions of successive agents, it is difficult to know whether all of the agents in the regimen are absolutely necessary without an off-drug clinical trial.	+
5. We advocate such a tapering approach when an agent appears to be adding to the side effects burden and is only an ambiguous contributor to overall clinical efficacy.	+
6. However, in the relative absence of side effects in patients who have been ill for many years, we would often conservatively advise maintaining the full complement of complex combination treatments to try to maintain and extend euthymia over the long term.	+
7. This rationale is illustrated in the next chapter, where even with maintenance of triple anticonvulsant therapy, episodes again began to break through.	+

8. Presumptive olanzapine-related weight gain was approached by the switch to ziprasidone in September 2001 (Figure 53.1, bottom right), and this was not associated with a loss of therapeutic benefit.　　+

9. Conversely, in the absence of substantial therapeutic benefits of a given complex combination treatment regimen, it appears prudent to begin to taper and discontinue a substantial group of the ineffective agents in order to begin an entirely new treatment strategy.　　±

10. As noted previously, it is clear that a new sequential clinical trials methodology for more rationally developing optimal algorithms for patients with highly treatment-refractory illness such as this is clearly needed.　　+++

11. In the absence of such systematic information and guidance from the literature, careful charting of mood and side effects is, in our experience, one of the most important components of developing individual treatment algorithms that are both successful and well tolerated.　　++

12. If the increase in depressive chronicity and severity upon gabapentin taper (in 1999, Figure 53.1, second arrow) were recognized, one might have considered a retrial with this agent.　　+

TAKE-HOME MESSAGE

Even the most rapidly cycling, long-term, treatment-resistant patients can achieve symptom remission, although sometimes this requires great patience (and heroism) on the individual's part and a willingness to carefully explore the range and combination of treatment options that extend well beyond conventional approaches to the illness.

54

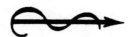

Complex Combination Therapy for the Reestablishment of Euthymia in a Bipolar II Patient

CASE HISTORY

This case example is a patient with bipolar II illness and comorbid PTSD who achieved euthymic status for a number of months after having been ill virtually her entire life, as described in Chapter 66. This chapter is a continuation of her prospective life chart illustrating a series of minor to major breakthrough depressive episodes that improved with the addition of another set of medications (Figure 54.1, top right and lower left). Another subsequent depressive episode (August 2001) again responded to the addition of several other agents, which led to the reestablishment of her euthymic baseline on a total of nine drugs.

As illustrated in the top right portion of the figure, a succession of depressive bursts, first of low, then of moderate and high severity broke through this patient's ongoing prophylaxis with gabapentin (1,800 mg/day), lamotrigine (300 mg/day), and carbamazepine (800 mg/day; Chapter 66). It is noteworthy that the more severe depression broke through at a time when the dose of carbamazepine was being reduced from 600 to 200 mg in order to avoid sedative side effects and the decreases in white blood cell count (WBC) it caused. With the onset of this depression (top right), benzodiazepines were administered for anxiety, and treatment with the serotonin and norepinephrine reuptake inhibitor

venlafaxine was begun. Lithium carbonate was added as an adjunctive treatment when venlafaxine showed little evidence of initial response. Lithium was also given in an attempt to boost the patient's WBC count (which it is known to do) and to counter the WBC-suppressive effects of carbamazepine. Note that on the bottom line of Figure 54.1, the time line is changed so that 1 rather than 2 years is represented, in order to illustrate some of the details of this patient's responsivity.

As the dose of venlafaxine was slowly increased to 200 mg and then to 300 mg, along with increases in carbamazepine to 900 mg/day, the patient's severity of depression began to lessen (Figure 54.1, bottom left). In November 2000, she reachieved her euthymic baseline, which was sustained for another 8 months (i.e., the longest period of wellness in her entire life). The dotted vertical line on Figure 54.1 in June 2001 suggests the possible increased vulnerability to the following depression with the tapering and then discontinuation of gabapentin.

With the onset of the next depression in August 2001, gabapentin treatment was reinitiated in addition to small doses of the atypical antipsychotic risperidone (0.5 mg/day) for mild paranoia, and donepezil initially at 5 mg and then increased to 10 mg for a sense of cognitive cloudiness.

The gabapentin had been tapered 2 months

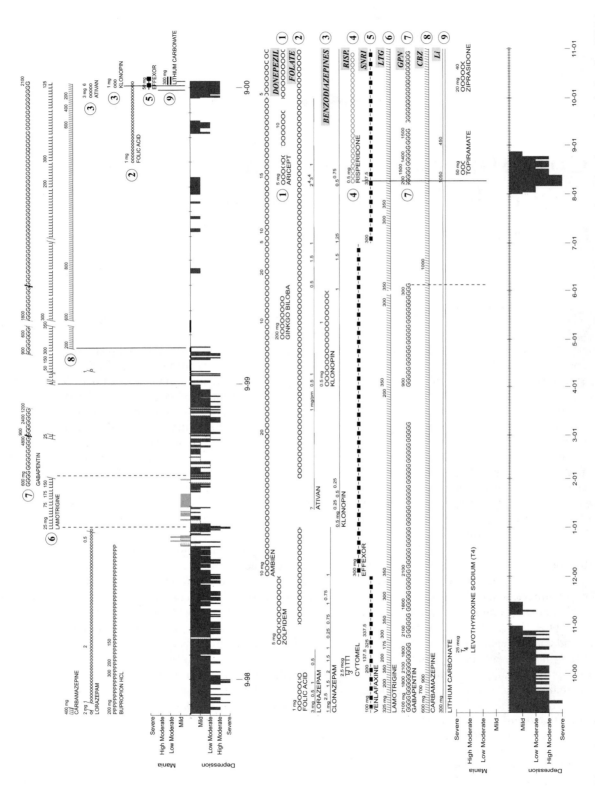

Figure 54.1 Mood stabilization with complex combination therapy. After achieving a remission with lamotrigine, gabapentin, and carbamazepine in October 1999 (top middle), this patient experienced breakthrough brief mild depressions, then an episode of moderate severity, and finally a severe recurrence (top right and bottom left). This recurrence required a new set of treatments: folate, clonazepam, venlafaxine, and lithium, yielding a 9-month remission (bottom). Another severe depression in August 2001 broke through treatment with six drugs (bottom right) and required additional treatment interventions to reachieve euthymia, which continued during treatment with nine separate drugs.

previously in an attempt to reduce the patient's overall burden of drugs contributing to weight gain, but with the reemergence of a severe episode, the patient was willing to reinitiate this treatment in August 2001, as well as begin risperidone, despite their potential for further weight gain. Donepezil was also added in an attempt to facilitate the patient's cognitive processing, which had become slow and problematic in the face of her severe renewed depressive symptoms. It is not clear which of these three agents (started within several days of each other to target different components of her depression) was most responsible for the patient's clinical improvement, but she did reestablish euthymia in September 2001, which was maintained for the several years we remained in contact.

Thus, the patient's regimen (Figure 54.1, bottom right) not only included the three initial anticonvulsants (carbamazepine, lamotrigine, and gabapentin) that were critical to her achieving her first well state (top middle), but relatively high antidepressant doses of venlafaxine, as augmented by lithium and folate. Benzodiazepines and risperidone were used to treat residual anxiety and paranoia, respectively, with donepezil for enhancing cognitive clarity.

It is noteworthy that in August 2001 a brief clinical trial was attempted with topiramate to try to assist her efforts to lose weight. In October 2001, ziprasidone treatment was attempted to see if it might prove an alternative to risperidone without weight gain liability. However, neither of these drugs was well tolerated, and the original regimen of nine separate agents was left in place, and the patient continued to do well except for the development of severe obesity.

BACKGROUND LITERATURE

Despite exercise and diet, the patient gained a considerable amount of weight on this complex regimen. Drugs with the potential for weight gain included lithium, gabapentin, carbamazepine, and risperidone, each of which alone have only mild to moderate weight gain liabilities.

Topiramate (Chapter 29) can be associated with considerable weight loss and was tried in this instance also because McIntyre and associates (2002) suggested that this drug can augment antidepressant efficacy, equal in magnitude to that of the antidepressant bupropion but with greater weight loss. Disappointingly, the patient did not tolerate the cognitive side effects of even low doses of this weight loss agent.

Folic acid was added (Figure 54.1, top right) because the patient began to show occasional breakthroughs of mild depression. Coppen and Bailey (2000) had reported that folic acid could successfully augment the antidepressant effects of other antidepressant agents and also potentiate the effects of lithium prophylaxis (Coppen et al., 1986).

It is noteworthy that the first prolonged depressive recurrence (top, right) after a series of depressive flurries and breakthroughs of moderate severity (suggestive of a tolerance pattern) occurred in the context of a reduction in the dose of carbamazepine. This observation, and the relapse in August 2001 after the tapering and discontinuation of gabapentin, continue to illustrate (although not definitively in either instance) the idea that patients often need to be treated prophylactically with full doses of the treatments to which they responded acutely in order to maintain their clinical response.

This patient also illustrates the point that breakthrough episodes can sometimes occur in patients who are initially well stabilized on a given regimen, suggesting a tolerance phenomenon. Here we would also emphasize the opposite: that is, renewed response can usually be acquired with different or additional augmenting strategies such as those initiated in September 2000 and then again in August 2001.

Despite the use of nine psychotropic medications, the patient had few side effects other than profound weight gain, which had already become an intractable problem. In the face of this patient's intolerance of topiramate, one could now consider zonisamide as a possible alternative for both mood stabilization and the positive side effect of weight loss (McElroy et al., 2005).

The addition of donepezil is worthy of further note. An open study by Burt, Sachs, and Demopulos (1999) reported that this drug, which is approved for the treatment of Alzheimer's disease, had positive effects on mood in an open series. Jacobsen and Comas-Diaz (1999) reported improvement in cognition when donepezil was added to other routinely used (primarily antidepressant) treatments when patients did not feel as cognitively clear as usual on these medications. However, a later double-blind, placebo-controlled, randomized study in patients with mania found no added benefit of donepezil (Evins et al., 2006). Further controlled clinical trials are required to assess the efficacy of donepezil and the growing series of related drugs for Alzheimer's disease (cholinesterase inhibitors) for alleviating depression.

It is noteworthy that this patient's PTSD symptomatology, which had been severe and persistent over many years (Chapter 66), remained in remission despite the breakthrough of several severe depressive episodes. These data support the idea that even a very long history of PTSD, although it can complicate therapeutic approaches to bipolar illness, does not preclude an eventual complete remission in all of the multiple facets of PTSD symptomatology, including nightmares, sleep disturbance, flashbacks, hyperstartle, and numbness and withdrawal as experienced by this individual.

Thus, this patient illustrates another interesting set of observations that although the serotonin-selective antidepressants are the only ones approved by the FDA for the treatment of PTSD, a number of the anticonvulsants have shown promise in small, usually open studies. In this patient, the combination of three different anticonvulsants—lamotrigine, gabapentin, and carbamazepine—was sufficient not only to bring the persistent depressions and hypomanic mood fluctuations to a period of sustained euthymia, but also to completely suppress essentially all of her PTSD symptoms. Thus, some patients will need other approaches in addition to SSRIs in order to more adequately treat sleep disturbance associated with PTSD, as well as the paroxysmal breakthrough of sleep-related nightmares or daytime flashbacks.

PRINCIPLES OF THE CASE / **STRENGTH OF EVIDENCE**

1. While attempts at tapering medications in the face of side effects is often warranted, this patient's course suggests that it can also have hazards. ±

2. Dose reductions in two separate instances of just one of several agents possibly involved in an effective therapeutic regimen may have been associated with the vulnerability to breakthrough symptoms. ±

3. The increasing severity of breakthrough depressions (Figure 54.1, top right) suggests a tolerance pattern. +

4. In the face of a good clinical response and a lack of side effects, the most conservative course is to continue prophylaxis with full-dose pharmacotherapy. ++

5. If there are difficult side effects, attempts to lower doses, taper the offending medications, or replace them with others with a more benign side effects profile are indicated. +++

6. Sometimes extremely complex combination therapy with multiple agents from multiple different drug classes is required, either to achieve initial mood stabilization or to reacquire it after breakthrough episodes. ++

7. This patient worked hard to build an excellent support system with her new friends and family and maintained an extremely close working relationship with her treating psychiatrist; both appeared helpful in facilitating her recovery from

the two intercurrent severe depressive recurrences (see Miklowitz, 2002, for further suggestions for building a support system).   ++

8. Miklowitz et al. (2007) provide strong evidence for the efficacy of several different types of focused psychotherapeutic interventions compared to treatment as usual. Psychotherapy and psychoeducational approaches should be part of the treatment for the majority of patients with bipolar illness.   +++

9. Also noteworthy is the fact that the episode occurring in August 2001 was associated with a very difficult set of psychosocial stressors threatening to disrupt the patient's newly acquired support system (Chapters 5 and 7).   +

10. As in many instances in clinical medicine, it is difficult to factor out the precise cause-effect relationships in multiple domains that lead to instances of increased illness vulnerability, symptom breakthrough, and therapeutic restabilization.   +++

TAKE-HOME MESSAGE

Even for patients with the most difficult treatment-refractory and comorbid courses of illness, a multidisciplinary and multimodal treatment approach (including psychotherapy and very complex pharmacotherapeutic regimens) can be associated with striking therapeutic successes.

55

The Addition of Clozapine and an Antidepressant to Lamotrigine and Valproate in the Treatment of Ultrarapid Cycling

CASE HISTORY

This patient is a 36-year-old with bipolar I disorder and an ultrarapid cycling course. His first depressive episode occurred at age 14, and his first mania at 16. Shortly after, he developed a rapid-cycling course with mood switches every 14 days and no well interval. Combination treatment with lithium and carbamazepine led to symptom remission for almost 9 years. During that time, the patient was able to complete an apprenticeship and work for several years.

The ultrarapid cycling then recurred despite the combination treatment in an apparent tolerance process. In addition, he developed the co-morbid symptoms of kleptomania, panic attacks, and binge eating. Attempts to stabilize his mood with valproate, lamotrigine, and different anti-depressants failed. He was unable to work any longer due to his rapid mood switches and was given a disability pension.

When he first visited a European outpatient clinic, he was taking a combination of lithium,

This chapter was modified from Dittmann, S., Forsthoff, A., Thoma, H., & Grunze, H. (2002). Clozapine as an add-on in the maintenance treatment of rapid cycling bipolar disorder. *Clinical Approaches in Bipolar Disorders, 1*, 31–33, with permission of the authors.

valproate, lamotrigine, and venlafaxine, with no change to the rapid-cycling course of his illness (Figure 55.1, left side). Both his depressive and manic episodes ranged from moderate to severe. Particularly during his depressed phases, he had strong suicidal ideation. Initially, the physicians switched venlafaxine to paroxetine because they felt it was not possible to taper the antidepressant component of his treatment due to his strong suicidal thoughts, and data suggest that venlafaxine is more likely to be associated with manias than the SSRIs (Post, Altshuler, et al., 2006). Due to ongoing mood instability, lithium was gradually tapered and treatment with clozapine was started.

After the titration phase, the daily dose of clozapine was 225 mg/day. In the subsequent 6 months, his manias subsided completely, but his depressive episodes were only minimally improved. Paroxetine was then replaced with omega-3 fatty acids, which improved the depressive symptoms somewhat after open treatment was initiated in April 2001. Suicidal ideation was no longer present, although moderate depressive episodes still occurred. The authors decided to start treatment with the norepineph-rine-selective antidepressant reboxetine and discontinue omega-3 fatty acids. Reboxetine is a

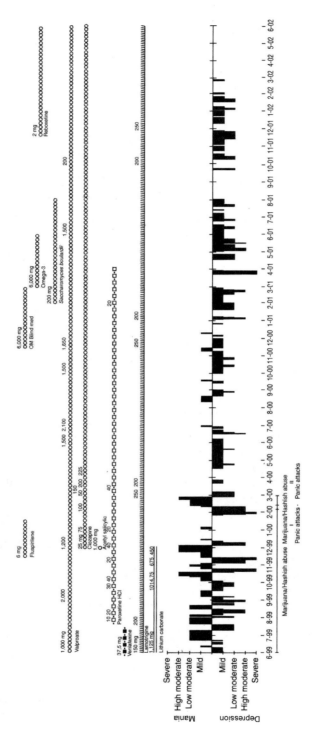

Figure 55.1 Clozapine augmentation (in 12/1999) of the effects of lamotrigine and valproate dramatically improved manic recurrences but was less effective on depressions that required the addition of an antidepressant (reboxetine).

442

selective reuptake inhibitor of norepinephrine not yet available in the United States, similar to atomoxetine. At the time of the case presentation, no depressive symptoms had occurred for over 3 months, and the patient was again able to work part time.

The combination treatment of valproate, clozapine, lamotrigine, and reboxetine was effective in this patient. The only side effects were weight gain, fatigue, and mild salivation, all of which subsided after some weeks of treatment. Now better able to control his eating habits, the patient lost 14 kg and experienced no manias for 1 year and no severe depressions for several months. Comorbid symptoms and suicidal ideation were no longer present.

BACKGROUND LITERATURE

Though several mood stabilizers, such as lithium, valproic acid, and carbamazepine, are available for the maintenance treatment of bipolar disorder, a number of patients are still unresponsive to their monotherapy or combination treatment (Banov et al., 1994). The treatment of rapid-cycling bipolar patients still presents a particular challenge for clinicians. It is estimated that 33% of patients with classical bipolar disorder do not respond to lithium (Prien & Gelenberg, 1989), and this proportion may double in patients with mixed episodes, rapid-cycling, multiple comorbidities, and various other illness patterns (Dunner, Patrick, & Fieve, 1977; McElroy, Keck, Pope, Hudson, Faedda, et al., 1992).

Many bipolar patients continue to be treated with typical antipsychotics in acute manic phases of their disorder (especially in Europe) and then continue these as maintenance treatment, despite the high risk of tardive dyskinesia (Kane, 1988; McElroy, Keck, & Strakowski, 1996). A longitudinal study suggested that long-term use of typical antipsychotic agents could be associated with increased depression and cycle acceleration (Kukopulos et al., 1980). In another study, in which double-blind lithium monotherapy was compared with the combination treatment of lithium and flupenthixol for 2 years, patients randomized to combination treat-

ment suffered from an increased number of depressive episodes, whereas the frequency of manic episodes did not differ significantly (Ahlfors et al., 1981).

Whether rapid-cycling bipolar patients should be treated with antidepressants in the depressive phase remains controversial (Chapters 34–38). U.S. authorities often recommend that antidepressants be avoided wherever possible (el Mallakh & Karippot, 2002), whereas European specialists do not exclude their use, particularly if depressive episodes are severe or suicidal ideation occurs (Moller & Grunze, 2000). Atypical antipsychotics, such as clozapine, olanzapine, risperidone, quetiapine, ziprasidone, and aripiprazole are considered relatively safe alternatives or adjuncts to mood stabilizers when used as add-on medication in the maintenance treatment of bipolar and schizoaffective disorders (Ghaemi, 2000). Several authors have reported even greater efficacy of clozapine in schizoaffective (Leppig, Bosch, Naber, & Hippius, 1989; Naber, Leppig, Grohmann, & Hippius, 1989; Owen, Beake, Marby, Dessain, & Cole, 1989) and bipolar disorder (Tohen & Zarate, 1998; Zarate, Tohen, & Baldessarini, 1995; Zarate, Tohen, Banov, Weiss, & Cole, 1995) than in schizophrenia (see Chapter 46).

However, few controlled trials of clozapine in maintenance treatment have been performed (Suppes et al., 1999). This lack of data might be due to clozapine's potential to induce agranulocytosis, but there is also a lack of commercial interest in this relatively old drug. Here we report on a well-characterized patient with rapid-cycling bipolar disorder who was followed up. Clozapine was administered in combination with reboxetine as add-on medication, which led to complete remission of symptoms. This case has appeared previously as part of a case series (Hummel et al., 2002).

PRINCIPLES OF THE CASE	STRENGTH OF EVIDENCE

1. Atypical antipsychotics (administered either alone or in

combination) are being used increasingly in bipolar and schizoaffective disorders for patients unresponsive to mood stabilizers. ++

2. This case report is in agreement with other reports (Chapter 46) and trials that show clozapine to be effective in patients with rapid cycling and dysphoric mania. ++

3. When clozapine was added to his mood stabilizer treatment, this patient's manic symptoms subsided completely while depressive recurrences persisted. ++

4. Therefore, as the general literature would suggest, clozapine appears more effective on manic than depressive symptoms. +

5. In the sequence of clinical trials in the United States, most clinicians would try several of the other atypical antipsychotics prior to clozapine because of its need for weekly white blood cell count monitoring and its less than ideal side effects profile. ++

6. Given the data on the striking antidepressant effects of quetiapine by Calabrese, Keck, and associates (2005), one would wonder whether it would have been as good as or better than clozapine in this patient. ±

7. Lamotrigine and valproate are often complementary and well tolerated in combination, despite increased risk of rash (as valproate doubles lamotrigine levels); either drug is helpful in preventing clozapine seizures, although lamotrigine would add less weight gain risk to clozapine. ++

8. Addition of an antidepressant (reboxetine) to the two anticonvulsants and clozapine appeared necessary to treat recurrent depressive symptoms completely. +

9. Reboxetine is norepinephrine selective in its blockage of reuptake like desipramine, nortriptyline, maprotiline, and the more recently approved atomoxetine. ++

10. No agranulocytosis occurred in this patient despite the 1–3% risk on clozapine (which necessitates close, usually weekly, monitoring of white blood counts). +++

11. Side effects were manageable, but included fatigue, increased salivation, and weight gain during the clozapine titration phase, but were less of a problem thereafter. +

12. The patient was able to lose more than 10 kg of weight during the continuation treatment with clozapine and valproate (once his mood improved, allowing more exercise and better adherence to a proper diet). +

13. When to treat the depressive phase of rapid-cycling bipolar disorder with an antidepressant as an adjunct to one or more mood stabilizers or atypical antipsychotics remains controversial, but in this case appeared necessary. +

14. After an initial remission on lithium and carbamazepine lasting 9 years, different drugs in a complex combination approach became necessary to restabilize this patient. ±

15. Returning to this previously effective combination after a pe-

riod of time off might also be a clinically useful option in instances of tolerance development. +

TAKE-HOME MESSAGE

A patient who had lost responsiveness to lithium and carbamazepine and experienced ultrarapid cycling with mood switches about every 14 days and no euthymic intervals despite aggressive pharmacotherapy was partially restabilized with the addition of an atypical antipsychotic (clozapine) and two anticonvulsant mood stabilizers (lamotrigine and valproate). A subsequent addition of the antidepressant reboxetine yielded a complete remission. A complex pharmacotherapeutic regimen change including drugs with many different mechanisms of action is sometimes required to restabilize an ultrarapid-cycling patient.

Part XI

ELECTROCONVULSIVE THERAPY

56

Role of Electroconvulsive Therapy in Acute Depression and Long-Term Prophylaxis of Bipolar Illness: Preliminary Risk-to-Benefit Analysis

CASE HISTORY

Mr. Z is a 36-year-old with a history of multiple psychiatric hospitalizations for depressive episodes associated with bipolar I disorder, which was first diagnosed in 1989 following a full-blown manic episode of 3 months duration meeting *DSM-IV* criteria (Figure 56.1). Family history of psychiatric illness was positive only for a father with alcoholism.

Prior to his first admission, Mr. Z was working successfully as an architectural engineer. His first psychiatric hospitalization was in November 1989 for depression with anhedonia, delusions, selective mutism, and severe anorexia requiring intravenous hydration and forced nutrition by feeding tube. Treatment with high-dose antipsychotics and multiple tricyclic antidepressants was unsuccessful. The episode responded dramatically to electroconvulsive therapy (ECT). Unilateral (UL) electrode placement was used initially to prevent memory loss and then replaced by bilateral (BL) ECT for greater efficacy.

Subsequent episodes, each precipitating inpatient psychiatric admission and all characterized by the same clinical features of major depression over the next 5 years (Figure 56.1, 1989–

1993) occurred despite preventive maintenance therapies with lithium, valproic acid, and carbamazepine with periods of concurrent administration of bupropion or antipsychotics for mood and psychotic symptoms. Good compliance with medication regimens was confirmed by the patient and his relatives. These pharmacologically refractory episodes all responded well to BL ECT in the inpatient setting. However, each hospitalization was costly and represented a significant disruption in the patient's ability to return to steady work and routine social pursuits.

After an inpatient admission in 1993, the patient was enrolled in a 10-month course of outpatient maintenance ECT receiving a total of 11 BL treatments, the last 9 of which were given at monthly intervals. During the first 6 months of outpatient ECT, he was on a tapering dose of haloperidol (from 10 to 2.5 mg) and benztropine (1 mg b.i.d.) with no recurrence of symptoms after discontinuation.

During the ECT treatments, the patient experienced no adverse medical complications and minimal cognitive side effects, and was able to complete college-level night courses. Scores on the Hamilton rating scale for depression ranged from 2 to 4 throughout the course of treatment. In addition to maintenance ECT treatments, he

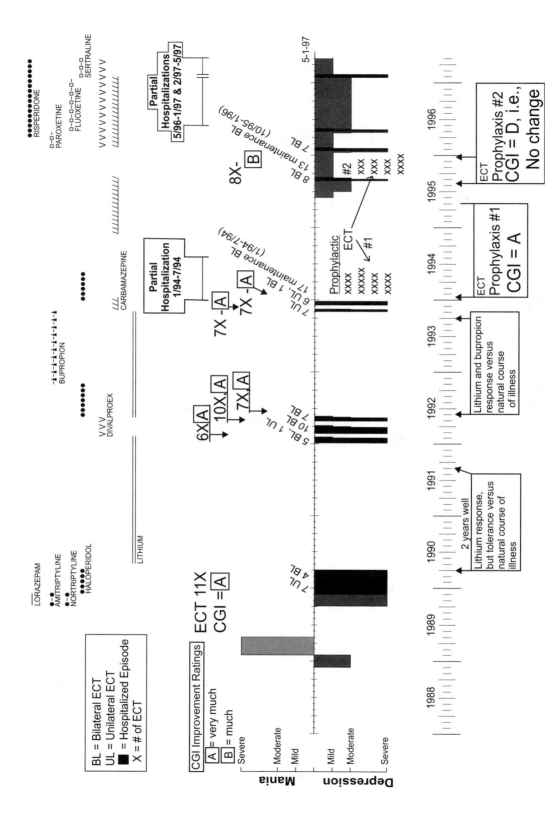

Figure 56.1 Complete acute and prophylactic response and failure of prophylactic ECT. Six remissions (CGI = A) achieved with ECT (X). Then lack of complete response to acute ECT in 1995 (i.e., baseline dysthymia persists) and the failure of ECT prophylaxis in 1996.

450

was enrolled in a partial hospitalization program immediately following discharge and then engaged in bimonthly supportive psychotherapy with a resident physician, which he continued. Prophylactic ECT response in 1994 on the Clinical Global Impressions scale (CGI) was A or very much improved, that is, a complete remission.

Upon termination of maintenance ECT, maintenance therapy with carbamazepine was initiated (in 1995) with a final dose of 800 mg/day. At 4-month follow up, he remained free of depressive symptoms and reported that the mild memory deficits related to ECT had resolved. However, depressions again broke through pharmacological treatment, requiring 8 acute and then 13 maintenance ECT treatments. Depression again recurred despite continuation ECT treatment, and a full euthymic baseline was not achieved after another 7 BL ECT treatments in 1996. Follow-up pharmacotherapy with an atypical antipsychotic (risperidone), a selective serotonin reuptake inhibitor (paroxetine or sertraline), valproate, and carbamazepine initially did not prevent recurrences.

This patient in 1994, and the patient in Chapter 35, illustrate good acute antidepressant responses to ECT. However, the excellent response to maintenance ECT was not unambiguous in 1994 because the well interval achieved was not substantially longer than the previous well intervals in 1990–1991 and 1992–1993 during lithium treatment. Moreover, the acute ECT response in 1995 was only partial (CGI score of B or much improved), and the second prophylactic series was not effective because the patient had a full-blown relapse requiring rehospitalization in January 1996 (CGI score of D or no change) in the course of recurrent episodes.

BACKGROUND LITERATURE

In this chapter, we do not have a very dramatic illustration of the efficacy of continuation ECT in the long-term treatment of bipolar illness because, with our limited experience with this modality, we have not had the opportunity to observe sustained long-term responses. However, a number of colleagues have indicated that ECT has occasionally played a useful preventive role and sometimes has been used when a variety of other treatment strategies have failed.

The acute efficacy of ECT has been clearly established in controlled trials in the scientific literature and in case studies. For example, the use of ECT to treat the recurrent major depressions of Senator Eagleton was so effective that his congressional colleagues and the rest of the nation were initially unaware of his problems with recurrent depression. Thus, we support the use of ECT on occasion when other pharmacological modalities are inadequate for an acute life-threatening depression; what is less certain is the use of ECT in long-term prophylaxis. Prophylaxis has not been systematically studied in controlled comparative trials in bipolar illness, nor have the best intervals between treatments been well established. The second patient illustrated in this chapter (Figure 56.2) had a complete response to ECT after two prior partial responses with rapid relapses, leaving it ambiguous as to what the best prophylactic regimen might be (several options are offered in the figure).

The patient discussed in Chapter 35 had an immediate response to a single ECT treatment, which ended her refractory depression as an inpatient at the NIMH. However, when another depression occurred shortly thereafter while she was an outpatient in New York City, a new series of ECT treatments was ineffective in achieving a remission. The patient in this chapter responded less well over time, and apparent prophylactic success with ECT in 1994 eventually became ineffective in 1995. These two failures to sustain response (Chapter 35 and Figure 56.1 here) raise the question of whether, in some patients, tolerance can develop to the therapeutic effects of ECT in the long-term treatment of the illness, just as tolerance can occur with other modalities such as lithium, carbamazepine, and valproate, as discussed in Chapters 12, 19, and 24, respectively. Whether suitable intervals of ECT administration can be found for the individual patient with rapid or continuously cycling bipolar depression that would help maintain long-term response remains to be demonstrated.

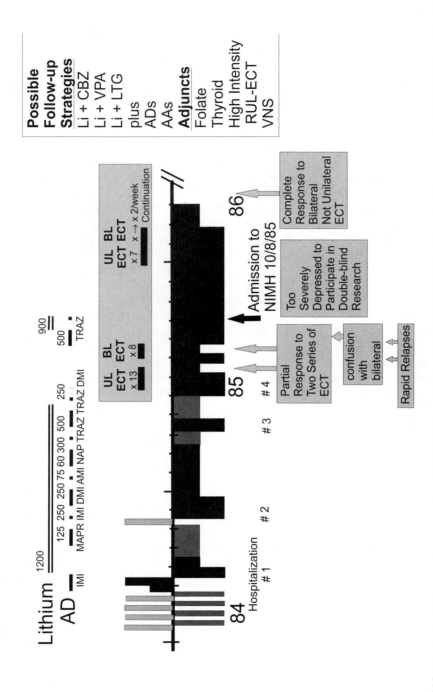

Figure 56.2 Transient antidepressant responses to unilateral (UL) and bilateral (BL) ECT in 1985 and a complete response to BL ECT with continuation in 1986. This patient failed to respond to lithium and to a variety of antidepressants. Given the rapid relapses in 1985 after two prior ECT series, a sequence of potential alternative follow-up treatment strategies is offered that might better help sustain the response.

History of ECT

Convulsive therapy was first used in the middle of the 20th century, administered in a chemical form with either insulin shock or pentylenetetrazol (Metrazol) injections, and shortly thereafter with the application of electricity, but in each of these instances without anesthesia. This old procedure had a number of negative consequences, and the history of this phase of ECT continues to have a negative impact on the clinical acceptance and stigma of this therapy to the present. Without suitable pretreatment anesthesia, many patients became extremely anxious, particularly with the administration of chemically induced seizures. Moreover, the muscle contractions associated with the seizures were sometimes of sufficient severity to be associated with bone fractures.

Both of these problems were mitigated with the use of more modern techniques, which involved first the application of a rapidly acting intravenous general anesthetic (usually a short-acting benzodiazepine), and then brief paralysis of the muscles (with curare or related compounds). This removed the anxiety, muscle soreness, and bone fractures that accompanied the seizure but also necessitated artificial respiration of the patient for the several minutes of induced paralysis during the seizure.

With modern techniques of anesthesia, the ECT procedure is now very different from its original form. Patients fall asleep and awaken a short time later largely unaware that they have had a seizure at all. The medical complications of ECT are thus essentially those of general anesthesia, with the risk of a serious or fatal outcome in approximately 1 in 10,000 patients.

Memory Loss One of the areas of greatest persisting concern in ECT, however, is the nature of the side effect of memory loss. This side effect appears to be highly dependent on the type of ECT administered. With traditional BL frontal ECT, confusion and memory loss are usually transient, typically lifting in 1 or 2 hours post-ECT. Both memory loss and post-ECT confusion are reduced with the use of right UL ECT. Sackeim and colleagues (1993) found that low-dose right UL ECT is not a particularly effective treatment modality. However, with higher intensity and brief pulses, the efficacy of right UL ECT (when the current is administered at 500% of the seizure threshold) is more like BL ECT and yet associated with lesser degrees of memory loss (Sackeim et al., 1993, 2000).

Sienaert et al., (2007) like Sackeim et al (2001) used ultra brief pulse (0.3 msec) ECT with good clinical effect and little memory loss. They found that this stimulation bifrontally at 1.5 times the seizure threshold and unilaterally at 6 times the seizure threshold were equally effective and neither caused mental impairment on the standardized Mini-Mental State exam.

Although memory loss with ECT has been intensively studied with a variety of formal psychometric tests, its severity and duration remain controversial. It is clear that ECT often induces a retrograde memory loss such that events occurring during the prior several weeks (often during the entire series of ECT treatments) are largely forgotten.

More problematic is when the retrograde memory loss extends further backward in time, so that events some months previously and, rarely, some years previously are difficult to access and essentially need to be relearned. There is very little evidence for an anterior grade amnesia, that is, the inability to lay down and access new memories (Rami-Gonzalez et al., 2001). These data on ECT-induced seizures mirror those of patients with epilepsy who have repeated grand mal or major motor seizures without evidence of major cognitive decline.

However, a few patients experience a considerable degree of retrograde memory loss, and we have seen a number of instances—in patients ranging in age from their early 20s to their 60s without any apparent special risk factor—in which retrograde memory loss has been quite substantial and profound. In these patients, the memory loss unfortunately involved considerable periods of time, ranging from 6 months to many years. For example, one patient had trouble navigating in her own household and had to relearn much of her musical technique as a pianist. This severity of memory loss is unusual, and its incidence has not been established. We have also seen a 45-year-old previously high-functioning business executive with a profound retrograde amnesia extending back about 8 to 10 years following a series of 24 BL ECT treatments. Even simple calculations and tasks are now a problem for this patient, suggesting that in extremely rare instances an anterograde problem with new learning can occur as well.

A study of Sackeim and colleagues (2007) of patients followed in different hospital settings in New York City has clarified some of the potential variables involved. Patients treated with a sine wave form of stimulation had more cognitive problems than those who received brief or ultra brief pulse stimulation. Based on these results and prior recommendations of an APA committee on ECT, it is clear that there is no longer any rationale for using this wave form and it should not be given. Individualizing the intensity of stimulation required to an individual's specific seizure threshold was also important to minimizing cognitive side effects.

The study also clarified that bilateral compared to unilateral electrode placement carried much greater risks for acute and persistent (at 6 months) retrograde memory loss. This was measured with a sensitive test of autobiographical memory. Strikingly, the severity of retrograde memory loss (the amount of time involved) was directly proportional to the number of bilateral ECT treatment received.

Experiments in animals also show that the memory loss is of the retrograde amnesia type and is associated with the inability to access previously constructed memory traces (rather than memory loss per se). Animals that have learned to run a maze are unable to find their way after acute electroconvulsive shock treatments (Beatty, Bierley, & Rush, 1985). If, however, they are tested while they are still under the influence of the convulsive seizure, they are able to perform the task without difficulty. These observations indicate that an aspect of the memory loss relates to state-dependent effects and, under appropriate circumstances, the memory traces can, in fact, be retrieved.

Mechanisms of Action The mechanism of ECT effectiveness remains a partial mystery, much like that of the exact mechanisms of action of the effective pharmacoprophylactic agents such as lithium, carbamazepine, and valproate, especially because so many central nervous system effects of these drugs and ECT have been delineated. However, there is a clear indication that ECT is also an anticonvulsant modality, and its application is able to inhibit not only amygdala-kindled seizures in animals (Post, Putnam, Contel, & Goldman, 1984) but also other types of seizures.

In patients, this anticonvulsant effect of ECT is evidenced by an increase in seizure threshold and increasing difficulty in achieving a seizure using the same amount of current in the same individual repeatedly over time. One study has indicated that this degree of seizure threshold increase was related to the degree of clinical efficacy, although this has not been replicated by all investigators (Sackeim, Decina, Portnoy, Neeley, & Malitz, 1987).

Two questions then emerge: (1) what is the mechanism of the ECT-induced anticonvulsant effects, and (2) is this mechanism related to its positive effects in the treatment of mania and depression? ECT induces a variety of acute and longer-lasting biochemical effects, which could be involved in both its psychotropic and anticonvulsant effects. It enhances catecholaminergic and indoleaminergic mechanisms and increases the mRNA and levels of a variety of brain neuropeptides, such as thyrotropin-releasing hormone (TRH), which are thought to be both endogenous anticonvulsant substances and possibly endogenous antidepressant and mood stabilizer substances as well (Chapters 9, 61, 62).

Opiate peptides are also induced and released by ECT. Studies in animals reveal that a dynorphin-like opiate peptide is released into spinal fluid after ECT seizures, such that spinal fluid of an animal that has had ECT will prevent seizures in other animals. This transferable effect can be blocked with the appropriate blockers of kappa opiate receptors (which block the effect of dynorphin, but not morphine; Tortella & Long, 1985).

ECT also induces the expression of immediate early genes (Nakajima et al., 1989) and neurotrophic factors such as brain-derived neuro-trophic factor, which has been closely linked to the effects of the unimodal antidepressants (Chapter 9). ECT's induction and production of neurotrophic and neuroprotective substances may account for the fact that seizures in patients with epilepsy normally terminate spontaneously without major neurocognitive defects.

Risk-to-Benefit Analysis in the Use of ECT in Bipolar Illness: A Focus on the Long-Term Course of Illness

Many clinicians and investigators, such as Max Fink (2001a, 2004) and Charles Kellner (2004), feel that the underuse of ECT in the treatment of refractory major depression and bipolar depression is medically irresponsible given its high degree of efficacy and general safety. We would take a more cautious approach for many of the reasons already stated and others noted below.

We agree that ECT is one of the fastest acting and most effective acute antidepressant modalities available, and thus should be used in patients with greater psychopharmacological treatment refractoriness, particularly when there is a serious risk of suicide or when there are medical contraindications to the use of pharmacological agents. It also may be life saving in instances of mania associated with malignant hyperthermia or lethal catatonia.

However, ECT's outstanding record, often stated as approximately 80% effectiveness in nonselected patients with serious major or psychotic major depression, appears to drop to approximately 50% in those with treatment-refractory recurrent major depression, as studied by Sackeim and colleagues (Prudic et al., 1996). Presumably, there would be a similar reduction in efficacy given the high degree of psychopharmacological refractoriness in patients with bipolar illness as well, and this presumption has been shown indirectly to be true in the case series of Grunhaus, Schreiber, Dolberg, Hirshman, and Dannon (2002), who saw equal effi-cacy (about 50%) in treatment-resistant unipolar and bipolar depressed patients.

An article by Prudic, Olfson, Marcus, Fuller, and Sackeim (2004) gives a more negative picture of the efficacy of ECT when used for either unipolar or bipolar depression in real clinical practice in seven hospitals in the New York City area (see Table 56.1). In this chart survey, they found only an approximate 30–47% remission rate from acute ECT treatment, and a substantial relapse rate (40%) over the next 10 days. This amounted to a rate of relapse of 4% per day after the last ECT session. By 6 months, 99 of 154 remitters had relapsed (64.3%), yielding a final total remission rate in the original 347 patients of 22.5%.

The relapse rate in this study by Prudic et al. was not related to the strength of the pharmacotherapy or whether or not continuation ECT (prophylactic ECT) was used. In those who relapsed, 44% had continuation ECT, and in non-relapsers, 49% had continuation ECT. As illustrated in Table 56.1, over the average 1 year of follow-up, a very low percentage of patients actually remained in clinical remission. These new statistics on the relatively poorer performance of ECT in real world settings, compared with what had been expected based on the previous literature, also needs to be calculated into the risk-to-benefit analysis of the use of ECT.

The Sackeim group has published a follow-up article on the degree of cognitive side effects experienced in this same patient population (Sackeim et al., 2007), as noted above. However even not considering these data about persisting problems with retrograde amnesia, the moderate initial response rates and the very rapid and high relapse rates, despite attempts at pharmacological or ECT continuation strategies, further slants the risk-to-benefit ratio for ECT toward greater risk because of this less-than-expected benefit. Moreover, the Prudic et al (2004) investigation followed up patients with both unipolar and bipolar depression receiving ECT, and in a cohort of only bipolar patients one might expect even less satisfactory long-term outcomes, based on the inherently higher relapse rate in bipolar illness compared with unipolar patients. Thus, Prudic et al.'s (2004) pessimistic figures on re-

Table 56.1 *Effectiveness of ECT in the Real World (7 hospitals in New York City): Results Do Not Match Up with Expectations (Prodic, Sackeim et al., 2004)*

Acute Response N = 347* (Intent to treat)	Completers	Relapse During 24 week follow-up	Final Remission Rates
46.7% remitted (Ham < 10)	(55.7%)	99/154 (64.3%) relapsed	22.5% (Ham < 10)
30.3% complete remission (Ham < 7)	(38.1%)	Relapse not related to strength of pharmacotherapy Continuation ECT not related to relapse Relapsers: 43.9% continuation ECT Non-relapsers: 49.0% had continuation ECT Acute relapse rate: 4% per day after last ECT	16.1% (Ham < 7)

ECT bottom line: 1) Remission rates that dissipate quickly
2) Extremely low remission rates at 6 months follow up
3) Lower ratio of benefit to risk than expected

*UP or BP

lapse may nonetheless represent an overly optimistic portrayal of the typical degree of responsivity that one might expect in bipolar illness.

How to Follow Up on an Acute Response: Which Pharmacotherapy? Assuming there is a good acute clinical response to ECT in the refractory bipolar patient with either chronic persistent depression or repeated intermittent major depressions, the question becomes: What pharmacological strategies can be used to maintain ECT-related clinical improvement for the long term? We would argue that systematic exploration of the potential efficacy of a variety of pharmacological approaches in long-term prophylaxis should be pursued in a given patient prior to resorting to ECT, if possible. In this way, an acute remission may be achieved with medication that would yield information about the most promising drug regimens for long-term prevention for that patient (to be confirmed later with more extended treatment). Most of the chapters in this book on dual and complex combination treatment indirectly address this approach and suggest that acute response is a good guide to what will work in the long term.

ECT is usually administered in the context of a drug holiday (a period of time without medications) and, in instances of loss of response to pharmacological treatment that had shown prior effectiveness (i.e., the development of tolerance), such a period of time off medications may assist in achieving a renewed period of responsiveness to the formerly effective agents. The likelihood remains, however, of another round of gradual loss of efficacy occurring in the reapplication of that previously effective regimen. Some investigators feel that ECT with its multiplicity of mechanisms may be sufficient to reset some neurochemical systems such that a patient who was nonresponsive to a previous drug regimen may become responsive to it. We are not aware of any anecdotal reports or systematic clinical literature that supports this perspective, however, other than the possible reversal of a tolerance process. Moreover, it would contradict the general theme established in the follow-up of ECT in unipolar depression that prior nonresponsivity to a given agent appeared to predict the ineffectiveness of that agent when used in the post-ECT prophylactic phase (Sackeim et al., 1990).

ECT Versus rTMS Surprisingly, as reviewed in Chapter 57, many studies have now revealed that rTMS, when administered over left prefrontal cortex at 10 Hz at 90–110% of motor threshold is as effective as ECT, at least in patients without psychotic depression. Although rTMS is not yet clinically available in the United

States, the relevant literature should be monitored to see whether ECT could be avoided with an rTMS series if and when it does become available. However, even in the instance of response to rTMS, one would have the same questions about long-term follow-up.

The long-term prophylactic efficacy of rTMS has not yet been systematically explored, and it is unclear what frequency of rTMS treatments may be required to maintain clinical improvement. If rTMS became an available clinical alternative, it is our opinion that it would be worth a try in advance of a course of intended ECT (if patient safety is not a pressing immediate issue), because of the greater convenience and decreased cost of rTMS as an outpatient procedure that does not require general anesthesia, and because problems with memory loss have not been observed.

Prophylactic ECT In the acute ECT responder with more chronic or recurrent depressions, prophylactic ECT may become a consideration (Andrade & Kurinji, 2002). It is our impression that most colleagues would essentially taper the frequency of ECT from its traditional three times per week to once or twice weekly and then attempt to spread out the seizures to once every 2 to 3 weeks to ascertain whether remission can be maintained with these longer treatment intervals.

A controlled study of the efficacy of prophylactic ECT in unipolar depression suggests that continuation ECT is not superior to pharmacotherapy with lithium and nortriptyline (Kellner et al., 2006). In both instances (maintenance ECT and lithium plus nortriptyline), only 46% maintained their improvement after 6 months of treatment. It is also disappointing that patients with bipolar depression were specifically excluded from that study, so that any inferences about prophylaxis in bipolar disorder would be indirect and tenuous.

The literature is mixed as to whether ECT can be given during an ongoing course of lithium prophylaxis, with some investigators proceeding in this fashion without stopping lithium, but most feeling that this practice is associated with increased cognitive side effects. Blunting

an ECT seizure with anticonvulsants or benzodiazepines that achieves a less effective outcome has been reported in the older literature, although anecdotal case reports suggest that ECT can be given with some mood-stabilizing anticonvulsants.

One European group has reported substantial success in maintaining patients with treatment-refractory bipolar illness on a regimen of clozapine and intermittent ECT (Kupchik et al., 2000). Clozapine has proconvulsant liabilities which, when used with ECT, would help achieve a maximally effective seizure, because each ECT treatment tends to increase the seizure threshold and make a full seizure more difficult to induce. Should levetiracetam, as discussed in Chapter 31, prove to be useful in bipolar illness, it could theoretically be used together with ECT because levetiracetam should not interfere with the ECT seizure, as it is ineffective against this traditional model of maximal electroshock in animals.

Given the panoply of new potential prophylactic therapies and combinations for bipolar patients discussed in previous chapters, one might wish to pursue a number of these pharmacological approaches prior to the use of ECT in the hope of achieving a successful remission. This strategy is full of ambiguity, however. Often a protracted series of clinical trials is required to achieve a remission, many times requiring extremely complex combination therapy as well (as illustrated in Chapters 49–55).

Finding the appropriate continuation pharmacotherapy regimen after a successful course of acute ECT is critical, but the choice is not always obvious. In one study by Sackeim, Haskett, and collaborators (2001), in those patients with unipolar depression who remitted on ECT and then were placed on placebo for follow-up, 84% relapsed over the subsequent 24 weeks, while 60% relapsed during antidepressant continuation with nortriptyline, and only 39% relapsed on the combination of lithium plus nortriptyline. Based on these data and other considerations, it would appear optimal to find a new prophylactic regimen following successful ECT rather than just returning to previously used antidepressant strategies in the hope that the ECT series would somehow enable the new level of responsivity.

ECT Versus Vagus Nerve Stimulation Another uncertainty is where to place the relative merits of vagus nerve stimulation (VNS), which has been widely used in patients with treatment-refractory seizure disorders and has been approved in the United States for treatment-refractory depression. As discussed in Chapter 58, initial studies show promise for those with treatment-refractory depression, and several investigators are pursuing the efficacy of this approach in cyclic bipolar patients. VNS has a unique time course of clinical efficacy in achieving an increased percentage of responders over the first 6 months to 1 year of treatment, rather than the more usual liability of most drugs (and ECT) showing a pattern of either steady effectiveness or a lessening of response via a tolerance process. Thus, the literature should be closely monitored to determine the eventual role of VNS in patients with treatment-refractory bipolar illness.

In the initial studies of VNS in bipolar patients (Nahas et al., 2005; Rush, Sackeim, et al., 2005), those with bipolar depression were as responsive as those with unipolar depression, and whether VNS will also modulate the manic side of the illness and prevent recurrent episodes remains to be established. Several promising case reports of VNS in bipolar disorder have been noted by others. Should VNS prove efficacious, it would also have a number of advantages over prophylactic ECT in terms of convenience, tolerability, and lack of memory loss.

Magnetic Seizure Therapy Versus ECT Magnetic seizure therapy (MST) involves many procedures similar to those used in ECT, including anesthesia and respiratory paralysis. However, the stimulation delivered to induce a full-blown seizure can be made much more focal with MST than ECT, because it is induced indirectly by rapidly oscillating magnetic fields that are not impeded by scalp and skull the way electrically induced seizures are. Initial studies of MST by Lisanby and associates (Kosel, Frick, Lisanby, Fisch, & Schlaepfer, 2003; Lisanby, Luber,

Schlaepfer, & Sackeim, 2003) indicated that it achieves clinical efficacy similar to that of ECT but with substantially less retrograde amnesia.

Based on studies in primates (Dwork et al., 2004), this improvement in amnesia is likely based on less involvement of the hippocampus with MST seizures and less induction of hippocampal dentate granule cell sprouting as assessed with Timm's stain. These investigators also measured the number of new cells produced in the CSF ventricular lining that then migrate up into the hippocampus.

As noted previously, this index of neurogenesis is increased by both lithium and the antidepressants and is also substantially increased with ECT. However, MST does not increase neurogenesis. Thus, to the extent that MST continues to show efficacy, its lack of effect on hippocampal neurogenesis would further suggest that the two phenomena are separable. It had been suggested by some investigators that antidepressant-induced neurogenesis was related to the behavioral effects of antidepressants based on the observations that when neurogenesis in antidepressant-treated animals was inhibited by X-ray, some of the behavioral responses associated with antidepressant efficacy in rodent models were inhibited (Santarelli et al., 2003). However, other investigators have found that antidepressant-induced neurogenesis is not necessary for antidepressant effects in other animal models, and these data would converge with the preliminary MST data in suggesting that neurogenesis is not directly linked to antidepressant effects.

In terms of clinical availability, ongoing efficacy and tolerability studies are being conducted with MST using a new machine that delivers very high-frequency stimulation (120 Hz); MST is not likely to become clinically available (even if it proves efficacious) until 2008 or thereafter. Therefore, in the use of physiological alternatives to drugs, one is left with different clinical modes of delivering conventional ECT at present. If right, brief-pulse high intensity UL ECT is used, the results are equal in efficacy to BL ECT at 150% of seizure threshold, and both are highly superior to the degree of efficacy achieved with 150% of seizure threshold with right UL ECT (Sackeim et al., 2000; but see McCall, Dunn, Rosenquist, & Hughes, 2002). Since the effects on memory are less problematic with right UL compared with BL ECT, it would appear that this should be the treatment of choice among current ECT techniques. One could also switch to BL treatments if the right UL treatments were not effective. The option of high-intensity brief pulse right UL ECT should at least be discussed with physicians by patients considering initiating a course of ECT, and either UL or bifrontal ultra brief pulse ECT should also be considered (Sienaert et al., 2007; Sackeim et al., 2001).

PRINCIPLES OF THE CASE	STRENGTH OF EVIDENCE
1. ECT can be as rapidly effective in bipolar depression as in unipolar depression.	+++
2. Modern ECT is medically safe, with the risk of death essentially equal to that of any other instance of anesthesia or surgery (approximately 1 in 10,000 individuals).	+++
3. ECT may be particularly indicated in instances of high suicide risk, medical necessity, or very high treatment refractoriness.	+++
4. Given the panoply of effective antimanic agents, ECT is rarely indicated for treatment of acute mania, except in instances of well-established treatment resistance or in malignant hyperthermia.	+
5. If used for mania, ECT should be given bilaterally, since right UL ECT has been reported to be ineffective in mania in one study.	++
6. Post-ECT confusion usually dissipates rapidly (1–2 hours), and retrograde amnesia typically encompasses the time period during the series of ECT treatments.	+++
7. The establishment of new memories is almost never impaired after ECT, and learning and memory may even be substantially improved with the clearing of the depression.	++
8. Reports and observations of more protracted ECT-related retrograde amnesia extending back months to years are relatively rare, but the severity of retrograde amnesia assessed after 6 months has now been found to be directly proportional to the number of bilateral treatments received (Sackeim et al., 2007).	++
9. Relapse into a depression after a successful series of ECT occurs rapidly at a rate of several percent per week such that the minority of patients remain well at 6 months (Prudic et al., 2004).	+++
10. This occurs whether or not continuation ECT is utilized.	++
11. An unresolved problem with the use of a course of ECT in bipolar illness is that it leaves one at a loss as to the best way to proceed with follow-up pharmacoprophylaxis.	++
12. Continuation or prophylactic ECT has been reported to be successfully used in some case series but not others, and it remains to be studied more systematically.	+
13. If prophylactic ECT is instituted, it is often begun with a tapering of the three times per week frequency used acutely to once per week and then a	

lengthening of intervals between ECT treatments toward a goal of one ECT treatment per month, if this is adequate for maintaining individual responsivity.   ±

14. Right UL brief pulse high-intensity (500% of seizure threshold) ECT is preferred by some investigators (Sackeim et al., 2000, 2007) and leaves one with the option of switching to BL treatments if needed because of lack of efficacy.   +

15. Others claim that supramaximal right UL ECT is equal to minimally suprathreshold BL ECT on both efficacy and memory (McCall et al., 2002).   +

16. At least five studies report equal efficacy of rTMS to ECT in patients with nonpsychotic depression, but rTMS is not currently available for general use outside of specific research protocols, and its continuation and prophylactic utility have not been assessed.   +

17. In the face of increasing duration of post-ECT confusion, one may wish to reevaluate the risk-to-benefit ratio of continuing ECT, because it could be a potential warning sign of an ensuing more profound memory loss.   ±

18. Because of systematic (Sackeim et al., 2007) and anecdotal evidence of problematic memory loss from ECT, one might alternatively consider new trials of pharmacoprophylaxis with complex combination therapy (Chapters 49–55) or a VNS implant if available in the future.   +

TAKE-HOME MESSAGE

An acute series of ECT treatments can be effective and potentially life saving in certain circumstances, but relapse in the first month is common, loss of autobiographical memory is proportional to the number of bilateral ECT, and its overall utility in continuation treatment and the long-term prophylaxis of bipolar illness remains obscure.

Part XII

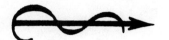

OTHER SOMATIC
TREATMENTS

57

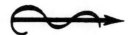

Repeated Response to 20-Hz but Not to 1-Hz Repetitive Transcranial Magnetic Stimulation

CASE HISTORY

This patient's illness onset began with a severe depressive episode requiring two hospitalizations that appeared to respond to tricyclic antidepressants (TCAs) and psychotherapy. However, upon discontinuing antidepressant prophylaxis in 1989, another major depressive episode occurred, which showed a partial response to the monoamine oxidase inhibitor phenelzine, but was associated with mood cycling; another severe depression occurred in 1991 that required hospitalization. As discussed in Chapter 37, one can only wonder whether continuation of the initial TCAs in 1989 and beyond would have prevented this and the subsequent course of recurrent major depressions.

In 1991, lithium and phenelzine continuation treatment appeared to be associated with improvement, and the patient was discharged from the hospital. Bupropion and then fluoxetine were substituted for the phenelzine, and valproate was continued with fluoxetine and augmented with T_3 and benzodiazepines as needed in much of 1991 and 1992. Despite this regimen, another severe depression emerged that was acutely responsive to ECT, but then she relapsed with another severe depression and was rehospitalized. The patient had inadequate response to two further courses of ECT (Chapter 56). While she was hospitalized at the NIMH in

1994, her depression continued, but was remarkably ameliorated with an infusion of thyrotropin-releasing hormone (TRH) in January 1994, as part of an endocrine testing protocol and as part of the intrathecal infusion paradigm (Chapters 61 and 62). However, upon further reassessing the response to TRH (after the carbamazepine trial), the patient failed to show as robust a response as initially demonstrated. During a double-blind clinical trial with the calcium channel blocker nimodipine (Chapter 32), the patient showed substantial clinical improvement, but mild depression and mood instability persisted, which was further treated with carbamazepine augmentation. Following discontinuation of nimodipine, carbamazepine alone was insufficient to hold this partial degree of improvement, and the patient began to experience more severe depressions.

This depression responded initially to repetitive transcranial magnetic stimulation (rTMS) acutely, and then with the institution of daily 20-Hz treatment the patient entered a complete remission for the first time in approximately 4 years (Figure 57.1, 1994). Given the prior response to the calcium channel blocker nimodipine and her lack of response to more traditional agents (illustrated at top of Figure 57.1), the patient was discharged on a regimen of another dihydropyridine L-type calcium channel blocker, isradipine, which is similar to nimodipine (Chap-

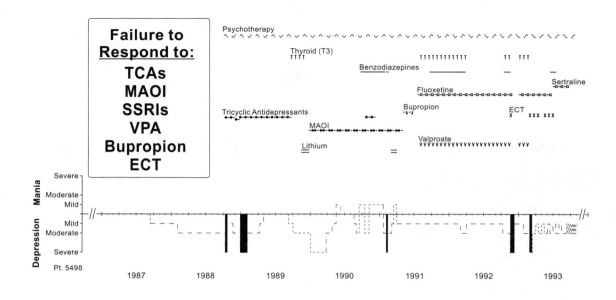

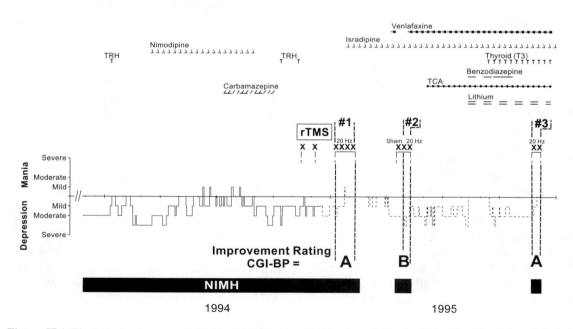

Figure 57.1 Three acute responses to 20-Hz rTMS in a treatment-refractory bipolar II female. The patient failed to respond to multiple trials with tricyclic antidepressants, monoamine oxidase inhibitors, second-generation antidepressants, mood stabilizers such as lithium and valproate, and electroconvulsive therapy prior to her NIMH admission. After admission, she did have a partial response to nimodipine but failed to respond to carbamazepine augmentation. On two occasions in 1995 and a third in 1996, the patient showed substantial improvement or remission while receiving rTMS of the brain at 20 Hz but not at 1 Hz.

ters 32 and 33), with the hope that it would provide effective prophylaxis. She did well for several months before experiencing a breakthrough depression; she was rehospitalized at the NIMH, and entered a randomized, crossover protocol comparing sham treatment versus 1-Hz versus 20-Hz rTMS.

In the 1-Hz rTMS phase (between the sham and 20-Hz phases) the patient's depression increased in severity, but with the crossover to the 20-Hz phase, a substantial improvement was again achieved (life chart depression rating improved from high moderate to mild severity). The patient was discharged on a more aggressive prophylactic regimen of the dual-targeted (norepinephrine and serotonin) antidepressant venlafaxine in addition to isradipine.

Again, her treatment regimen was not sufficient to prevent further depression of high moderate severity, even with TCA augmentation at night for sleep. Following lithium augmentation, another brief period of remission occurred, but the patient then showed breakthrough depression despite T_3 supplementation, and she returned to the NIMH. She responded to 20-Hz rTMS for the third time and was discharged on the full pharmacological regimen noted above.

In the 3 years following her third trial on rTMS, the patient continued to experience a moderate (but not complete) degree of improvement with this regimen of lithium, isradipine, venlafaxine, and T_3 augmentation with TCAs at night for sleep. The patient's responses to 20-Hz rTMS on three occasions and not to 1-Hz rTMS or sham strongly suggests the selective ability of high-frequency stimulation of the left frontal cortex to achieve an antidepressant response in this patient.

BACKGROUND LITERATURE

rTMS of the brain is a new technology borrowed from neurologists who were using it to discretely stimulate the brain over the motor cortex. Stimulation over that area induced contralateral arm or leg movements depending on the ventral or dorsal area of the motor cortex

stimulated, respectively. One is able to achieve this focality of brain stimulation because of several factors. The rapid onset and offset of magnetic fluxes generate rapidly changing magnetic fields that are not inhibited by the scalp or skull. These rapid changes are associated with the induction of electrical current perpendicular to the magnetic field which, with the use of a figure 8-shaped magnetic coil, can be relatively focal in stimulating a discrete area of the cortex and tissue several centimeters beneath it (George et al., 2003; Hallett, 1996; Pascual-Leone, Grafman, Cohen, Roth, & Hallett, 1997).

rTMS has been used to probe other brain regions; for example, when stimulation is applied over the occipital (visual) cortex, flashes of light are induced. When rTMS is used over the speech areas of frontal and temporal cortex, speech difficulties or speech arrest can be achieved using higher frequency and intensity of stimulation (George et al., 1996).

Given the extensive literature indicating that relative frontal hypometabolism often correlates with the severity of depressions (Ketter et al., 1997), George and colleagues (1995) in our group decided to move the area stimulated by rTMS to the prefrontal cortex in an effort to affect mood. Initial studies in normal volunteers demonstrated excellent tolerability of the procedure. Mild increases in happiness and decreases in sadness (on a 100-mm line rating) were reported with stimulation over the right frontal cortex, with the converse over the left frontal cortex (George et al., 1996; Pascual-Leone et al., 1996a).

However, when the same rTMS parameters were applied to depressed patients, several patients felt better when the left rather than right side was stimulated (George et al., 1995; Pascual-Leone, Rubio, Pallardo, & Catala, 1996). Thus, we proceeded to study patients with 20-Hz stimulation over the left frontal cortex for approximately 20 minutes, five times per week.

Two of the first six patients showed relatively dramatic clinical responses (including the patient reported here) and one patient did so in association with the improvement of her substantial baseline hypometabolism on positron emission tomography (PET) scan (George et al., 1995). Pascual-Leone, Rubio, et al. (1996) followed up these observations with a study in which they found responses in 11 of 17 patients given four days of 10-Hz stimulation over left frontal cortex. Interestingly, they did not see this degree of improvement with right frontal, occipital, posterior, vertex (top of head), or sham stimulation.

In a series of randomized crossover studies, we explored the different effects on mood of high (20 Hz) versus low (1 Hz) rTMS versus sham rTMS on improvement in depression. As illustrated in Figure 57.2, in two of the studies—one at 80% of motor threshold (MT) intensity and the second at 100% MT—we found that patients tended to improve on one frequency and worsen on the other during the 10 days of once-daily rTMS for 20 minutes over

the left prefrontal cortex (Kimbrell et al., 1999; Speer et al., 2000).

These data led us to speculate as to whether there could be predictors of which patients might respond best to high- versus low-frequency rTMS. Speer and colleagues (2000) observed that 20-Hz rTMS increased brain blood flow (which parallels neural activity) on PET scans, persisting for at least 48 hours after the series of 10 rTMS stimulations. Conversely, 1 Hz produced less robust but significant decrements in activity, particularly in frontal areas of the brain.

Thus, we were interested in determining whether depressed patients with low baseline neural activity in frontal cortex (the classic presentation of depression on PET scanning) would respond better to the high-frequency stimulation (which would increase brain activity) and whether those with the atypical pattern of in-

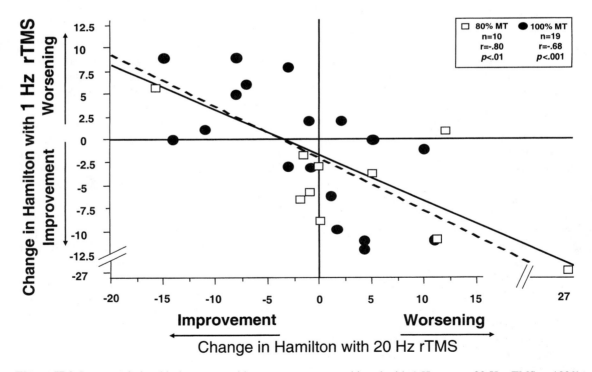

Figure 57.2 Inverse relationship between antidepressant response achieved with 1-Hz versus 20-Hz rTMS at 100% MT in each patient. Individual patients respond better to either high- or low-frequency rTMS, as illustrated by the significant negative correlation between patients' degree of improvement on high- versus low-frequency rTMS.

creased metabolism associated with their depression would do better on 1 Hz (which would decrease frontal activity). Initial exploration of this hypothesis by Kimbrell and associates (1999) suggested that this was the case when baseline PET scans were examined for degree of baseline metabolism measured with 2-deoxyglucose. In a subsequent analysis, Speer and colleagues (in press) found using PET that regional cerebral blood flow at baseline appeared to be a better predictor of rTMS response than regional metabolism.

Nonetheless, these preliminary data point to the possibility of using brain activity measured on PET scans to assist in the choice of the best frequency of rTMS for a given patient. We have also raised this conjecture on the choice of different drug treatments for depression (i.e., using carbamazepine in instances of baseline hypermetabolism, and nimodipine for hypometabolism, as discussed in Chapter 33).

In attempts to find more robust antidepressant effects with rTMS, we followed the study of 1-Hz versus 20-Hz rTMS at 80% of MT with another study of the same frequencies, but at 100% of MT (Speer et al., 2000), and most recently at 110% of MT (Speer et al., 2006), in an attempt to increase the intensity of rTMS to achieve better, more lasting effects. This approach is promising, as both high- and low-frequency rTMS at 110% MT was more effective than sham rTMS. The most consistent reports of clinical improvement in the literature appear to result from the use of intermediate frequencies of stimulation (10 Hz) over the left prefrontal cortex at moderate to high intensities between 90% and 110% of MT.

As noted in the previous Chapter, using these parameters six studies have indicated that severely depressed patients randomized to either ECT or rTMS showed approximately equal degrees of responsivity (about 60% response rates) to either treatment (Dannon et al., 2002; Grunhaus et al., 2000, 2003; Janicak et al., 2002; Pridmore et al., 2000; Schulze-Rauschenbach et al., 2005). However, in one study there was a clear superiority of ECT over rTMS for those with psychotic depression, as might be expected

(Grunhaus et al., 2000). Also, when Dr. Grunhaus crossed over rTMS nonresponders to ECT, many improved, but ECT nonresponders rarely subsequently fared well with rTMS. Eranti et al. (2007), in a 6-month study of 46 depressed patients randomized to ECT or rTMS, found that ECT was substantially more effective for the short-term treatment of depression (after 15 days of treatment).

Some investigators have reported that low-frequency stimulation over the right prefrontal cortex was also effective in the treatment of depression (Nahas, Kozel, Li, Anderson, & George, 2003). Another study reported that the distance between the scalp and the underlying brain may be an important parameter for rTMS effectiveness, and higher intensities of stimulation may be needed for those (particularly older individuals) in whom the brain is further away from the underlying scalp and skull (Kozel et al., 2000).

The anatomical location of stimulation and intensity, the number of stimulations and their wave form, and the amount of time on versus off stimulation trains all need to be further explored to ascertain the most optimal parameters that can be used safely. If high frequencies and intensities are used with rTMS, it is possible to generate a seizure, which is most clearly a major issue and one to be absolutely avoided in the application of rTMS to control subjects. Since the purposeful induction of a major motor seizure, that is, ECT, is a known treatment for severe depression, the unintended induction of a seizure in a depressed patient would not have the same adverse implications as in a normal volunteer. Around the world, almost a thousand depressed patients have been studied with rTMS, and only one or two seizures have been induced, because of the use of carefully planned safety parameters.

Although some studies have not found statistically significant improvement in the active phases of rTMS compared with sham stimulation, summaries of the literature using meta-analytic statistical techniques have indicated that there is an overall superiority of active compared with sham rTMS (Burt, Lisanby, &

Sackeim, 2002; Holtzheimer, Russo, & Avery, 2001; Kozel & George, 2002; McNamara, Ray, Arthurs, & Boniface, 2001). However, because of the ambiguities of the exact optimal parameters of rTMS and the lack of multiple large comparative studies similar to those used in drug evaluations, rTMS has not achieved wide acceptance as an efficacious treatment in the scientific literature. A large multicenter study of rTMS at 120% of MT was highly efficacious compared with placebo (Avery et al., 2006, 2007), and the machine used has been submitted for approval by the FDA.

Currently in the United States, rTMS remains an experimental antidepressant approach worthy of further exploration and study but not available to the general public. This contrasts with rTMS availability in Canada, Australia, and some European countries.

Should rTMS eventually be approved and widely available in the United States, it would obviously have a considerable range of advantages over ECT, such as not requiring anesthesia in a hospital suite, nor the induction of a seizure or the associated decrements in cognitive functioning (such as memory loss) that sometimes occur with ECT. The ability to have an rTMS session in a practitioner's office would also carry none of the stigma currently associated with ECT, despite the many modern revisions of the ECT procedure. Moreover, since the patient remains fully awake and able to converse with others during the procedure, it may be possible to enhance psychotherapeutic procedures with concurrent rTMS (Post & Speer, 2007).

One group has combined high-frequency rTMS over left prefrontal cortex with low-frequency rTMS over right prefrontal cortex, in an attempt to enhance antidepressant efficacy, with some apparent reported success (Garcia-Toro et al., 2006). Another group has preliminarily explored the possible antimanic effects of low-frequency stimulation over the prefrontal cortex (Fitzgerald, Huntsman, Gunewardene, Kulkarni, & Daskalakis, 2006) in an effort to suppress the high levels of neural activity seen in several PET studies in mania. These studies remain to be confirmed, as does the possible utility of rTMS for patients with cyclic bipolar presentations, where different frequencies of rTMS could be used in different mood phases of illness.

PRINCIPLES OF THE CASE

	STRENGTH OF EVIDENCE
1. Stopping effective medication (as in 1989, Figure 57.1, and as discussed in Chapter 13) may be associated with more difficult-to-treat relapses.	+
2. It is possible to become tolerant (lose responsiveness) to many treatments, including ECT, as appeared to happen to this patient in 1992–1993.	++
3. rTMS can work in some patients initially responsive to ECT, but is less effective in ECT nonresponders in our experience and in the literature.	++
4. Six randomized studies have shown approximately equal effectiveness of ECT and rTMS. ECT is more effective for psychotic depression and more rTMS nonresponders respond well to ECT than ECT nonresponders do to rTMS.	++
5. This patient was among the best of our rTMS responders at 80% of MT; most of our patients even at 100% of MT have had only partial responses.	++
6. Use of higher intensities (110–120% of MT) and longer duration of treatment is associated with the best response.	++
7. Some patients respond better to high- (20 Hz) compared to low-frequency (1 Hz) rTMS over left prefrontal cortex, and some show the opposite pattern.	+++

8. This differential esponse may be related to the degree of frontal cortical activation seen on PET scans. +

9. Twenty-Hz rTMS for 10 days increases blood flow (neural activity) in frontal cortex, anterior cingulate, and other areas of brain implicated in depression, whereas 1-Hz rTMS decreases frontal cortical activity; these change are observed 72 hours after the last treatment. ++

10. Depressed patients with low baseline activity of prefrontal cortex may respond better to high-frequency rTMS. ±

11. Patients with high baseline activity may do somewhat better with low-frequency rTMS. ±

12. These generalizations are not yet well documented enough to be used clinically, and rTMS is currently not available as a treatment (outside of research protocols) in the United States, but is available in Canada, Australia, and some European countries. ±

13. rTMS induces many biochemical changes in animal brains consistent with other effective antidepressant modalities including increasing BDNF. ++

14. Unlike ECT, rTMS has few cognitive side effects and does not require anesthesia nor the induction of a seizure. ++

15. Studies of long-term continuation rTMS have yet to be conducted but are clearly needed. ++

16. The optimal rTMS frequencies for depressed patients or subgroups have not yet been clearly defined. +

17. Most of the rTMS studies reporting good response rates have used 10-Hz stimulation of left prefrontal cortex at 90–120% of MT. Motor threshold is the amount of current needed to produce a thumb twitch when stimulating over the motor cortex. Stimulation over the prefrontal cortex produces no movement or acute subjective response. ++

18. This intermediate (10 Hz) rTMS frequency may be more effective than either high (20 Hz) or low (1 Hz) frequencies, which could push neural activity too strongly above or below baseline, respectively, and which could engender compensatory responses in the brain and loss of response. ±

19. When rTMS becomes widely available in the United States, a trial of rTMS prior to using ECT may be effective and has fewer side effects. ++

20. Given the current limited literature, 10-Hz rTMS may be the best frequency to try first, along with higher intensities (110–120%) of MT for longer duration of treatment (3–6 weeks). +

21. Like ECT, the nature of follow-up with rTMS procedures and/or prophylactic drug treatment (as seen in this patient) need to be further clarified. +++

TAKE-HOME MESSAGE

While not yet generally available in the United States, rTMS may ultimately be further developed and become a beneficial treatment alternative or adjunct to medications for unipolar and bipolar patients with difficult to treat depressions.

58

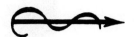

Vagus Nerve Stimulation in the Treatment of Bipolar Depression

CASE HISTORY

One patient whom we know well from a prior hospitalization later responded to vagus nerve stimulation (VNS) after failing multiple conventional and experimental approaches to the illness (Figure 58.1). He suffered from severe incapacitating depression (seven hospitalizations) and would swing dramatically into frustratingly irritable and dysfunctional hypomanias. Trials with the SSRIs (fluoxetine, sertraline, paroxetine), the SNRI venlafaxine, the MAOIs (tranylcypromine and phenelzine), lithium, and valproate were not successful.

At the NIMH he responded to neither gabapentin nor lamotrigine and wished to return home to South Carolina, where he was initially lost to follow-up. Some years later we learned from Dr. M. George that the patient was doing well and was now able to work for the first time in many years. The improvement began following VNS, and the patient had a sustained remission that lasted 1.5 years. He then had some loss of response but continued to be improved over baseline.

BACKGROUND LITERATURE

Stimulation of the vagus nerve is an approved treatment for patients with epilepsy whose seizures are inadequately treated by anticonvulsant drugs and are not candidates for curative epi-

lepsy surgery (Ben-Menachem et al., 1994). From the outset, our neurological colleagues told us that we should try VNS in affectively ill patients because they repeatedly saw that patients felt better during VNS treatment for their seizures, whether or not there was a dramatic clinical reduction in seizure frequency (Elger, Hoppe, Falkai, Rush, & Elger, 2000).

These empirical observations and a variety of theoretical rationales outlined by George and colleagues (2000) led Rush et al. (2000) to conduct an open clinical trial of VNS in patients with treatment-refractory unipolar and bipolar depression. The results were very provocative, in that not only did 40–50% of patients show evidence of a good response, but the responder rate appeared to improve over the course of the first year of treatment, and a number of patients achieved remission of their symptoms for the first time in many years. The side effects profile was relatively benign, with hoarseness and cough being prominent in an initially small percentage of patients and then dissipating in severity over the course of treatment.

These promising initial open observations led to the conduct of a double-blind, randomized trial wherein all patients were implanted, but only one-half the patients on a randomized basis received active treatment in the initial 12 weeks. Following this, all patients had active treatment. On the primary outcome measure of the Hamilton depression rating scale, there was no evidence for a significant advantage of active treat-

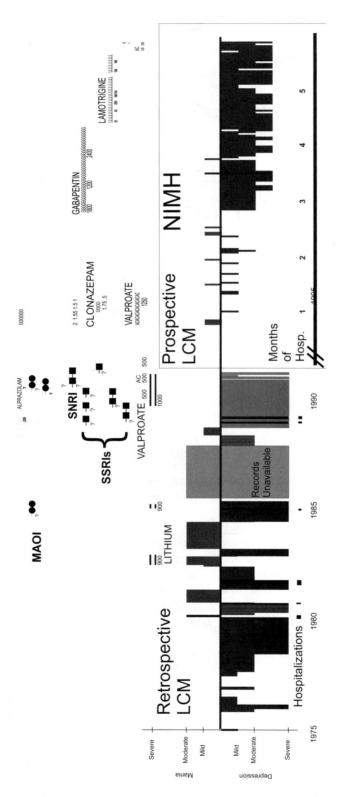

Figure 58.1 The patient was virtually continuously ill from 1980 to 1995. He had a 20-year history of incapacitating depressions requiring seven hospitalizations. He failed to respond to lithium, valproate, four SSRIs, two MAOIs, venlafaxine, benzodiazepines, gabapentin, and lamotrigine. No precise data were available from 1988 to 1991, although the patient remained ill. He continued to do poorly until a vagus nerve stimulation device was implanted, and sustained a remission for 1.5 years (not illustrated).

ment over inactive VNS (apparatus implantation), although on a secondary outcome measure of the Inventory of Depressive Symptomatology there was a significant difference (Rush, Marangell, et al., 2005).

As in the first open clinical trial, 40–50% of highly treatment-refractory patients responded to VNS (with a 50% improvement in their Hamilton depression rating scale scores) and the procedure was again well tolerated.

A group headed up by John Rush and Loren Marangell are now attempting to assess in open clinical investigations whether VNS is appropriate for those with more treatment-refractory cyclic bipolar affective disorders, although only a small number of patients have been studied to date and no clear statements can be made at this juncture.

What Is VNS and How Might It Work?

Perhaps the easiest way to conceptualize VNS is like a cardiac pacemaker with the wire leads attached to the vagus nerve in the left part of the neck instead of to the heart. The stimulating part of the device is about 3 inches in diameter and less than an inch thick and is implanted under the skin on the upper left front part of the chest just below the left clavicle. In this minor surgical procedure, the stimulating wires are then attached to the left part of the vagus nerve in the neck in order to avoid fibers in the right vagus nerve that affect cardiac induction.

The vagus nerve is not only the main sensory afferent pathway conveying messages from the stomach and internal abdominal organs to the brain, but also carries efferent messages from the brain back down to the heart and internal organs. When the vagus nerve in the neck is stimulated, many fibers that synapse in the brain stem nucleus of the tractus solitarius fire and then activity proceeds forward to a variety of forebrain anatomical sites.

In this way, VNS can modulate noradrenergic and serotonergic tone in a large area of the forebrain. It is of interest that lesions that deplete norepinephrine in the forebrain prevent the anticonvulsant effects of VNS in animal seizure models (Krahl, Clark, Smith, & Browning, 1998). In humans with refractory epilepsy, VNS appears to activate a number of forebrain structures, as seen on PET scans (Henry et al., 1998). This would theoretically be of use, particularly for the subgroup of patients who have depression associated with hypometabolism or hypoactivity in a number of forebrain structures, including the prefrontal and temporal cortices.

VNS stimulation frequency and intensity can be adjusted from outside of the body so that the stimulation is barely detectable. If a patient experiences hoarseness with the stimulation, it occurs only when the VNS is in the on mode for a second or two but not in the off mode for 5 to 10 seconds at a time. The patient is given a magnet that can turn off the stimulator completely at any time should VNS become uncomfortable.

Most of the patients implanted for refractory epilepsy and those more recently implanted for refractory depression have continued to leave the VNS apparatus in place over a considerable period of time without untoward effects. If it does not work or if it is so wished, it can be removed with a minor surgical procedure. Both this and the implantation can be performed by a neurosurgeon or a skilled head and neck surgeon with few immediate or postoperative complications.

Clinical Correlates of Response

In the first open series studied by Rush and colleagues (2000), patients were extremely treatment-refractory and had been in a depressive episode for an average of 2 years despite multiple medication treatment regimens. However, when numbers of prior clinical trials for the given depressive episode were assessed in relationship to ultimate VNS response, it was ascertained that those who had the largest number of unsuccessful prior trials within the current depressive episode were among those who showed no response to VNS at all.

None of the seven patients with seven or more trials meeting strict adequacy criteria (more like a total of 15 medication trials) responded. Therefore, in the second (controlled) study, these patients were excluded. As has also been documented by Grunhaus et al. (2002) for antidepressant response to ECT, both bipolar and unipolar depressed patients appeared to show equal degrees of responsiveness to VNS in the first open study. In general, most patients were maintained on their previously inadequately effective medications when treatment with VNS was begun. Thus, VNS has been used as an adjunctive treatment in these preliminary clinical studies in affective disorders, just as it has been used as add-on to anticonvulsants in treatment-refractory epilepsy.

In the patients with refractory epilepsy, only a relatively small percentage (20%) achieved full remission with the addition of VNS (DeGiorgio et al., 2000), and a similar percentage (17%) achieved a complete remission (as opposed to a response of 50% reduction in Hamilton depression rating scale score) with VNS for depression (Rush et al., 2000).

Implications for Future Clinical Therapeutics

VNS has been FDA approved for treatment of refractory depression. It is an interesting question where rTMS and VNS might fall in the sequential algorithm for those with treatment-refractory unipolar disorders and, ultimately, bipolar disorders as further information is gleaned about this population. Without further input from the literature, our personal current sequence would be to explore a variety of complex drug combination therapies first, as discussed in previous chapters, followed by a clinical trial of rTMS in an attempt to avoid the potential problems, costs, and side effects of ECT (Prudic et al., 2004; Sackeim et al., 2007).

In many instances we would also choose VNS over ECT, particularly in terms of evaluation of the relative risk-to-benefit ratio for long-term response. ECT has acute efficacy, but in the highly recurrent unipolar or bipolar affective disorders, relapse often requires either a new series of ECT treatments or consideration of a se-

ries of unknown pharmacological explorations in the interim in an attempt to avoid using maintenance ECT, the effectiveness and tolerability of which has not been systematically studied or proven (Prudic et al., 2002).

VNS has the convenience of not requiring new treatments other than ongoing monitoring. Thus, after initial implantation, office or hospital visits for repeated induction of ECT, including anesthesia, muscle paralysis, and ventilation, would not be required. The potential for impairment of cognitive function would also be obviated (Sackeim, Keilp, et al., 2001; Sackeim et al., 2007).

Obviously, such an approach is highly provisional and a new round of data in both acute bipolar depression and refractory cycling is eagerly awaited. Given the current lack of availability of rTMS and limited access to VNS in the United States, we encourage patients to volunteer for experimental protocols for further examining efficacy. There appears to be minimal risk with either procedure and the possibility of ultimate clinical benefit, particularly if one volunteers for a protocol that involves all subjects eventually receiving an active treatment arm.

PRINCIPLES OF THE CASE	STRENGTH OF EVIDENCE
1. VNS is currently an FDA approved adjunctive treatment for patients with refractory epilepsy, where the results are statistically positive and clinically significant but not overwhelming.	++
2. Preliminary open clinical trials in patients with highly treatment-refractory unipolar and bipolar illness reveal an approximately 50% response rate in the first 6 months to 1 year of treatment, with a smaller percentage of patients achieving remission.	++
3. With more extended treatment, several more patients became responsive or entered remission,	

thus making it one of the very few treatments in psychiatry that appears to acquire rather than lose treatment responders over time. +

4. This time course of effects makes a placebo response less likely, but it does not rule it out completely. +

5. As some anticonvulsant drugs have emerged with mood-stabilizing effects (lamotrigine, valproate, and carbamazepine), it is hoped that this newest anticonvulsant modality VNS will achieve similar positive effects in the affective disorders. ±

6. However, a number of anticonvulsant compounds have been shown not to possess acute antimanic efficacy (i.e., gabapentin, tiagabine, and topiramate), clearly indicating that all anticonvulsant modalities as a class will not necessarily have antimanic or mood-stabilizing effects. +++

7. It is of interest that the seizures of ECT exert anticonvulsant effects, but the lack of need for a seizure with the brain stimulation techniques of rTMS and VNS raises the possibility that antidepressant and perhaps mood-stabilizing effects could can be achieved without the requirement of a seizure and its potential liabilities and inconvenience. ++

TAKE-HOME MESSAGE

The patient illustrated failed a large number of routine and experimental clinical trials of medications and was incapacitated by his severe recurrent depressions. Following his volunteering for a VNS protocol in South Carolina as an experimental subject, he entered a remission that lasted about 1.5 years but then began to have some breakthrough episodes. VNS is a promising, moderately invasive treatment for difficult to treat affective disorders. Its ultimate utility in maintenance treatment of bipolar disorder remains to be better defined.

59

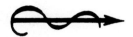

Sleep Deprivation:
A Useful Facilitator of the
Switch Out of Depression

CASE HISTORY

Patient 1

This bipolar patient had a history of severe recurrent immobilizing and incapacitating depressions unresponsive to many traditional antidepressant and mood-stabilizing modalities (Figure 59.1). When the patient was asked if he wished to stay up all night with the ward staff to see whether such a night of total sleep deprivation (SD) would trigger the end of his depressions earlier than ordinarily expected, he was initially reluctant and quizzical about the potential efficacy of such a paradoxical treatment approach. How could staying up all night improve the situation when he was already feeling extremely tired and fatigued all of the time?

After explaining to the patient that the odds were about 50–50 for a good response, he was willing to try. He showed no response the first time, at Day 20 but, surprisingly to him, felt all better and somewhat hypomanic following the next attempt. When SD was given again closer to times when his depressions would ordinarily be stopping (i.e., Days 400, 570, and 670), SD appeared to trigger the end of his depressive episode. Earlier in an episode, SD had no or only partial effects on his depressed mood.

Patient 2

The second patient suffered from recurrent disabling depressions in the context of bipolar II illness. The depressions began to take on the form of ultrarapid cycling, often accompanied by a pattern of recurrent brief depression (Figure 59.2, shaded area below baseline). Whenever this patient was near the end of his depressive episode, he responded with a dramatic remission on multiple occasions. However, when we attempted to apply the sleep deprivations repeatedly, they appeared to exacerbate the patient's mood instability, and ultradian cycling (multiple switches within a single day) became manifest.

BACKGROUND LITERATURE

Pflug and Tolle (1971) were the first to suggest that one night of SD would paradoxically improve mood in severely depressed patients. Their initial observations were greeted with skepticism until many groups around the world began to replicate these observations.

Usually, after having the most difficulty staying awake in the early hours of the morning (4–6 A.M.), patients begin to note an improve-

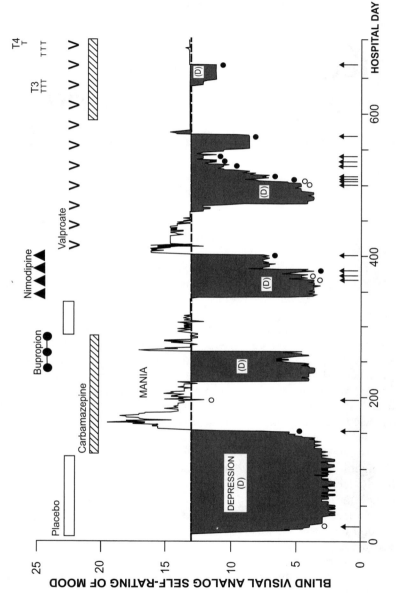

Figure 59.1 Effect of sleep deprivation in recurrent bipolar II depression: relationship to duration of episode and number of inductions. The response to sleep deprivation was robust and dramatic when applied toward the end of a bipolar depression (shaded circles: see approximately Days 150, 400, 570, and 670), but it showed little evidence of clinical effect when utilized early in an episode or prior to one starting (open circles: see approximately Days 20, 370, and 500). Each arrow and circle indicates one night of sleep deprivation. Open circles: Early in or before an episode, sleep deprivation was ineffective 6 of 6 times. Shaded circles: Late in episode, sleep deprivation was effective 10 of 10 times. (See Chapter 15 for a discussion of this patient's medication response.)

478

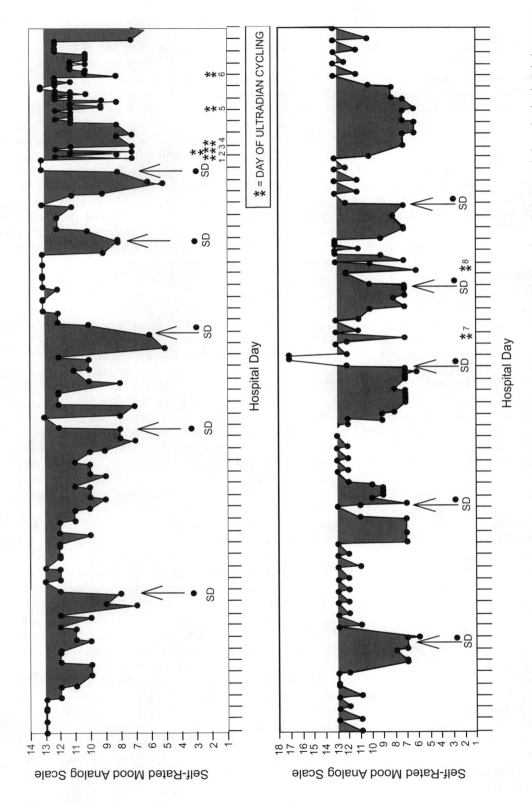

Figure 59.2 Marked antidepressant efficacy of sleep deprivation in a bipolar II patient with recurrent brief depressions: Did repeated sleep deprivations induce more ultradian cycling? A patient with a pattern of recurrent brief depressions in the context of bipolar II illness showed repeated responses to one night's total sleep deprivation (SD, see arrows), but these may have disorganized circadian rhythms and increased proneness to days with faster ultradian cycling (indicated by * for days 1 to 8).

479

ment in mood, often leading to a complete remission of their depressive symptoms over the late morning and early afternoon of the SD day. In most instances, however, a full night's recovery sleep would be associated with a return of full-blown depressive symptomatology. Baxter (1985) was the first of several other investigators to report that concurrent treatment with lithium was able to block this sleep-related relapse.

It was found that one night of SD improved mood in those with both insomnic and hypersomnic presentations of their depression, and that those with greater initial severity of depressive symptoms and the most marked circadian diurnal variation in mood were among those who responded best.

The mechanisms of SD-induced mood improvements have been studied but not clearly elucidated. One of the most consistent findings is that lack of sleep increases nighttime TSH secretion in both depressed patients and normal volunteers (likely reflecting an increased release of TRH, which is normally suppressed during sleep). A substantial number of studies have reported that the degree of improvement is related to the degree of increase in TSH experienced with the SD (Parekh et al., 1998) These observations are thus consistent with the suggestions noted in Chapters 9 and 62, that TRH may be an endogenous antidepressant substance.

In addition to lithium cotreatment, another attempt at maintaining the overnight SD-induced improvement in depressed mood has been to slowly change the patient's circadian sleep-wake cycle (Benedetti et al., 2001). After mood is improved on the SD day, it is suggested that the patient go to sleep at 5 P.M. and awaken by alarm at 1 A.M. the first night after SD, and then at 6 P.M. to 2 A.M. the next, at 7 P.M. to 3 A.M. the next, etc., until the patient achieves the usual hours of sleep (approx. 11 P.M. to 6 A.M.). How often this will sustain the SD-induced mood improvement in patients with bipolar illness is not known, but is worth a trial in those who show a good initial acute response to this manipulation.

Many have asked why a night of SD should be helpful when complaints about sleep loss and fatigue are such a prominent part of the depressive syndrome in the first place. One counterintuitive way of viewing this procedure is to suggest that the mechanisms associated with sleep loss are compensatory and associated with those in the body that are actually attempting to bring about an improvement in mood and remission of a depressive episode. In this fashion, if they can be further encouraged with a complete night of SD, this could be connected with more substantial clinical antidepressant effects. Although it is not clear whether this or other mechanistic explanations are correct, the consistency of the observations across many laboratories does suggest that the mood improvement is a meaningful phenomenon in about 50% of severely depressed patients.

It is also interesting that SD of the first half of the night is not effective, whereas that of the second half of the night (3 A.M. to 7 A.M.) is helpful. If one naps during the SD night, this is often sufficient to obscure or inhibit a positive response. Moreover, during the SD day, if one systematically studies napping after clinical mood improvement, it appears that longer naps, particularly those associated with the presence of rapid eye movement (dreaming) sleep, are the ones that are most likely to be associated with the return of depressive mood immediately after the end of the nap (Riemann, Wiegand, Lauer, & Berger, 1994).

Altogether, these data suggest the importance of sleep and wakefulness and their timing in depression and its improvement. Neurochemical and physiological mechanisms that arise during sleep may be, to some extent, depressogenic. This view would be consistent with the observations that many patients with bipolar depression have exacerbations of their mood and the most difficulty in awakening in the morning hours, even after a full night's sleep.

It is noteworthy that patients with primary anxiety disorders tend to be worse after one night's SD, which is similar to the response of normal volunteers, who also tend to feel more irritable, fuzzy-headed, and fatigued following a night of SD (Roy-Byrne, Uhde, & Post, 1986). It is also of interest that SD can be a precipitant of seizures in those with epilepsy, again suggesting another inverse relationship between seizures and mood.

The SD response appears to be state dependent in unipolar and bipolar depressed patients; mood improves when a patient is in a depressed state, but shows little change or mild worsening when the individual is in a normal (euthymic) state (i.e., see approximately Day 195 in Figure 59.1). This illustrates the principle that one cannot always extrapolate from responses in normal volunteers to those in depressed individuals, and vice versa.

Wu et al. (1992) and Ebert, Feistel, Barocka, and Kaschka (1994) found that patients with evidence of baseline limbic hyperactivity on PET or SPECT scans show better response to SD than those with a normal or hypoactive pattern.

PRINCIPLES OF THE CASE	STRENGTH OF EVIDENCE
1. Total deprivation of one night's sleep may be associated with dramatic improvement in mood the next day in those with severe depressions.	+++
2. Partial deprivation of sleep in the last half of the night (i.e., 2 A.M.–6 A.M.) appears more important than SD in the first part of the night (i.e., 11 P.M.–3 A.M.) for this mood improvement.	++
3. Sleep suppresses TRH secretion and SD increases TRH. Such an increase in TRH could be related to the antidepressant effects of SD (Chapters 61 and 62).	++
4. In some studies, the degree of increase in TRH (assessed indirectly by increases in plasma TSH) is related to the degree of improvement in mood.	+
5. SD may work more robustly and trigger the end of a depressive episode when it is applied near the end of an expected episode, as opposed to episode outset or midphase (see Figure 59.1).	+
6. Four studies document that concomitant treatment with lithium may help maintain SD-induced mood improvement and prevent relapse following a night of sleep.	+++
7. A phase change in hours of sleep following SD may also help sustain mood improvement (i.e., sleeping 6 P.M. to 1 A.M. the next night, 7 P.M. to 2 A.M. the next, 8 P.M. to 3 A.M. the next, and so on, until normal hours of sleep are achieved).	+
8. The SD improvement indicates that depressed mood can literally improve overnight, even though our effective antidepressant treatments often take weeks to become fully effective.	+++
9. While the SD procedure (± a phase change) is widely used in many European centers, it is rarely used by practitioners in the United States, and the overall clinical utility of accelerating antidepressant response is still controversial.	±

TAKE-HOME MESSAGE

One night of sleep deprivation can be associated with a rapid-onset (next-day) dramatic improvement in depressed mood in about 50% of depressed patients, and this acute response can sometimes be maintained by concurrent treatment with lithium or phase changes in the sleep-wake cycle.

Part XIII

DIETARY AND OTHER
SUPPLEMENTS

60

Omega-3 Fatty Acids in Depression Prophylaxis?

CASE HISTORY

In late 1996, this patient showed a pattern of recurrent hypomanias despite cotreatment with valproic acid, lithium, thyroid hormone, and clonazepam. A major manic episode occurred following the start of bupropion treatment, was ameliorated with olanzapine, and was followed by an extended depression. The action of gabapentin (600–900 mg/day) in 1998 appeared to partially lessen the severity of depressive recurrences. The patient chose to enter a 4-month, double-blind, placebo-controlled trial of omega-3 fatty acids.

After the blind randomized 4-month phase, which had little impact on the depressive recurrence, open omega-3 fatty acids with 6 g of eicosapentanoic acid (EPA) was initiated with apparent attenuation of the depressive severity. In 2002, only short periods of time with minimal depression occurred. The patient remained virtually well in all of 2001 (Figure 60.1, bottom line).

Thus, prior to the initiation of omega-3 fatty acids, the patient experienced substantial periods of low to high moderate depressions each year. In contrast, the first year on omega-3 fatty acids with 6 g of EPA (Figure 60.1, top right) was characterized by occasional mild depressive recurrence, and in the second year (bottom mood line), essentially complete euthymia.

BACKGROUND LITERATURE

Based on a variety of theoretical and empirical rationales, a number of studies have begun to examine the potential salutary effects of omega-3 fatty acids in recurrent unipolar and bipolar depression (Stoll and associates, 1999). Part of the rationale was suggested by Dr. Joe Hibbeln, who found a very high inverse relationship between the amount of omega-3 fatty acids in the diet and the incidence of depression, suicide, and postpartum depression across a large number of countries throughout the world (Hibbeln & Salem, 1995). Low levels of omega-3 fatty acids compared with normal controls also began to be reported in blood elements of patients with affective disorders and schizophrenia (Peet, Murphy, Shay, & Horrobin, 1998).

These findings, in conjunction with the membrane-active effects of omega-3 fatty acids, began to stimulate interest in their potential therapeutic utility. These agents also share some of the biochemical effects of the mood stabilizers lithium and valproate, such as the ability to block protein kinase C. In addition, these drugs and omega-3 fatty acids have the ability to inhibit phospholipase C and increase arachidonic acid, which have also been postulated to play a role in the therapeutic efficacy of lithium carbonate.

An initial 4-month, double-blind study of

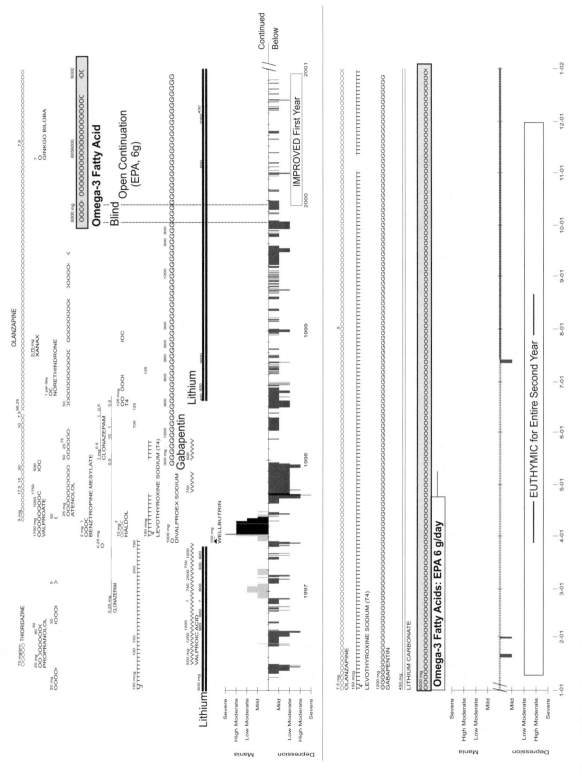

Figure 60.1 Possible sustained response to open EPA (6 g/day). In late 1996–1997, this patient had recurrent major depressions, two hypomanias, and one manic episode despite treatment with lithium, valproate, and T4. In 1997, olanzapine attenuated and prevented further manic episodes. Gabapentin, in 1998, attenuated depressive severity, but mild to moderate recurrences remained. Following open addition of omega-3 fatty acids (EPA 6 g/day), depression ratings were minimal (top right) and the patient remained virtually asymptomatic in all of 2001 (bottom line).

omega-3 fatty acids by Stoll and associates (1999) suggested that 9.6 g of a mixed product of omega-3 fatty acids (with both EPA and docosahexanoic acid, DHA) was more effective than placebo (olive oil) in preventing mood episodes in treatment-refractory bipolar patients. A small ($n = 20$) 4-week, double-blind, placebo-controlled study of 2 g of the ethyl ester of EPA (E-EPA) in patients with major depressive disorder by Nemets, Stahl, and Belmaker (2002) found highly significant benefits of the addition of E-EPA compared with placebo after 4 weeks. A larger double-blind, placebo-controlled, dose-ranging study was completed by Peet and Horrobin (2002); doses of 1, 2, or 4 g/day of E-EPA or placebo were given to 70 patients with persistent depression in addition to their usual medication. The 1 g/day E-EPA group showed a significantly better outcome than the placebo group on all three rating scales.

Six double-blind, placebo-controlled studies of omega-3 fatty acids have been conducted in patients with schizophrenia. One study was negative, but the other five were moderately to strongly positive in their assessment of the benefit of omega-3 fatty acids.

We completed a study of more than 120 patients (ages 18–65) who were randomized to 6 g of E-EPA or placebo for 4 months, followed by an 8-month open continuation phase. About half were in an acute depression and half were cycling. Preliminary analyses of the double-blind phase of this study did not suggest any overall positive results compared with placebo. However, in a post hoc analysis of the cycling patients, the younger patients did better on active EPA than placebo, while the older patients did worse on active EPA than placebo (Keck, Mintz, et al., 2006). One also needs to ascertain whether the few apparent responders in the blind continued to respond in the open phase of the study, as suggested by the isolated positive example in this case report. In regard to better effects in younger patients in the study of Keck, Mintz, et al., Nemets, Nemets, Apter, Bracha, and Belmaker (2006) reported positive effects of low-dose EPA and DHA compared with placebo in child- and adolescent-onset depression.

As illustrated in the life chart (Figure 60.1),

this patient had substantial cycling and residual depression despite multimodal treatments of her illness. When omega-3 fatty acids were started in an open fashion, the patient achieved almost a complete remission for the first time in many years.

The question remains as to whether the patient's remission was directly related to omega-3 fatty acids, was a natural course-of-illness phenomenon, or possibly merely a continuation of previously partially effective agents that gradually induced the remission. One possible explanation for the divergent findings in the literature are the initial suggestions of Horrobin and colleagues that lower doses of E-EPA in the range of 1–2 g/day may be more beneficial than higher doses, which appear to have a paradoxical effect on levels of arachidonic acid in the cell membranes of blood elements. Horrobin believes that increasing arachidonic acid in the body is crucial to the efficacy of the omega-3 fatty acids. In the dose-ranging study of 1, 2, or 4 g of E-EPA per day versus placebo in schizophrenic patients (Peet & Horrobin, 2002), the 1 and 2 g doses increased arachidonic acid levels, whereas the higher dose (4 g EPA) decreased these levels. Thus, the lack of positive effects in our latest randomized study (Keck, Mintz, et al., 2006) may be because we used too high a dose of EPA. Consistent with this view are the data of Frangou, Lewis, and McCrone (2006) where low doses 1 and 2 g EPA did not differ from each other, but were superior to placebo.

An alternative explanation has been suggested by Hibbeln. He and his colleagues conducted a study of 3 g of E-EPA in patients with schizophrenia and found no overall positive effects. However, those who had the intended increases in membrane DHA (thought to be the active endogenous component of omega-3 fatty acids) showed significant improvement over placebo. In contrast, those who did not achieve this effect of increasing DHA with the omega-3 fatty acids showed clinical worsening compared with placebo. However, when Hibbeln assayed our patients, he found no evidence of a similar relationship (Fenton, Dickerson, Boronow, Hibbeln, & Knable, 2001). Thus, while age, dose, and preexisting membrane deficits could affect response, we have no definitive evidence of the subgroups of patients who might be particularly responsive.

It is also noteworthy that a number of studies in animals, and one study in humans (Schlanger, Shinitzky, & Yam, 2002), suggest the potential efficacy of omega-3 fatty acids in seizure disorders, a finding of considerable interest in relationship to the psychotropic properties of a variety of other anticonvulsant compounds (discussed in previous chapters). In addition to omega-3 fatty acids' possible effects in affective disorders, the drug is thought to exert beneficial effects in a variety of medical syndromes, including rheumatoid arthritis and cardiovascular disease, such as myocardial infarction (heart attack) and stroke.

As the scientific field has not conclusively determined the optimal use (if any) of omega-3 fatty acids or other supplements noted in Tables 60.1 & 60.2 in the mood disorders, how should a particular physician and patient team consider the use of these agents? We give the following suggestions based on personal opinion only; these opinions are highly provisional, and patients and their doctors should check both the existing and future literature for new data and revision of these preliminary suggestions. In the Tables we have attempted to integrate the evaluation of efficacy and risk into an overall rating of utility or practicality of considering such an option. More details are given in Post (2005).

It is important to note that almost all of the positive studies in psychiatry have been reported with the use of omega-3 fatty acids as an adjunct, and consideration of using omega-3 fatty acids alone in the treatment of bipolar illness would not (at this time) appear wise. On the contrary, the use of omega-3 fatty acids or other nutraceuticals alone may lead one to avoid prescription medication approaches with known treatment efficacy.

It would appear from the literature that lower doses of pure E-EPA may be more effective than those employed in the study of Keck, Mintz, et al. (6 g). Most of the positive studies with omega-3 fatty acids used 1 or 2 g of E-EPA. Pure DHA supplementation increases blood levels of DHA; pure EPA does not con-

sistently increase DHA. Thus pure DHA may be preferable over EPA. Perhaps the best approach is using several grams per day of the more readily available mixed preparations, although Stoll et al. (1999) used 9 g/day. The course of illness over 1 to 2 months should be examined for treatment response, as in some studies it takes time for supplemental omega-3 fatty acids to change membrane composition. Use in children, adolescents, and young adults has more support in the literature than for older individuals, and may be worthy of a careful clinical trial.

More definitive studies in the scientific literature have indicated that omega-3 fatty acids are effective for cardiovascular health and perhaps in the treatment of rheumatoid arthritis. None of the studies in psychiatry or in these other medical areas revealed serious or life-threatening side effects.

Thus, the risk-to-benefit ratio of using omega-3 fatty acids would appear to be relatively favorable, as it is possible that there could be positive effects either on the affective components of the illness or on the secondary health benefits in other medical areas. Aside from the moderate cost, the inconvenience of taking a large number of gel capsules per day, and mild gastrointestinal side effects associated with these preparations in some patients, there appear to be few other major negatives to considering the use of this approach as a possible augmentation strategy.

PRINCIPLES OF THE CASE	STRENGTH OF EVIDENCE
1. Little evidence of a clinical response was noted in the double-blind phase of this patient's clinical trial. This would be consistent with this phase being a randomization to placebo, with initiation of active treatment in the open phase. However, it is also possible that the initial phase was also active treatment and that some number of months are required to show an optimal therapeutic effect.	+

Table 60.1 *Vitamins and Other Nutraceuticals in Refractory Depression*

Supplement	Doses/Day	Target	Evidence	Liabilities	Risk Rating	Utility/ Practicality
Vitamins and minerals						
Folate	2 mg (males) 1 mg (females)	Mood	+++	NK	A	I
		Birth defects	++			
		↓Homocysteine	+++			
		↓Homocysteine on VPA	?			
Ascorbate (Vitamin C)	3000 mg	Vigour, mood, DA, colds (flu)	+	NK	A	II
Vitamin D		Osteoporosis	+++	NK	A	II
Calcium		Osteoporosis	+++		A	II
Zinc	25 mg	↑Mood	±	Can deplete copper	C	IV
Zinc plus selenium	25 mg 50 mg	↓VPA alopecia	(±)		C	II
Hypercholesterolaemia						
Diet		↓Cholesterol and triglycerides	++	Rebound weight gain	A−	I
Exercise	20 min three times weekly	↓HDL and ↓LDL	+++		A	I
Statin drugs		↓Cardiovascular risk	+++	Rare liver and muscle problems	B	II
Overweight/insulin resistance						
Diet		↓Cardiovascular risk	+++	Rebound weight gain	A−	I
Exercise		Well-being	+++		A	I
Cinnamon		↑Insulin receptor sensitivity	+		A	II
Topiramate		Weight loss	+++		C	II
Zonisamide		Weight loss	++		B	II
Glucocorticoid excess						
RU-486		Mood, psychosis, cognition	+	Expense? Availability	B	IV
Ketoconazole		Mood	+	↑drug-drug interaction	C	IV
CRH antagonist		Mood, anxiety	NA	None available	NA	NA
Thyroid						
Cytomel (T$_3$)	25–37.5 μg	Mood Cognition on Li	++		B+	I
Synthroid (T$_4$)	25–100 μg	Mood	+	Long half-life	B	II
Supraphysiological (T$_4$)	300–500 μg	Refractory depression	+	Possible hyperthyroidism	D	III

CRH: Corticotropin-releasing hormone; DA: Dopamine; HDL: High-density lipoprotein; LDL: Low-density lipoprotein; NA: Not available; NK: Not known; VPA: Valproate.

Strength of evidence key: +++, Strong evidence; ++, Good evidence; +, Some evidence; ±, Positive and negative evidence; ?, Unknown; —, No evidence.

Risk Rating: As in school grades. Utility rating: I, very high; II, high; III, moderate; IV, low.

Table 60.2 *Other Nutraceuticals in Refractory Depression*

Type	Dose	Intended Effect	Evidence	Assets	Liabilities	Risk/ Benefit for BP
SAMe*	400–2400 mg/ day	Antidepressant (>20 mg/day)	+++	Few side effects Repairs liver damage ↓ Gall stones	Can induce mania Must be in blister pack to prevent oxidation	V
		Antioxidant	+++			
		Fibromyalgia (6 mg/day)	++			
*Rhodiola rosea** (Golden Root)	100 mg/day to start, ↑ to one capsule every 3–14 days to 300–900 mg	Antidepressant	±	May help Parkinsomism? Oestrogen binding (could help regress breast cancer)	Unstudied in bipolar depression Excessive stimulation Vivid dreams Mild GI upset (not with MAOI)	IV
		Focus	++			
		Exam stress	+			
		Reverse SSRI sexual dysfunction	±			
		Fibromyalgia	±			
Inositol	12–18 g	Antidepressant	(++)	↓ Cycling in animal models ↓ OCD, ↓ anxiety	Huge dose Expense	III
Choline	6 g	Antidepressant	+	Theoretical reversal of brain deficit	Expense Smell (fish)	III

*Based on overview of Richard P. Brown, M.D., in the 12th Annual Course: Advances in the Treatment of Depression, June 26 (2004) Albert Einstein College of Medicine.

BP: Bipolar depression; GI: Gastrointestinal; MAOI: Monoamine oxidase inhibitor; OCD: Obsessive-compulsive disorder; SAMe: S-adenosyl-L-methionine; SSRI: Serotonin-selective re-uptake inhibitors.

Strength of evidence key: +++, Strong evidence; ++, Good evidence; +, Some evidence; ±, Positive and negative evidence; ?, Unknown; —, No evidence.

2. This supposition would be consistent with some observations that it takes several months to reverse the low levels of omega-3 fatty acids in the cell membranes of blood elements (and presumably also neurons) following dietary adjunctive treatment. ++

3. Although this patient was one of the few who showed an outstanding apparent response to 6 g EPA, this response could just as well be a natural course-of-illness variation. ++

4. For patients considering taking omega-3 fatty acid preparations, products that have 1–2 g of pure EPA or similar or higher doses

of mixed EPA and DHA would appear to be most promising. ±

5. Younger adults (less than 35 years old) and children and adolescents may respond better than older individuals. ±

6. Omega-3 fatty acids are safe and may help with cardiovascular and joint health even in the absence of a significant effect on mood. +

7. The addition of the atypical neuroleptic olanzapine appeared associated with a better antimanic than antidepressant response, consistent with the literature. +

8. The initial period of treatment with adjunctive gabapentin ap-

peared to be associated with a diminution of both the frequency and severity of depressive episodes. This has also been documented in one placebo controlled trial (Vieta et al., 2006), and anti-anxiety effects of the drug have been confirmed in those with primary anxiety disorders.   +

9. Since alternative explanations for the improved course of illness following the institution of omega-3 fatty acids in open treatment (e.g., simply a longer duration of treatment with the olanzapine-gabapentin-lithium combination) cannot be ruled out, the real efficacy of omega-3 fatty acids in this individual cannot be more definitively established without an off-drug trial period.   ++

10. Given the benign nature of the side effects profile of omega-3 fatty acids and its potential salutary effects on cardiovascular and arthritic symptomatology, it would not appear clinically urgent that such a trial be undertaken in this individual (i.e., when things are going well, leave well enough alone).   +

11. However, if the potential for adverse side effects was moderate to high, one might want a more definitive answer. Close monitoring on a systematic mood chart such as the one illustrated may help in the decision-making process, along with the ability to rapidly restart the drug if the initial signs of a recurrence were emerging.   ++

12. Stoll indicated that freshly caught Atlantic and Pacific salmon

(which eat other fish) possess substantial amounts of omega-3 fatty acids, in contrast to those that are farm grown and fed with grain and vegetable-based food containing little of the omega-3 fatty acids thought to be valuable for their psychotropic effects. (Thus, if omega-3 fatty acids prove to be effective in bipolar illness, one might want to stick with wild salmon over farm grown.)   +

13. Arctic brown bears like to eat just the skin of the salmon because it is so full of fat, and it helps them hibernate through the winter. However, you might want to stick with the meat rather than the skin, especially if you are not planning a winter-long hibernation. EPA helps lower total cholesterol and triglycerides, however.   ++

TAKE-HOME MESSAGE

The diet of Eskimos, rich in fish containing omega-3 fatty acids, could help account for their low level of depression and suicide. Taking omega-3 fatty acid supplements may be more convenient than moving to Alaska for most individuals living in more temperate climates. Whether some doses and formulations of omega-3 fatty acids actually improve mood in the general population of patients with bipolar illness remains to be determined; 6 g EPA for 4 months in our study of 120 patients was not more significantly beneficial than placebo (despite the promising result in the patient illustrated here). Lower doses of EPA or the combination of EPA and DHA in younger individuals may be worthy of a clinical trial.

61

Acute Antidepressant Response and Tolerance to Thyrotropin-Releasing Hormone (TRH)

CASE HISTORY

The presentation of this patient's (Figure 61.1) severe depressive crises as graphed and described in Chapter 40 made his acute responsiveness to TRH administration all the more remarkable. One day following the administration of TRH, the patient repeatedly showed dramatic clinical improvement, that is, essentially complete amelioration of his depression, anxiety, and profound suicidality. Interestingly, this persisted for less than 1 day after intrathecal administration, but was more long-lasting after intravenous TRH administration. Despite attempts to sustain the patient's mood with increasingly frequent intravenous dosing schedules, the patient eventually lost responsiveness completely to TRH administered intravenously (Figure 61.1), similar to the patient illustrated in Figure 61.2, who developed tolerance to subcutaneous TRH.

BACKGROUND LITERATURE

Theoretical Implications of Acute Complete Response to TRH

This acute (24 hour) dramatic responsiveness to TRH, similar to the response to sleep deprivation (Chapter 59), indicates that depression is not inherently unresponsive within a time frame of hours to 1 day; that is, it does not always require the 2 to 3 weeks of daily drug administration that is the usual time frame for most of the currently available antidepressant treatments to work. On the contrary, response to TRH would suggest that under appropriate circumstances, depression can be ameliorated more rapidly (essentially overnight), but the critical issue is how to extend the duration of the response and prevent acute relapses. The rapid onset of response to ketamine (Zarate et al., 2006) in unipolar depression is also consistent with this view of the feasibility of an immediate response, in this instance suggesting that glutamate mechanisms are important to this time course.

There has been some success in sustaining the antidepressant response to sleep deprivation with lithium augmentation (Baxter, 1985; Szuba et al., 1994) or circadian phase changes, and other strategies deserve to be considered in an attempt to maintain the acute response to TRH administration. Dr. Mark Frye has proposed a study to determine if TRH would be able to accelerate the onset of antidepressant effect of venlafaxine faster than T_3 augmentation, and thus see whether TRH would be able to induce an acute improvement that would then bridge the time until venlafaxine began to exert its full effect (usually requiring 2 to 4 weeks or more).

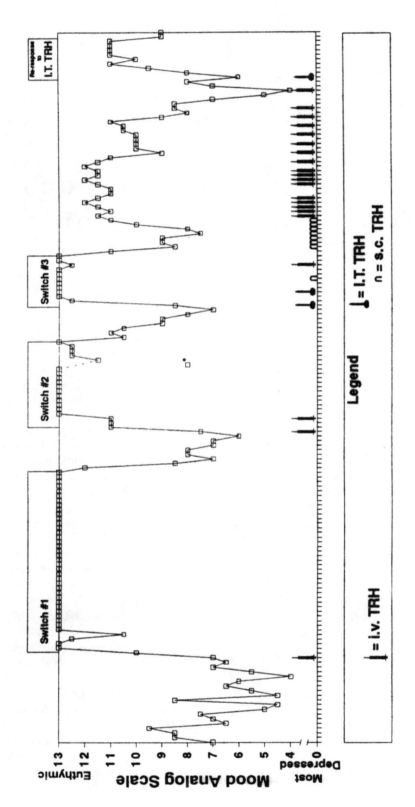

Figure 61.1 Initial TRH-induced switches out of depression with eventual tolerance: reresponse to intrathecal (I.T.) TRH. This patient's severe depression remitted following 500 μg of intravenous (i.v.) TRH (shaded syringe image) at Switch 1 and following intrathecal (I.T.) TRH (switch3). Attempts to replicate acute responses with TRH (500 μg subcutaneously ∩) were not successful, and ultimately the patient's severe depression returned despite repeated i.v. TRH. He still responded to I.T. TRH (far right) despite tolerance to the i.v. route. *Episode of viral labrynthitis.

494

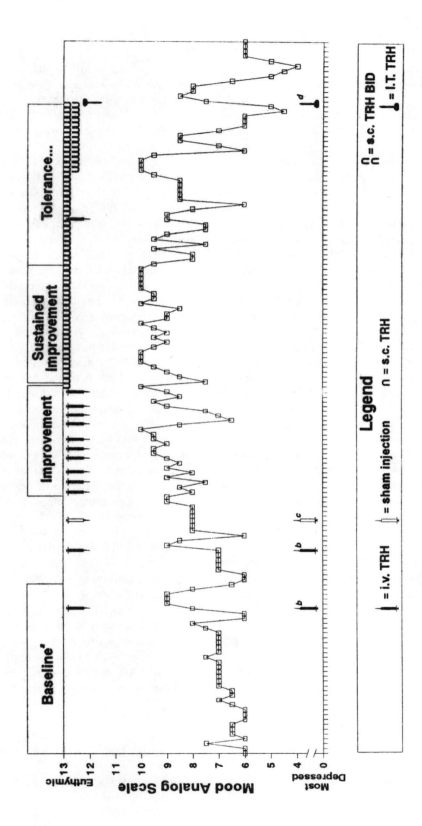

Figure 61.2 Response to repeated parenteral TRH and eventual treatment resistance: reresponse to I.T. TRH. This second patient, discussed in more detail in Chapter 62, repeatedly responded, but only partially, to 500 μg intravenous (i.v.) TRH (shaded syringes at top), but not to saline (sham injection, unshaded syringe). In contrast to the patient in Figure 61.1, she responded to and maintained her improvement on 500 μg subcutaneous (s.c.) TRH (∩ daily s.c.). However, despite doubling the dose with twice-a-day administration of s.c. TRH (top right), depression returned in a tolerance-like pattern. She also reresponded to I.T. TRH, and her improvement lasted 4 to 5 days. As repeated I.T. administration of a drug had never been attempted in psychiatry, further I.T. injections during spinal taps were not given (but see Chapter 62). [a]Inadequate response to nimodipine. [b]Acute response to i.v. TRH stim test. [c]Use of an active placebo for TRH with i.v. procaine showed no response. [d]Reresponse to I.T. TRH.

495

Reasons for Efficacy of Venlafaxine in This Individual

The fact that venlafaxine is a dual amine reuptake blocker with potent effects on both noradrenergic and serotonergic mechanisms is the likely reason that it was eventually effective in this individual (Chapter 40), when other serotonin-selective and more traditional antidepressant modalities were not. This finding is now supported by several meta-analyses in the general literature, that is, that venlafaxine can be more effective than SSRIs in the treatment of unipolar depression (Stahl et al., 2002).

It is also possible that drugs may be more likely to work at different phases of a depressive episode, as is also seen with sleep deprivation. For example, with the extremely long duration of the last depressive episode in this individual, perhaps endogenous adaptive changes that normally help patients cycle out of depression build up to the point that a drug like venlafaxine could now be effective.

We have postulated that TRH is one of a number of endogenous antidepressant substances in the brain (Chapters 9 and 10). The patient also had repeated trials with synthetic TRH given intravenously prior to the successful treatment with venlafaxine. This raises the possibility that episode-driven internal adaptive mechanisms such as increases in TRH were, in this case, supplemented by the exogenous (outside) administration of TRH and together were sufficient to achieve a therapeutic response. It is also possible that intravenous or intrathecal TRH was sufficient by itself.

Loss of Efficacy via Tolerance

The apparent loss of effectiveness via development of tolerance to multiple treatment approaches (i.e., to lithium, ECT, and TRH) in this patient perhaps deserves highlighting in relationship to the more focal discussion of this phenomenon in other chapters (12, 19, 24, 27). It is worth noting that it could be conceptualized that the patient became tolerant to prophylactic treatment with lithium (and antidepressant and

T_3 augmentation), which were maintained for both the 1991 and 1992 episodes (see Figure 40.1). In addition, it is apparent that he became tolerant to the effects of ECT and showed a complete lack of responsiveness during the second ECT series in 1993.

At the NIMH as well, we observed tolerance to the mood-elevating effects of TRH with relapses following TRH-induced remissions occurring at successively shorter intervals (Figure 61.1), finally culminating in a complete lack of responsiveness to IV TRH (Callahan et al., 1997). Some of the potential mechanisms underlying the development of tolerance are alluded to in other chapters and the potential differential treatment approaches to the illness in the face of the development of tolerance to a drug after initial responsiveness compared with drug non-responsiveness from the outset are suggested, but remain to be directly tested. It is noteworthy that while both patients in Figures 61.1 and 61.2 became tolerant to chronic TRH via the intravenous or subcutaneous route, they were still responsive when it was administered intrathecally (directly into the cerebrospinal fluid). This different rate of tolerance development as a function of a different route of internal drug administration, or different external or environmental context, has also been seen with other substances such as morphine.

One possible approach to tolerance is returning to the initially effective drug after a period of time off it (Pazzaglia & Post, 1992). We did use the principle of returning to a previously effective treatment agent when we used lithium to augment the effects of venlafaxine (Chapter 40). Since lithium had previously been effective in long-term maintenance in this patient, we and the patient remain hopeful that this new regimen will provide a much longer period of remission than he has otherwise experienced.

PRINCIPLES OF THE CASE	STRENGTH OF EVIDENCE
1. A complete lifting of even the most severely depressed mood can occur within a day (as	

seen here with TRH), or overnight, as seen with sleep deprivation (Chapter 59). +++

2. Thus, depression can theoretically be alleviated rapidly, even though our currently available antidepressant drugs and mood stabilizers often take many weeks to exert maximum effects. +++

3. These immediate-onset effects are often difficult to capture and maintain for clinical benefit, and may be associated with tolerance development (although there are ways of sustaining sleep deprivation response; Chapter 59). +

4. TRH is a cotransmitter in many serotonergic neurons in the raphe nucleus in the brain stem (Chapter 9). +++

5. This coexistence could be related to TRH's efficacy, but this has not been verified. ±

6. Substance P is also a cotransmitter in some serotonin neurons and there are unconfirmed reports that substance P antagonists exert antidepressant properties. ±

7. We postulate that TRH is an endogenous substance (natural chemical in the brain) that can exert antidepressant effects and may be part of the brain's own adaptive mechanisms for alleviating depression. +

8. Blocking the effects of a peptide such as CRH, thought to be involved in driving some of the primary pathological aspects of depression, is also a new therapeutic that is being explored by several different drug companies. +

9. In some patients, illness progression may be evident in increasing duration or severity of episodes, if not in increasing frequency (see Chapter 40). Illness progression and treatment resistance can also be evident in the eventual loss of effectiveness of treatment (tolerance) such as that which occurred with lithium, ECT, and TRH in this individual and to most treatments (see Chapter 62) in the patient in Figure 61.2. ++

10. A return to a previously effective therapy in the face of tolerance, and switching to new drugs with different mechanisms of action may be useful therapeutic approaches if tolerance develops. +

TAKE-HOME MESSAGE

In some individuals, recurrent depression can run a course of increasing illness severity and duration. However, despite this overall pattern of worsening of illness and loss of response to several treatments, continued psychopharmacological exploration can result in a complete remission. Making use of neuropeptide mechanisms (i.e., TRH agonism or CRH antagonism) may provide a new avenue to therapeutics in the future.

62

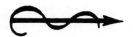

Overcoming Repeated Tolerance Development: Use of More Treatments in Combination, More Adjunctive Strategies, and a Question of the Ultimate Role of TRH

CASE HISTORY

The patient whose course of illness and treatment is shown in the life chart is a middle-aged married white female (Figure 62.1). Her hyperthymic (energetic) temperament switched to dysthymia during long-term butalbital treatment of her migraines. Major depressions began to emerge (1987–1988) with six hospitalizations in the next five years (Figure 62.1). These depressions did not adequately respond to mood stabilizers (lithium or valproate); antidepressants (desipramine, fluoxetine, bupropion, nortriptyline, or venlafaxine); benzodiazepines (temazepam, oxazepam, diazepam, lorazepam, or clonazepam); neuroleptics (trifluoperazine or thioridazine); or adjunctive estrogen and levothyroxine (T_4).

In many instances, the patient showed evidence of initial response to a variety of protocol treatments at the NIMH, only to slowly develop treatment resistance in an apparent tolerance pattern (loss of efficacy while maintaining appropriate treatment doses and blood levels) over

a period of weeks to 1–2 months (Figure 62.2). These treatments included repetitive transcranial magnetic stimulation (rTMS; 20 Hz) daily, then twice daily; thyrotropin-releasing hormone (TRH) 500 µg daily, intravenously and subcutaneously (see euthymic period in late 1994); lamotrigine; lamotrigine and bupropion; lamotrigine, bupropion, liothyronine sodium (T_3), and T_4; and lastly lamotrigine, bupropion, T_3, T_4, and TRH 500 µg in the morning.

She was readmitted in 1996 after a near-lethal suicide attempt as her depression returned during treatment with the last set of drugs noted above. In consultation with Drs. M. Szuba, A. Winokur, and M. Frye, and based on the observations of Philpot (1993), we decided to use small doses of TRH (50 µg) in the evening. With this regimen the patient's mood remained relatively stable, with only brief periods of depression for the last several years (Figure 62.3).

This case and that of Philpot (1993) are the only instances of which we are aware that suggest the possible utility of low-dose parenteral TRH as an adjunctive treatment. Essentially, the

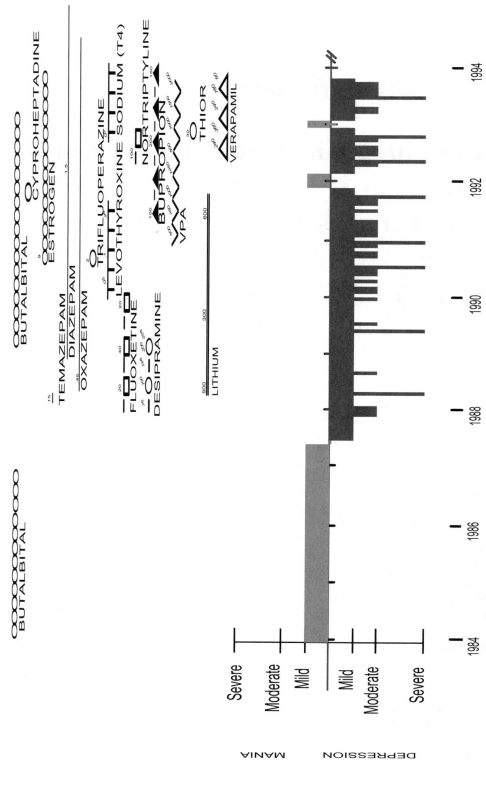

Figure 62.1 Retrospective life chart. Recurrent severe bipolar II depressions, emerging off a dysthymic baseline were highly resistant to treatment with mood stabilizers, antidepressants, benzodiazepines, antipsychotics, estrogen, and thyroid supplementation.

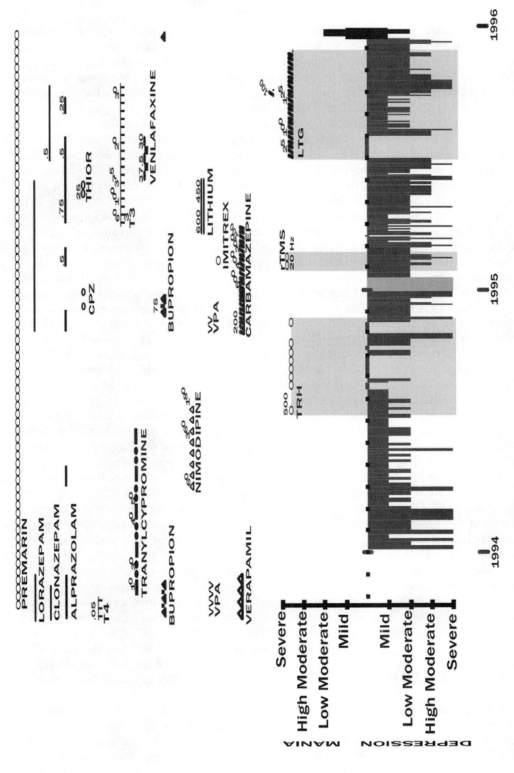

Figure 62.2 Prospective life chart. Hospital course at NIMH showed initial but unsustained responses to multiple treatments (see shading) including repeated parenteral administration of TRH (also see Figure 61.2) and the combination of lamotrigine, bupropion, T₃, T₄, and benzodiazepines.

same treatment regimen without the TRH (i.e., lamotrigine, bupropion, T_3, and T_4) was associated with a severe breakthrough depression in early 1996. It was only after two changes were made that her mood remained normal or only mildly depressed: (1) very low doses of TRH (50 μg subcutaneously) were used, and (2) these were administered at bedtime rather than in the morning (Figure 62.3).

Whether the low doses or evening doses of TRH were the critical ingredient in her sustained response remains to be more clearly delineated. Systematic double-blind clinical trials of TRH augmentation versus placebo are required to document or refute these preliminary case observations. Moreover, it also remains for further exploration to ascertain whether a positive mood response to 500 μg TRH during an endocrine challenge TRH test (as shown by this patient) is predictive of a subsequent positive long-term response to low-dose adjunctive TRH.

This case report is presented only for its academic interest and potential implications for future work and research, because TRH is not generally clinically available. This patient was able to use subcutaneous TRH because a family member was a physician. Moreover, the company making intravenous TRH in the United States transiently removed it from the market for fear of contamination in its production. Drs. A. Winokur and M. Kubek are among the few physicians in the United States who continue a major interest in TRH research, both for its direct clinical implications and also to attempt to develop a long-acting TRH preparation. Up to this point, this goal has been hampered by a lack of interest by the pharmaceutical industry, but Winokur and Kubek continue to press forward (Gary, Sevarino, Yarbrough, Prange, & Winokur, 2003; Kubek, Liang, Byrd, & Domb, 1998).

BACKGROUND LITERATURE

TRH is a hypothalamic peptide that controls the release of thyroid-stimulating hormone (TSH) from the pituitary, which then circulates through the blood and increases secretion of hormones (T_3 and T_4) from the thyroid gland in the neck.

Similar to the hypothalamic-pituitary-adrenal axis modulating cortisol production, which is overactive in approximately half of all severely depressed patients, this hypothalamic-pituitary-thyroid axis modulating thyroid hormone production is overactive in many depressed patients as well. Several studies, but not all, have reported increased TRH in the spinal fluid of depressed patients (Banki, Bissette, Arato, & Nemeroff, 1988; Loosen, 1988). When TRH is given as an endocrine stimulation test and TSH is measured in the blood, a blunted TSH response to TRH is thought to indicate downregulation of the system because of initial TRH overactivity. Thyroid hormone is often high in depression and decreases with remission.

Early work of Prange, Lara, Wilson, Alltop, and Breese (1972) using intravenous and subcutaneous TRH suggested acute antidepressant effects, but these were not always replicated in subsequent studies. One possible confounding factor is that only small amounts of TRH given by these routes reach the central nervous system, and the second is the possible development of loss of responsiveness or tolerance over time. If this latter observation is taken into consideration, many of the initial controlled studies of TRH would appear more positive than the overviews in the literature suggest.

One study even suggested antimanic effects (Huey, Janowsky, Mandell, Judd, & Pendery, 1975), raising the possibility that TRH could be an endogenous mood stabilizer substance. This possibility is further supported by the findings of TRH in animals. TRH is able to cause hyperactivity and awakening of animals from torpor or hibernation when it is given in either the cerebrospinal fluid system of the ventricles or in a discrete area of brain such as the hippocampus (but not in other brain regions; Stanton, Winokur, & Beckman, 1980). At the same time, in animals that experience baseline hyperactivity, TRH has the ability to reduce this hyperactivity toward normal.

As noted in Chapter 9, we postulated that TRH might be an endogenous anticonvulsant substance that helps terminate seizures and is important to the anticonvulsant effects of some drugs such as carbamazepine. In support of this

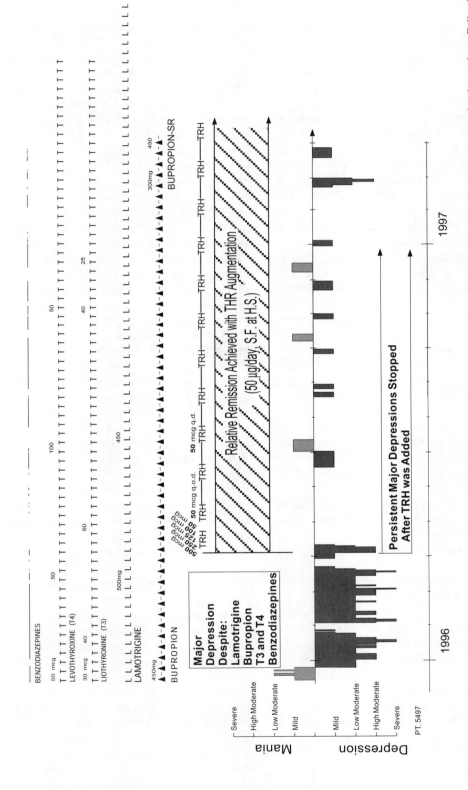

Figure 62.3 Following a near-lethal suicide attempt after hospital discharge, the patient was readmitted and continued to have recurrent major depressions. Following the addition of minute doses of TRH administered subcutaneously at bedtime, her illness moderated remarkably and she has remained relatively unimpaired for the past 10 years.

notion, when animals have become tolerant to the anticonvulsant effects of carbamazepine, the breakthrough amygdala-kindled seizures are no longer capable of increasing the messenger RNA for TRH as they usually do (Weiss et al., 1995); TRH, when administered directly to the hippocampus bilaterally, is also able to attenuate amygdala-kindled seizures (Wan, Noguera, & Weiss, 1998).

Just as we think that TRH may be an endogenous anticonvulsant substance, as revealed in the amygdala kindling model, the clinical data available suggest that it may be an endogenous antidepressant substance as well. The dramatic initial response of the patient discussed here to intravenous and subcutaneous 500-µg TRH is discussed in a paper by Callahan et al. (1997). This patient also had a robust response to TRH administered directly into the cerebrospinal fluid as compared with a sham control procedure, as reported by Marangell et al. (1997). What was noteworthy about her TRH response to TSH (500 µg intravenously or subcutaneously) was that, like many other initially effective therapeutic approaches in her treatment (rTMS, lamotrigine alone, lamotrigine plus bupropion, and lamotrigine plus several other augmentation strategies), the positive antidepressant effects could not be sustained with increasing doses and frequencies of TRH administration (Figure 61.2).

The same thing happened during her clinical trials of rTMS wherein she had an initial dramatic response over several weeks but could not sustain it with increasing frequencies of rTMS administration (including twice daily). Several studies have reported that rTMS increases the levels of TSH in blood, suggesting that it could be releasing TRH (Cohrs, Tergau, Korn, Becker, & Hajak, 2001; Szuba et al., 2001). More clearly, using positron emission tomography scan methodology in normal volunteers (Strafella, Paus, Barrett, & Dagher, 2001) shows that unilateral rTMS increases dopamine release in striatal portions of the midbrain, thought to be intimately involved in motor modulation and perhaps mood. It is also of interest that antidepressant effects of sleep deprivation may be mediated, in part, by increases in TRH secretion,

as implied by the increases in plasma TSH (Chapter 59).

This patient also had a good initial response to lamotrigine, and this drug has received considerable attention because of controlled evidence for its acute and prophylactic effects in depressive phases of bipolar illness. Lamotrigine was FDA approved in 2003 for the prevention of a depressive, mixed, or manic episode. Lamotrigine was augmented by bupropion which, interestingly, increases dopamine levels not only in the motor part of the striatum (dorsal caudate nucleus) but also in the ventral striatum (the nucleus accumbens), which is thought to be most intimately involved in mood, activity, reward, and drug self-administration. Thyroid augmentation was attempted in the hope of sustaining her initial antidepressant effects to these compounds, but was not successful.

This patient thus appears characteristic of a small group of patients who have initial good responsivity to a variety of treatments but then lose this response by the development of treatment resistance or tolerance. Loss of responsiveness has been recognized as a potential liability in a small subgroup of patients who are on long-term maintenance treatment with a variety of antidepressant and mood-stabilizing regimens, including lithium, carbamazepine, and valproate, as noted in previous chapters. The best maneuvers for preventing or reversing tolerance development have not been systematically studied, and one can glean only hints about these processes from preclinical data on anticonvulsant tolerance development and on a few case studies.

It is thought that tolerance development may be delayed by (1) using sustained moderate doses of drug rather than only the minimally effective dose, (2) using several mechanistically different drugs in combination, (3) treating the illness earlier rather than later in its development, and (4) finding other ways of reducing factors that drive the primary illness. How these findings derived from observations in the amygdala-kindling preparation (where higher stimulation intensities result in faster tolerance development and lower stimulation intensities slow tolerance) translates into clinical practice in the psychopharmacology of bipolar illness is not known.

However, one might suggest that one could reduce bipolar illness drive not only by treating and preventing episodes earlier in the course of illness and not stopping effective treatments, but also by attending to and ameliorating potentially precipitating or exacerbating life events, as discussed in Chapter 6. Moreover, avoiding or stopping alcohol and drug abuse comorbidities that could additionally exacerbate the illness and some of its basic pathophysiological mechanisms would likely equate to lowering illness drive. Use of multiple treatments in combination is also thought to reduce the development of tolerance, as discussed in Chapters 49 to 55.

PRINCIPLES OF THE CASE	STRENGTH OF EVIDENCE
1. Migraine is not an infrequent comorbidity in bipolar illness, especially BPII.	++
2. Curiously, this patient's migraines diminished when her periods of severe and sustained depression emerged and then reappeared in 1998 during a period of relative affective illness quiescence.	±
3. Although failure to respond to carbamazepine is a relative indicator of lamotrigine nonresponse (Obrocea et al., 2002), this patient showed a good initial response to lamotrigine prior to the development of tolerance. In the late 1980s and early 1990s, lithium was ineffective in preventing the progression of her illness and was also ineffective during an acute trial in 1995, yet she did show a good response to lamotrigine, suggesting that there are differential subgroups of patients responsive to lithium or lamotrigine.	+
4. TRH may be an endogenous antidepressant substance based on this and other patients' initial responsivity to intrathecal TRH and to more sustained subcutaneous administration (Figure 61.2) and, finally, a sustained response to low-dose TRH, as illustrated (Figure 62.3).	+
5. The use of different timing during the day of drug administration is sometimes helpful in approaching the circadian rhythm disturbances accompanying the illness. In this instance, it is not clear whether the evening dose of TRH was an important ingredient of the patient's response.	±
6. Similarly, it is not clear whether decreasing the dose of TRH from the usual 500 µg used in TRH endocrine testing to the 50 µg used here was important to overcoming the tolerance phenomenon.	±
7. This patient made a nearly lethal suicide attempt in 1996 when her illness reemerged through initially successful treatment with lamotrigine, bupropion, and thyroid augmentation. Such breakthrough episodes can have lethal consequences and are another reason to endorse early, long-term, full-dose prophylaxis (Chapter 35).	++
8. It is important to protect the patient from such suicidal impulses because the apparent hopelessness of an individual's situation is often colored by the severity of depression, and in this case an effective treatment regimen was, in fact, found shortly after this period of complete hopelessness.	++
9. One should be encouraged by the many case reports presented in this volume indicating that illness progression of virtually every pattern and severity can ultimately be	

either substantially improved, as in this individual, or brought into full remission.   ++

10. The importance of persisting with therapeutic optimism and aggressive treatment approaches in the face of even the most incapacitating bipolar depressions is reemphasized.   +++

11. In this patient, the use of pramipexole in 2000 was based on the fact that maximum doses of bupropion (450 mg/day) were being used. Pramipexole is a direct dopamine D_2 and D_3 agonist, which Goldberg has reported to be effective in the treatment of bipolar depression (Goldberg et al., 2004). The target dose is approximately 1 mg/day, achieved with a very slow titration in order to avoid gastrointestinal and orthostatic hypotension side effects. The average dose in the Goldberg et al. study was 1.7 mg/day.   ++

12. The importance of keeping detailed records of medication trials in this life chart or a related format is again highlighted. It helped reveal the repeated tolerance patterns, which helped lead to an entirely new therapeutic approach.   ++

13. It is only the detailed consideration of prior treatment trials that either were ineffective from the outset or resulted in gradual tolerance phenomena that allowed physicians not to replicate clinical strategies already found lack-

ing, but rather to continue to explore new potential therapeutic options that were ultimately successful.   ++

14. This patient's husband was extremely supportive throughout her many years of treatment-resistant depression and, as in many other families, played a critical role in sustaining her through these most difficult and protracted periods of relentlessly recurring depression, even prior to his participation in the TRH administration.   +++

15. Support from friends and family is often critical to recovery and can be life saving.   +

16. If TRH were not available, in an attempt to sustain acute treatment response one might try a retrial of lithium augmentation, augmentation with several trials of different atypical antipsychotics, a GABA-active drug, high-dose T_4, and vagus nerve stimulation, among a great many other options.   ±

TAKE-HOME MESSAGE

Psychopharmacological, somatic, and psychotherapeutic approaches to bipolar illness are rapidly evolving, and one should sustain a hopeful attitude even in the face of the most difficult and hopeless-seeming circumstances of episode reccurence and in this case repeated tolerance development.

Part XIV

ILLNESS COMPLICATIONS AND COMORBIDITY

63

Alcohol in Bipolar Illness

CASE HISTORY

There is an excess of problems with alcohol abuse and dependence in patients with bipolar illness compared with the general population (Frye, Altshuler, et al., 2003). As illustrated in Figure 63.1, this exceeds the general population for males by a factor of 2.5 to 3. However, what is particularly striking is the more than seven-fold increased incidence of alcohol-related problems (abuse or dependence) in women with bipolar illness compared to women in the general population. Preliminary evidence suggests that females with more than four prior depressions, as well as a history of verbal abuse, social phobia, polysubstance abuse, and a family history of alcoholism, are at increased risk for use and abuse of alcohol. These data suggest the possibility that women are initially attempting to treat their affective disorder with alcohol and related substances and that early intervention may be of particular importance to these patients, not only to better treat and prevent the depressive phases of bipolar illness, but also to reverse the potential long-lasting added neurobiological abnormalities that accompany alcohol abuse.

Bipolar men with a history of alcoholism, compared to those without, had a more frequent history of physical abuse (40% vs. 14%), a past history of a suicide attempt, and a positive family history for alcohol abuse, drug abuse, and bipolar illness (Frye, Altshuler, et al., 2003).

Given these increased risks of a second complicating illness (alcohol abuse) in addition to an already difficult one such as bipolar illness, clinicians and physicians should be particularly alert to this issue. They should directly ask all individuals, and particularly women, about their use of alcohol and related substances so that therapeutic approaches can be instituted as soon as possible.

BACKGROUND LITERATURE

Alcohol initially acts as an anxiolytic, potentially moderating generalized anxiety, social phobia, and initially even panic. However, its sole use to self-medicate these conditions is associated with a number of serious hazards and liabilities. Tolerance develops rapidly not only to the subtle euphoria of alcohol intoxication but to its anxiolytic and anticonvulsant effects as well. Alcohol acts initially as an anticonvulsant by facilitating chloride influx through the benzodiazepine-GABA-chloride ionophore and by inhibiting calcium-related influx through the receptor for the major excitatory neurotransmitter in the brain (glutamate). Thus, if a patient is attempting to self-treat a primary anxiety disorder or an affective illness with comorbid anxiety components, the initially positive effects of alcohol may rapidly be transformed to negative ones as tolerance develops.

Drinking to the point of intoxication not only becomes therapeutically inadequate for its secondary effects on mood and anxiety but has the potential to be further incapacitating in its own right and in generating a new set of clinical difficulties (Figure 63.2, bottom). When a heavy

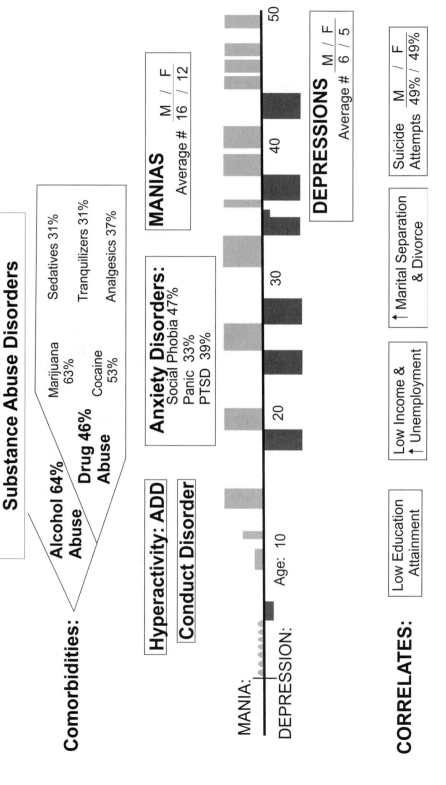

Figure 63.1 Comorbidities and their correlates in bipolar illness in epidemiological survey in the United States. Figure shows the high rates of anxiety and substance abuse comorbidities along with a hypothetical but median course of bipolar illness (based on the early studies of Kessler et al., 1996). Comorbid anxiety disorders may induce self-medication attempts with alcohol. Occasionally the causal links may be in the opposite direction, with substance abuse leading to anxiety disorder. Only 45% of bipolar patients were in any form of active treatment. ADD, attention deficit disorder.

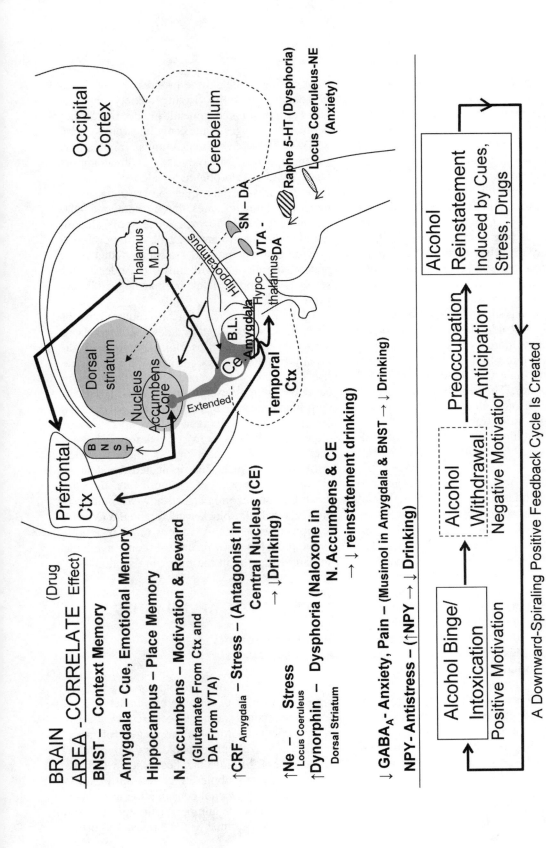

Figure 63.2 Neuroanatomy of alcohol dependence. Much preclinical work has characterized the neural and biochemical substrates (top) involved in the different phases of alcohol intoxication, withdrawal, and reinstatement and their progression via a positive feedback cycle (bottom). For the non-specialist, the general point is the complexity and multiplicity of neurochemical substances and neuroanatomical areas involved in many of the different components of the addiction process. However, many of these pathways overlap with those thought to be involved in the neurobiology of uncomplicated bipolar illness, revealing how comorbid alcohol abuse may complicate treatment. BNST, bed nucleus of the striaterminalis; Ctx, cortex; DA, dopamine; VTA, ventral tegmental area; CRF, corticotrophin releasing factor; CE, central nucleus; Ne, norepinephrine; NPY, nemopeptide Y; BL, basolateral nucleus of the amygdale; 5-HT, serotonin. After G. Koob, November 9, 2004.

drinker wakes up the next morning, he or she may begin to develop shakes and other minor symptoms of alcohol withdrawal. Binge drinkers may have more serious withdrawal reactions, with increases not only in bodily distress, but also in feelings of anxiety and panic themselves. This may, in part, help engender the vicious cycle of increasing the need for further alcohol, leading to another cycle of intoxication and withdrawal. Considerable progress has been made in understanding some of the details of the neurobiology of different components of alcohol addiction (Figure 63.2, top; Koob, 2006).

Dr. Jim Ballenger noticed that young individuals drinking even extraordinarily large amounts of alcohol did not go into full-blown delirium tremens (DTs), but older individuals who had experienced many more cycles of intoxication and withdrawal more often presented with full-blown DTs. The same was the case for alcohol withdrawal seizures. They rarely occurred even after the most serious initial intoxications and withdrawals, but after repeated bouts of intoxication and withdrawal, alcohol withdrawal-related seizures emerged with an increased frequency.

Based on these observations, Ballenger and Post (1978a) postulated the kindling theory of alcohol withdrawal episodes, suggesting that repeated episodes of alcohol withdrawal could produce progressive increases in excitability similar to those observed with direct administration of proconvulsant compounds themselves or with electrical stimulation of the amygdala, in the classic kindling model (Chapter 10). Subsequent preclinical data from a variety of laboratories and clinical observations from many investigators have basically validated the postulates of the kindling formulation (Pinel, 1980; Post, 2004c).

The laboratory studies, in particular, were able to demonstrate that repeated administration of even the same precise amounts of alcohol (achieving similar blood alcohol levels) were capable of producing increased behavioral and convulsive reactivity as a function of the number of withdrawal episodes (Gonzalez, Veatch, Ticku, & Becker, 2001; Matsumoto, Burke, Inoue, & Wilce, 2001; Ulrichsen et al., 1998). In

the kindling model, these progressive increases in neural excitability driving anxiety and seizures, are postulated to result in enduring, if not permanent, changes in the central nervous system.

These data have direct clinical implications for therapeutics. Not only is it of great importance to address problems of alcohol abuse up front and prevent the sequence of progression to more problematic states, but in someone who has already begun to experience some alcohol withdrawal symptomatology, it is important to provide pharmacological assistance—that is, to prevent the alcohol withdrawal episodes themselves with appropriate pharmacological intervention.

In the past, this has typically required use of diazepam or the high-potency anticonvulsant benzodiazepines such as clonazepam and lorazepam, but these drugs carried with them some risk for increased use and abuse. Thus, many patients' acute episodes were treated acutely with intravenous diazepam for DTs or seizures, but a less-than-systematic follow-up often left these individuals at increased risk for further severe withdrawal reactions if they resumed drinking. Preclinical data indicated that benzodiazepine treatment of withdrawals did not block the sensitization effect; however, interestingly, the calcium blocker nifedipine did (Veatch & Gonzalez, 1999). A variety of new options and approaches have recently become available and are discussed in the following section.

THERAPEUTIC APPROACHES

Treat Comorbid
Anxiety Disorders   + +

Some 40% of patients with bipolar illness carry a lifetime history of a comorbid anxiety disorder. One should attempt to directly address these anxiety disorders in the context of mood stabilization with pharmacological approaches to the illness. Lithium has been shown to have little primary anxiolytic effect and no real efficacy in reducing alcohol consumption in primary alcoholism. Thus, a number of the mood-stabilizing anticonvulsants would appear important to consider, particularly as alternatives to the benzodiazepines with their liability for misuse.

There is a very substantial although mostly European literature indicating the utility of carbamazepine for the acute management of withdrawal episodes, in both inpatient settings and long-term maintenance treatment for the accompanying anxiety and dysphoria (Agricola, Mazzarino, Urani, Gallo, & Grossi, 1982; Ballenger & Post, 1984; Myrick & Anton, 2000; Stuppaeck et al., 1992). To the extent that the sister compound of carbamazepine, oxcarbazepine, has a similar pharmacological profile, one would expect similar positive attributes of this newer and easier-to-use compound compared with carbamazepine. Given the failure of benzodiazepines to block alcohol withdrawal sensitization, one should increasingly consider alternatives such as carbamazepine.

Valproate has been reported to have efficacy in primary anxiety disorders such as panic attacks in open studies (Keck, Taylor, Tugrul, McElroy, & Bennett, 1993). A controlled study by Davis et al. (2005) documents valproate's acute antianxiety and antidepressant properties. Salloum et al. (2005) has also reported that valproate reduces alcohol use in those with bipolar disorder and comorbid alcoholism.

Some evidence suggests that gabapentin is helpful in acute alcohol withdrawal (Bozikas, Petrikis, Gamvrula, Savvidou, & Karavatos, 2002; Voris, Smith, Rao, Thorne, & Flowers, 2003), and this agent, which increases brain GABA, may be a particularly useful alternative and substitute for alcohol use in patients with affective disorders, since there is already a substantial literature on the adjunctive use of gabapentin for the refractory components of the illness.

Particularly helpful in this regard is the fact that gabapentin has few drug interactions, is easy to use, can be rapidly escalated, does not affect liver enzymes and function (which are often at risk in individuals with alcohol-related problems), and has a very wide range of tolerable therapeutic doses from several hundred milligrams at night to several thousand milligrams in divided doses per day. With gabapentin, it is important to note that doses need to be BID,

TID, or QID both because it has a relatively short half-life and because high levels of the drug can inhibit its own uptake and transport into the body. A number of the other putative mood-stabilizing anticonvulsant compounds may ultimately be shown to play a role in comorbid alcoholism similar to the compounds already mentioned. One candidate is topiramate which is not an antimanic agent, but shows efficacy in a number of comorbidities including alcohol abuse (Johnson et al., 2003, 2007).

Thus, a key principle in treating substance abuse comorbidity and other symptomatic areas emerging through ongoing therapy is to attempt to use one drug for two separate therapeutic targets. That is, choose a drug that might be helpful both as a mood stabilizer and with comorbid anxiety and related symptoms that might drive a further wish for alcohol intake. A number of the mood-stabilizing anticonvulsants noted above not only seem to fulfill these two roles but also improve sleep and symptoms of PTSD, which often can further be associated with an extremely high incidence of alcohol use and abuse.

Consider Anticraving Drugs Naltrexone and Acamprosate ++

New approaches are also currently available to potentially assist individuals in ameliorating the primary craving for alcohol should this not resolve on its own with adequate treatment of the other components of the affective disorder. The long-lasting opiate antagonist naltrexone, when administered in 50-mg doses in the morning, has been shown both to decrease subjective ratings of alcohol craving and to actually increase the number of clean urines on formal testing of outpatients in active therapeutic settings (Volpicelli et al., 1992).

What has not been systematically studied is how naltrexone would work as adjunctive therapy in patients with a primary bipolar illness, although even at this stage of initial relative ignorance in this regard, there do not appear to be any obvious clinical or theoretical contraindications. It is of interest that some investigators suggest, on the basis of case vignettes and uncontrolled observations, that naltrexone may also be of use in instances of cutting behavior and other acts of self-mutilation, as well as in other components of PTSD symptomatology.

Another pharmacological approach to the problem of alcohol craving is available in Europe and more recently in the United States as well. A substantial body of controlled investigation in Europe (16 controlled trials in 11 European countries in more than 4,500 outpatients) and more mixed results in the United States indicate that the compound acamprosate (calcium acetylhomotaurine) is more effective than placebo in reducing alcohol-related craving and actual imbibing (Mason & Ownby, 2000). This drug, like naltrexone, has relatively few side effects and may ultimately emerge as a useful adjunct in patients with bipolar illness, as well as those with primary alcohol abuse diagnoses.

Drs. Grunze and Walden in Germany, and Nolen and Kupka in the Netherlands have begun to assess the utility of acamprosate in those with concurrent alcohol problems in the context of bipolar illness. Their initial studies suggest that acamprosate may not be a primary mood stabilizer as initially hoped, and its role in the treatment of comorbid alcohol-related problems in bipolar illness are uncertain. Average doses in the European trial were 1.3 to 26 mg/day total with BID or TID dosing. Diarrhea or loose stools were the only side effects greater on acamprosate than placebo.

Positive Effects of Topiramate in Primary Alcoholism   +++

Topiramate has been reported to be highly effective in decreasing alcohol intake and craving compared with placebo in primary alcoholics (Johnson et al., 2003), and a replication study also achieved similar results (2007). Johnson et al. (2003) reported that topiramate (titrated from 25 to 300 mg/day) was markedly superior to placebo in a 12-week trial on virtually all measures of drinking behavior and alcohol craving. Given topiramate's possible positive effects on weight and in bulimia, PTSD, and cocaine abuse, as well as depressed mood in open aug-

mentation studies (Chapter 29), it is possible that topiramate will have a role in the treatment of bipolar illness comorbidities such as alcoholism and cocaine abuse, even if it is not a primary mood stabilizer in monotherapy.

Alcoholics Anonymous and Related 12-Step Programs   ++

A number of studies have documented the efficacy of systematic psychotherapeutic interventions in assisting patients to maintain themselves without alcohol. While this can sometimes be done in the context of an ongoing psychotherapeutic and pharmacotherapeutic relationship, often adjunctive use of a 12-step program such as Alcoholics Anonymous (AA) is of critical importance. This program provides additional motivation, group support, and individual access to another person who has struggled with and knows well the vicissitudes of remaining alcohol free.

One note of caution should be inserted in relationship to the issue of using AA in the context of other treatments for bipolar illness. While some groups are particularly enlightened about the use of ancillary medications for primary treatment of underlying medical and psychiatric disorders, there are still some groups within the AA framework who believe that any substance (including psychopharmacological agents) should be avoided. Thus, patients who do go to AA should be queried as to whether the group is pressuring them to stop taking medication and if they are, given appropriate instructions to circumvent that. Alcohol-related treatment should not place the bipolar patient at increased risk for relapse because of misguided AA-suggested alterations or cessation of the primary pharmacological approaches to the affective disorders.

Primary and Secondary Prevention   +

The adolescent with an initial diagnosis of bipolar illness should be given some early alerts about alcohol and substance abuse as part of their overall education about the course and treatment of bipolar illness. To the extent that specific approaches aimed at primary prevention can be instituted and are successful, it would be of great importance to the individual (who is already at high risk for a difficult outcome from an affective disorder) to be able to avoid another set of problems for which they are also at high risk.

Facing this problem may be particularly difficult for the adolescent and young adult for whom alcohol use appears to be increasingly viewed as a rite of passage, and on some college campuses drinking to intoxication and stupor is sanctioned or even applauded. Role-playing the type of responses that can be utilized when others are tempting the patient with alcohol and other substances may be particularly helpful in the depressive and euthymic phases of the illness.

Concurrent excellent treatment of the manic phase of the illness may also be of critical importance in this regard, to avoid the level of illness severity associated with poor judgment and an inability to recognize adverse consequences of one's actions. A specialized treatment setting wherein a variety of techniques are available, including the ability to routinely test for substances in bodily fluids, may at times be indicated.

PRINCIPLES OF THE CASE

STRENGTH OF EVIDENCE

1. Compared with their gender in the general population, women rather than men with bipolar illness are at increased risk for alcohol abuse (sevenfold greater incidence for women; threefold for men).   ++

2. Women may be self-treating their anxiety and depression, and these problems should be targeted earlier and more specifically with pharmacotherapy.   +

3. Alcohol may initially alleviate anxiety and social phobia, but with tolerance and dependence can backfire, increase depression, and deplete serotonin (which is already deficient in the illness).   +

4. Repeated bouts of ethanol intoxication and withdrawal can sensitize behavioral, neurochemical, and electrophysiological aspects of withdrawal.   +++

5. Treatment with benzodiazepines does not block this sensitization; treatment with the calcium channel blocker nifedipine, however, does.   +++

6. Alcohol use and abuse is easy to slide into, but very difficult to get out of.   +++

7. Therapy, 12-step, or a related program is a must for many.   ++

8. Ask women about substance use and treat their anxiety and depression symptoms early and aggressively.   +++

9. Engage adolescents with bipolar illness in education and primary substance abuse prevention programs.   ++

10. Carbamazepine and valproate help in alcohol withdrawal but should be used cautiously or avoided in those with liver damage.   ++

11. Depression in those with a prior history of alcoholism may be particularly responsive to carbamazepine.   +

12. Gabapentin is a possible substitute for benzodiazepines and will not affect the liver (because it is excreted by the kidneys).   ++

13. Topiramate (titrated to 300 mg) helps with alcohol craving and abstinence significantly more than placebo in both early- and late-onset alcoholism.   +++

14. Naltrexone is approved for alcohol craving in conjunction with therapy in primary alcoholism, but it has not been studied in bipolar illness with comorbid alcoholism. Its effects are greatest in those with early onset and a positive family history of alcoholism.   +

15. Acamprosate is available and well studied in Europe (but less so in the United States)

for helping with primary alcohol abstinence when used in conjunction with an active therapy program. How well it would work in those with bipolar illness is much less certain.   +

TAKE-HOME MESSAGE

Watch out for self-treatment of affective illness and anxiety syndromes with alcohol, especially in women; although alcohol may help a little initially, its effects are not sustained, and may make mood and anxiety worse. One should develop substance abuse preventive programs for adolescents with bipolar illness.

64

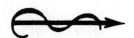

Cocaine and Related Psychomotor Stimulants in Bipolar Illness

CASE HISTORY

This patient had only isolated, intermittent episodes of mild depression and hypomania prior to 2000. At that time he took a trip to Columbia and began to cycle more rapidly and continuously, and the amplitude of manias and depressions increased considerably (Figure 64.1). Initially, this appeared to be the spontaneous course of his untreated bipolar illness, but the patient eventually reported that this occurred during substantial use of cocaine. Lithium may have helped avoid the full-blown manic episode in 2003, but others occurred despite lithium.

Although one can only speculate about the precise role that comorbid cocaine use played in this exacerbation of a previously mild mood disorder, there was a clear temporal coincidence of cocaine use and more regular and severe cycling. The patient attempted to decrease his cocaine use, but was initially unable to do so.

BACKGROUND LITERATURE

Bipolar illness is associated with more psychiatric comorbidities than all other major psychiatric illnesses, with the possible exception of PTSD. Across a wide range of epidemiological and clinical samples, the incidence of comorbid substance abuse typically ranges from 30% to 60% in patients with bipolar illness (Kessler et al., 1996; Regier et al., 1990). A substantial amount of this abuse involves alcohol and marijuana, but psychomotor stimulants are the next most widely abused drug category.

In the majority of instances, it appears that psychomotor stimulant use and abuse begins after the onset of an affective disorder. The sequence suggests that patients are, in part, attempting to enhance their manic euphoria or moderate their depression, fatigue, or anhedonia with the stimulant. However, only approximately one third of patients with major depressive disorders will have a positive or mood-elevating response to psychomotor stimulant administration with either amphetamine or cocaine (Post, 1975). Other individuals find that stimulant-induced activation engenders anxiety, dysphoria, tearfulness, irritability, and mood lability, and, in a few cases, panic attacks (Chapter 42).

In the depressive phase of bipolar illness, particularly with morning psychomotor retardation and an inability to focus and get motivated, psychomotor stimulants are sometimes used by physicians as an adjunctive treatment to other agents, while awaiting more robust primary antidepressant effects from the other medications. When stimulants are used by the patient, they may be associated with transient clinical improvement, but often there is rapid tolerance (tachyphylaxis) or slowly developing tolerance to the positive mood-elevating effects of the stimulants, while concurrently, the negative aspects such as dysphoric activation, anxiety, and irritability become more prominent.

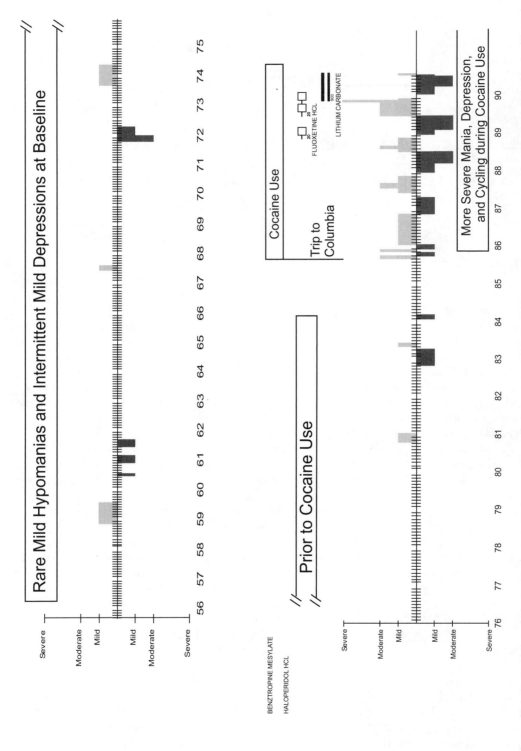

Figure 64.1 Comorbidity of bipolar illness and cocaine use. The patient showed a dramatic shift to a more severe pattern of manic and cyclic bipolar illness in 2000. He later revealed that this occurred following a trip to Colombia where he was able to acquire a considerable amount of cocaine that he continued to use thereafter. This patient illustrates that abuse of psychomotor stimulants (e.g., cocaine, amphetamine, methylphenidate) can exacerbate and complicate the course of bipolar illness.

Stimulant use can also occur in the hypomanic or manic phases of the illness in an effort to sustain and enhance it. Hypomania is often associated with poor judgment and an inability to anticipate negative consequences of actions, aspects that often draw the patient to individuals and places where drugs of abuse are readily available. Initial responses may, again, be highly positive and euphorigenic, but with chronic use and dose escalation, this process tends to be associated with more anxious and dysphoric components. In some individuals, this can progress to the development of transient paranoia or full-blown paranoid psychosis that can closely mimic psychotic mania or an acute schizophreniform reaction (Post, 1975).

These transitions from positive to negative effects with chronic use and dose escalation make cocaine particularly problematic because initial effects may appear pleasant and benign, but only later do the adverse aspects become more apparent. Animal studies reveal that even when the same dose is administered repeatedly in the same environmental context, increasing behavioral effects (motor hyperactivity and repetitive movements or stereotypy) are observed (Post, 1977).

This increasing response to the same dose over time is called stimulant-induced behavioral sensitization, that is, the opposite of tolerance, whereby effects lessen over time. The stimulants may possess the worst of both worlds, with tolerance developing to the euphorigenic components of the stimulants and sensitization occurring to some of the more adverse aspects such as dysphoria, anxiety, panic attacks, and paranoia.

These aspects can be problematic enough in their own right, but a variety of studies also indicate that cocaine sensitization can show cross-sensitization to stress (Antelman, Eichler, Black, & Kocan, 1980; Kalivas & Duffy, 1989). Some repeated stressors can also show sensitization, and stress can exacerbate cocaine effects. These preclinical data also suggest that not only will cocaine use make patients more vulnerable to some stressors, but that stressors can also repreciptate stimulant abuse in those who have been abstinent. Thus, there is the potential for a vi-

cious cycle effect whereby stress and affective illness-related variables exacerbate stimulant abuse problems and vice versa. Many of these alterations could be associated with cocaine and stress-related changes in BDNF in the nucleus accumbens and hippocampus as discussed in Chapter 10.

There are now overwhelming data from animals and humans that cocaine use and abuse can cause changes in gene expression that lead to long-term if not permanent deleterious neurobiological adaptations (Post & Weiss, 1997). For example, in both animals and humans, chronic cocaine use is associated with an increase in dynorphin mRNA and peptide levels, as well as increases in dynorphin receptors (Figure 64.2). Dynorphin is one of the opiate peptides in the brain. However, in contrast to the opiate peptide beta-endorphin, which is associated with euphoria, dynorphin administration to humans is associated with dysphoria and psychosis. The upregulation of dynorphin levels and receptors in the striatum following chronic cocaine use could thus represent one mechanism for the late occurrence of dysphoric and psychotomimetic effects of cocaine (Figure 64.2).

Other long-term adaptations with chronic cocaine administration appear to occur in the dopamine cell bodies in the ventral-tegmental area as well as the nerve endings in the striatum, which appear to release more dopamine. BDNF increases in this dopamine pathway with both cocaine and defeat stress, and the BDNF changes are essential to the occurrence of both cocaine sensitization and defeat-related behavior in rodents (Berton et al., 2006). There are also alterations in glutamate tone at several sites, and in the prefrontal cortex this alteration is associated with relative hypometabolism that can be seen in cocaine users on PET scans. The degree of frontal hypometabolism correlates with the severity of depression reported by former users of cocaine. Since endogenous depression is already associated with hypometabolism of the frontal cortex, this cocaine-related alteration could provide for additive effects on this regional pathology and further exacerbate the depressive condition, as is suggested by the illness course in the patient illustrated here.

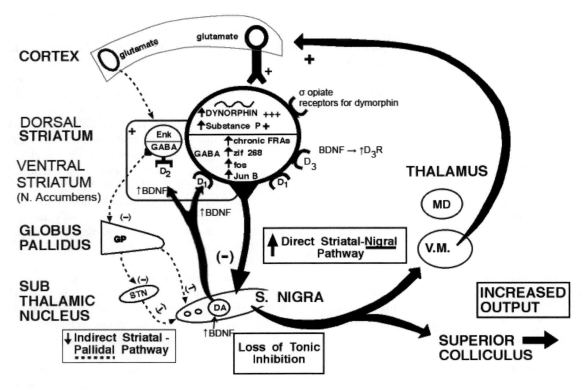

Figure 64.2 Cocaine reprograms the genetic machinery of the direct striatal output pathway, increasing manic severity and dysphoria. Cocaine causes animals to be more active in response to the same dose in the same environment
(called behavioral sensitization). This response is based on increased neural activity in the NA (nucleus accumbens)
dopamine pathway along with increases in BDNF as well as in the return pathway or the direct striatal-nigral
pathway. Chronic cocaine use also increases dynorphin levels in animals and humans, which could account for the
increasing dysphoria. Because chronic cocaine also increases the number of dynorphin (sigma opiate) receptors, and
dynorphin produces psychosis and dysphoria in humans, it is easy to see why the initial euphoric effects may become
much more unpleasant over time.

Because the frontal cortex also inhibits activity in the amygdala, cocaine further worsens the
problem of frontal hypofunction associated with
limbic (amygdala) hyperactivation. Female animals sensitize twice as readily to cocaine as
males. This may in part contribute to the difficulties some female users have in stopping cocaine use while pregnant. If in utero exposure
to cocaine were to occur, it could lead to potentially sequential and additive further adverse
outcomes, as schematized in Figure 64.3. Such
a potential downward-spiraling cascade of adversities again reemphasizes the importance of
primary prevention and absolute avoidance of

cocaine and related stimulants in already vulnerable individuals with affective disorders.
Myelination of neurons by glial cells increases in the adult brain until and beyond the
fourth decade of life. In long-term cocaine abus-
ers, this increased myelination fails to occur
(Bartzokis et al., 2002), suggesting further neural substrates for cocaine-induced dysfunction
that may be pertinent to the affective disorders
at the level of glial deficiency (glia are the
source of the myelin sheath that protects neurons). Bipolar illness in the absence of stimulant
use is already associated with deficits in neuronal and glial numbers and activity (Rajkow-

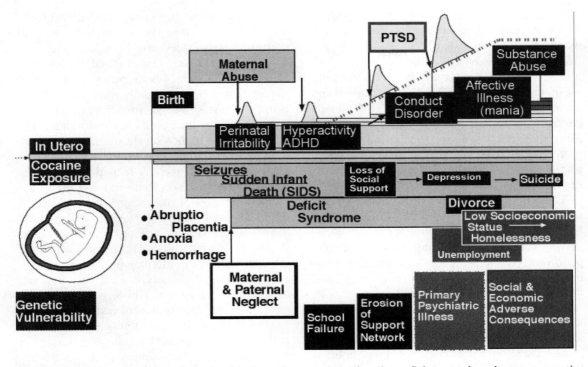

Figure 64.3 Nonhereditary transgenerational impact of maternal cocaine abuse. Substance abuse has some genetic components, but many of the effects of cocaine use can be environmentally transmitted across generations if the pregnant mother exposes the fetus to cocaine in utero (Yan et al., 2004). Such exposed infants have more birth and perinatal medical complications. Behavioral sensitization generated in utero may be compounded by maternal neglect and abuse if the addicted mother continues to use cocaine during the child's infancy. Cocaine also cross-sensitizes to stress, putting the infant at further risk for PTSD or affective illness, with many progressive and unfolding negative consequences, including loss of social supports, school failure, and ultimate adoption of alcohol and substance abuse patterns. Conversely, cross-fostering studies in rodents indicate that many presumably genetically transmitted traits not only can be ameliorated by different parental rearing behaviors, but also the positive characteristics can then be transmitted to the next generation as well.

ska, 2000, Post et al., 2003), data which also suggest that cocaine-induced neural and glial deficits could interact and be additive with those of the primary illness.

Another type of pathological process that can occur with repeated cocaine administration is pharmacological kindling (Chapter 42). For example, in electrical kindling of the brain, repeated once-daily stimulation of the amygdala for just 1 second will evoke increasing electrophysiological responses and behavioral abnormalities, culminating in the occurrence of full-blown seizures in response to a stimulation that was previously subthreshold (Goddard, McIntyre, & Leech, 1969). With enough electrically

kindled stimulations, spontaneous seizures may begin to occur.

The local anesthetic property of cocaine, which is approximately equal to that of the local anesthetic lidocaine, is capable of causing kindling-like progression of both abnormal behaviors and, ultimately, full-blown seizures. With repeated lidocaine administration in animals, we have also observed the same progressive responsivity to the same dose over time. A given dose that is previously subconvulsant will come to evoke seizures, and with enough induced seizures, spontaneous seizures also occur in the absence of drug administration (Post, Kopanda, & Lee, 1975).

In contrast to lidocaine-induced seizures, which are relatively well tolerated by the majority of laboratory animals (rats) even for long periods of time, cocaine-induced seizures are highly lethal in animals and humans. Virtually all of the rodents die after the first or second cocaine-induced kindled seizure. The famous basketball star Len Bias of the University of Maryland, celebrating being drafted into the professional ranks by the Boston Celtics, had a single cocaine-related seizure and died almost immediately.

Thus, in addition to the problematic aspects of the stimulant components of cocaine, which lead to behavioral sensitization, cross-sensitization to stress, and increasing amounts of dysphoria and paranoia, the local anesthetic components of cocaine may produce an increased likelihood for panic attacks and seizures with repeated use. It is not clear which individuals who experiment with cocaine will become addicted and which will be able to put the drug aside. Therefore, avoidance of this problem from the outset would appear to be the best policy.

Inasmuch as adolescents in general are already at a high risk for experimenting with drugs of abuse, the even higher risk of such experimentation in association with the diagnosis of bipolar illness (a sevenfold increase; Wilens et al., 2004) should lead to attempts at primary prevention of substance abuse in any adolescent diagnosed with bipolar disorder. Education about the risks of cocaine abuse, several of which are enumerated above, is certainly in order. More specific psychotherapeutic approaches to drug avoidance may be appropriate as well. This approach could involve role playing about how to say no to a "friend" offering a free smoke of marijuana or a hit of cocaine and then teasing the youngster who is trying to say no. This might be a difficult enough interpersonal interaction for a healthy adolescent but likely even more problematic for someone with bipolar disorder already struggling with issues of self-esteem in depression, poor judgment in mania, and wanting closer friendships in any phase of the illness.

There is overwhelming evidence from animal studies and some supporting clinical evidence that those who have had particularly stressful early life experiences may be at increased risk for substance abuse. For example, in neonatal rat pups, a single 24-hour period of maternal deprivation or repeated daily maternal deprivation for 3 hours (but not for 15 minutes) in the first 10 days of life results in these animals not only showing higher levels of the stress hormone corticosterone (the rat equivalent of human cortisol) and anxiety-related behaviors as adults, but also makes them more prone to the adoption of alcohol and cocaine self-administration compared with littermate controls (Huot, Thrivikraman, Meaney, & Plotsky, 2001; Meaney, Brake, & Gratton, 2002). The animals who were not stressed early in life may press a lever to receive cocaine (or alcohol) on a few occasions and then stop, but those with a history of early stress go on to a full-blown alcohol addiction or nonstop cocaine use. If access to cocaine is not limited (by either removing the lever or lowering the dose of cocaine), many animals will self-administer cocaine continuously until it kills them.

Perhaps, in some parallels to these experimental observations that have been replicated in many laboratories, we found that bipolar patients who have experienced extremely traumatic events in childhood (i.e., physical and sexual abuse) were significantly more likely to have a history of prior or current substance abuse compared with bipolar patients without such early traumas (Leverich, Perez, Luckenbaugh, & Post, 2002; Leverich & Post, 2006). Significantly more of these individuals had also made medically serious suicide attempts prior to study entry. Therefore, it would appear to be highly prudent to have a heightened awareness of the potential for an increased incidence of substance abuse in adolescents and adults with bipolar illness in general. In particular, special attention should be paid to the subgroup who have also experienced traumatic events as children.

For those unlucky enough to be unable to avoid cocaine use in the first place, a number of placebo-controlled studies show positive results. Referral to a 12-step program is of great value and provides many different types of crucial

Table 64.1 *Treatments for Bipolar Comorbidities: Evidence from Primary Substance Use/Abuse Disorders*

Alcohol		Cocaine	Nicotine	Food/Bulimia
Abstinence	Withdrawal			
Naltrexone (A)B	Benzodiazepine (A)C	Topiramate (A)A	Bupropion (A)A	Topiramate (A)A
Acamprosate (A)C	Carbamazepine (A)A	Modafinil (A)A	Nicotine Patch (A)A	Zonisamide (A)A
Disulfiram (A)C	Valproate (C)A	12 Step (A)A	Rimonabant (A)D	
Topiramate (A)A	Gabapentin (D, E)B	Disulfiram (A)C		
12 Step (A)A		Carbamazepine (A)A		
Valproate (A**)A		N-Acetylcysteine (A)A		
		Baclofen (A)D		

First letter = Level of Evidence (A–E) in (primary syndrome or ** in bipolar patients). (A), controlled clinical trials; (B), large case series; (C), smaller open studies; (D), not effective; or (E), worse.

Second letter = Utility Grade A–D. A, highly compatible with use in bipolar patients; B, may be helpful; C, possibly useful; D, not recommended.

programs and supports. Topiramate, the anticonvulsant that is not a primary antimanic agent, appears to decrease cocaine intake and craving (Kampman et al., 2004), in addition to its positive effects on alcohol abstinence (Johnson et al., 2003) and PTSD (Berlant & Van Kammen, 2002). Carbamazepine was more effective than placebo, but only in cocaine users with a comorbid mood disorder. Modafinil also has been reported in controlled trials to assist in abstinence. Modafinil would appear to have considerable utility, since we have also found it significantly better than placebo in the treatment of residual depression, fatigue, and inability to focus in bipolar depressed adults (Frye et al., 2007). Thus to the extent that a patient was using cocaine to self medicate depression, modafinil may be particularly helpful.

Disulfiram apparently makes the cocaine high quite unpleasant and thus may also assist with cocaine abstinence as it also does with alcohol abstinence, although the intensity of the adverse effect of alcohol with disulfiram is much greater than that with cocaine (Suh, Pettinati, Kampman, & O'Brien, 2006.) Although baclofen also helps reduce cocaine use in those with primary cocaine addiction, it would appear to have little potential utility in those with bipolar illness. Baclofen (a $GABA_B$ agonist) exacerbated depressions in our study of affectively ill patients without substance abuse problems (Post et al., 1991).

PRINCIPLES OF THE CASE

STRENGTH OF EVIDENCE

1. Bipolar illness appears to be a substantial risk factor for substance abuse. +++

2. Comorbid abuse of psychomotor stimulants can exacerbate bipolar illness and appears associated with an increased incidence of dysphoric components of mania. ++

3. Goldberg and Whiteside (2002) reported an increased incidence of antidepressant-induced switches into hypomania and mania in those with a history of substance abuse compared to those without. Cocaine users may show cross-sensitization to stressors, as well as to manic induction with antidepressants. +

4. Being free of substance abuse problems by avoiding drugs in the first place would appear to be far easier than the remediation of an already full-blown drug addiction. This may be particularly true for patients

who are already troubled by a
major affective disorder.   ++

5. Bipolar affective illness and
cocaine abuse are both associated with long-term changes
in gene expression.   +++

6. Both may also involve structural and chemical alterations
in neurons and glia in the cen-
tral nervous system.   ++

7. Some of the changes in gene
expression induced by cocaine
may directly interact with neuropathological mechanisms in
bipolar illness and further complicate bipolar illness course
and response to treatment.
This could include:

   a. Prefrontal cortical hypome-
      tabolism   +

   b. Amygdala overactivity   +

   c. Cortisol hypersecretion   +

   d. Unexplained hyperintensi-
      ties on MRI   +

8. Those who use psychomotor
stimulants appear to have a
less benign course of bipolar
affective disorder than those
without such abuse problems.   ++

9. Those with early-onset bipolar
illness are more prone to develop substance use and also
have more dysphoric mania
and ultra-ultrarapid (ultradian)
cycling.   ++

10. Participation in a 12-step treatment program may be ex-
tremely helpful in facilitating
abstinence.   +

11. Conditioned cueing, that is,
specific cues or the return to

the environmental context
where one has used a drug previously, may precipitate crav-
ing, relapse, or paranoia.   +

12. Cocaine cues activate the limbic system, as seen on positron emission tomography in
those with abuse problems.   +

13. The amygdala response on
positron emission tomography
to the local anesthetic procaine is enhanced in stimulant
(cocaine) users, possibly reflecting local anesthetic kindling, while the amygdala
response to procaine is attenuated in patients with affective
illness.   +

14. Current potential treatment options for cocaine abstinence include carbamazepine, topiramate, modafinil, disulfiram,
and possibly aripiprazole or
quetiapine. None are as yet
well studied in bipolar illness
with cocaine abuse comorbidity or FDA approved for this
indication, however.   ++

TAKE-HOME MESSAGE

Having one difficult-to-treat neuropsychiatric
illness (bipolar illness) is vastly less complicated than having to contend with a second difficult-to-treat illness (such as stimulant addiction) as well. If there is any way this potential
complication (which could add to the downward
spiral of stress sensitization, affective illness
progression, and poor response to therapeutics)
can be avoided, it should be strongly encouraged and sought.

65

Anger Attacks: A High Incidence in Childhood- and Adult-Onset Bipolar Illness

CASE HISTORY

We present a case without a life chart of a 15-year-old female with escalating anger attacks and initial response to carbamazepine. This patient was born of a mother who was a polysubstance abuser (not bipolar), and who not only neglected but also physically abused the infant for her first 3 months of life, until she was adopted by another family. Her new caring adoptive parents reported increasing anger and tantrumlike behavior with biting, hitting, kicking, and screaming upon minor provocation. This behavior initially responded well to treatment with carbamazepine, but progressively emerged following additional provoking circumstances despite ongoing treatment. New added stressors included a move, being teased at school, and losing a part-time job. In a tolerance-like pattern, mild, then moderate and severe anger attacks emerged following only minor provocation.

BACKGROUND LITERATURE

Impact of Neonatal Stressors on Brain Development and Behavior

Data in experimental animals indicate that exposure of the fetus to stimulants via a pregnant mother results in long-lasting increased behavioral responsivity to stimulant challenge during adulthood of the animal. Infants exposed to cocaine via the maternal route during their prenatal life are also at a substantially higher risk for the development of a seizure disorder and for sudden infant death syndrome (Fares, McCulloch, & Raju, 1997; Keller & Snyder-Keller, 2000). Because repeated exposure to high-dose local anesthetics in experimental animals kindles seizures, it is possible that repeated exposure to cocaine could also kindle seizures in the developing human fetus, as well as sensitize it to psychomotor stimulant and stressor-induced behavioral reactivity.

Repeated maternal separation stress in the neonatal rat pup is also associated with lifelong increases in the stress hormone equivalent of cortisol in rodents, and with anxiety-like behaviors (Ladd et al., 2000; Plotsky & Meaney, 1993). Even a single day of separation from the mother can produce the above effects, along with decreases in hippocampal brain-derived neurotrophic factor and calcium calmodulin kinase-II (necessary for cell survival and long-term memory) and increases in the rate of preprogrammed cell death in the brain (Smith, Kim, van Oers, & Levine, 1997; Zhang, Xing, Levine, Post, & Smith, 1998; Zhang et al., 2002).

It is also well documented in humans that parental neglect can lead to the syndrome of psychosocial dwarfism based on a failure of adequate levels of growth hormone to activate enzymes necessary for normal central nervous system growth and development. In an animal model of this syndrome in the rodent, maternal separation can induce a lack of responsiveness of the enzyme ornithine decarboxylase to growth hormone stimulation in the neonatal rat pup (Kuhn, Butler, & Schanberg, 1978). This enzyme dysfunction can be reversed by appropriate stroking of the ventral surface (tummy) of the separated rat pup's stomach with a soft toothbrush in a way that mimics the licking of the mother's tongue (Pauk, Kuhn, Field, & Schanberg, 1986). Thus, touch appears to be a crucial modality for cementing many infant-maternal bonds necessary for adequate growth and development.

Anger Attacks in Children

Anger attacks may be an accompaniment of bipolar disorder over the entire developmental spectrum. They are very common in childhood-onset bipolar illness, with severe attacks (temper tantrums) lasting as much as an hour or more triggered by even trivial provocations. They can often be among the earliest or major presenting symptom of childhood-onset bipolar illness that otherwise emerges with more classical sets of affective symptoms as the child develops (Fergus et al., 2003). Early more specific differentiators of prepubertal onset bipolar illness and ADHD are the occurrence of brief and extended periods of mood elevation and decreased need for sleep. Marked increases in irritability and poor frustration tolerance also occur in about 50% of ADHD children, but are more prevalent (90%) and more severe in the youngest children with bipolar disorder.

These attacks can emerge in the most caring of environments and in the face of unbelievable degrees of maternal equanimity. However, temper tantrums and other related apparently purposeful behavior associated with bipolar illness could also evoke negative or harsh disciplinary reactions that may not be helpful and in some instances may be counterproductive.

Anger Attacks in Adult Bipolar Depression

Anger attacks can also be a prominent accompaniment of both unipolar (Fava & Rosenbaum, 1999) and bipolar depressive disorder in adults. Perlis and associates (2004) reported that among depressed individuals, those with bipolar illness had a 62% incidence of anger attacks, and unipolar patients a 26% incidence rate, in an otherwise pure depressive (not mixed) episode. Moreover, in a multivariate statistical analysis, anger attacks themselves emerge as a significant predictor of bipolarity in patients presenting with a pure depressive episode.

The anger attacks in the Perlis et al. (2004) study were identified on the basis of a questionnaire, indicating a background of irritability and a tendency to overreact to minor annoyances, including at least one episode of excessive or situationally inappropriate anger, with four or more associated features, which may be physical (such as sweating or fast heart rate); psychological (the desire to attack or shout at others); or behavioral (actually attacking others, throwing or destroying objects, etc.).

The Perlis et al. study also needs to be put in the additional context that patients with mixed and manic episodes are often definitionally characterized by increased irritability, anger, and aggression, such that the overall incidence of anger attacks in bipolar illness may be markedly underestimated when based solely on those observed during depressive phases of the illness. Thus, untreated or inadequately treated bipolar illness in a parent can be associated with an increased tendency toward anger attacks in general and the possibility of an increased incidence of those directed at their children, especially those showing (but even in those not showing) provocative and frustrating behavior and temper tantrums.

It is noteworthy that anger attacks that occur in the context of unipolar depression respond very well to antidepressants, especially those of the selective serotonin reuptake inhibitor (SSRI) class (Fava et al., 1991, 1996). A more recent study of the SSRI citalopram in bipolar depressed patients found a significant reduction in anger attacks (from 38.6% to 14.6%; Mammen,

Pilkonis, Chengappa, & Kupfer, 2004). However, given the ambiguities of the appropriate place of antidepressants in the overall therapeutic armamentarium of bipolar depression (Chapters 34–38), it is important to note that many of the other treatment options available in mood disorders show substantial degrees of efficacy for anger attacks and aggression.

Lithium, carbamazepine, and valproate all have an extensive literature base supporting their use in a variety of anger, aggressive, and dyscontrol syndromes, and one would encourage the addition of one or more of these types of agents to the treatment of an individual with bipolar illness and anger attacks that were not adequately responsive to his or her current therapy.

Anger attacks in patients with bipolar illness can also escalate to overt aggression in the context of alcohol and substance abuse or comorbid PTSD. Therefore, it is important to identify and treat this symptom cluster adequately, particularly in households in which children are at a high risk of being the subjects of anger attacks. If a parent with anger attacks has young children at home, special attention should be paid to the intensive treatment of this individual's affective illness . To the extent possible, such parents should receive more comprehensive treatment and more intensive support to prevent any potentially increased adverse consequences for their children. Although not necessarily a medical emergency, such a situation should be treated with the utmost care and sensitivity. Weissman et al (2007) have also observed that the children of unipolar depressed mothers whose depression has been treated to remission have fewer behavioral problems and psychiatric diagnoses compared to those whose mothers' depression is only partially treated.

Psychological and Pharmacological Treatment Principles

The utility of avoiding unnecessary confrontations that may precipitate frequent anger attacks in the child with bipolar and related illnesses has been outlined by Ross W. Greene (1998) in his book *The Explosive Child*. A holding technique may be appropriate for some preschool children. Arnold Meyersberg (personal communication, 1985) has described how a child during a tantrum can be placed sitting on the lap of the holding person (child's back to the adult's chest), with the child's hands crossed in front and the wrists gently but firmly held so that the child is protected from hitting, kicking, screaming, or biting self or others. On the first occasion, holding may be necessary for as long as 30 to 90 minutes. Subsequently, holding is required for shorter periods of time as the child begins to rapidly de-escalate from the anger or tantrum attack. After three to five such holding sequences, the anger attacks will likely cease altogether and, instead, the parental figure may be approached by the child for verbal assurance or for voluntary physical holding in the face of frustrations that previously would have triggered anger attacks.

The physiological and psychological aspects of this type of literal and figurative holding should be carefully explained and worked through with the parents, and they should be given enough support to maintain the holding intervention long enough to be successful. The need for such holding instead of just leaving the child to his or her own devices should be recognized, especially when issues of abandonment are prominent and techniques for calming oneself not well developed.

Carbamazepine is useful in the treatment of a variety of anger syndromes independent of psychiatric diagnosis (Roy-Byrne, Uhde, et al., 1984) and can inhibit the paroxysms of different types of attacks, including facial pain in trigeminal neuralgia, epileptic symptoms in temporal lobe epilepsy with complex partial seizures, and affective symptoms in manic-depressive illness. In each of these treatment instances, it is recognized that in a percentage of initially responsive patients, tolerance to positive medication effects can develop. The exact treatment algorithms for preventing or reversing this tolerance are not entirely known, but a variety of suggestions are presented in Chapters 8 & 19. In cases of anger attacks, we would suggest a similar array of choices in augmenting carbamazepine with lithium or other mood-stabilizing anticonvulsants such as valproate. A period of time off carbamazepine and then reinstitution of treatment may also be worthy of consideration in the face of tolerance development because this approach has been reported to be successful in some patients with affective or trigeminal neuralgia disorders (Pazzaglia & Post, 1992).

As previously noted, anger attacks are also highly responsive to treatment with the SSRIs in those with unipolar and bipolar depression. Mood stabilizers and the entire class of atypical antipsychotics may also be helpful in bipolar depression both to prevent anger and anxiety attacks and possible switches into hypomania or mania in the presence of antidepressant augmentation.

PRINCIPLES OF THE CASE	STRENGTH OF EVIDENCE
1. Anger attacks in adults are common in patients with bipolar depression, as well as in mixed states and mania.	+++
2. Lithium and the mood stabilizer anticonvulsants carbamazepine and valproate can have positive effects on anger, aggression, and dyscontrol syndromes.	++
3. The atypical antipsychotics are also likely to be highly effective for anger attacks.	+
4. Severe, prolonged, inconsolable temper tantrums can be among the first presenting signs of the bipolar prodrome in very young children, but are clearly not diagnostic.	++
5. Temper tantrums are nonspecific and their strength as a predictor of later bipolar illness remains unclear.	±
6. Treatment of childhood tantrums and anger attacks often requires multiple therapeutic modalities including psychotherapy for the child, adults, or families involved, as well as pharmacotherapy.	++
7. Specifically targeted therapeutic approaches, such as those of Ross W. Greene (1998) in *The Explosive Child,* may be useful.	++
8. In physically size-appropriate preadolescents, the holding approach of Meyersberg and others described here may also be a treatment option.	+
9. Anger attacks can be manifest in bipolar children, even with the most compassionate, restrained, and calming parental approaches.	+++
10. It is important to view these attacks as illness-related behavior and not readily under a child's control, that is, much like an epileptic seizure. This viewpoint helps maintain parental equanimity.	+
11. Parents or children with uncontrolled anger attacks should get intensive support and treatment if they have a psychiatric diagnosis and are symptomatic.	++
12. A depressed mother (with or without anger attacks) of a neonate or toddler most often needs and should be offered additional support, whether or not it is specifically requested.	++
13. Mechanisms for increased rest, time-outs, group support, and ready access to phone and personal contact systems should be developed.	++
14. If a child of parents with active affective illness has a difficult bipolar-like presentation, intensive therapeutic intervention with the entire family will likely be needed.	++

TAKE-HOME MESSAGE

Parents with inadequately treated unipolar and bipolar illness often have anger attacks as part of the illness, and may need extra support, especially if they have a difficult youngster who is displaying prolonged and uncontrolled tantrums. Anger attacks in children with bipolar illness are not uncommon and are nonspecific, but still require very conserted treatment intervention.

66

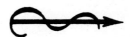

Remission in a Patient
With Severe Bipolar Illness and
Post-Traumatic Stress Disorder

CASE HISTORY

Retrospective Course

This patient's retrospective life chart history (Figure 66.1) is striking for the occurrence of a series of extreme stressors, including a history of early physical and sexual abuse, many other psychological and physical assaults in her youth and adulthood, and an adult episode of sexual assault in 1982. In addition to her mania and depression, the patient had classic PTSD symptoms, including an almost lifelong sleep disturbance with insomnia, nightmares, and frequent awakenings; evidence of hyperstartle; spontaneous flashbacks; and a considerable degree of withdrawal and numbing. These symptoms, along with evidence of a single stressor or a series of severe stressors, yield the PTSD diagnosis.

After a delay of 15 years in the onset of treatment following her initial major depression, the patient had an inadequate response to a variety of mood stabilizers, antipsychotics, and antidepressants for both bipolar and PTSD symptoms (Figure 66.2). These treatments included antidepressants (bupropion, sertraline, fluoxetine, paroxetine, and venlafaxine); benzodiazepines (zolpidem, temazepam, lorazepam); mood stabilizers (lithium, carbamazepine, valproate); antipsychotics (thioridazine, thiothixine, risperidone,

olanzapine); two courses of ECT; and ongoing psychotherapy.

Inpatient Treatment

As illustrated in Figure 66.3, the extreme incapacitation (seen from 1995 to 1998) continued to be observed at the NIMH. The patient was often unable to leave her bed or room, overwhelmed by extreme anxiety, flashbacks, and associated depressive symptoms. She volunteered to participate in a clinical trial of repeated transcranial magnetic stimulation (rTMS) of the brain. This trial involved 1 month of randomly assigned treatment with either sham or 1 Hz (active) rTMS over the right prefrontal cortex, with a frequency of one stimulation per second for 20 minutes per day and a crossover to the other treatment. Because 1 Hz rTMS dampens overactive neural activity as seen on positron emission tomography scans, and there is evidence of right frontal hyperactivity in patients with PTSD, it was postulated that low-frequency rTMS might normalize this activity or improve PTSD symptomatology.

Disappointingly, the patient failed to improve to any substantial degree in either phase of the rTMS trial, and was offered the opportunity to participate in a double-blind, randomized controlled trial of lamotrigine, gabapentin, and pla-

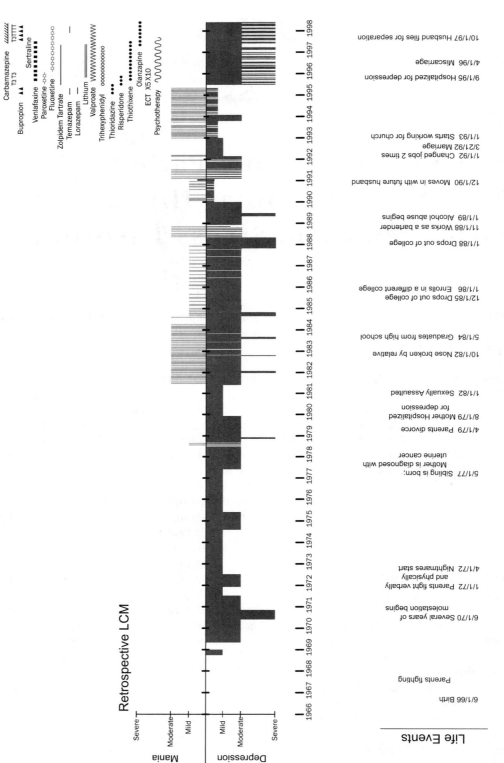

Figure 66.1 Retrospective mood chart showing a 25-year history of untreated bipolar illness and ultrarapid cycling, as well as comorbid PTSD (see Figure 66.2). Initial treatment attempts in 1995 to 1998 were unsuccessful.

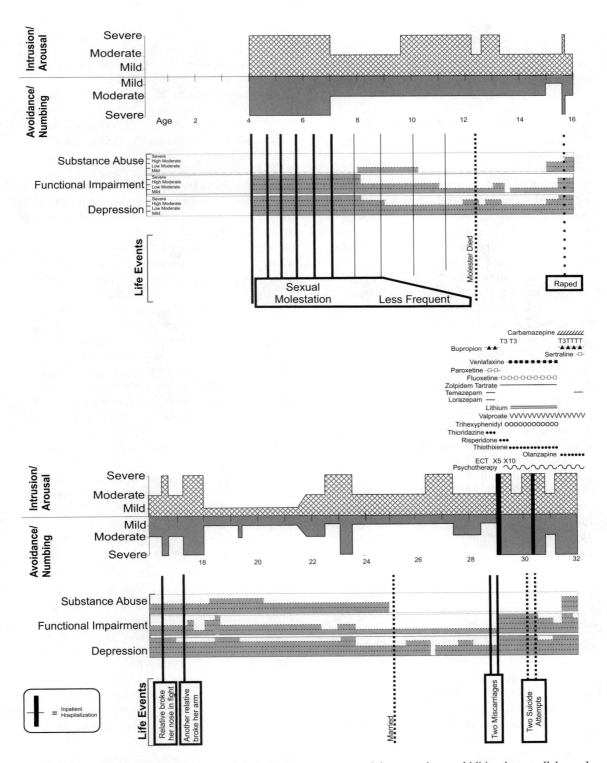

Figure 66.2 Graphic depiction of the severity of PTSD symptoms, precipitants, and comorbidities that parallel mood symptoms illustrated in Figure 66.1. Intrusion and arousal symptoms are graphed above baseline and avoidance and numbing symptoms below. Severity of substance abuse, functional impairment, and comorbid depression are shaded in dark bars where height reflects severity. Selective stressful life events are noted below the graphs. The PTSD symptoms completely remitted in 2000 (see Figure 66.3).

cebo, with each phase lasting about 6 weeks, as previously described by Frye, Ketter, Kimbrell, et al. (2000; Chapters 25 and 26).

On the Phase I drug (later revealed to be lamotrigine), the patient showed substantial improvement in her depression and PTSD symptoms and became slightly hypomanic. This improvement continued to some extent in phase II (revealed to be gabapentin; Figure 66.3). However, her symptoms worsened over the course of the trial, convergent with a series of recurrent stressors, and the patient had to return home for an important event in the family. Phase III (revealed to be placebo) was associated with a continuation of her initial symptomatology, and was therefore terminated early. The patient then chose to be (blindly) reexposed to the Phase I agent (lamotrigine) associated with the greatest initial improvement.

When gabapentin was added to lamotrigine (because of a lack of sustained effect), the patient continued to be moderately symptomatic, experiencing a recurrence of sleep disturbance, nightmares, and flashbacks.

Carbamazepine was added to the two other anticonvulsant drugs, and remission of both PTSD and affective symptoms was dramatic, complete, and maintained for the rest of her inpatient hospital stay. The patient was able to experience positive affect, enjoy herself, and return to work for the first time in many years. Her subsequent course is further discussed in Chapter 54.

BACKGROUND LITERATURE

Bipolar illness is often associated with a variety of other comorbid conditions. Of bipolar patients in the Stanley Foundation Bipolar Network, 40% have experienced an anxiety disorder, and 40% have also suffered from an associated substance abuse disorder (either alcohol or other substances of abuse; Suppes et al., 2001). In this life chart highlight, we discuss the pharmacotherapy of a patient with bipolar disorder who also suffered from PTSD and comorbid alcohol use (see also Chapter 6 on the co-occurrence of PTSD and bipolar illness).

Because of these two conditions, the patient had been almost completely incapacitated for several years and had not responded to a variety of conventional pharmacotherapies. As illustrated, she experienced a full remission on the combination of lamotrigine, gabapentin, and carbamazepine.

The life chart illustrates a number of important principles in the treatment of bipolar illness and PTSD. Despite many unsuccessful clinical trials, new medications or combinations of drugs may still produce remarkable clinical improvement. Lamotrigine has emerged as a significant treatment option for patients whose illness has not responded to other treatments (Calabrese et al., 1999; Frye, Ketter, Kimbrell, et al., 2000). In 2003, lamotrigine was approved for the prevention of depressive, manic, or mixed episodes. However, lamotrigine must be used carefully and dosages increased very slowly, because rapid dose escalation appears to increase the risk of a very severe rash associated with exfoliative dermatitis (sloughing off of the skin), requiring emergency medical treatment and hospitalization (in approximately 1 in 5,000 adults and 1 in 2,500 children; Guberman et al., 1999). Nonetheless, if one proceeds slowly, there is a reduced chance of developing a severe rash, and other side effects of the drug tend to be minimal, making it a generally well-tolerated and highly effective medication.

A range of anticonvulsants may be effective in the treatment of PTSD. A preliminary report suggests that lamotrigine may be effective in PTSD (Hertzberg et al., 1999), as it was in the patient illustrated (Figure 66.3). Previous studies suggested that both carbamazepine and valproate also helped some PTSD symptoms, particularly insomnia, sleep disruption, and nightmares (Ford, 1996; Keck, McElroy, & Friedman, 1992). The serotonin-selective antidepressants are the only agents currently approved for the treatment of PTSD; in this patient, a variety of such antidepressants had previously failed to produce any amelioration of her symptoms, however. The combination norepinephrine- and serotonin-active drug mirtazapine is also promising (Davidson et al., 2003), as is direct blockade of overactive norepineph-

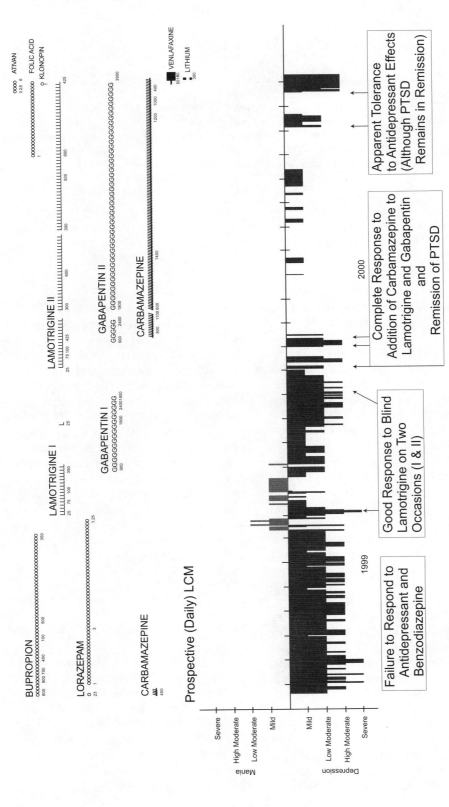

Figure 66.3 Prospective life chart showing excellent antidepressant response to lamotrigine and worsening of depression on gabapentin. A dramatic remission of both affective and PTSD symptoms was achieved when carbamazepine was added to lamotrigine and gabapentin combination therapy. Depressions of increasing severity began to emerge (as discussed in Chapter 54) that required increasingly complex treatment.

Table 66.1 *Potential Treatments for Comorbidities: Anxiety Disorders*

Social Phobia	Panic/Agrophobia	PTSD	OCD
Gabapentin (A)A	Gabapentin (A)A	SSRIs (A)B	SSRIs (A)B
Clonazepam (A)A	Clonazepam (A)A	Atypical antipsychotics (A)A	Atypicals (A)A
Antidepressants (A)B	Antidepressants (A)B	Lamotrigine (B**)A	Lamotrigine (D)A
	Valproate (B)A	Topiramate (C)A	Carbamazepine (D)A
	Lamotrigine (B**)A	Carbamazepine (C)A	Gabapentin (D, E)B
	Carbamazepine (C)A	Benzodiazepine (E)C	

First letter = Level of Evidence (in primary disorder only): (A) = Double blind clinical trial; (B) = Large case expense; (C) = Much open study; (D) = Few cases; (E) = Ambiguous; (F) = Worse.
** = Studied in bipolar disorder.
Second letter = Utility in bipolar disorder grade A–D. A, highly compatible with use in bipolar patients; B, may be helpful; C, possibly useful; D, not recommended.

rine alpha-1 receptors with the antihypertensive drug prazosin (Raskind et al., 2003, 2007). Topiramate also shows considerable promise (Chapter 29).

Carefully charting a course of illness and response to treatment facilitates the optimal development of pharmacotherapeutic regimens, which, in some cases, are complex. This patient was extremely diligent in charting both her bipolar illness and PTSD symptoms (Osuch, Brotman, et al., 2001). Life charting allows one to delineate subtle degrees of improvement or deterioration with the addition or subtraction of a different drug, and provides important clues to an overall assessment of the risk-to-benefit ratio of a given drug in the context of the entire treatment regimen. A separate form has also been developed for charting the retrospective and prospective longitudinal course of PTSD symptoms (Osuch, Brotman, et al., 2001), which we would recommend for patients with PTSD.

Adjunctive gabapentin may play a role in some components of bipolar illness, despite several negative placebo-controlled studies of gabapentin in mania or in monotherapy in highly treatment-refractory affectively ill patients, including our own at the NIMH (Frye, Ketter, Kimbrell, et al., 2000; Chapter 25). Gabapentin has a very benign side effects profile even at high doses and shows positive effects in anxiety disorders and social phobia (in controlled trials), and in open studies of pain syndromes, tremor, restless leg syndrome, and perhaps also obses-

sive-compulsive symptoms, Parkinson's disease, and alcohol withdrawal.

Carbamazepine remains a drug with considerable utility in the treatment of bipolar disorder, even though it is often the fourth choice after lithium, lamotrigine, and valproate, largely because of the possibility of multiple drug interactions and the fear of exceedingly rare but serious hematological side effects. While oxcarbazepine appears to share carbamazepine's psychotrophic profile and is safer and easier to use (Chapter 20), whether it will mirror all of carbamazepine's (Chapter 17) therapeutic effects remains to be seen. When an attempt was made (see Chapter 54) to substitute oxcarbazepine for carbamazepine in this patient (to avoid suppression of white blood cells), it was not successful, and her mood slipped.

PRINCIPLES OF THE CASE

STRENGTH OF EVIDENCE

1. Bipolar illness co-occurs with a traumatic childhood history of physical or sexual abuse in about 20% of Stanley Foundation Bipolar Network outpatients (which is roughly similar to the rate in the general U.S. or Canadian population).   ++

2. Full syndromic PTSD occurs

in less than 10% of patients with bipolar illness, however. +

3. When there is a history of early childhood trauma, bipolar illness shows an earlier age of onset and a more adverse course, including increased suicide attempts compared with bipolar patients without such traumatic life events. ++

4. Although the SSRI antidepressants are FDA approved for PTSD, they are often insufficient for achieving a complete response. ++

5. Lamotrigine improved this patient's depression. ++

6. Gabapentin did not help depression in this case but did decrease anxiety. +

7. Both mood and PTSD symptoms remitted with the addition of carbamazepine to the other two anticonvulsants (lamotrigine and gabapentin), despite the fact that the patient was previously resistant to carbamazepine in conjunction with valproate, benzodiazepines, and olanzapine. +

8. The anticonvulsants, although not yet systematically tested in PTSD, may be an important treatment approach to both bipolar illness mood stabilization and relief of PTSD symptomatology. ±

9. Also promising are drugs active on norepinephrine and serotonin, such as mirtazapine, which would also help sleep, but may be overly sedating for some and cause weight gain. +

10. Prazosin, a drug for high blood pressure that directly blocks norepinephrine alpha-1 receptors, dramatically decreased nightmares and other PTSD symptoms in controlled studies (Raskind et al., 2003, 2007). +++

11. Thus, a range of new options beyond the SSRIs are available for PTSD. When it is comorbid with bipolar illness, a number of anticonvulsants may be helpful as primary treatments of both the bipolar disorder and the symptoms of PTSD. These anticonvulsants might include carbamazepine, valproate, lamotrigine, gabapentin, and topiramate. +

12. The atypical antipsychotics have not been formally tested in bipolar disorder with comorbid PTSD but show considerable promise for both syndromes. ++

13. The utility of the opiate antagonist naltrexone remains to be further explored for treatment of repeated cutting and self-harm. ++

TAKE-HOME MESSAGE

Even the most severe treatment-resistant mood disorder can usually be successfully treated; this patient struggled heroically with her traumatic history, comorbid PTSD, and bipolar illness, and finally achieved remission of both, in this instance with three anticonvulsants in combination: lamotrigine, gabapentin, and carbamazepine. More of her subsequent clinical course appears in Chapter 54.

Part XV

CHILDHOOD ONSET
OF BIPOLAR ILLNESS

67

Affective Dysfunction From Ages 3 to 11 and Improvement at Age 12 After Sequential Clinical Trials: Background on Pediatric Psychopharmacology of Bipolar Disorder

CASE HISTORY

The graphic depiction of the course and evolution of a child's activated and withdrawn behaviors (Figure 67.1) is derived from extensive typewritten notes of the patient's mother. Additionally, several lengthy telephone interviews with the mother were used to further clarify and evaluate the observed behaviors and their impact on her child's ability to continue to interact and function at home, with friends, at school, and in after-school activities (see Appendix 3, last section). The mother related that there was a history of mood disorders in the families of both parents for two or more generations.

As an infant, the child slept most of the time for the first 3 months of life and was very hard to awaken even to be nursed. When awake she was generally smiley. At 5 months, however, she developed very disturbed sleep with multiple awakenings attributed to ear infections, but this also seemed to herald further difficulties and ongoing sleep disruption.

Sporadic tantrums began to emerge when she was 9 months old, and she seemed to crave constant interaction with her mother. In her second and third years, her tantrums increased in severity and frequency and were, at times, accompanied by unusually aggressive behaviors toward her mother. The child was also remarkably fearless on the playground when using the equipment or going down slides.

After her third birthday, her tantrums decreased in frequency and she seemed somewhat better overall. However, in October 1991 (age 4.5) she had an extraordinarily severe tantrum, tried to jump out of the car, fiercely attacked her mother, and wished her dead. Kindergarten and first grade were much better years for her, and her mother thought that she had outgrown her previous difficult and troubling behaviors.

Another severe tantrum occurred in October

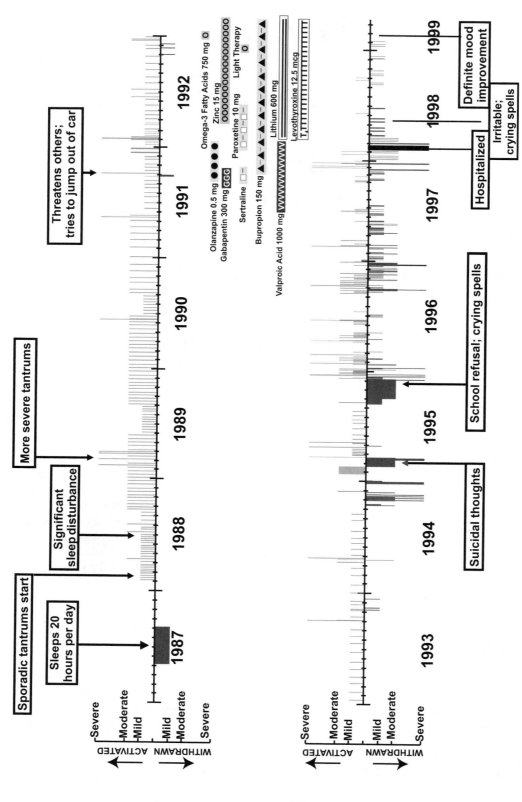

Figure 67.1 Kiddie Life Chart (K-LCM): marked response in a 12-year-old with early-onset bipolar illness. The patient's affective lability, irritability, and dyscontrol, including severe and very prolonged tantrums, characterized the earliest presentation of the illness (1988–1994). Classic manic and depressive episodes developed only later at age 7 and 8 (1994–1995). Apparent response to valproate plus other agents was not sustained. Response to lithium plus bupropion, T₃, and omega-3 fatty acids was dramatic and sustained for several years.

1993, accompanied by suicidal thoughts and homicidal threats toward others. The child had thoughts of her own death in November 1993, and the fall of 1994 marked the reemergence of tantrums, more severe and frequent than before, and now with distinct depressive behaviors, suicidal thoughts, great sadness with crying spells, and school refusal, as well as extreme irritability and angry, threatening outbursts toward others. Between times she could be cheerful, cooperative, friendly, very creative, and playful, with many expressions of love and affection for her mother and others. The summer of 1995, like summers before, was a calmer and better time, only to be followed by a return in the fall of the previous episodic severe symptoms and functional impairment.

In 1997, the child was finally diagnosed with bipolar illness, and in June the mood stabilizer valproate was instituted, starting with 125 mg and eventually titrated to 1,250 mg/day. This helped ameliorate the most severe tantrums, which were now reduced to short, angry outbursts. In September 1997, a brief trial of sertraline for continuing depressive symptoms brought too much sedation in the morning and too much activation in the evening. After tapering sertraline, bupropion was started in October and increased to 300 mg/day, and it remained in the regimen when valproate (1,000 mg/day) was discontinued in February 1998 after her hospitalization for depression.

Although somewhat improved, the remaining symptoms of her bipolar illness still caused some difficulties in functioning. The patient finally became well on a combination of bupropion, lithium, cytomel (T_3), and adjunctive omega-3 fatty acids. She was now an A student, finished the 10th grade, and was happy with friends and family. However, several years later, renewal of marijuana smoking resulted in a major relapse.

BACKGROUND LITERATURE

With few exceptions, the treatment principles of childhood- and adolescent-onset bipolar illness are indirectly derived from the knowledge base in treating adults with bipolar illness (Table 67.1). Relatively few controlled clinical trials specifically relating to children are available, but are generally consistent with the view that many of the inferences from the adult literature will be applicable.

Geller, Cooper, Watts, Cosby, and Fox (1992) studied lithium versus placebo in young children with bipolar illness and comorbid substance dependency. Compared with placebo, lithium was significantly more effective in ameliorating their symptomatology. The drug was generally well tolerated with no unexpected side effects beyond those anticipated from the adult literature.

One of the most informative studies was that of Kowatch and collaborators (2000) comparing young children with *DSM-IV*-diagnosed mania with treatment randomized among the three choices most commonly used in adults, that is, lithium, valproate, and carbamazepine. These investigators found approximately 40–50% response rates in acute mania with each of the drugs, and again, all were reasonably well tolerated. The authors observed that relatively few patients responded completely to any of these drugs as monotherapy, and often, combinations of treatment over a period of months were required for the achievement of solid mood stabilization. In addition, they found that following this satisfactory treatment of the mood fluctuations of bipolar illness, many patients required the addition of small doses of psychomotor stimulants in order to treat residual ADHD symptomatology and establish a complete remission of all symptomatology.

Biederman et al.'s (1999) retrospective observations support this viewpoint, and there is a general consensus in the literature that mood stabilization needs to be achieved prior to the effective use of psychomotor stimulants (Kowatch et al., 2005). In many investigators' experience, these children are too often treated in the community with psychomotor stimulants alone (Chapter 68) or antidepressants alone, prior to the use of mood stabilizers. These initial trials are typically without success, and in many instances may result in illness exacerbation and an increased level of dysphoria and manic psychosis.

Calabrese, Shelton, and associates (2005)

Table 67.1 *General Profiles of Mood Stabilizers and Atypical Antipsychotics (AA) in Adult Bipolar Disorder*

Mood Stabilizaers	Acute			Prophylaxis				Child Utility
	Mania	Depression	Tolerability	Mania	Depression	Tolerability	Utility	
Mood Stabilizers								
Lithium	+++[FDA]	++	B+	+++[FDA]	+++	B	A	B+
Carbamazepine (Tegretol, ER-Equetro)	+++[FDA]	++	B	++	+++	B+	A−	B
Valproate (Depakote)	+++[FDA]	++	B+	+++	++	B	A	B+
Lamotrigine (Lamictal)	0	(+++)[a]	A−	++[FDA]	+++[FDA]	A	A	B(−)
Other Anticonvulsants								
Oxcarbazepine (Trileptal)	++	+	A−	(++)	(+)	A−	B	B
Topiramate (Topamax)	0	+	B+	(±)	(±)	B	B+	B[wt. loss]
Zonegram (Zonisamide)	+	(+)	B+	(+)	(±)	A−	B+	B[wt. loss]
Atypical Antipsychotics								
Aripiprazole (Abilify)	+++[FDA]	++	A−	+++[FDA]	(++)	A	A	A
Quetiapine (Serquel)	+++[FDA]	+++[FDA]	B	(+++)[b]	(+++)[c]	B	A	A−
Ziprasidone (Geodon)	+++[FDA]	(+)	B	(++)	(+)	A	A	B+
Risperidone (Risperidol)	+++[FDA]	±	B+	(++)	(+)	A	B+	B+
Olanzepine (Zyprexa)	+++[FDA]	++	B	+++[FDA]	+	B	B	B
Clozapine (Clozaril)	+++	(+)	B−	+++	++	C	C	C

0, no effect; ±, possible effect; +, likely or small effect; ++, moderate effect; +++, marked effect; ( ), some ambiguity.
[FDA], FDA approved; [a], metaanalysis is positive; [b], positive unpublished data; [c], positive unpublished data.
Child utility (last column), subjective integration of effectiveness and tolerability data.

found only a remarkably small group of adult patients with rapid cycling who responded to the combination of two of the most widely used agents in the illness, lithium and valproate. The response rate was under one quarter of the observed patients (who stayed in the study) and was only 17% in the intent-to-treat analysis (all those who entered). This indicated that the majority of adult patients with rapid-cycling bipolar illness were unable to be stabilized well enough to enter a proposed randomization to monotherapy. Moreover, in those who did achieve a good enough response to the combination and were randomized, there was a very high incidence (about 50%) of dropouts for mood exacerbation prior to the intended 1 year of monotherapy. These data further suggest that combination treatment may be required to maintain stability even in adults with responsive illness.

In contrast to these disappointing observa-tions in adults with rapid cycling, Findling and associates (2005) observed somewhat higher rates of mood stabilization (43%) with the combination of lithium and valproate in childhood-onset bipolar illness. However, upon randomization to monotheray with either lithium or valproate, about two thirds of the children relapsed. The vast majority did rerespond to the combination, but often required adjunctive treatment of comorbid ADHD with psychomotor stimulants and other agents (Findling et al., 2006)

These data have several important implications. Mania in children is difficult to treat and often requires combination treatment to achieve and maintain stability. Monotherapy may be the ideal, but in children (average age 12) meeting strict DSM IV criteria for mania, is rarely achieveable. Stimulants and other agents are often also required. Whether a larger percentage of children (compared with the very few adults in the Calabrese, Shelton, et al., 2005, study) will be able to achieve sustained improvement following combination treatment with valproate and lithium remains to be clarified. If it is a reliable experience, it could suggest that early treatment with mood stabilizers of bipolar illness in children (before the illness gains momentum) may be more effective than treatment in adults with rapid cycling who have already experienced multiple episodes.

While Geller et al. (2002) described a difficult and poor prognosis course in a cohort of children with bipolar illness treated in the community, the data of Findling et al. (2006) on the lithium-valproate combination suggest that this might, in part, be related to less aggressive mood stabilizer treatment these patients received in the community. However, the study of Birmaher et al. (2006) also revealed the children with BP I and BP II illness took about 9 months to stabilize, and those with BP NOS took on average more than 2½ years! BP NOS comprised about 35% of the patient group, almost always meeting the same diagnostic criteria of the others with the exception of the required 4 day duration needed for a diagnosis of BP II. About 30% of the BP NOS children converted to BP I or II during the follow up and this increased to 50% in those with a positive family history of bipolar disorder in first degree relatives. Thus, while the most diagnostic controversy surrounds the BP NOS subtype, the data of Birmaher and colleagues (2006) are very edifying. Those with BP NOS are common, are quite ill, cycle the fastest, take the longest to remit, and often are a precursor to the more accepted BP I and II subtypes.

At the University of Cincinnati, Melissa DelBello and colleagues (2002) conducted the first controlled clinical trial of an atypical neuroleptic in childhood- and adolescent-onset bipolar illness. These investigators compared adjunctive quetiapine and placebo to ongoing treatment with a mood stabilizer such as lithium or valproate. Quetiapine's addition was associated with a higher incidence and more rapid rate of improvement than with the mood stabilizer alone. A second study of quetiapine monotherapy also was more effective than valproate on

some measures (DelBello et al., 2006; see Figure 47.1). These data support an emerging series of observations in children, indicating that the atypical neuroleptics are as effective in treatment of childhood-onset bipolar illness as they are in the adult variety. Tohen et al (2007) reported that olanzepine was as highly effective in child and adolescent mania, but was associated with even more side effects in the metabolic syndrome domain than in adults.

A number of investigators have observed that children have somewhat more problematic experiences with extrapyramidal side effects to the atypical antipsychotics than expected from experience with adults. These extrapyramidal side effects can include Parkinson-like syndrome based on blockade of dopamine receptors, with tremor, rigidity and stiffness, mask faces, drooling, and slowness to initiate movement. Also, problems with restless or jumpy legs and an inability to sit still (akathisia) are seen in some children as well. One of the more striking problems in children in the U.S. population in general, and in children treated with a variety of psychotropic agents that are prone to cause weight gain, is the current pandemic of childhood obesity, sometimes associated with type 2 (usually adult-onset) diabetes mellitus, hypercholesterolemia, and hyperlipidemia, predisposing to later cardiovascular risk. The atypical neuroleptics and other drugs are classified according to their relative weight gain liabilities in Table 45.1, and in the absence of further systematic information based on direct studies in children, one can only assume that these general proclivities for weight gain will also be relevant when these drugs are used in childhood-onset bipolar illness. Thus, weight gain can be rather striking with clozapine and olanzapine, somewhat less with risperidone and quetiapine, and, importantly, ziprasidone and aripiprazole appear to be weight neutral in adults, but not necessarily in children. Many have observed some weight gain in children on aripiprazole, but perhaps less gain with ziprasidone.

Tolerability in terms of weight gain should thus be considered in a child's regimen, because this can be not only socially disabling but medically problematic as well. In this regard, one should also be alert to the possibilities of weight gain on lithium and valproate in the child and adolescent and be aware that some of lithium's other effects can be difficult for a child to accept, such as acne and gastrointestinal distress, and the need for regular blood level monitoring.

Considerable controversy has occurred around whether adolescent and young adult women treated with valproate for their bipolar illness will be prone to polycystic ovary syndrome (PCOS), as are many individuals who are so treated for their epilepsy (Isojarvi, Tauboll, et al., 2001). Preliminary data suggest that PCOS occurs at an increased rate in patients with epilepsy and is not a high-risk problem in those with bipolar illness. However, some elements of PCOS can occur with valproate; weight gain and increased levels of testosterone are reported in some series (Joffe et al., 2006), but not others (Rasgon et al., 2005). Menstrual irregularities are part of the syndrome, and while these may be present in young women with bipolar illness even prior to starting valproate, they occur more frequently after valproate treatment. Increased facial hair (hirsutism) is also part of PCOS, although this has not been reported to be a problem in patients with bipolar illness.

Virtually all of the symptoms of PCOS can be prevented with concurrent treatment with birth control pills, which also makes the concern about this potential valproate side effect a moot point in those so treated. Should any of the elements of PCOS emerge during valproate treatment, it is noteworthy that they are reversible off drug and when patients with epilepsy are crossed over to another anticonvulsant without this liability, such as lamotrigine.

Data of Findling et al. (2005, 2006) noted above indicate that many children require the combination of lithium and valproate for good mood stabilization. However, most still required additional treatment with stimulants to treat residual ADHD symptoms, and several children also required additional atypical antipsychotics. In children at high risk for full syndromal bipolar disorder who had prodromal or early symptoms of the illness, Findling et al (2007) did not find valproate monotherapy more effective than placebo, however.

As noted in Chapter 25, lamotrigine appears to have better antidepressant than antimanic mood-stabilizing effects in adults and a particularly user-friendly side effects profile, with the possible exception of the risk of a medically serious and life-threatening rash (Chapters 25 and 26). This is of particular importance because one of the risk factors for this rash is thought to be young age. If one is considering using lamotrigine in late adolescent and early adult onset bipolar illness, one should begin the drug at very low levels and titrate upward extremely slowly, preferably even more slowly than in the guidelines outlined in the *Physician's Desk Reference*.

The incidence of serious rash with this slow titration schedule is thought to be much lower than previously reported, based on more aggressive dosing strategies. In children it is estimated to be 4 cases in 10,000, or 1 patient in 2,500 individuals exposed. Given lamotrigine's excellent profile as an antidepressant and in terms of side effects tolerability, it is likely that individuals will carefully consider this risk-to-benefit ratio and in many instances decide in favor of a clinical trial with lamotrigine because this drug does not possess many of the typical side effect liabilities of lithium or valproate, including weight gain, sedation, and the possible dermatological problems of acne, alopecia, or hirsutism.

As many youngsters with bipolar depression have the typical reverse vegetative symptoms of depression (i.e., hypersomnia, increased appetite, slowness, and apathy rather than agitation) and weight gain rather than weight loss, lamotrigine would be an excellent treatment approach to this type of depressive presentation, even given the rash risk. Chang and associates (2007) reported good antidepressant effects of lamotrigine in adolescents, in marked contrast to his experience with antidepressants which either uncomfortably activated them or switched them into hypomania or mania in a high proportion of instances.

As noted previously in Chapter 20, oxcarbazepine is a close structural relative of carbamazepine, differing by only the addition of a single oxygen molecule in the middle ring of the compound. This changes its side effects profile in a more favorable direction. Compared with carbamazepine, which has a multitude of drug-drug interactions with other compounds because of metabolism by liver enzymes (CYP450, 3A4), oxcarbazepine has fewer of these interactions because of minimal degrees of enzyme induction. The only side effect more prominent with oxcarbazepine than with carbamazepine is low serum sodium (hyponatremia), which occurs in about 3% of patients exposed, although it is higher in some series. Oxcarbazepine has been shown to be no more effective than placebo in the treatment of child and adolescent-onset mania, however (Wagner et al., 2006).

In those children with psychotic presentations or those not responsive to initial treatment with one or more mood stabilizers, the addition of an atypical neuroleptic may be considered. Weight gain liability should be one factor in the choice of potential therapeutic agents in this class. Many clinicians will start treatment with an atypical antipsychotic alone or in combination with a mood stabilizer. If, after mood stabilization has been achieved, residual symptoms of ADHD remain prominent, most authorities would then recommend adjunctive use of psychomotor stimulants, but only in low doses as necessary (Kowatch et al., 2005).

PRINCIPLES OF THE CASE	STRENGTH OF EVIDENCE
1. Although not common, significant sleep disturbance with insomnia (or rare hypersomnia) in the first years of life is a possible clue to bipolar illness.	±
2. Severe tantrums in the context of extreme mood lability, irritability, poor frustration tolerance, and aggression are quite typical of the earliest presentations of bipolar disorder, but can also occur to a lesser extent and severity in ADHD (Luckenbaugh et al 2006; Figure 67.2).	++
3. Brief or extended periods of mood	

elevation, along with decreased need for sleep, are among the strongest early differentiators of children with a prepubertal on of bipolar disorder from children with ADHD (Figure 67.2). ++

4. A homicidal threat toward the mother or a threat to jump out of a car with suicidal intent are also highly consistent with a bipolar diagnosis and inconsistent with that of ADHD, as are the presence of hallucinations or delusions. ++

5. The more classical and discrete periods of depression and hypomania characteristic of most adult presentations may not begin until years 8 or 9 of the child's life, as illustrated in the current case presentation and seen in Fergus et al. (2000). ++

6. Despite the severe dysfunction that this child suffered most of her childhood, eventually including the presence of classic discrete episodes of either manic or depressive symptoms in 1994 and 1995, the diagnosis of bipolar illness was not made and treatment was not initiated until age 9.5. This pattern of long delays in diagnosis and treatment of childhood-onset bipolar disorder is all too common. +++

7. The mood stabilizer valproic acid with antidepressant augmentation was not effective in maintaining this patient's initial improvement. +

8. It was not until she switched to lithium with thyroid and bupropion augmentation that more marked improvement was observed. This illustrates the principle that lack of adequate response to one mood stabilizer (valproate) is not necessarily indicative of lack of response to another (lithium). ++

9. In many instances, a combination

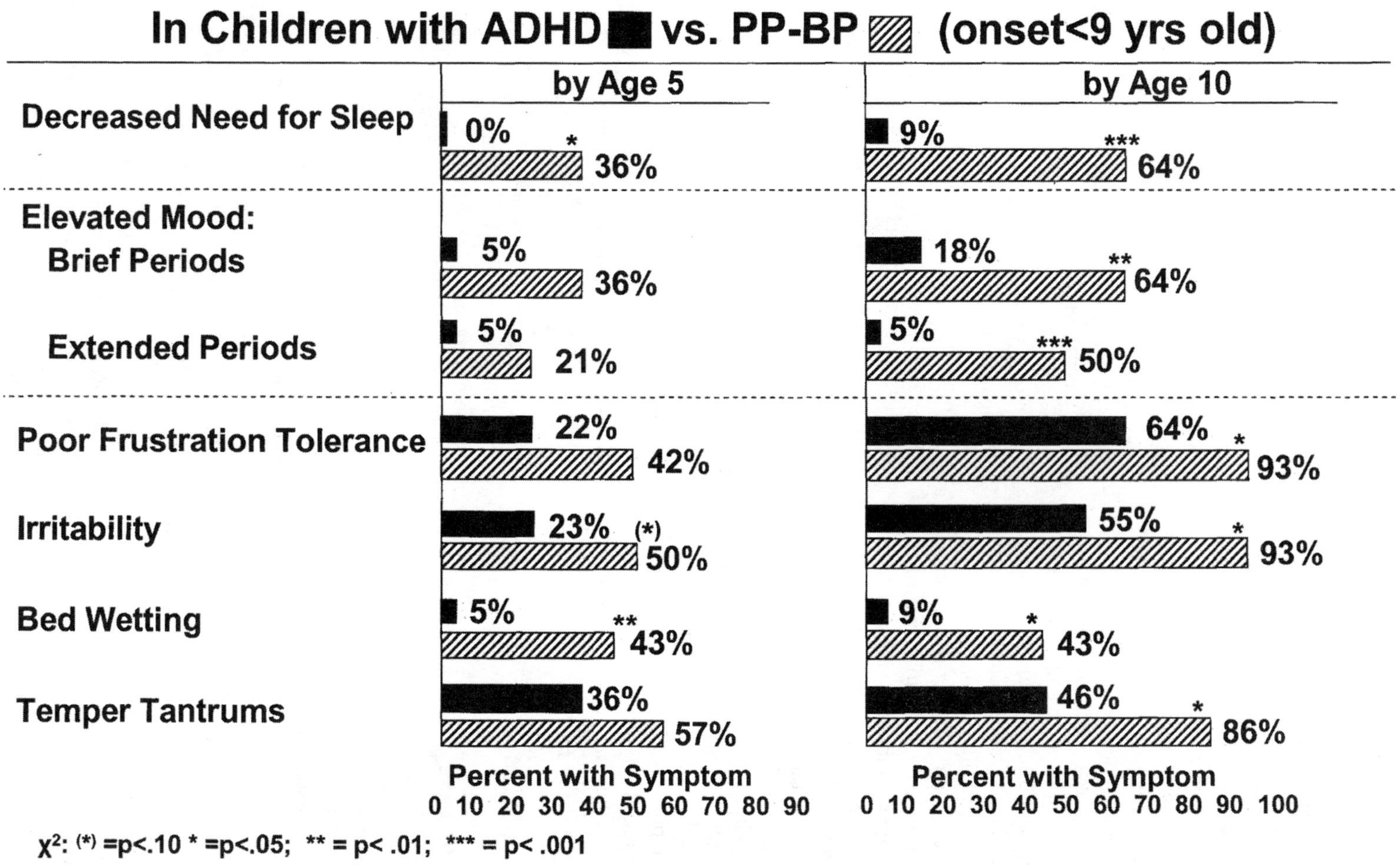

In Children with ADHD ■ vs. PP-BP ▨ (onset<9 yrs old)

by Age 5

Symptom	ADHD	PP-BP
Decreased Need for Sleep	0% (*)	36%
Elevated Mood: Brief Periods	5%	36%
Extended Periods	5%	21%
Poor Frustration Tolerance	22%	42%
Irritability	23% (*)	50%
Bed Wetting	5% (**)	43%
Temper Tantrums	36%	57%

Percent with Symptom
0 10 20 30 40 50 60 70 80 90

by Age 10

Symptom	ADHD	PP-BP
Decreased Need for Sleep	9% (***)	64%
Elevated Mood: Brief Periods	18% (**)	64%
Extended Periods	5% (***)	50%
Poor Frustration Tolerance	64% (*)	93%
Irritability	55% (*)	93%
Bed Wetting	9% (*)	43%
Temper Tantrums	46% (*)	86%

Percent with Symptom
0 10 20 30 40 50 60 70 80 90 100

χ²: (*) =p<.10 * =p<.05; ** = p<.01; *** = p<.001

Figure 67.2 Differential incidence of symptoms reported retrospectively in each year by parents of children (average age 11) diagnosed with prepubertal onset bipolar disorder (PP-BP) versus attention deficit hyperactivity disorder (ADHD) by Findling and associates at Case Western Reserve Hospital in Cleveland using the K-SADs interview of both parents and the children. The percentage of children having symptoms of moderate or greater severity (dysfunction) cumulatively by age 5 and by age 10 are illustrated. Decreased sleep and periods of elevated mood are highly differential, while other symptoms listed were only relative differentiators. The typical ADHD symptoms of hyperactivity, inattention, and impulsivity were virtually identical in both groups.

of two mood stabilizers may be required. ++

10. In adults, thyroid augmentation is often helpful in potentiating response to traditional antidepressant compounds. It has also been reported in the literature that T_3 (25 to 37.5 µg/day) may improve not only mood on lithium, but also cognition. Whether these observations will prove consistent in children remains to be seen. +

11. The addition of omega-3 fatty acids stems from the positive reports of efficacy reviewed in Chapter 60. The confound of initiating this agent and several other pharmacological changes in a similar time frame makes it difficult to determine which of these agents was most critical to the patient's remission. The low risk and benign side effects profile make omega-3 fatty acids particularly appealing for children, even in the absence of systematic data on efficacy in children. 1 to 2 gms/ day doses are probably preferable to higher doses. +

12. While the academic question noted above as to which were the critical elements for the child's response remains unanswered, the youngster and her family were extremely delighted with the virtual cessation of what had been a disabling bipolar illness course. Therefore they were not interested in more definitively answering the question with sequential discontinuation trials that might lead to a simplified regimen but could also be associated with illness exacerbation. ++

13. Acquiring a full remission often requires a substantial series of sequential clinical trials to establish an optimal treatment regimen. ++

14. Clinical trials, such as those of val-

proate and others in this case, although not associated with very sustained improvement, can nonetheless be considered worthwhile because of the information gleaned for the patient and her family (i.e., one can view it as positive information about a negative response, so that other strategies could be considered and initiated in the future as successfully done here). ++

15. A positive family history of bipolar illness on one or both sides of the parents' families is not unusual in such instances of very early onset bipolar illness. This should trigger earlier consideration of this diagnosis and, if verified, early treatment. +++

16. If such children are first seen in a primary care setting, the family history and a presenting kiddie LCM should help the practitioner arrive at the correct diagnosis. ++

17. The presence of symptoms noted in principles 1 to 5 above should further alert families and physicians to the likelihood that a child may not just have ADHD, requiring stimulants alone, but bipolar disorder plus comorbid ADHD, where mood stabilizers are required prior to the use of stimulants (if needed at all for residual ADHD symptoms). ++

TAKE-HOME MESSAGE

No matter how severe, protracted, and apparently treatment resistant a child or adult's affective disorder appears, one should not give up hope that marked improvement can still be achieved. In the study of Birmaher et al. (2006), it took more than 2 1/2 years before those with bipolar disorder NOS presentations remitted, whereas those with bipolar I and II illness reached remission faster (in less than 1 year).

68

Nimodipine Treatment of an Adolescent With Ultradian Cycling Bipolar Affective Illness: Some Practical Treatment Principles for Parents of Children With Bipolar Illness

CASE HISTORY

Exacerbation of Mania by Antidepressants and Panrefractoriness to Standard Adult Agents

In preschool, the patient illustrated in the life chart (Figure 68.1; Davanzo, Krah, Kleiner, & McCracken, 1999) was described as aggressive and cruel to animals. He was also noted to have difficulties learning to read and was diagnosed as dyslexic (Figure 68.1). At the age of 6 he was diagnosed with ADHD and treated with methylphenidate for a period of 9 months (Figure 68.1, right), followed by dextroamphetamine for a period of 14 months. On stimulants he continued to experience difficulty concentrating and developed noticeable rebound, rapid speech, and occasional stomachache.

In January 1991, at age 9, he was diagnosed with chronic fatigue syndrome (likely a first depression) by his pediatrician and treated for symptoms of depression a year later with fluox-

etine 20 mg/day for a period of 2 weeks. After 10 days on fluoxetine, the patient became acutely manic, requiring his first inpatient psychiatric admission in October 1992, at the age of 10.

At that time, he presented with severe agitation and dyscontrol and was diagnosed with bipolar disorder and ADHD. After 3 weeks, he was discharged on lithium and clonidine. In March 1993, at the age of 10 years, 7 months, he had a second manic episode. He was treated with adjunctive neuroleptics as an outpatient for approximately 8 months, in addition to lithium and clonidine in adjusted doses. During this episode, he suffered from intermittent periods of depression (e.g., lack of energy, wanting to watch TV all day), anhedonia, melancholia, and lack of appetite, lasting 2 to 3 months and remitting spontaneously.

He was hospitalized for a second time in November 1993 at age 11, with the diagnosis of bipolar I disorder, most recent episode manic, with psychotic features, and rapid cycling. This (his third) manic episode manifested with severe

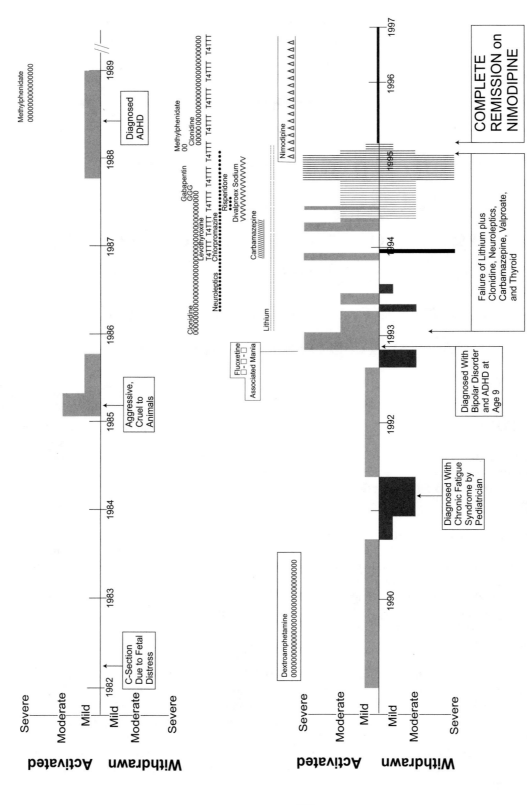

Figure 68.1 Mood stabilization with nimodipine in an adolescent with bipolar ultradian cycling illness. The life chart shows: (1) a poor response to stimulants (age 7–8, for a presumptive diagnosis of ADHD); (2) a fluoxetine-related switch into mania (at age 11 after two major depressions); (3) inadequate response to lithium, plus adjunctive neuroleptics, carbamazepine, divalproex sodium, gabapentin, levothyroxine, and clonidine (age 11–13, for now clearly evident bipolar illness); and finally (4) an excellent response to the nimodipine (age 14–15, for ultradian cycling that began at age 13).

irritability, cruelty to animals, impulsivity (crossing the street without looking), grandiosity (believing nothing could happen to him), hypersexuality (increased masturbation), suicidal ideation, and abnormal perceptions (reports of seeing a monster in his room).

Daily behaviors charted by staff showed an alternating pattern of lethargy, introversion, and depressed mood in the mornings, followed by hypertalkativeness, poor impulse control, agitation and irritability, and suicidality at bedtime, almost on a daily basis. Carbamazepine was started and titrated to a level of 8 µg/dl. Decreased suicidal ideation, irritability, and overall mood swings were documented after 2 weeks. In addition to medication, the patient received weekly individual psychotherapy and parent training.

Four months later, in March 1994, despite compliance with lithium and carbamazepine, the patient was readmitted to the hospital. He appeared manic and reported depressed mood with suicidal ideation, as well as visual and auditory command hallucinations. Carbamazepine was switched to divalproex sodium, and a therapeutic level of 93 µg/dl was achieved after 10 days. By the third week of treatment he became less pressured in speech, more redirectable, and less hyperactive and irritable. He voiced no suicidal ideation and was discharged on lithium carbonate, divalproex sodium, levothyroxine (T$_4$), and clonidine.

The patient remained in remission for approximately 2 months but was soon readmitted to the hospital for a fourth time in a manic psychotic state. His lithium level was 0.8 mm and his valproate level was 124 µg/dl (i.e., the normal range for lithium and normal to high range for valproate). Standard chemistry laboratory values were normal. The lithium dosage was increased, and chlorpromazine was added, resulting in partial resolution of symptoms. He was discharged on chlorpromazine, divalproex sodium, levothyroxine, lithium, and clonidine. On this regimen he gained weight and developed an intention tremor in both hands. He was reported to have low energy and difficulty walking.

One month later he was noted to be "more creative, fearful and hyperactive," and had hit a peer in school. The patient was unable to tolerate an increase in levothyroxine (T$_4$) and chlorpromazine or clonazepam due to the intolerable side effects of tachycardia, heat intolerance, and sweating. He also failed trials of risperidone and gabapentin due to side effects (Figure 68.1, bottom row, right).

Inpatient Observations: Response to Nimodipine

The patient was admitted in a manic state, intermittently depressed and agitated. Daily behaviors charted by staff revealed a chaotic pattern of introversion, depressed mood, and suicidality interspersed with periods of hypertalkativeness, hypomania, poor impulse control, agitation, and severe irritability. These shifts occurred within 24-hour periods and therefore were considered to satisfy criteria for an ultradian cycling type of bipolar affective illness (Kramlinger & Post, 1996).

After written informed parental consent, nimodipine was started at 30 mg at bedtime. The drug was ultimately titrated up to 60 mg orally three times daily over a period of 12 days, with daily monitoring of blood pressure and heart rate. The patient entered the trial taking lithium 450 mg twice daily, levothyroxine 200 µg/day, and chlorpromazine 25 mg twice daily. These medications were held constant, except for lithium, which was decreased by half the dose on Day 10, and discontinued on Day 13. By Day 3, the patient showed decreased severity of depression, although he continued to experience repeated, rapid, and clinically significant changes of mood.

Nimodipine was increased to 30 mg three times daily on Day 4. On Day 6, although still manic, the patient slept well for the first time in months, followed by two days of hypersomnia and sedation. On Day 9 the patient's mood stabilized. His nimodipine dosage was 30 mg twice daily and 60 mg at bedtime. He reported "feeling better than ever before in his life." He appeared calm and participated appropriately in ward activities. On Days 9 through 12 he was generally euthymic.

Several days later, an attempt was made to taper levothyroxine, which resulted in increased hyperactivity. This was attributed to comorbid ADHD, and methylphenidate was initiated. By discharge on Day 18, the patient's mood remained stable, with no evidence of cycling for nine days. He was discharged on the following medications: nimodipine 60 mg three times daily, levothyroxine 200 μg every morning, methylphenidate 10 mg twice daily, and chlorpromazine 25 mg twice daily. One month after discharge, clonidine was substituted for methylphenidate due to the development of persistent motor tics on methylphenidate.

The patient remained in remission for three years and had not required hospitalization from 1995 through 2005. He remains compliant with medication treatment and denies significant side effects. In the spring of 1998 when his nimodipine dosage was reduced from 180 mg/day to 150 mg/day, he developed signs of hypomania, prompting a return to the original dose.

This patient illustrates a response to the L-type calcium channel blocker nimodipine in combination with T_4, methylphenidate, and chlorpromazine when many other mood stabilizer regimens had failed. Illness exacerbation with fluoxetine (1992) and lack of adequate response to stimulants until after the mood was stabilized are not unusual. Other dihydropyridine calcium channel blockers such as isradipine and amlodipine may also be effective, but not at all well studied. Amlodipine is the easiest of the dihydropyridines to use because of its long half-life allowing once daily dosing, but we are not aware of published cases suggesting its efficacy.

PRINCIPLES OF THE CASE	STRENGTH OF EVIDENCE

1. Extremes of irritability, aggressiveness, and poor frustration tolerance are often among the symptoms of childhood-onset bipolar illness, as indicated in Figure 68.1 (1985), but they do not discriminate the disorder from ADHD in the first years of life as well as decreased need for sleep and brief and extended periods of mood elevation (Figure 67.2).   ++

2. It is not uncommon for individuals with bipolar illness to be diagnosed with ADHD and then treated unsuccessfully as this individual was, with stimulants such as methylphenidate and dextroamphetamine. Luckily, this patient did not experience major exacerbations of his illness from these agents, as do some bipolar children given these drugs without being cotreated with a mood stabilizer.   ++

3. Prolonged unsuccessful treatment with a stimulant is not an uncommon history in a child with bipolar disorder (as in this case for 23 months without a good effect). When these drugs are ineffective (or worse), they should be carefully monitored and rapidly abandoned (or avoided altogether if possible) until after mood is stabilized.   +++

4. Many child psychiatry experts in bipolar disorders recommend not continuing more than about 2 weeks with a stimulant if an inadequate response is observed. Positive responses to stimulants occur rapidly in the first day or two of use so that months of ineffective treatment should be relatively easy to avoid. More problematic to evaluate would be when stimulants help the comorbid ADHD symptoms but do nothing for the other aspects of bipolar illness that impair functioning. This occurrence should lead to the rapid consideration of adding a mood stabilizer or atypical antipsychotic rather than changing stimulants or pushing their dose higher.   ++

5. The 1990 diagnosis of chronic fa-

tigue syndrome in this child is also typical of many children with bipolar disorder, who will be given almost any psychiatric or medical diagnosis instead of bipolar illness. Until recently, bipolar disorder had been a diagnosis of exclusion and last resort in children. Instead, especially in children at high risk by virtue of a positive family history, the diagnosis should be actively looked for and appropriately ruled in or out.   +

6. This patient's major depression in 1992 at age 10, treated with fluoxetine, resulted in a switch into full-blown mania. This switching on antidepressants occurs in about 35% of prepubertal-onset major depression or dysphoria when treated with antidepressants. A much higher switch rate occurs in depressed children with a bipolar disorder, such that some investigators recommend lamotrigine in such instances (of course with an exquisitely low and slow dose titration to reduce the risk of serious rash).   ++

7. The failure to respond to lithium, carbamazepine, and divalproex sodium can occur in about 50% of instances with each drug individually in adults and children.   ++

8. However, it is quite unusual that a patient such as this would fail to respond to combination therapy with all three agents, particularly with adjunctive use of typical and atypical antipsychotic agents, thyroid potentiation, clonidine, and ultimately, the addition of gabapentin.   ±

9. The stable remission observed when the dihydropyridine calcium channel blocker nimodipine was substituted for lithium and valproate (with the continuation of the previously unsuccessful clonidine and T_4) is both dramatic and

rare (since this class of agents is very infrequently used for bipolar illness, even in adults). Thus, the generality of this type of response to other youngsters with the illness is not known.   ±

10. The dihydropyridine calcium channel blockers, such as nimodipine, isradipine, and amlodipine, are used for vasodilation and primarily for elevated blood pressures and are thus rarely given to children, although a modicum of data support their use in some treatment-refractory bipolar adults (Chapters 32 and 33).   ++

11. The dihydropyridine type of calcium channel blocker may have better antidepressant and mood-stabilizing properties than the closely related phenylalkylamine calcium channel blocker·verapamil (see Chapter 32).   +

12. In our studies in adults, nimodipine was documented to be effective (usually in double-blind off-on-off-on designs) in about 30% of treatment-resistant adults, although usually the response was not complete and other adjunctive agents were required.   ++

13. Several of these responsive patients also responded to another related dihydropyridine, isradipine, but not to the phenylalkylamine verapamil, suggesting different effects on mood and behavior of these two subclasses of L-type calcium channel blockers (Chapter 33).   ++

14. Nimodipine is FDA approved only for subarachnoid hemorrhage and is thus inordinately expensive (about $20,000–30,000 per year) at the moderate to high doses required. The other dihydropyridines that are approved for treatment of blood pressure are less expensive, and

may be able to substitute for nimodipine, as seen in several individuals
in double-blind crossover trials.   +

15. Amlodipine has a long half-life, allowing easy use and once-daily
dosing (in contrast to multiple
doses required with isradipine and
nimodipine). Whether it will have
the same effects as nimodipine has
not been systematically tested.   ±

16. In the same vein, given the excellent side effects profile of aripiprazole in adults with schizophrenia
and schizoaffective illness (about
equivalent to placebo), and two
positive studies in mania (one
showing better efficacy than placebo and one better efficacy than
haloperidol), we would suggest
consideration of the use of this or
other atypical antipsychotics prior
to resorting to the dihydropyridines
discussed above.   ++

17. Parenthetically, aripiprazole has
just begun to be studied in childhood bipolar disorder with promising results (Findling et al., unpublished data). Drugs such as this
with little danger of serious side effects in adults would be excellent
drugs to consider for use in early intervention studies for children at
high risk of an affective disorder because of one or two parents (or
sides of family) with bipolar illness. ++

TWELVE PRELIMINARY DIAGNOSTIC AND TREATMENT SUGGESTIONS FOR PARENTS WITH CHILDREN WHO LIKELY HAVE BIPOLAR I, II, OR NOS DISORDER (modified from the *Bipolar Network News* newsletter, vol 5, issue 2, pg 6)

The diagnostic controversies involved in the
presentation of childhood bipolar illness and the
disagreements about diagnostic thresholds make
it particularly important for parents to have an
approximate set of guidelines from which they
may begin to pursue treatment options. The
book *The Bipolar Child*, by Papolos and Papolos (1999) is available, as are books by Findling, Kowatch, and Post (2002), Geller and
Delbello (2003), and Birmaher (2004). A new
edition of the Findling et al book will be published by the APA Press, Inc. and will include
Dr. Mary Fristadt who is an expert on the psychotherapeutic approaches to the illness. Kowatch et al (2005) presented consensus guidelines for children with BP I disorder only
because so little evidence was available for
those with BP II or NOS.

We have decided to make a series of preliminary suggestions and recommendations based
on the minimal evidence available to date in the
field. We acknowledge that these are only the
roughest outlines and should rapidly be sup-
planted by those more empirically based as further studies are completed and new information
is gained from the various NIMH and other research initiatives in children.

It should also be stated from the outset that
the following recommendations are only preliminary views drawn from a group of individual
investigators, each of whom agrees with the
general principles as stated, but many of whom
would have different approaches in different patients in their own clinical practices. In addition,
they do not represent the views of many others
in the field who believe the syndrome is over-
diagnosed and would advise more conservative
approaches while awaiting a more systematic
database upon which to build such recommendations. They do not represent the views of the
NIMH or the guidelines of any other group or
agency. We appreciate the input and edification
of Drs. Kiki Chang (Stanford), Robert Kowatch
and Melissa DelBello (Cincinnati), Robert Findling (Cleveland), and Barbara Geller (St.
Louis), who helped us write an editorial about
the diagnosis of bipolar disorder in children
(Post et al., 2004) and continue to contribute
their wisdom.

Whether or not there is a positive history of
bipolar illness on one or both sides of the fam-

ily, one should be open to the possibility that a child or your child does (or does not) have bipolar illness. Moreover childhood onset bipolar illness is often associated with multiple other co-existing (comorbid) diagnoses such as ADHD, oppositional defiant disorder, school phobia, and other anxiety disorder diagnoses; and in adolescence, with conduct and eating disorders and alcohol and substance abuse. These and the differing ages of children and changes in symptom severity and quality as a function of course of illness further complicate the diagnostic process.

1. A critical element in approaching your child's illness is to not get discouraged. As frustrating as it might be, one should note that the child in this chapter and in Chapter 67 are examples of remissions achieved, even after very long and difficult courses of childhood-onset bipolar illness. One should remain hopeful. Moreover, no matter how severe, frustrating, or apparently willful your child's behavior appears, try to view it as part of the symptoms of a bipolar-like illness and out of the child's volitional control.

2. The earliest presentations of the illness may involve marked mood lability, irritability, aggression, poor frustration tolerance, and prolonged tantrums. Early robust differentiators of prepubertal-onset bipolar disorder from ADHD include decreased sleep and a period of brief or extended mood elevation(see Figure 67.2). Only later (after age 5) will increased somatic complaints (body aches, pains, and feeling ill), decreased appetite, periods of sadness, suicidal thoughts, and inappropriate sexual behavior begin to occur, and then these will help distinguish bipolar illness from ADHD as well (Luckenbaugh, Findling, Leverich, Pizzarello, & Post, 2006). However, the typical symptoms of ADHD such as hyperactivity, impulsivity, inattention, and distractability do not differentiate prepubertal onset bipolar disorder from ADHD, particularly since ADHD is highly comorbid with the earliest onsets of bipolar disorder. Hallucinations or delusions in a very young child clearly differentiate and are much more likely associated with bipolar disorder than childhood onset schizophrenia.

3. Chart the course of your child's mood swings on a daily basis, preferably in a systematic graphic format. One format of a systematic Kiddie Life Chart is available on the Internet at www.bipolarnews.org and is also published in Leverich and Post (1998) and in Appendix 3. This or some other daily assessment tool will be essential from several perspectives: (1) it will be extremely helpful in arriving at the appropriate diagnosis based on longitudinal observations; 2) it will track the symptomatic presentation of the illness, which will help engender more effective treatment efforts from professionals; and 3) it will help you and clinicians develop optimal treatment approaches, by showing even small consistent changes with treatment, and facilitate consultation if needed. Other hints about diagnosis are in Chapter 67.

4. If the diagnosis is bipolar illness (even BP NOS where very rapid mood fluctuations within a day may occur), initiate treatment with mood stabilizers or an atypical antipsychotic rather than antidepressants or stimulants (Kowatch et al., 2000, 2005). Kowatch found in an open randomized study that lithium, carbamazepine, and valproate are each effective in approximately 40–50% of children with early-onset bipolar mania (average age about 12). Because these drugs are accepted and effective mood stabilizers in adult illness, they likely will have long-term efficacy in preventing both manic and depressive episodes in children and adolescents as well (based on indirect inferences from the modicum of acute antimanic efficacy data in this age group). The details of the side effects profiles and potential range of efficacy of these well-accepted mood stabilizers for adults are readily available and discussed in detail elsewhere. Antidepressants and stimulants may exacerbate or destabilize the illness if used without a mood stabilizer (see 1992 in Figure 68.1).

5. If one mood stabilizer is not effective, a second mood stabilizer or atypical antipsychotic may be tried as an alternative or may be added to the regimen. If this is not effective, a revision of the mood stabilizer-atypical regimen should be considered, or a third drug added.

6. All of the drugs currently being evaluated as potential mood stabilizers are in a position

similar to carbamazepine in its first 30 years of
use in adult-onset bipolar illness, in that it was
FDA approved for use as an anticonvulsant in
patients with epilepsy or in those with trigeminal neuralgia, but not for bipolar illness. Moreover, no drugs are as yet approved specifically
for childhood-onset bipolar illness (Kowatch et
al., 2005). Use of alternative drugs should generally be explored after the more traditional options of lithium, carbamazepine-ER, or valproate and the atypical antipsychotics have been
tried.

If residual manic or psychotic symptoms remain after otherwise partial efficacy with one or
more mood stabilizers in combination, one could
consider augmenting with one of the newer
atypical antipsychotics that do not require
weekly blood monitoring, as opposed to clozapine, which does require intensive (weekly)
monitoring. These drugs, which include risperidone, olanzapine, and quetiapine, may not be
quite as benign in children and adolescents as
originally conceptualized in adults because substantial degrees of weight gain (especially on
clozapine and olanzapine) and, more rarely, a
moderate amount of extrapyramidal motor side
effects such as parkinsonism (tremor, rigidity,
slowness, or masked faces) or akathisia (need
to move one's legs) can occur. In contrast, the
atypical antipsychotics ziprasidone and aripiprazole may be somewhat better tolerated, and less
prone to weight gain and related problems. If
aripiprazole is administered, it should be started
at a very low dose (such as 2.5 mg/day) and
titrated upward (as a function of age) to target
doses ranging from 5 mg/day in the very young
to 8–10 mg/day in older children. Another
newly approved add-on treatment for refractory
epilepsy is topiramate. Open studies with add-
on topiramate in adults not adequately responsive to their previous regimen suggest possible
mood-stabilizing effects of this agent in augmentation. It is also associated with moderate
degrees of weight loss. It has no antimanic efficacy in monotherapy in adults, although the one
study conducted in adolescents was positive on
some measures (Chapter 29). Acute antidepressant effects in adults were not consistently observed, but were equal to those of bupropion in

one study. Topiramate may also be useful in migraine prevention and the treatment of bulimia,
PTSD, and alcohol and cocaine abuse, although
there are few studies in youngsters with bipolar
disorder.

The potential for weight loss can be a positive side effect of topiramate for some individuals, and contrasts with some of the currently
available atypical antipsychotics and, to some
extent, lithium and valproate. This side effect
may give topiramate, even with unproven efficacy in affective illness in either adults or children, a rationale for the patient with drug-
related weight gain.

A problematic side effect of this agent in
some 5–10% of patients is speech or word-finding difficulties, which may occur more often in
patients already on complex medication regimens and if topiramate is added rapidly or used
in high doses. Thus, a conservative regimen for
this agent is to start with one 25-mg pill per day
and increase the dose by one pill on a weekly
basis in an attempt to avoid confusion and memory problems. Zonisamide may be an alternative
to topiramate with the potential for positive effects on mania, depression, sleep, and weight
loss. Another approach to limiting weight gain
and the potential for type 2 diabetes on atypicals
is metformin with doses starting at 850mg/day
and increasing to 2550mg/day, possibly as am-
plified with sibutramine (Baptista et al., 2006;
Henderson et al., 2005; Uzcategui et al., 2007).

Oxcarbazepine, with its lower potential for
serious side effects (except low serum sodium)
and drug-drug interactions, may be an alternative to carbamazepine, but not as convenient for
once-nightly dosing as the long acting preparation of carbamazepine sold as Equetro. Moreover, Wagner et al. (2006) found equal efficacy
of oxcarbazepine and placebo in childhood onset mania, Carbamazepine may be more effective in those with more severe mania at baseline
and oxcarbazepine in less severe illness.

Among the newer anticonvulsants, gabapentin has a good safety profile in adults, but its
efficacy in controlled studies of adult mania and
cycling did not exceed that of placebo (Chapter
26). Formal studies in pediatric populations of
patients with mood dysregulation remain to be

performed. There are anecdotal reports that gabapentin may, at times, exacerbate dyscontrol symptoms in children particularly in those with preexisting brain damage, but its potential effects on anxiety, social phobia, and depressed mood, as well as in chronic pain syndromes when used as an adjunctive agent deserves further exploration. Although in our larger NIMH study of 6 weeks of monotherapy gabapentin response did not exceed that of placebo, those who did have a good to excellent response were younger adults with shorter durations of illness.

Another unproven but promising class of agents for adult bipolar illness are the dihydropyridine L-type calcium channel blockers (Chapters 32 and 33), which are used primarily for high blood pressure, arrhythmias, subarachnoid hemorrhage, and migraine. These agents include nimodipine, isradipine, and amlodipine. Amlodipine has a longer half-life than either nimodipine or isradipine and is suitable for single nighttime dosing, but its effectiveness in bipolar disorder has not be explored. The case reported here (Davanzo et al., 1999) shows an excellent response to nimodipine in an adolescent bipolar patient, and this whole class of agents (which may have a more benign side effects profile than lithium) deserves further investigation and controlled trials in children and adolescents with bipolar-like syndromes.

The role of omega-3 fatty acids is also beginning to be studied in adults with unipolar and bipolar illness (Chapter 60). Further clinical trials in larger numbers of adult subjects are exploring this promising approach, which has few serious side effects. Systematic data on efficacy in children are not yet available, beyond ambiguous case reports such as that in Chapter 67.

Another anticonvulsant is lamotrigine. Initially lamotrigine was not recommended by the FDA for anyone younger than 16 years of age because of the risks of a severe rash, but is now approved for use in 2 year olds with some seizure subtypes. Lamotrigine is FDA approved for the prevention of depressive, manic and mixed episodes in adults, and its effects in acute depression are promising (Chapter 25). Lamotrigine is associated with an approximately 5–8% risk of a benign rash (red, itchy, and goes away with stopping the drug), but with about 1 in 5,000 cases in adults progressing to a severe and potentially life-threatening type where some of the skin sloughs off called Stevens-Johnson syndrome (SJS) or toxic epidermal necrolysis (TENS). It appears that the risk for this uncommon medical complication is increased with rapid dose increases, a combination of lamotrigine with valproate (which doubles lamotrigine levels), a history of severe rashes on other drugs, and younger age. The incidence of severe rash in children is about 1 in 2,500.

If one were to use this drug in patients below age 16, starting at 12.5 mg every other day and then proceeding exquisitely slowly (after getting good written informed consent from the child and parents) would be prudent. A 2 mg tab is available from drug company representatives, and some epileptologists start with this dose in the youngest children. For the depressed adolescent, this drug may be a good alternative to a traditional mood stabilizer plus an antidepressant, because of its excellent side effects profile (in the absence of rash) of being nonsedating and weight neutral.

7. Additional augmentation of the mood stabilizer or atypical antipsychotic treatment regimen can be targeted to residual symptoms with one of the following options.

If ADHD symptoms remain after optimal mood stabilization has been achieved, augmentation with a psychomotor stimulant may then be considered, such as methylphenidate, amphetamine, or pemoline. The longer acting compounds of this class may simplify use in children. The approval of atomoxetine for ADHD also raises this as a possibility, but we are not aware of studies in bipolar children with comorbid ADHD, and its norepinephrine effects may increase risk of switching (Chapter 40). Three very positive reports of modafinil efficacy for ADHD were presented at the 2005 American Psychiatric Association meeting.

If persistent depressive elements of the syndrome remain particularly severe, one might consider augmentation of the mood stabilizers with the antidepressant bupropion. In addition to the promise of antidepressant effects, bupropion might also target concurrent ADHD symptoms, because one study reported that bupropion and methylphenidate showed equal efficacy on ADHD symptoms in children without comorbid depression (Barrickman et al., 1995).

The utility of adding one of the SSRIs, such as fluoxetine, paroxetine, sertraline, fluvoxamine, and citalopram, also requires further examination. Tricyclic antidepressants should be avoided because of ambiguous efficacy and safety in children and the high lethality in overdose. The SSRIs can be useful for comorbid anxiety, panic, and obsessive-compulsive symptoms, but only as an adjunct to mood stabilizers or atypical antipsychotics.

Thyroid potentiation of an antidepressant or mood-stabilizing regimen is often considered in adults in light of positive effects of T_3 (25–37.5 ìg/day) in studies independent of whether or not there are abnormalities in thyroid function; no systematic efficacy data exist in children, however.

8. We suggest a focused search for a compatible doctor who is willing to be sympathetic, exploratory, and creative in his or her treatment approaches, and willing to listen to you and the nature of your child's side effects and responses to treatment or initial lack thereof. This doctor could be an adult psychiatrist specializing in psychopharmacology, if an appropriate child psychiatrist cannot be easily located. Adult and pediatric neurologists may also be very familiar with a wide range of the drugs potentially needed. As with adult-onset bipolar illness, where talk therapy alone does not appear sufficient, individual or family treatment may be very helpful in early-onset bipolar illness, but, almost universally, medications are required as well. As with any medical illness, you should feel free to obtain a second opinion. If you and your only available physician disagree about whether your child has bipolar disorder, ask about his or her alternative diagnoses, and press for treatments that will nonetheless address your child's symptomatic presentation. Continue bringing the mood chart of your child's difficulties because this may help in treatment initiation, evaluations, and revisions.

9. If you as a parent have unipolar or bipolar illness, consider making use of your own treatment team for advice, suggestions, and support about your child's treatment, and let your child's doctor know which medications have been particularly helpful for you or other family members, because drug responses often replicate within a family.

10. If you have a child with bipolar illness, request regular child or family sessions with a knowledgeable therapist. Any managed health care system should recognize that this treatment is very much in their as well as your child's long-term best interest, because helping to prevent major difficulties, hospitalizations, and special placements will save money in the long term. Insist that therapy, in addition to psychopharmacological intervention, be endorsed by your insurance company.

11. Finding a support group, with the help of advocacy groups such as the Depression and Bipolar Support Alliance or the National Alliance for the Mentally Ill, may be helpful as well. Some support groups are specifically directed at the problems of children with bipolar illness, and the Child and Adolescent Bipolar Foundation has an interactive Web site at www.cabf.org.

12. Parents may want to consider some approaches to managing your child during difficult times as suggested by Dr. Ross Greene at Massachusetts General Hospital in his book *The Explosive Child* (Greene, 1998, pp. 133–173). He proposes a framework in the form of three "baskets" into which your child's behaviors can be placed during times of conflict between you and your child with bipolar disorder. This is not as simple as it sounds, and you will likely need the help of an experienced psychotherapist.

Basket A, the Safety Basket, would contain a very few behaviors that are not allowed and are not negotiable because they relate to safety, that is, behaviors that could be harmful to your child, other people, animals, or property. For Basket A you are the authority figure who makes the decision about the safety of behaviors. Very few things go in Basket A.

Basket B Greene calls the Compromise Basket, into which behaviors fall that are a high priority, but over which you do not want to induce a meltdown in your child based on your interventions. Basket B provides the opportunity for communication (rationales and altered conceptualizations), negotiation, and compromise between yourself and your child. Greene notes that this may be a very difficult and slowly developing process, however, and not that much would go into Basket B initially. We would add that it is much easier to get to communication and negotiation on more areas of troubling behavior after substantial improvement and more stability have been achieved with medication.

Basket C is the Reduction of Frustration Basket wherein most of your child's behaviors should be placed. In Basket C you ignore the behavior or sidestep or circumvent any intervention around it. Even behaviors you once considered a high priority should initially be dumped into Basket C because they are something that can be put aside, at least for now.

If you actively choose to downgrade a whole host of your child's inappropriate behaviors to Basket C, it is not giving in or showing lack of discipline. Placing as many things as possible initially in this basket recognizes that your child may not have good (or much of any) control over his or her irritability, impulsivity, and frustration tolerance, and it is desirable to avoid as many unnecessary confrontations as possible that may lead to meltdowns. It will ultimately allow you to more readily begin to put a few items in Basket B as improvement in mood stability and communication occurs.

Initially making Basket C huge may be difficult for most parents and requires practice, as well as considerable support from a therapist. Ask yourself about deferring a Basket B behavior for a while and making it a Basket C item. Will it really harm anything if the bedroom is not cleaned up and left a mess for a while longer, or if the child wants to eat under the table instead of at the table?

When you do eventually work on one or two things placed in Basket B, remember that your child may have the equivalent of an emotional learning disability. Papolos and Papolos (1999) emphasize the difficulty these children have with labeling or even recognizing emotions in themselves or other children even more than in adults. New positron emission tomography scan data confirm these deficits at a neurobiological level. You may have to help the child to slowly build such a repertoire of recognizing emotions before reaching the stage wherein they can identify external triggers, label internal states, and verbalize feelings rather than acting on them and reacting to emotional situations.

Be a coach and practice being a coach for the few items placed in Basket B. Imagine two different types of baseball coaches, Coach X and Coach Y described by a knowledgeable psychiatrist colleague. A child in the outfield in a baseball game misses a fly ball, and Coach X screams, "How can you let that keep on happening? If you don't wake up out there and pay attention, you'll cost us the game and you'll never get anywhere. Just concentrate harder!" On the other hand Coach Y says, "This is a common problem. When the ball is hit high and hard (sometimes you can tell by the sound), start running back right away. It is easier to come in for the ball if it looks like it will land short than to run backward if it looks long. Also, if it falls in front of you, that's okay; it will only be a single, not a triple or a home run. Try that out and see if it helps next time." Ask yourself which would be the more helpful approach. As you can imagine, Coach Y will win the day every time. You may need as much practice at being like Coach Y as your child needs practice to begin to view situations differently and respond in a more appropriate fashion.

Children with a learning disability in school need a lot of time, special techniques, practice, and tutoring to begin to deal with, for example, their inability to recognize words or read (dyslexia). Similarly, a child with bipolar illness has a learning disability pertaining to emotional recognition and regulation. With practice, the deficits can be overcome or circumvented. There is evidence that a key structure in emotional regulation, the amygdala, is too small in youngsters with bipolar disorder, but too big in older adults with long-term bipolar illness. This may help with the view that the child with bipolar illness is like the child with cerebral palsy where there are easily seen deficits in motor control, usually based on injury to the parts of the brain controlling motor behavior—the motor cortex and extrapyramidal systems (such as dorsal caudate, globus pallidus, and putamen). This child often cannot run and play with other kids without years of rehabilitation effort.

The child with bipolar illness may have a temporary cerebral palsy of the brain systems likely involved in emotion regulation (amygdala), in social interactions (anterior cingulate), and in holding concepts from long-term memory at the forefront while deciding what actions are appropriate (i.e., working memory, involving the prefrontal cortex). However, with time and appropriate practice and rehabilitation techniques as well as medications, these deficits can be overcome. It is worth reemphasizing that many of the major medications for bipolar illness (lithium, valproate, and antidepressants) increase the production of new neurons (neurogenesis) and cell survival via neurotrophic factors, such as brain-derived neurotrophic factor. Thus,

medications may not only help restore normal behavior, but they could also facilitate the brain's own compensatory and repair mechanisms for some of the deficits underlying bipolar disorder.

TAKE-HOME MESSAGE

Children and adults with apparently even the most treatment-refractory forms of bipolar illnesses should remain hopeful and continue the sequential clinical trial approach with careful longitudinal monitoring of mood and side effects, because ultimate mood stabilization will likely be achieved with the use of a new medication, class of medications, or novel combination approaches, as this individual dramatically illustrates.

Part XVI

CONCLUSION

69

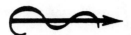

Getting Well and Staying Well: Guidelines for Patients and Families

You may have just perused several chapters in this book and read about patients with severe and recurrent episodes of mania and depression, and feel frightened or anxious about recently receiving the diagnosis of bipolar illness and the implications for your functioning in the future. It is important to emphasize that the overall message of this book is extraordinarily positive about the potential for reaching full mood stabilization and maintaining it. While patients with extremely adverse prior courses of illness are described in many of the chapters, the end result and the message of almost every chapter is that marked improvement or remission can still be achieved, although in some instances this may take a considerable period of time and require many medication revisions.

It is important to begin to address the treatment of this illness from the positive perspective that the glass is half full and that improvement can ultimately be achieved, rather than the perspective that the glass is half empty and periods of disability are likely to occur and recur over the lifetime of an individual with this diagnosis. This attitudinal approach to the illness is of considerable importance to patients and their families. If the illness is approached with some degree of optimism and acceptance and consequent activism in the course of its treatment, the outcome is more likely to be positive. Conversely, if the illness is denied and ignored, complications are much more likely to occur.

With early recognition and treatment, there is a very high likelihood that the illness will not ultimately have a major impact on one's functioning. Thus, if one is dealing with an initial episode or the acute symptoms of a second or third affective episode, the goal should be directed at obtaining help early and aggressively working to achieve symptom remission. Once this has been accomplished in whatever time necessary, the next goal becomes sustaining or maintaining this remission of manic and depressive episodes and symptomatology.

However, while this phase of the illness quiescence would appear to be easier to manage, it is at this juncture that, in our experience, one is in the greatest danger of not achieving the ultimate goal of sustained remission. Some of the danger pertains to the attitude toward the remission itself; it is often associated with a feeling that the illness is at bay, no longer a problem, can be managed readily, and therefore medications are not really necessary. One may begin to feel that will power and motivation will be sufficient to carry the day and prevent untoward consequences from further symptomatology.

This view initially appears reasonable enough, given individuals' return to the apparent safety of feeling that they are back to their usual selves. As weeks or months of wellness then ensue, the idea that the illness is gone appears to be reinforced by each day's additional experience of wellness. Medications that were taken regularly often start to be taken less regularly, and eventually many patients decide to try their luck and see if they can manage without them altogether.

However, this approach and attitude fail to account for the realities of bipolar illness. It is almost invariably recurrent. The patient should know that this is the case, even if the first episode had many unusual extenuating circumstances, such as being triggered by sleep deprivation, long' airplane flights with major time zone shifts, periods of substance abuse, or even prescribed antidepressant medications. One should not feel secure in the notion that if one avoids these apparent precipitating circumstances, the illness will not recur. While it may have been triggered or precipitated by these or other unusual circumstances or psychosocial stresses, even in the absence of these conditions episodes are highly likely to subsequently recur.

So, how should one proceed? We recommend that one use this time of remission to become educated about the illness and to educate friends and family members that maintenance and preventive drug treatment approaches are essential to one's remaining well. We agree that this is often an extremely difficult sell when one is no longer feeling ill (i.e., apparently cured), but the facts are quite different. At the moment there are no cures, only suppression and prevention of symptoms and episodes (Table 69.1). This invariably requires the use of maintenance or preventive medications. The view of the illness is a little like that for blood pressure or hypercholesterolemia, both of which one of the authors (RMP) has and each require two different medications in combination to control. Everyone knows what will happen if I stop these drugs; my hypertension and high cholesterol will return making me more vulnerable to another heart attack. It would not happen right away, but likely would in the near future. So bipolar illness in remission is like the status of these two conditions. Do I now have high blood pressure and cholesterol? No, but I do have the condition (illness), and it will return if I am silly enough to try and prove it to myself again. Even if I didn't have a heart attack, the new level of high blood pressure might damage my kidneys and achieve a new set point that would make it forever more difficult to control. The analogies to well controlled bipolar are obvious, but somehow are more difficult for people to apply to themselves.

How do we really be so sure that medications are absolutely required? The clinical experiment has already been conducted tens of thousands of times, and the answer is quite clear. In the middle of the last century there were extensive attempts to treat bipolar illness intensively without medications. Even when patients entered the most prestigious hospitals, with the best programs of psychotherapy, with family and social support, the illness continued to recur and inflict severe damage on individuals and their families. This was the repeated experience in places like Chestnut Lodge in Rockville, Maryland, the Institute of Living in Hartford, Connecticut, the Yale Psychiatric Research Institute in New Haven, Connecticut, the Menninger Clinic in Topeka, Kansas, and so on.

Regardless of the intensity or duration of treatment, motivation of the individual, expertise of the staff and hospital, psychoanalytic other conceptual psychotherapeutic approaches to the illness, the overall outcome was disappointingly the same. The illness invariably recurred and in many instances progressively worsened. There did not appear to be much difference in the frequency or severity of episodes compared with baseline, or that expected from observations in patients with the illness and no treatment at all.

Thomas Sczaz wrote about the "myth of mental illness." Seymour Kety countered the entire book with the statement that it is the only

Table 69.1 *Types of Vulnerability to Bipolar Illness*

A. *Constant*
   I. Genetic endowment (multiple SNPs)
   II. Perinatal insults → lifelong altered set points
B. *Interactive*
   Genetic × environmental impact on gene expression
C. *Progressive increases*
   III. Stress sensitization
   IV. Episode sensitization
   V. Substance abuse sensitization

Vulnerability does not dissipate; it may accumulate.

myth he knows with a genetic vulnerability. Moreover, when Dr. Sczaz acted on his beliefs, which were contrary to those of the general medical community, and took a patient off lithium maintenance treatment and the patient subsequently committed suicide, a large monetary settlement was offered in lieu of the case going to a jury trial for malpractice. The dangers of relapse or worse are very real, even when the illness is managed by "true believers" of the opposite persuasion.

Thus, if it is at all possible, try to adopt a positive and proactive attitude about the long-term treatment of the illness. With careful monitoring and good consistent treatment, the illness can have a relatively minor impact on one's life, much like that in other chronic medical illnesses such as diabetes or epilepsy when they are well controlled.

The diabetes example is particularly relevant because, with this life-threatening medical illness, the patient can play a major role in assisting the physician to keep it under control as closely as possible. Patients learn how to assess their glucose levels and change their medication accordingly, as recommended by their physicians. In the end, this prevents the early onset of a host of medical problems associated with poorly controlled blood sugar levels, including retinal injury, heart attack, kidney dysfunction, and painful neurological and vascular compromise of the legs, sometimes requiring amputation. Similarly, careful monitoring of both medication and side effects can be a key factor in keeping bipolar illness under optimal control and avoiding many problems occurring secondary to it.

There is a consistent and widely replicated literature demonstrating that people with bipolar illness are overrepresented among writers, poets, and other occupations needing high levels of creativity. Many of our most famous composers, artists, and successful businesspersons have struggled with bipolar illness as well. This is not in any way to minimize the suffering that can occur with this illness, but only to emphasize that, in many instances, the obstacles it presents can be overcome and one can lead a rich, successful, and creative life.

At the same time, if bipolar illness symptoms are ignored and major episodes accumulate, with their toll on family, friends, employment opportunities, and associated social and economic supports, the results can be devastating. All too disappointingly, many individuals with bipolar illness are overrepresented among those who are homeless or incarcerated in our penal system rather than in active treatment. Dave Miklowitz's (2002) primer, *The Bipolar Disorder Survival Guide: What You and Your Family Need to Know*, has many useful and practical approaches to assist in the process of generating an active, positive approach to bipolar illness, and minimize its impact on the individual, family, and related support systems.

It is often crucial to have a very active two-way partnership between family or friends and the individual patient, as well as the partnership of clinicians and physicians with the patient against the illness. Friends and family can play a key role in encouraging the depressed patient to seek treatment and stay with it until it is successful, and assist in the even more difficult task of encouraging a hypomanic or manic patient to seek and stay in treatment.

If a patient has undergone repeated experiences of escalating into full-blown hypomania or mania and losing insight into need for treatment, it might be useful for the patient to work out (in a nonmanic state) specific mechanisms with supporters, providing advance directives for how the patient wishes to be coaxed or, at the other end of the continuum, forced into treatment and committed for hospitalization. Building these kinds of family and social supports when the patient is relatively stable may be invaluable in preventing some of the more dire consequences of full-blown episodes should they recur.

Such agreements in advance may also be critical in dealing with the specific characteristics of both depressive and manic phases of the illness, which inherently conspire to prevent such helpful contact. In the depressed phase, patients not only do not seek contact and support but withdraw from it and often have a sense of guilt and hopelessness about their current circumstances that render them immobile and unable even to be open to the possibility of support from others. Similarly, the manic phase of the illness is optimally designed to alienate friends, family members, employers, and even hospital staff, should the manic individual be lucky enough to understand the need for hospitalization or be committed involuntarily.

As outlined by Janowsky and Davis in their classic article "Playing the Manic Game," a manic individual often has unusual insight into the most vulnerable areas of others' psyches and is incredibly adept at exploiting staff members' weakest and most raw points, and generally raising the level of havoc in almost any treatment system. Adding to this argumentative, in-your-face, interpersonal insensitivity is a unique knack for a variety of other adverse consequences, including overspending (sometimes to

the point of bankruptcy), getting oneself fired, dissolving an otherwise healthy and successful marriage, and engaging in substance abuse and indiscreet sexual encounters that could even result in the acquisition of lethal illness such as AIDS.

Given this range from potential minor discomfts to catastrophic consequences, one can easily see the rationale for the repeated emphasis throughout virtually every chapter in this volume for both early symptomatic intervention and, most crucially, early institution and long-term maintenance of pharmacoprophylaxis (continuous drug treatment that prevents episodes). Yet it is all too common that the individual and family system not only miss these opportunities but fail to enact and stick with a treatment plan once it has begun to be developed.

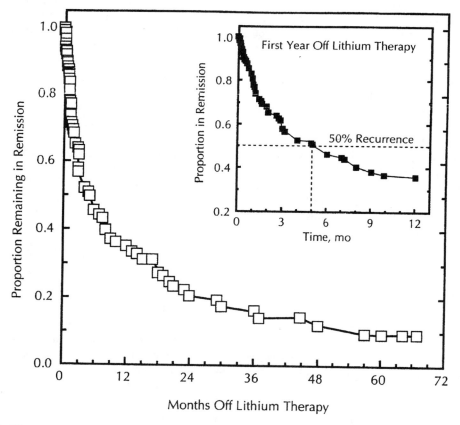

Figure 69.1 Ninety percent of patients relapse after stopping effective lithium treatment; fifty percent relapse in the first five months (see insert). (Data from Suppes et al., 1991, with permission).

How can one begin to change the odds in favor of maintenance of remission over repeated exacerbations? Education is a critical ingredient, and a full frontal assault is needed against the subtle to severe societal barriers to adequate care based on stigma or inadequate health care access for this serious central nervous system disorder. Knowing and seeing the facts and numbers will often help in making a well-informed decision.

For example, one should know the odds that even after long-term successful prophylactic treatment with lithium, stopping treatment results in 50% of individuals relapsing within the first 5 months off treatment and an 80–90% relapse rate within the first year and a half off treatment (Suppes, Baldessarini, Faedda, & Tohen, 1991) (Figure 69.1). While some studies suggest that a slow taper of lithium may lower this relapse rate, more recent studies have questioned that idea.

Moreover, one should imagine and visualize, when assessing the risk-to-benefit ratio for maintenance treatment, what the potential consequences of a new episode might be for a given individual, including the possibility, as described in Chapters 8 and 13, that the response might not be as good if treatment is restarted after a relapse has occurred. If one has the ability to avoid some of the devastating personal stories of illness and loss told in this volume, that should also be factored into risk-benefit discussions about starting or maintaining preventive drug treatment (pharmacoprophylaxis). We hope this book helps some patients avoid such disasters.

Another reason to maintain preventive treatment is the new data that lithium and valproate are neuroprotective and increase cell survival factors such as brain-derived neurotrophic factor (BDNF) and Bcl-2 (Table 69.2). The antidepressants all increase BDNF, which is important to both cell survival and long-term memory. The antidepressants (and the atypical antipsychotics quetiapine and zaprisidone) also prevent stress-induced decreases in BDNF. The antidepressants, as well as lithium, also increase the generation of new nerve cells in the brain (i.e., neurogenesis). Thus, many of our treatments not

Table 69.2 *Brain Derived Neurotrophic Factor (BDNF) is Involved in Each Type of Vulnerability*

A. *Constant*
  I. Val 66 *val* proBDNF → early onset, rapid cycling
     Val 66 *met* proBDNF →↓ working memory
  II. Repetitive Perinatal Stressors
     ↓ BDNF in adult prefrontal cortex and hippocampus
     ↓ BDNF (in serum in humans)
B. *Interactive*
  Val 66 met BDNF decreases 5HT-T$_{ss}$ mediated brain volume deficits
C. *Progressive*
  III. Repeated stressors → decrease BDNF (hippo)
  IV. Each episode → decreases serum BDNF
     (greater severity → greater BDNF lowering)
  V. Repeated defeat stress and cocaine both
     Decrease BDNF in hippocampus
     Increase BDNF in VTA/N. accumbens

only help prevent affective episodes but help protect the brain, potentially repairing, reversing, or preventing cell loss (Table 69.3)

We encourage the patient and family to attempt to use the shock and dismay of a bipolar diagnosis as a positive motivation for developing and maintaining an action plan. We have used the term *malignant transformation* to describe how the illness may progress in frequency (Chapter 2), severity (Chapter 3), or treatment resistance (Chapter 8) if adequate treatment measures are not brought to bear.

Table 69.3 *Therapeutic Strategies May Act to:*

  I. Repair or ameliorate deficits in basal BDNF:
     Lithium, VAP, CBZ, O-3-FA, antidepressants increase BDNF
  II. Prevent further BDNF decreases by
     A. Stressors directly
     B. Indirectly by preventing episodes of mania and depression
     C. Helping avoid substance abuse
  III. Protect the brain from further insult from
     A. Ageing and
     B. Medical cormorbidities (such as stroke and M.I.)

In this regard, we also think it is appropriate to extend the cancer analogy to the notion of early and aggressive intervention. The initial stage of anxiety (and perhaps terror) of a man's diagnosis of prostate cancer or a woman's diagnosis of breast cancer is typically weathered and rapidly transformed into a search for optimal therapeutic approaches. For both of these types of cancers, a wide range of options is available and many different physicians can be found who have the heartfelt and secure conviction that their particular recommended treatment paradigm is the most optimal.

This diversity of potential approaches is also a potential problem at the outset of treatment of bipolar illness, but it is not the crucial problem. Individuals with cancer almost always make a well-informed decision based on available evidence and choose an aggressive action plan to best avoid the possibility that this illness will recur, progress, or eventually take their life. This kind of rapid transformation from shock and disbelief to active treatment all too often does not occur in the case of bipolar illness, often because of an inadequate appreciation for the potential adverse consequences of the illness and the subtle or not-so-subtle consequences of stigma about the "mental" illnesses of the brain, as opposed to neurological or neurodegenerative illnesses. There is no empirical rationale for this distinction.

In the epilepsies, for example, as in bipolar illness, there are no pathognomonic lesions, although there may be funny squiggles on the EEG, and that appears to be enough to make the difference. Everyone agrees that seizures should be treated and prevented; access to health care is unlimited, and even complex and costly neurosurgical diagnostic and therapeutic procedures are paid for by insurance coverage without question.

In stark contrast, in bipolar illness there is public (but not academic) controversy about the absolute need for preventive intervention; health care access is limited even though the morbidity of the illness can be devastating; and the lethality rate of the illness is as high or higher than that of epilepsy. Long-term prevention of seizures is the accepted goal of treatment of epilepsy, and few fail to initiate such treatment or

stop it on their own. If you get in trouble, you can even call an ambulance to ensure that you get appropriate medical attention. Few of these treatment-facilitating factors pertain to bipolar illness. One must, instead, carefully negotiate the multiple road blocks to adequate treatment even when it is highly desired and sought.

We suggest that it is useful for families to think of the diagnosis of bipolar illness as being like that of a seizure disorder, with the well-recognized need for long-term preventive treatment, or like malignancy, wherein early intervention is seen as a life-saving necessity. Diabetes is even a better example as long term treatment is invariably needed. Moreover, in bipolar illness there is now unequivocal evidence that manic and depressive episodes are associated with decreases in neurotrophic factors such as BDNF and increases in oxidative stress both of which can endanger the cells of the brain (Table 69.2). Therefore, the candidate mechanisms for episodes increasing the vulnerability to future episodes are no longer just hypothetical constructs but very real changes that we should do our best to prevent (Table 69.3).

Individuals write inspirational books about their fights with and triumphs over cancer. The community rallies support, holds marches for additional research funding, and sends cards, flowers, and well wishes to the ill individual. While few of these tremendous endorsements, supports, and overt well wishes occur for individuals with bipolar illness, these patients are no less worthy of such support, and perhaps even more heroic because of the added adversities, shame, and stigma that they have to overcome in their struggles with this illness.

Given this great array of potential impediments to acquisition of adequate treatment, we wish each patient and every family having a member with bipolar illness all the best in acquiring a good start, and obtaining excellent education and treatment to minimize the impact of this illness. We urge the development of a positive attitude, building a good treatment team and support system, and sticking with treatments that are working for long-term prevention. If episodes break through, one should revise treatment and keep on aggressively going after the illness until one gets rebalanced. One of the primary take-home messages of this book should be that no matter how severe the prior course of bipolar illness, one can almost always find an effective treatment approach.

Keep up the search until effective treatment regimens are found, then cherish the remission, and follow the medically wise and advised course to maintain the well interval with consistent, long-term prophylactic treatment.

Part XVII

APPENDICES

1

Medication Names and Classes

SELECTED PSYCHOTROPIC DRUGS BY GENERIC NAME

Generic Name	Brand Name	Use
Alprazolam	Xanax ER	Antianxiety; high potency benzodiazepine
Amantadine	Symmetrel, Symadine	Antiparkinsonian; antiviral
Amitriptyline	Elavil, Endep, Enovil	Antidepressant (tricyclic); sedative
Amlodipine	Norvasc	Antihypertensive; anticycling?
Amoxapine	Asendin	Antidepressant (tricyclic); sedative
Aripiprazole	Abilify	Atypical antipsychotic; D_2 receptor partial agonist
Benztropine	Cogentin	Anticholinergic; antihistamine
Biperiden	Akineton	Anticholinergic; antiparkinsonian
Bromocriptine	Parlodel	Dopamine (D_2) receptor agonist
Buprenorphine	Buprenex	Antiaddiction; partial agonist at opiate receptor
Bupropion	Wellbutrin	Antidepressant, dopamine active
Buspirone	Buspar	Antianxiety
Carbamazepine	Tegretol, Equetro	Anticonvulsant; antimanic; mood stabilizer
Carbidopa/levodopa	Sinemet	Dopaminergic agent for parkinsonism
Chlordiazepoxide	Librium, Libratabs	Benzodiazepine; sedative-hypnotic
Chlorpromazine	Thorazine, Ormazine	Antipsychotic (phenothiazine)
Chlorprothixene	Taractan	Antipsychotic (thioxanthene)
Citalopram	Celexa	Antidepressant (SSRI)
Clomipramine	Anafranil	Antidepressant (tricyclic)
Clonazepam	Klonopin	Benzodiazepine (high potency); anticonvulsant
Clonidine	Catapres	Antihypertensive
Clorazepate	Tranxene	Antianxiety; benzodiazepine; anticonvulsant
Clorgyline		Antidepressant (MAOI type A)
Clozapine	Clozaril	Atypical antipsychotic (dibenzazepine)
Cyproheptadine	Periactin	Antihistamine; antiserotonergic
Dantrolene	Dantrium	Antispasticity; for malignant hyperthermia
Desipramine	Norpramin; Pertofrane	Antidepressant (tricyclic)
Dexfenfluramine	Redux	Antiobesity
Dextroamphetamine	Dexadrine, Adderall	Sympathomimetic
Diazepam	Valium	Antianxiety; benzodiazepine
Dihydroergotamine	Migranal	Migraine
Diltiazem	Cardizem	Calcium channel blocker
Diphenhydramine	Benadryl	Antianxiety; histamine; parkinsonism

Generic Name	Brand Name	Use
Disulfiram	Antabuse	Antiaddiction (alcohol induces nausea)
Divalproex	Depakote	Anticonvulsant; antimanic, mood stabilizer
Donepezil	Aricept	Boosts level of acetylcholine; a cholinesterase inhibitor
Doxepin	Adapin, Sinequan	Antidepressant (tricyclic)
Duloxetine	Cymbalta	Antidepressant; serotonin-norepinephrine uptake inhibitor (SNRI)
Estazolam	ProSom	Hypnotic (triazolobenzodiazepine)
Excitatory amino acid		Glutamate; aspartate involved in CNS diseases
Felbamate	Felbatol	Therapy-resistant onset seizures
Fenfluramine	Pondimin	Appetite suppressant (nonamphetamine)
Flumazenil	Romazicon	Benzodiazepine receptor antagonist (inverse agonist)
Fluoxetine	Prozac	Antidepressant (SSRI)
Fluphenazine	Prolixin	Antipsychotic (phenothiazine)
Flurazepam	Dalmane	Hypnotic
Fluvoxamine	Luvox	Antidepressant (SSRI)
Fosphenytoin	Cerebyx	Anticonvulsant
Gabapentin	Neurontin	Anticonvulsant; antipain
Galantamine	Reminyl	Anti-Alzheimer's; a cholinesterase inhibitor
Haloperidol	Haldol	Antipsychotic (butyrophenone)
Hydroxyzine	Atarax, Marax, Vistaril	Antianxiety; antihistamine
Imipramine	Tofranil	Antidepressant (tricyclic)
Isocarboxazid	Marplan	Antidepressant (MAOI)
Isradipine	DynaCirc	Antihypertensive
Ketamine	Ketalar	Rapid onset antidepressant; anaesthetic
Lamotrigine	Lamictal	Anticonvulsant; mood stabilizer
L-dopa, levodopa	Atamet, Larodopa	Antiparkinsonian
Levacecarnine (acetyl-L-carnitine)	Alcar	Cognition enhancer; neuroprotective
Levetiracetam	Keppra	Anticonvulsant
Lithium	Eskalith, Lithobid	Antimanic, mood stabilizer
Lorazepam	Ativan	Antianxiety; benzodiazepine
Loxapine	Loxitane, Loxapine	Antipsychotic (dibenzoxapine)
Maprotiline	Ludiomil	Antidepressant (tetracyclic)
Mementine	Namenda	Anti-Alzheimer's via glutamate blockade
Mesoridazine	Serentil	Antipsychotic (phenothiazine)
Methadone	Dolophine	Antiaddiction
Methylphenidate	Ritalin	Stimulant
Midazolam	Versed	Sedative; benzodiazepine
Mirtazepine	Remeron	Antidepressant
Moclobemide	Aurorix	Antipanic; antidepressant (MAOI)
Modafinil	Provigil	Antinarcolepsy
Molindone	Moban	Antipsychotic (dihydroindolone)
Nalmefene	Revex	Antagonist to narcotics; antiaddiction
Naloxone	Narcan	Opiate antagonist, antiaddiction
Naltrexone	ReVia, Trexan	Opioid antagonist (long acting); antiaddiction (alcohol)
Naratriptan	Amerge	Serotonin receptor antagonist for migraine
Nefazodone	Serzone	Antidepressant
Neurotrophin-3 (NT-3)		Neurodegenerative diseases and injury
Nimodipine	Nimotop	Calcium channel blocker; anticycling

Generic Name	Brand Name	Use
Nortriptyline	Pamelor, Aventyl	Antidepressant (tricyclic); Norepinephrine selective
Olanzapine	Zyprexa, Zydis	Atypical antipsychotic
Ondansetron	Zofran	Antianxiety; antinausea
Oxazepam	Serax	Antianxiety; benzodiazepine
Oxcarbazepine	Trileptal	Anticonvulsant; likely antimanic
Paroxetine	Paxil	Antidepressant (SSRI)
Pemoline	Cylert	Stimulant
Perphenazine	Etrafon, Triavil, Trilafon	Antipsychotic (phenothiazine)
Phenelzine	Nardil	Antidepressant (MAOI)
Phenobarbital	Arco-Lase Plus, Donnatal	Anticonvulsant; sedative; barbiturate
Phentermine	Adipex-P, Fastin	Antiobesity
Phosphatidylserine	BC-PS	Anti-Alzheimer's; cognition enhancer
Physostigmine	Synapton SR	Cholinergic; cognition enhancer
Pindolol	Visken	Antidepressant augmentor; blocks $5HT_{1A}$ receptors
Pramipexole	Miapex	Antiparkinsonian; antidepressant; D_2, D_3 agonist
Prochlorperazine	Compazine	Antinausea
Propranolol	Inderal	Antihypertensive; antitremor; blocks NE beta receptors
Protriptyline	Vivactil	Antidepressant (tricyclic)
Quetiapine	Seroquel	Atypical antipsychotic; dopamine and serotonin receptor antagonist
Riluzole	Rilutek	Anti-ALS drug; antidepressant
Risperidone	Risperdal	Atypical antipsychotic
Ropinirole	Requip	Antiparkinsonian; D_2, D_3 agonist; restless legs
Secobarbital	Seconal	Sedative-hypnotic; barbiturate
Selegiline, L-deprenyl	Eldepryl, Carbex, Ensam	Antidepressant (MAOI type B)
Sertraline	Zoloft	Antidepressant (SSRI)
Sibutramine	Meridia	Antiobesity
Tacrine	Cognex	Anti-Alzheimer's; cognition enhancer
Temazepam	Restoril	Hypnotic; benzodiazepine
Thioridazine	Mellaril	Antipsychotic (phenothiazine)
Thiothixine	Navane	Antipsychotic
Tiagabine	Gabitril	GABA reuptake inhibitor; anticonvulsant
Topiramate	Topamax	Anticonvulsant; weight loss
Tranylcypromine	Parnate	Antidepressant (MAOI)
Trazodone	Desyrel	Antidepressant; sedative
Triazolam	Halcion	Hypnotic; benzodiazepine
Trifluoperazine	Stelazine	Antipsychotic
Triflupromazine	Vesprin	Antipsychotic (phenothiazine)
Trihexyphenidyl	Artane	Anticholinergic
Trimipramine	Surmontil	Antidepressant (tricyclic)
Valproate	Depakene, Depakote	Anticonvulsant; mood stabilizer; antimigraine
Venlafaxine	Effexor	Antidepressant; NE & 5HT active
Verapamil	Calan, Isoptin	Calcium channel inhibitor for blood pressure
Vigabatrin	Sabril	Refractory epilepsy
Yohimbine	Yocon, Dayto Himbin, Yohimex	Sympatholytic; blocks NE α_2 receptors
Ziprasidone	Geodon	Atypical antipsychotic
Zolpidem	Ambien	Hypnotic (imidazopyridine)
Zomatriptan	Zomig	Antidepressant (SSRI)
Zonisamide	Zonegran	Anticonvulsant; weight loss

MEDICATIONS BY BRAND NAME

Brand Name	Generic Name
Abilify	Aripiprazole
Achromycin	Tetracycline
Aciphex	Histamine (H-2) blocker
Adalat	Nifedipine
Adapin, Sinequan	Doxepin
Adipex-P, Fastin	Phentermine
Airet	Albuterol
Akineton	Biperiden
Alcar	Levacecarnine
Ambien	Zolpidem
Amitril	Amitriptyline
Anafranil	Clomipramine
Antabuse	Disulfiram
Arco-Lase Plus	Phenobarbital
Aricept	Donepezil
Artane	Trihexyphenidyl
Asendin	Amoxapine
Atamet, Larodopa	L-dopa, levodopa
Atarax, Marax, Vistaril	Hydroxyzine
Ativan	Lorazepam
Aurorix	Moclobemide
BC-PS	Phosphatidylserine
Benadryl	Diphenhydramine
Buprenex	Buprenorphine
Buspar	Buspirone
Calan	Verapamil
Campral	Acamprosate
Cardizem	Diltiazem
Catapres	Clonidine
Celexa	Citalopram
CCK	Cholecystokinin
Centrax	Prazepam
Cerebyx	Fosphenytoin
Clozaril	Clozapine
Cogentin	Benztropine
Cognex	Tacrine
Compazine	Prochlorperazine
Cylert	Pemoline
Cymbalta	Duloxetine
Cytomel	Liothyronine, triiodothyronine (T_3)
Dalmane	Flurazepam
Daloxin	Loxapine
Dantrium	Dantrolene
Depakote, Depakene	Divalproex, valproic acid, valproate
Desyrel	Trazodone
Dexedrine, Adderall	Dextroamphetamine

Brand Name	Generic Name
Diamox	Acetazolamide
Dilantin	Phenytoin
Dolophine	Methadone
DynaCirc	Isradipine
Edronax	Reboxetine
Effexor	Venlafaxine
Elavil	Amitriptyline
Eldepryl, Carbex	Selegiline, l-deprenyl
Equetro	Carbamazepine-ER
Eskalith, Lithobid	Lithium
Etrafon, Triavil, Trilafon	Perphenazine
Eutonyl	Pargyline
Felbatol	Felbamate
Feldene	Piroxicam
Gabitril	Tiagabine
Geodon	Ziprasidone
Halcion	Triazolam
Haldol	Haloperidol
Hydropres	Reserpine
Imigran	Sumatriptan
Imitrex	Sumatriptan
Inderal	Propranolol
Kemadrin	Procyclidine
Keppra	Levetiracetam
Klonopin	Clonazepam
Lamictal	Lamotrigine
Lanoxin	Digoxin
Librium, Limbitrol	Chlordiazepoxide
Lithobid	Lithium
Loxitane	Loxapine
Ludiomil	Maprotiline
Luvox	Fluvoxamine
Lyrica	Pregabelin
Marplan	Isocarboxazid
Mellaril, Millazine	Thioridazine
Meridia	Sibutramine
Mirapex	Pramipexole
Migranal	Dihydroergotamine
Moban	Molindone
Narcan	Naloxone
Nardil	Phenelzine
Navane	Thiothixene
Neurontin	Gabapentin
Nimotop	Nimodipine
Norpramin, Pertofrane	Desipramine
Norvasc	Amlodipine
Orap	Pimozide
Pamelor, Aventyl	Nortriptyline
Parlodel	Bromocriptine
Parnate	Tranylcypromine

Brand Name	Generic Name
Paxil	Paroxetine
Periactin	Cyproheptadine
Pondimin	Fenfluramine
Prolixin	Fluphenazine
ProSom	Estazolam
Provigil	Modafinil
Prozac	Fluoxetine
Redux	Dexfenfluramine
Regitine	Phentolamine
Relefact TRH	Protirelin
Remeron	Mirtazepine
Reminyl	Galantamine
Requip	Ropinirole
Restoril	Temazepam
Revex	Nalmefene
ReVia, Trexan	Naltrexone
Risperdal	Risperidone
Ritalin	Methylphenidate
Romazicon	Flumazenil
Sabril	Vigabratrin
Seconal	Secobarbital
Serax	Oxazepam
Serentil	Mesoridazine
Seroquel	Quetiapine
Serzone	Nefazodone
Sinemet	Carbidopa/levodopa
Sinequan, Adapin	Doxepin
Stelazine, Suprazine	Trifluoperazine
Strattera	Atomoxetine
Surmontil	Trimipramine
Symbyax	Olanzapine and fluoxetine
Symmetrel	Amantadine
Synapton SR	Physostigmine
Synthroid	Levothyroxine (T_4)
Tagamet	Cimetidine
Taractan	Chlorprothixene
Tegretol	Carbamazepine
Temgesic	Buphrenorphine
Thorazine	Chlorpromazine
Tofranil	Imipramine
Topamax	Topiramate
Tranxene	Clorazepate dipotassium
Triavil	Amitriptyline and perphenazine
Trilafon	Perphenazine
Trileptal	Oxcarbazepine
Trivastal retard 50	Piribedil
Valium	Diazepam
Vasotec	Enalapril
Versed	Midazolam
Vesprin	Triflupromazine

Brand Name	Generic Name
Visken	Pindolol
Vistaril	Hydroxyzine
Vivactil, Neoactil	Protriptyline
Wellbutrin	Bupropion
Xanax	Alprazolam
Yocon	Yohimbine
Zantac	Ranitidine
Zarontin	Ethosuximide
Zeldox, Geodon	Ziprasidone
Zithromax	Azithromycin
Zofran	Ondansetron
Zoloft	Sertraline
Zomig	Zomatriptan
Zonegran	Zonisamide
Zyprexa, Zydis	Olanzapine

MEDICATIONS BY DRUG CLASS

Anticonvulsants

Clonazepam (Klonopin)
Carbamazepine (mood stabilizer; Tegretol, Equetro)
Felbamate (Felbatol)
Gabapentin (Neurontin)
Lamotrigine (mood stabilizer; Lamictal)
Levetiracetam (Keppra)
Lorazepam (Ativan)
Phenytoin (Dilantin)
Topiramate (Topamax)
Divalproex sodium (mood stabilizer; Depakote)
Valproic acid (mood stabilizer; Depakene)
Vigabatrin (Sabril)
Zonisamide (Zonegran)

L-Type Calcium Channel Blockers

Dihydropyridines
    Isradipine (DynaCirc, Prescal)
    Nifedipine (Adalat, Procardia)
    Nimodipine (Nimotop)
    Felodipine (Plendil)

Diphenylalklamine
    Verapamil (Calan, Isoptin)

Benzothiazepine
    Diltiazem (Cardizem)

Lithium Salts

Lithium carbonate (mood stabilizer; Eskalith, others)
Lithium citrate (mood stabilizer; Cibalith-S)
Lithium sustained release (mood stabilizer; Eskalith CR, Lithobid)

Antidepressants

Tricyclics (TCAs)
Amitriptyline (Elavil, Endep)
Bupropion (Wellbutrin)
Clomipramine (Anafranil)
Desipramine (Norpramin, Pertofrane)
Doxepin (Adapin, Sinequan)
Imipramine (Tofranil, Janimine)
Mirtazapine (Remeron)
Nortriptyline (Aventyl, Pamelor)
Protriptyline (Vivactil)
Trazodone (Desyrel)
Trimipramine (Surmontil)

Tetracyclics
Amoxapine (Asendin)
Maprotiline (NRI; Ludiomil)

Monoamine Oxidase Inhibitors (MAOIs)
Isocarboxazid (Marplan; no longer made)
Phenelzine (Nardil)
Tranylcypromine (Parnate)
Clorgyline (NIMH, investigational)
Selegeline (Ensam)
Moclobemide (Aurorix)

Triazolopyridines (Serotonin Modulators)
Trazodone (Desyrel)
Nefazodone (Serzone)

Selective Serotonin Reuptake Inhibitors (SSRIs)
Citalopram (Celexa)
Fluoxetine (Prozac)
Fluvoxamine (Luvox)
Paroxetine (Paxil)
Sertraline (Zoloft)
Escitalopram (Lexapro)

Serotonin Norepinephrine Reuptake Inhibitors (SNRIs)
Venlafaxine (Effexor)
Duloxetine (Cymbalta)

Selective Noradrenaline Reuptake Inhibitors
Reboxetine (Edronax)[a]
Atomoxetine (Strattera)

Thyroid Hormones

Levothyroxine, T_4 (Synthroid, others)
Liothyronine, T_3 (Cytomel)
Liotrix, T_4-T_3 combo (Thyrolar, Euthroid)
Thyrotropin-releasing hormone injection, protirelin (Relefact, Thyrel)

Benzodiazepines

Clonazepam (Klonopin)
Clorazepate (Tranxene)
Diazepam (Valium)
Flurazepam (Dalmane)
Lorazepam (Ativan)
Oxazepam (Serax)
Temazepam (Restoril)
Triazolam (Halcion)
Alprazolam (Xanax)

Azapirones (Anxiolytics)

Buspirone (Buspar)

Antipsychotics

Typicals (Older)
Chlorpromazine (Thorazine, others)
Mesoridazine (Serentil)
Trifluoperazine (Stelazine)
Fluphenazine (Prolixin)
Pimozide (Orap)
Perphenazine (Trilafon)
Haloperidol (Haldol)
Thioridazine (Mellaril)
Thiothixene (Navane)
Loxapine (Loxitane)

Atypicals (Newer)
Clozapine (Clozaril)
Olanzepine (Zyprexa)
Risperidone (Risperdal)
Sertindole (Serdolect)[b]
Quetiapine (Seroquel)
Ziprasidone (Geodon)
Aripiprazole (Abilify)

Anticholinergics

Benztropine (Cogentin)
Diphenhydramine (Benadryl)
Trihexyphenidyl (Artane)

Beta-Blockers

Atenolol (Tenormin)
Labetalol (Normodyne, Trandate)
Metoprolol (Lopressor)
Propranolol (Inderal)
Pindolol (Visken)
Nadolol (Corgard)

Anorexigenics

Fenfluramine (Pondimin)
Dexfenfluramine (Redux)[b]
Phentermine (Fastin, others)

Also see anticonvulsants
Topiramate, Zonisamide

Stimulants

Dextroamphetamine (Dexadrine)
Dextroamphetamine-amphetamine mixture (Adderall)
Methylphenidate (Ritalin)
Pemoline (Cylert)

Anti-Narcolepsy

Modafinil (Provigil)

[a]not approved in United States
[b]removed from the market

2

Life Charting:
A. Personal Calendar; B. Adult Forms;
C. Childhood Forms

A. Instructions for Filling Out a Personal Calendar (available from Depression and Bipolar Support Alliance)

A Brief, Compact, Easy Way to Monitor Your Mood and Clinical Response

We recommend that each patient or family member (if the patient is unable) complete a daily LCM rating form that includes mood, functional impairment, sleep, medication side effects, and other target symptoms. This will facilitate the evaluation of the effectiveness of each medication and help in the goal of achieving and maintaining a remission of symptoms in the relative absence of side effects. Should a consultation be needed, such a record will be invaluable.

It is useful to link completing the LCM each night to a given activity to make it a more automatic habit. For example, do not brush your teeth (or take nighttime medications) before completing your ratings. Show these ratings to your prescribing doctor and therapist at each visit.

Rate Mood First

The patient self-rating has a 0–100 mood analog scale to allow for fine discrimination of the daily mood changes rated by the patient (0 = the most depressed the patient can imagine being, 50 = balanced or level mood, and 100 = most activated, energetic, or manic the patient could ever be).

Rate Dysfunction Caused by Mood

The patient is then asked to chart depressed or manic episode severity at the four possible levels of episode severity (mild, low moderate, high moderate, or severe) based on functional impairment driven by mood dysregulation.

Depression Severity based on degree of depression related difficulty in usual activities:

- *Mild depression* represents a distinct low mood, but *no impairment* in the patient's usual (normal) level of functioning.
- *Low moderate* depression means that *some extra effort* is needed to function in the patient's usual social and occupational roles and interactions at home, work, or school.
- *High moderate* depression denotes that the patient is functioning only with *great extra effort* and has marked difficulty in usual roles and routines.
- *Severe* depression indicates essential incapacitation, that the patient is largely *unable to function* in any of the usual social and occupational roles, and needs caretaking at home or hospitalization.

Hypomania Severity based on altered functioning:

- *Mild hypomania* is described as feeling very mild symptoms such as increased energy, decreased need for sleep, irritability, or euphoria with *little or no functional impairment* and possible *enhancement* of functioning.

- *Low moderate* mania represents *some difficulty* with goal-oriented activity (resulting from symptoms such as substantial increase in energy, distractibility, hypertalkativeness, racing thoughts, etc.), and the patient might get some feedback that the behavior is different or odd.

- *High moderate* mania indicates *great difficulty* with goal-oriented activity (because of manic mood symptoms). The patient gets much feedback that this behavior is difficult or outlandish. Others appear angry or frustrated with the patient's behavior, and they are concerned about the patient's ability to look after self or others.

- *Severe* mania represents essential incapacitation and *inability to function* in any activity. Family and friends see such patients as out of control and want them in the hospital or another controlled environment.

Dysphoric Mania or Hypomania Dysphoric mania exists when the patient has increased energy, decreased need for sleep, racing thoughts, and so on, but is uncomfortable, irritable, angry, and has a sense of being unpleasantly overdriven. If hypomania is dysphoric, check the designated box (above the mania ratings) to differentiate it from the more euphoric and expansive form of mania.

Ultra-ultrarapid or Ultradian Cycling Sudden, distinct, and large mood changes within a single day are rated by the patient as a split mood rating, indicating the lowest mood for the day (e.g., 27), and the most activated or manic mood for the day (e.g., 69), and is entered in the mood box (below the depression ratings) as 69/27. Each time the mood crosses from one state to another (i.e., from depression to mania or from mania to depression within one day), this is counted as one mood switch. The number of times that the mood switches polarity (or switches from moderate to severe depression back to baseline euthymia) is entered in the mood switches/day box.

These switches within a day can also be charted on the mood-related functioning scale (mild, low moderate, high moderate, severe) according to the most extreme changes in functioning experienced that day.

For women, menses are tracked by checking the days of the menstrual period at the bottom of the rating form.

Hours of Sleep (From Previous Night)

The patient form has a daily box for hours of sleep for nighttime sleep, rounded to the full hour. Note that when a patient rates mood each night, the hours of sleep is from the previous night. (Naps taken after getting up are not added into the total nighttime sleep but can be circled above the hours of sleep line.)

Medications

Enter medication names in the allocated spaces. Write in the number of pills taken each day for each medicine. The dose of one pill should be listed, so you only have to write in the number of pills taken each day.

Life Events

Life events can be entered in the appropriate space, with a severity of impact rating of very negative (−4) to very positive (+4) estimating the potential impact the event might have according to its desirability, controllability, and degree of unexpectedness.

Side Effects

List side effects of medications and check off whether they were mild, moderate, or severe.

Comorbid Symptoms

Cormorbid symptoms are any other prominent symptoms that a patient might have, such as anxiety, irritability, or urge to drink. These can be rated 0 to 10, where 0 is none or not at all and 10 is the most extreme ever. Number of panic or anger attacks or drinks per day can also be listed so the physician can see the effect of medications on these kinds of target symptoms and occurrences.

Bottom Line

Use this personal calendar mood chart on a daily basis and it will remarkably facilitate your treatment.

Note: The further details in Section B can be ignored and are only for those wishing more complete instructions and forms for both retrospective mood charting of the prior course of illness and the prospective daily ratings already discussed here.

B. Adult Prospective (1.) and Retrospective (2.) Mood Charting: From a Special Issue of the Bipolar Network News (BNN); Available online at www.bipolarnews.org

Life Chart Highlight

1. Prospective Life Chart - Self Version

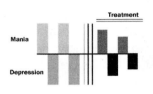

Introduction

We hope that learning how to chart your own course of illness will be useful and will make it easier for you and your physician to evaluate how well a medication or treatment works for you and which are the most effective for you in the short and long-term management of your illness.

Starting your daily ratings now as part of your current treatment while also constructing a retrospective Life Chart of your past course of illness (as your time allows, p. 8), will create a *Portable Psychiatric History* that is available to you and your physician at all times as a comprehensive overview of the course of your illness and its response to treatment. Also, life charts can be very valuable should you transfer to a different treatment setting or wish to obtain a consultation regarding further treatment options.

This life chart guide introduces you to the current, daily (*i.e., prospective*) charting of your mood and functioning and provides guidelines for using the NIMH-LCM™ Self-Rated Prospective form (LCM- S/P) on a daily basis.

Think of the life chart as a way of sketching an outline of your past and current course of illness in the form of a simple, continuous graph that can visually record manic and depressive episodes and hospitalizations you have experienced, medications you have taken, and important things that have happened in your life.

Charting Your Illness

The LCM- S/P uses daily ratings of mood and functioning along with entry of the total number of tablets of medications taken each day to track the course and treatment of your affective illness. Each box on the form represents one day and each form pro-

vides for ratings for one month. An example of a completed prospective life chart is given on page 5 as a guide.

The daily rating, which is done at the end of each day, will only take a minute or two and can easily be completed together with taking your evening medications. This is useful not only in tracking the daily course of illness, but can also help you remember to take all your prescribed medications for the day. A blank prospective form is given on page 6 for you to fill out if you choose to do so. Consider making copies of the blank form before you fill it out, so you can continue your mood charting in the future. You can also find blank copies of the form at our website at **www.bipolarnews.org.**

Graphing Episodes:

❶ The time line in the middle of the chart, (which also marks the **Days of the Month**), is called the baseline, which indicates a level or balanced mood state, i.e., no depression, hypomania or mania.

Episodes of depression are drawn below the baseline and episodes of hypomania or mania are drawn above the baseline at four severity levels (mild, low moderate, high moderate, or severe). Severity is based on the level of functional impairment due to depressive, hypomanic, or manic mood symptoms in your usual social, educational, and occupational roles. Any hospitalization for mania or depression is rated at the most severe level and blackened in.

Mood Scale:

❷ The prospective rating form provides a **mood scale** (on the left lower corner of the form) to assist

you in rating your daily mood with fine gradations. The scale is from 0-100 (0 = most depressed you could imagine being; 50 = balanced or level mood; 100 = most energetic/activated/manic you could ever be).

After you have rated your mood on this scale, you record the number you chose for the day in the row marked **Mood (0–100)**. For example, if today you felt moderately depressed you might rate your mood as 32 or 35, or if you felt mildly hypomanic, you might rate your mood as 54 or 57.

You then assess how much your mood has affected your ability to function (for that day) in your usual roles at home, work, school or with friends. The level of functional impairment based on mood symptoms determines the severity of your episode, as described in detail in the following section.

Assessing Episode Severity:

❸ **Functional impairment resulting from manic or depressive mood symptoms** has been employed as an effective and more consistent way of **measuring episode severity.** Episode severity has been categorized at four levels prospectively and for ease of use we have preceded the levels of episode severity at the left margin of the form. Tables with key words indicating the corresponding episode severity level are provided on page 7 to help you assess your level of hypomania, mania, or depression.

The following guidelines have been established for rating the four levels of episode severity for the daily prospective life chart ratings. After you have determined the level of episode severity for that particular day, draw

■ **Tip:**
It may help to identify and develop a short list of your typical symptoms associated with depressed and manic episodes. For example, for some people the best marker of hypomania may be increased energy, for others decreased need for sleep, for others increased sociability, phone calling or spending. Likewise, for depression, some people feel slow or apathetic while others feel agitated, some sleep more while others can't sleep much, some have the feeling that their mind is blank while others are plagued with depressive thoughts. Having your own list of your typical symptoms can serve as your own **Early Warning System** to help you and your doctor be more aware of any signs of re-emergence of your illness.

■ If you feel comfortable sharing your key symptom list with selected people in your usual environment, such as family, friends, or a trusted co-worker, it can significantly contribute to your ability to stay well. Early warning symptoms of an impending breakthrough episode are sometimes ignored (possibly in the hope that things will get better on their own) or simply not recognized (particularly an impending manic breakthrough).

Prospective Life Chart

a solid line along the dots according to that level (mild, low moderate, high moderate, severe). For hypomania or mania, use the top edge of the box for the day you are rating; for depression, use the bottom edge of the box. For days you are euthymic (no hypomania, mania, or depression), draw a straight line through the day of the month, as shown in the example on page 5 (days 1–4, 12–14, and 28–31).

Hypomania and Mania:

At the **mild level** of hypomania you may experience very mild symptoms such as decreased need for sleep, increased energy, some irritability or euphoria (elated, very happy mood), or an increase in the rate of thought, speech or sociability. At the mild level these symptoms have no negative impact and might even initially enhance your ability to function.

At the **low moderate level** of mania you have some of the above symptoms to a somewhat greater degree with some added symptoms, you may begin to be less productive and more unfocused, and you get some feedback from family, friends, or coworkers that your behavior is different from your usual self.

At the **high moderate level** of mania you may experience very significant symptoms such as very decreased need for sleep (or you may not sleep at all), a greatly increased level of energy, feeling all powerful or out of control, extremely rapid thoughts and speech, and a lot of feedback that your behavior is different or difficult. Friends, family, or coworkers express great concern about your ability to look after yourself or others, and others may appear angry or frustrated with your behavior.

At the **highest or severe level** of the manic mood state there is an even greater increase in the above symptoms with much insistence by family and friends that you need medical attention, that your behavior is out of

control, or they might take you to the hospital concerned that they and you cannot keep you safe any longer.

Dysphoric Hypomania or Mania:

If you experience increases in energy, activity, your rate of thinking and interactions (typical of hypomania or mania), but also with anger and irritability in the context of decreased need for sleep, you may be experiencing what is known as dysphoric hypomania or mania, which is experienced, at times, by about 40% of patients. On the high side of the mood scale (i.e., above 50 to 100), even if the activation feels driven, unpleasant, and is accompanied by anxiety, irritability, and anger, you are not slowed down or fatigued. Anxiety, irritability, anger and decreased sleep can also occur with agitated depression with pacing and ruminations, however, there is usually a sense of fatigue and slowness in responding.

On days that you may experience such a dysphoric, unhappy, irritable hypomania or mania, please put a checkmark in the **Dysphoric Mania** box above the mania section of the life chart form (right below the **Hours Of Sleep** box.)

Depression:

Mild depression represents a subjective sense of distress, a low mood, some social isolation, but you continue to function with little or no functional impairment.

Low moderate depression indicates that functioning in your usual roles is more difficult due to depressive mood symptoms and requires extra time or effort (you have to push yourself to get things done).

High moderate depression indicates that functioning is very difficult and requires great extra time or great extra effort with very marked difficulty in your usual routines.

Severe depression means that you are unable to function in any one of your usual social and occupational roles, i.e., you are unable to get out of bed, go to school or work, or carry out

any of your routine functions, and you require much extra care at home, or need to be hospitalized.

Ultradian Cycling:

4 At times you may experience what is called very fast, "ultradian" cycling within a day by switching mood states (A) or by experiencing significant switches within the same mood state (B) as described below.

(A) Cycling (switching) within a day between hypomania or mania and depression:

Sudden, distinct, and large mood changes within a single day are rated as a split mood rating indicating the most energized/manic mood for the day (for example 75), and the lowest mood for the day (for example 16). This split mood rating is entered in the **Mood (0 - 100)** box (located below the depression ratings) as 75/16. Each time the mood crosses from one mood state to another (i.e., from depression to hypomania or mania or from hypomania or mania to depression) within one day, this is counted as one mood switch. The number of times that the mood switches from one mood to the other is entered in the **Number of Mood Switches/Day** box.

(B) Cycling (switching) within a day within the same mood state:

Sudden, sharp and dramatic mood switches within a single day within one mood state (such as from very mild hypomania to mania and back) are also counted as a mood switch. The greatest amplitude (or range) of a sudden switch, for example, 85/54 for a switch within the manic range, (or, for instance, 41/12 for a switch within the depressive range), is recorded as a split mood rating and is entered in the **Mood (0 - 100)** box. The number of switches is then entered in the **Number of Mood Switches/Day** box.

Please note that typical diurnal mood variation, i.e., worse in the

NIMH-LCM™ Self/PROSPECTIVE Ratings: The LCM-S/P™

Name: **My Chart**   Month **OCTOBER**   Year **1994**

Days of Month — 1·2·3·4·5·6·7·8·9·10·11·12·13·14·15·16·17·18·19·20·21·22·23·24·25·26·27·28·29·30·31

❺

Medication Name	DOSE per tablet	UNIT (mg, mcg gm)	Enter total # of tablets TAKEN per day
Lithium			
Tegretol	200	mg	4 4 4 4 4 4 4 4 4 4 4 4 4 4 4 4 4 4 4 4 4 4 4 4 5 5 5 5 5 5 5 5 5 5 5 5 5
Depakote			
Prozac	10	mg	3 3 3 3 3 3 3 3 3 3 3 3 3 3 3 3 3 3 2 2 2 2 2

Please track all medications that you are currently taking.

Days of Month — 1·2·3·4·5·6·7·8·9·10·11·12·13·14·15·16·17·18·19·20·21·22·23·24·25·26·27·28·29·30·31

EXAMPLE

❻

| Hours of Sleep | 7 7 8 7 8 8 9 9 10 9 7 7 7 7 6 4 4 3 0 1 4 6 4 8 8 10 7 6 6 7 7 |
| Dysphoric Mania (√) if Yes | ✓ ✓ |

❸ **Mania**

SEVERE — Essentially Incapacitated or Hospitalized
MODERATE high — GREAT Difficulty with Goal-Oriented Activity
MODERATE low — SOME Difficulty with Goal-Oriented Activity
MILD — More Energized & Productive with Little or No Functional Impairment

Days of Month — 1·2·3·4·5·6·7·8·9·10·11·12·13·14·15·16·17·18·19·20·21·22·23·24·25·26·27·28·29·30·31 — Baseline

MILD — Little or No Functional Impairment
MODERATE low — Functioning with SOME Effort
MODERATE high — Functioning with GREAT Effort
SEVERE — Essentially Incapacitated or Hospitalized

❸ **Depression** *TRACK COMORBID SYMPTOMS HERE*

❽ anxiety

❹
| Number of Mood Switches / Day | | 2 | | | 6 3 | |
| Mood (0 - 100) | 50 50 50 50 40 35 50/30 25 30 40 40 50 50 55 60 60 70 75 75 60 60 56/28 54/26 30 30 40 40 50 50 50 |

❷
0 — Most Depressed Ever
50 — Balanced
100 — Most Manic (Activated) Ever

Impact (-4 to +4): +1   +2   -3

❾ **Life Events**
Trip to the beach   Job interview   Death of pet

Please circle the days of your menstrual period.

❼ **Days of Month** — 1·2·3·4·(5)(6)(7)(8)(9)·10·11·12·13·14·15·16·17·18·19·20·21·22·23·24·25·26·27·28·29·30·31

NIMH-LCM™ Self/PROSPECTIVE Ratings: The LCM-S/P™

Name _____ Month _____ Year _____

LCM-SP™ Version 2-02

Days of Month — 1 2 3 4 5 6 7 8 9 10 11 12 13 14 15 16 17 18 19 20 21 22 23 24 25 26 27 28 29 30 31

Medication Name	DOSE per tablet	UNIT (mg, mcg, gm)		*Enter total # of tablets TAKEN per day*
Lithium				
Tegretol				
Depakote				

Please track all medications that you are currently taking.

Days of Month — 1 2 3 4 5 6 7 8 9 10 11 12 13 14 15 16 17 18 19 20 21 22 23 24 25 26 27 28 29 30 31

Hours of Sleep

Dysphoric Mania (✓) if Yes

Mania

SEVERE	Essentially Incapacitated or	Hospitalized		SEVERE
high	GREAT Difficulty with Goal-Oriented Activity			MODERATE
MODERATE				
low	SOME Difficulty with Goal-Oriented Activity			
MILD	More Energized & Productive with Little or No Functional Impairment			MILD

Days of Month — 1 2 3 4 5 6 7 8 9 10 11 12 13 14 15 16 17 18 19 20 21 22 23 24 25 26 27 28 29 30 31 Baseline

MILD	Little or No Functional Impairment			MILD
low	Functioning with SOME Effort			MODERATE
MODERATE				
high	Functioning with GREAT Effort			
SEVERE	Essentially Incapacitated or	Hospitalized		SEVERE

Depression *TRACK COMORBID SYMPTOMS HERE*

Number of Mood Switches / Day

Mood (0 - 100)

Impact (-4 to +4)

0   50   100
Most   Balanced   Most
Depressed   Manic
Ever   (Activated)
Ever

Life Events

Please circle the days of your menstrual period.

Days of Month — 1 2 3 4 5 6 7 8 9 10 11 12 13 14 15 16 17 18 19 20 21 22 23 24 25 26 27 28 29 30 31

Prospective life chart form for daily tracking

Prospective Life Chart

morning and a very gradual improvement during the day (or better in the morning with a gradual worsening as the day goes on) should not be counted as a mood switch.

After counting and entering the number of mood switches per day you then rate how much your worst hypomanic, manic, and depressive symptoms of this day have affected your ability to function. Indicate the greatest functional impact of these manic and depressive switches by drawing vertical lines to the most severe impairment level reached, following the guidelines on the margin of the life chart rating form. For an example, see page 5, the 22nd and 23rd days of the month.

Medications:

5 Record each **medication and dose** in the left margin of the Medication Section. Enter the daily total number of tablets taken of each medication in the appropriate box (e.g., lithium, 300 mg, 3 tablets). This can best be done in the evening when you chart your mood and episode severity for the day, and will help you track your medications and make sure that you haven't taken all your medications for the day. Three of the most common mood stabilizers (lithium, Tegretol® [carbamazepine], and Depakote® [valproate, valproic acid]) have already been entered in the medication section for your convenience.

Hours of Sleep:

6 **Hours of sleep** (rounded to the nearest whole hour) can be recorded in the appropriate box (above the mania section). If you slept, for example, 4.5 hours, round to the nearest whole hour, i.e., 5. Count only nighttime sleep and do not include naps you might have taken several hours after you got up.

Menses:

7 For premenopausal women, menses are tracked by **circling the days** of the menstrual periods at the bottom of the rating form (see example, bottom of page 5).

Comorbid Symptoms:

8 Record any other illness symptoms you may have experienced for days or all of this month, such as anxiety, number of panic attacks, alcohol use (i.e., number of drinks per day), binge eating, etc., in the space labeled **Track Comorbid Symptoms Here**. Please indicate start and stop dates of these symptoms with arrows pointing to the date line.

Life Events:

9 Record important life events you may have experienced on any of the days of the month in the **Life Events** section of the life chart.

Also rate the expected impact each key life event had on a scale from +4 (extremely positive) to 0 (neutral) to -4 (extremely negative) and enter your rating in the **Impact (-4 to +4)** box available for each day. When rating the impact of the event, please consider how desirable the event was, how much you felt the event was under your control, how expected or anticipated the event was (or how unexpectedly it happened), how potentially disruptive the event could be long-term, and how much it could potentially affect or lower your self-esteem. A list of life events is given in the left margin of page 4 to help you complete the life events section.

Summary

By completing your daily prospective ratings, you are generating an accurate and detailed picture of your illness and its response to treatment and relationship to stressors. This should be very helpful to you and your doctor in assessing the effectiveness of treatment and maintaining or changing it accordingly. ■

Sample key words for levels of DEPRESSION and associated functional impairment

Types of Mood and Vegetative Symptoms	Severity Level	Functional Impairment
subjective distress mild sad mood not sharp, sluggish "a bit off" mild disinterest sleep and appetite o.k.	MILD	• minimal or no impairment, continue to function well at work, school, and home
depressed mood hopeless lack of interest tearful anxious irritable decreased concentration decreased energy decreased self-esteem feelings of guilt, self-reproach unable to enjoy things no interest in pleasurable things suicidal ideation sleep disturbance appetite disturbance physically slowed down decreased sexual interest/activity agitated angry socially withdrawn isolates at home	LOW MODERATE ↓ HIGH MODERATE	• some extra effort needed to function • occasionally missing days from work or school • noticeable impairment at work, school, or home • much extra effort needed to function • very significant impairment at work, school, or home • missing many days from work or school, barely scraping by
immobilized lack of self care poor eating poor fluid intake unable to dress long speech delays, or mute very agitated, pacing very suicidal cannot think or remember false beliefs (delusions) sensory distortions (hallucinations)	SEVERE	• not working • not in school • not functioning at home • cannot carry out any routine activities incapacitated at home or • hospitalized

Sample key words for levels of MANIA and associated functional impairment

Types of Mood and Vegetative Symptoms	Severity Level	Functional Impairment
increased energy increased activity more social enthusiastic, exuberant irritable talkative feel more productive	MILD	• minimal or no impairment; continue to function well at work, school, and home • functioning may even improve in some areas
euphoric irritable intrusive hypertalkative disruptive insistent overinvolved decreased need for sleep increased energy pressured flight of ideas very distractible increased spending speeding uncomfortably driven increased sexual interest/activity promiscuous grandiose may be reckless	LOW MODERATE ↓ HIGH MODERATE	• difficulty with goal-oriented activity • feel productive but may not be (e.g., starting many projects without finishing) • get in trouble with work, school, family • others comment about behavior • can't focus • others angry/frustrated with you • poor judgment • great difficulty with goal oriented activities
need little or no sleep feel out of control explosive feel all powerful invincible angry potentially violent excessive energy extremely driven reckless see or hear things not there	SEVERE	• close supervision needed • asked to leave work or school • unable to function with any goal-oriented activity • bizarre behavior or decisions • family and friends insist that you get help • in trouble with the law • hospitalized

Life Chart Highlight

2. Retrospective Life Chart - Self Version

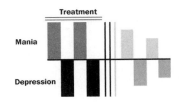

Introduction

In the past you have probably been asked many questions about your illness by doctors or therapists who have worked with you, and by family members or friends who were concerned about your well-being. The retrospective life chart can be a very valuable tool in helping you organize and visually present many important aspects of the past course of your illness.

Ask your family and friends to assist you with your retrospective life chart by helping you remember times you were depressed or hypomanic or manic, in recalling important events in your life that may have been associated with an episode, and medications you have taken. Many other sources of information, such as diaries, calendars, medical records, physician notes, pharmacy printouts, etc. will further help in the life-charting process and produce a life chart that is as accurate and representative of your prior course of illness as possible.

The retrospective life chart is very similar to the prospective life chart on page 3; however, there are some key differences:

1) Ratings are done by month, not daily, as in the prospective form;

2) There are only three levels of episode severity (mild, moderate, and severe hypomania, mania, or depression) in the retrospective life chart as opposed to four levels in the prospective life chart, because it was decided that it would be easier to distinguish low moderate and high moderate levels of episode severity when rating each day; a retrospective life chart is rated by month, where three levels of episode severity seemed more appropriate and easier to recall.

3) Hours of Sleep, Menses, and Mood (0 - 100) boxes have been eliminated.

We have developed a life chart form to make charting of past episodes and medications as easy as possible for you (page 9). The time frame for each form covers five years on each page and provides for episode severity coding (based on functional impairment resulting from mood symptoms) in the left margin of the form. Each space (or box) on the form represents one month and the months of each year are numbered within the dateline/baseline. Use dotted lines to graph episodes when details of timing cannot be reconstructed (estimated episodes), i.e., you are certain that an episode took place but you are not very sure when the episode started or stopped; this is still important information and should be recorded on the life chart with dotted lines.

Graphing Episodes:

1 The time line in the middle of the chart, (which also marks the **Months of Year**), is called the baseline, which indicates a level or balanced mood state, i.e., you are *not* depressed or hypomanic or manic.

Episodes of depression are drawn below the baseline and episodes of hypomania or mania are drawn above the baseline at three severity levels (mild, moderate, or severe). Severity is based on your level of functional impairment due to depressive or manic mood symptoms in your usual social, educational, and occupational roles. Any hospitalization for mania or depression is rated at the most severe level and blackened in.

Assessing Episode Severity:

Functional impairment resulting from manic or depressive mood symptoms has been employed as an effective and more consistent way of measuring episode severity. Episode severity has been categorized at three levels retrospectively and for ease of use we have precoded the levels of episode severity at the left margin of the form.

The following guidelines have been established for rating the three levels of episode severity for the daily prospective life chart ratings:

Hypomania and Mania:

At the **mild level** of hypomania you may experience very mild symptoms such as decreased need for sleep, increased energy, some irritability or euphoria (elated, very happy mood), or an increase in the rate of thought, speech or sociability. At the mild level these symptoms have no negative impact and might even initially enhance your ability to function.

At the **moderate level** of mania you have some of the above symptoms to a somewhat greater degree with some added symptoms, you may begin to be less productive and more unfocused, and you get some feedback from family, friends, or coworkers that your behavior is different from your usual self. As your mania accelerates you may experience very significant symptoms such as very decreased need for sleep (or you may not sleep at all), a greatly increased level of energy, feeling all powerful or out of control, extremely rapid thoughts and speech, and a lot of feedback that your behavior is different or difficult. Friends, family, or coworkers express great concern about your ability to look after yourself or others, and oth-

NIMH-LCM™ Self Ratings (RETROSPECTIVE)

Patient Name _____ PLEASE PRINT _____ Years 19___ - 19___

LCM-SR™ Version 2-02

Monthly Medication Dose (if available)

Other (
Other (
Other (
Thyroid (T3 or T4)
Benzodiazepine (
Neuroleptic (
MAOI (
Antidepressant II (
Antidepressant I (
Depakote
Tegretol
Lithium

Mania

Dysphoric Mania (✓)

SEVERE — Essentially Incapacitated or Hospitalized

MODERATE — Notable Difficulty with Goal-Oriented Activity

MILD — More Energized & Productive With Little or No Functional Impairment

Months of Year

SEVERE / MODERATE / MILD / Baseline / MILD / MODERATE / SEVERE

MILD — Little or No Functional Impairment

MODERATE — Functioning with Notable Difficulty

SEVERE — Essentially Incapacitated or Hospitalized

Depression

TRACK COMORBID SYMPTOMS HERE

Number of Mood Switches Per Month

Cycling Within A Day (✓)

Impact (−4 to +4)

Life Events

(Date)

Retrospective life chart form for monthly tracking

Retrospective Life Chart

ers may appear angry or frustrated with your behavior.

At the **severe level** of the manic mood state there is an even greater increase in the above symptoms with much insistence by family and friends that you need medical attention, that your behavior is out of control, or they might take you to the hospital concerned that they and you cannot keep you safe any longer.

Dysphoric Hypomania or Mania:

If you experienced increases in energy, activity, your rate of thinking and interactions (typical of hypomania or mania), but also with anger and irritability in the context of decreased need for sleep, you may have experienced what is known as dysphoric hypomania or mania, which occurs in about 40% of patients. Even if the activation felt driven, unpleasant, and was accompanied by anxiety, irritability, and anger, you were not slowed down or fatigued. Anxiety, irritability, anger and decreased sleep can also occur with agitated depression with pacing and ruminations, however, there is usually a sense of fatigue and slowness in responding.

In months that you may have experienced such a dysphoric, unhappy, irritable hypomania or mania, put a checkmark in the **Dysphoric Mania** box above the mania section of the life chart form.

Depression:

Mild depression represents a subjective sense of distress, a low mood, some social isolation, but you continue to function with little or no functional impairment.

Moderate depression indicates that functioning in your usual roles (work, school, or with family) is more difficult due to depressive mood symptoms and requires extra time or effort (you have to push yourself to get things done). You may miss days from work, school, or other regular activities or responsibilities.

Severe depression means that you are unable to function in any one of your usual social and occupational roles, i.e., you are unable to get out of bed, go to school or work, or carry out any of your routine functions, and you require much extra care at home, or need to be hospitalized.

In summary, the impairment in your ability to function that you experienced as a result of being hypomanic, manic, or depressed determines the severity rating of the episode when you graph the episode on your life chart.

Frequent Cycling:

2 If you were experiencing frequent cycling between a manic or depressive episode (or within a depressive or manic episode), indicate the range of the mood changes or switches, (i.e. the severity of the switch into the manic and depressive range using life chart episode severity criteria) by drawing vertical lines to the highest severity of hypomania or mania and depression you experienced.

If you had ultra-rapid cycling (one or more full episodes lasting a week or less), indicate this by frequent, spaced lines above and below the baseline (to the appropriate level of severity) and simply mark the approximate total number of episodes or mood switches per month in the box marked **Number of Mood Switches Per Month** (rather than trying to exactly match the number of vertical lines above and below the baseline to the ultra-rapid episode occurrence).

Ultradian cycling is defined by a clear shift between (or within) hypomanic or manic and depressive episodes within a day and is indicated by densely packed frequent lines above and below the baseline to the appropriate level of severity. If you recall such periods of ultradian cycling in the past, put a checkmark in the **Cycling Within a Day** box for any month you remember having experi-

enced such distinct, rapid mood cycling within a day.

If you experienced both patterns of cycling during a month (one or more full episodes lasting a week or less and periods of cycling within the day), continue to record the total approximate number of episodes or mood switches lasting a week or less in the **Number of Mood Switches Per Month** box and also put a check mark in the **Cycling Within a Day** box.

Please note that typical diurnal mood variation, i.e., worse in the morning and a very gradual improvement during the day (or better in the morning with a gradual worsening as the day goes on) should not be counted as a mood switch.

Medications:

3 Record each medication and dose you may have taken in the past in the **Medication** section. You can draw lines through each medication row for the medication that you have entered in the margin at the time point the medication was started. Be sure to indicate the dose at the start of a medication (if known) or any dose change that may have occurred over time.

Comorbid Symptoms:

4 Record any other illness symptoms you may have experienced, such as anxiety, number of panic attacks, alcohol use (i.e., number of drinks per day), binge eating, etc., in the space labeled **Track Comorbid Symptoms Here**. Indicate start and stop dates of these symptoms with arrows pointing to the date line.

Life Events:

5 Record important life events you may have experienced in any months in the **Life Events** section of the life chart.

Retrospective Life Chart

Also rate the impact each key life event had on you on a scale from +4 (extremely positive) to 0 (neutral) to -4 (extremely negative) and enter your rating in the **Impact (-4 to +4)** box available for each month. When rating the impact of the event, please consider how desirable the event was, how much you felt the event was under your control, how expected or anticipated the event was (or how unexpectedly it happened), how potentially disruptive the event was long-term, and how much it affected or lowered your self-esteem.

Summary

When you begin graphing your past episodes of mania and depression on the life chart it is generally easiest to start with the last year since this is probably the year you most clearly remember.

Graph last year's episodes at the appropriate severity level (i.e., at the level of functional impairment resulting from mood symptoms) following the instructions and examples given here. Record the medications with doses whenever possible, as well as important life events you remember took place, or any additional events that may not be on the list.

Be sure to draw the degree of episode severity on the appropriate line of episode severity as indicated in the margin rather than in the middle of the boxes. For hypomania or mania draw the line along the top edge of the box and for depression draw the line along the bottom edge of the box at the severity level you determined was correct.

When you are finished with recording episodes, medications, and events for the last year, try to go back to the beginning of your illness following the same method of graphing episodes, medications, and whenever possible, events. Try to record as much information as you can recall at this

time and don't be worried if you can't remember exact dates, or all the names of the medications. If you remember that you were on an antidepressant medication but have forgotten the exact name, record it under the class of antidepressant medication (as precoded in the left margin), without a specific name. This is applicable to any other medication where you cannot recall the name; knowing the class of the medication with which you were treated will provide important information in itself with regard to past treatment responses and what might be the best next step in your treatment.

Try to work forward in time from the onset of your illness but if you feel more comfortable working your way backward from the current time, or want to continue with a time period you remember well, proceed in that fashion. Many people work backward and forward in time on the life chart in a way that is most productive and helpful for them and provides them with the most information about their course of illness.

The life chart graph can be a very basic or a more detailed picture of your course of illness depending on the information available and the amount of time you can spend on it as well as your current mood.

Working on your life chart is easier when you are feeling better and it is generally helpful to review your chart again when you are well. Your personal records and recollections, insurance statements and bills, hospital or physician records, pharmacy printouts, performance reviews from work, school or college grades, disability statements, family and friends' recollections, all can assist you in recalling important times and possible mood episodes in your life. The life-charting process is open-ended so that further information can be added to the life chart at any time as more material is gathered or when you are able to spend more time on it, but it will

be most helpful to you and your doctor if as many episodes and medications as possible can be graphed out in the beginning even if they are only estimated in terms of timing (i.e., using dotted lines). ■

//www: bipolar

Websites on bipolar illness that may be helpful to you:

www.jbrf.org
Juvenile Bipolar Research Foundation

pn.psychiatryonline.org
American Psychiatric Association newspaper

www.nami.org
National Alliance for the Mentally Ill

www.ndmda.org
National Depressive and Manic-Depressive Association

www.narsad.org
National Alliance for Research on Schizophrenia and Depression

www.bpkids.org
The Child and Adolescent Bipolar Foundation

www.bpso.org
Bipolar Significant Others

www.nimh.nih.gov/health/topics/child-and-adolescent-mental-health/index.shtml
NIMH Child and Adolescent Mental Health

www.clinicaltrials.gov
NIMH Clinical Trial Database

www.stepbd.org
Systematic Treatment Enhancement Program for Bipolar Disorder

www.edc.gsph.pitt.edu/stard
Sequenced Treatment Alternatives to Relieve Depression

www.ncbi.nlm.nih.gov/entrez/query.fcgi
PubMed (National Library of Medicine)

www.nih.gov
National Institutes of Health

www.bipolarnews.org
Bipolar Network News

NIMH-LCM™ Self Ratings (RETROSPECTIVE)

Patient Name _____   *PLEASE PRINT*   **Years 19___ - 19___**

LCM-SR™ Version 2-02

Monthly Medication Dose (if available)

Other ( )
Other ( )
Other ( )
Thyroid (T3 or T4)
Benzodiazepine ( )
Neuroleptic ( )
MAOI ( )
Antidepressant II ( )
Antidepressant I ( )
Depakote
Tegretol
Lithium

Dysphoric Mania [✓]

Mania

SEVERE — Essentially Incapacitated or Hospitalized
MODERATE — Notable Difficulty with Goal-Oriented Activity
MILD — More Energized & Productive With Little or No Functional Impairment

Months of Year

MILD — Little or No Functional Impairment
MODERATE — Functioning with Notable Difficulty
SEVERE — Essentially Incapacitated or Hospitalized

Depression

TRACK COMORBID SYMPTOMS HERE

Number of Mood Switches Per Month
Cycling Within A Day (✓=yes)

Impact (-4 to +4)
Life Events
(Date)

SEVERE
MODERATE
MILD
Baseline
MILD
MODERATE
SEVERE

Retrospective life chart form for monthly tracking

NIMH-LCM™ Self/PROSPECTIVE Ratings: The LCM-S/P™

Name _____ Month _____ Year _____

LCM-SP™ Version 2-02

Days of Month — 1 2 3 4 5 6 7 8 9 10 11 12 13 14 15 16 17 18 19 20 21 22 23 24 25 26 27 28 29 30 31

Medication Name	DOSE per tablet	UNIT (mg, mcg gm)		
Lithium				*Enter total # of tablets TAKEN per day*
Tegretol				
Depakote				

Please track all medications that you are currently taking.

Days of Month — 1 2 3 4 5 6 7 8 9 10 11 12 13 14 15 16 17 18 19 20 21 22 23 24 25 26 27 28 29 30 31

Hours of Sleep

Dysphoric Mania (√ if Yes)

Mania

SEVERE	Essentially Incapacitated or Hospitalized		SEVERE
high MODERATE	GREAT Difficulty with Goal-Oriented Activity		
low	SOME Difficulty with Goal-Oriented Activity		MODERATE
MILD	More Energized & Productive with Little or No Functional Impairment		MILD

Days of Month — 1 2 3 4 5 6 7 8 9 10 11 12 13 14 15 16 17 18 19 20 21 22 23 24 25 26 27 28 29 30 31 Baseline

MILD	Little or No Functional Impairment		MILD
low	Functioning with SOME Effort		
MODERATE	Functioning with GREAT Effort		MODERATE
high			
SEVERE	Essentially Incapacitated or Hospitalized		SEVERE

Depression *TRACK COMORBID SYMPTOMS HERE*

Number of Mood Switches / Day

Mood (0 - 100)

Impact (-4 to +4)

Life Events

0 50 100
Most Depressed Ever   Balanced   Most Manic (Activated) Ever

Please circle the days of your menstrual period.

Days of Month — 1 2 3 4 5 6 7 8 9 10 11 12 13 14 15 16 17 18 19 20 21 22 23 24 25 26 27 28 29 30 31

Prospective life chart form for daily tracking

Life Chart Highlight

3. Kiddie Life Chart - Parental Prospective and Retrospective Versions

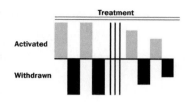

Introduction

At the turn of the twentieth century, the German psychiatrist Dr. Emil Kraepelin in his life chart graphs already showed early onset bipolar disorder in adolescents. The NIMH has developed a retrospective and prospective "Kiddie" life chart method for children and adolescents, to be completed by parents. Rather than defining illness phases as mania and depression, we categorized mood symptoms and behaviors (with associated functional impairment) as either activated or withdrawn.

The following is a list of suggested steps for completing daily prospective life chart ratings of your child or adolescent. For an example of a completed life chart, see page 5, as the adult prospective life chart is similar in many ways. A retrospective kiddie life chart form and instructions are given on pages 14–15.

Severity of Symptoms and Behaviors:

Assess how much the child's or adolescent's **Activated** or **Withdrawn** behaviors have affected his or her ability to function in usual social or educational roles or interactions at home, with peers, or at school. Check the most prominent symptoms and behaviors for the month (see top box of form at right) and rate the degree of dysfunction caused by these symptoms and behaviors in the Activated and Withdrawn sections of the rating scale.

Activated:

Draw a solid line along the dots according to the severity of impairment experienced; use the **top edge** of the **box for activated symptoms:**

Mild level: Very energetic, enhanced functioning or slightly disorganized; happier or more irritable than usual;

Low Moderate level: Some feedback and own observation that behavior is different or unusual; some problems with goal-oriented activities and social interactions;

High Moderate level: Much feedback and own observation that behavior is out of control, highly unusual, bizarre, excessive;

Severe level: Family and friends want child or adolescent in the hospital; he or she cannot be managed at home.

Normal/Usual

Draw a line through the dateline in the middle (marked **Days of Month** and **Baseline**).

Withdrawn

Draw a solid line along the dots according to the severity of impairment experienced; use the bottom edge of box for withdrawn symptoms:

Mild level: Low mood, might seem a little withdrawn but essentially no impairment in all areas of daily activities;

Low Moderate level: Some extra effort needed in usual roles, noticeable withdrawal, decrease in many activities;

High Moderate level: Much extra effort needed; marked difficulty in usual activities, missed days from school;

Severe level: Largely unable to function in any capacity.

If hospitalized for Activated or Withdrawn symptoms and behaviors, blacken in boxes. Do not draw a line through the middle of a box.

Hours of Sleep:

Rate the approximate number of **Hours of Sleep** (rounded to the nearest hour) that the child or adolescent had the night before. Do not count daytime naps.

Psychosis:

Put a check mark in the **Psychosis** box for any day the child or adolescent seems to exhibit psychotic symptoms such as paranoid thinking, hearing voices, bizarre behaviors, appearing mute and internally preoccupied, others.

Medication:

Enter the name and total dose taken per day in the **Interventions or Treatments** section. If your child participates in any type of therapy or other behavioral interventions, please record these in the same section and put a checkmark for the days the therapy occurred.

Number of Switches:

If behaviors and symptoms changed dramatically in the course of a day, indicate the greatest functional impact of these activated and depressive switches in the appropriate rating sections of the life chart by drawing vertical lines to the appropriate impairment level in the rating sections of the K-LCM (i.e., how much did the child's most activated and depressive/withdrawn symptoms of the day affect his or her ability to function). Estimate how often the behaviors and symptoms switched in a day and record the approximate number in the **Number of Switches/Day** box.

Important Events of the Day:

Record important events (and/or specific behaviors) in the **Life Events and Predominant Symptoms** section. Rate

K-LCM™/P: The Child Life Chart Method - *Parent Daily* PROSPECTIVE Ratings

Name _____   Month _____   Year _____

K-LCM™/P version 2-02

Please Check √ **ALL BEHAVIORS AND SYMPTOMS*** Observed in Your Child **THIS MONTH:**

ACTIVATED

___1 Impulsivity	___13 Stealing
___2 Irritability	___14 Disregard for authority
___3 Temper tantrums	___15 Fighting
___4 Sleeps less than usual	___16 Destruction of property
___5 Hyperactivity	___17 Excessive risk taking
___6 Increased aggression	___18 Trouble with the law
___7 Skips school	___19 Lack of remorse
___8 Decreased attention span	___20 Frequent lying
___9 Inappropriate sexual behavior	___21 Racing thoughts
___10 Unusually happy and enthusiastic	___22 Bizarre behavior
___11 Excessively talkative	___23 Other: _____
___12 Unreasonably and excessively self-confident	___24 Other: _____

WITHDRAWN

___25 Periods of sadness	___35 Suicidal gesture
___26 Low self-esteem/ sense of worthlessness	___36 Serious suicide attempt
___27 More withdrawn than usual	___37 Physical complaints
___28 Cries more easily than usual	___38 Sleeps more than usual
___29 Unusually clingy and dependent	___39 Obsessive thoughts
___30 Less active and energetic than usual	___40 Night terrors
___31 Excessive guilt	___41 Does not talk or respond
___32 More anxious (tense/worried) than usual	___42 Paranoid thinking
___33 Change in appetite	___43 Hearing voices
___34 Suicidal thinking	___44 Other: _____
	___45 Other: _____

Interventions or Treatments *(list below)*

For each **MEDICATION**, please enter the **total dose taken** per day.
For OTHER TREATMENT INTERVENTIONS (e.g., psychotherapy, behavior modification, etc.), please **check the days the treatment was received.**

Days of Month ➡ 1 · 2 · 3 · 4 · 5 · 6 · 7 · 8 · 9 ·10 ·11 ·12 ·13 ·14 ·15 ·16 ·17 ·18 ·19 ·20 ·21 ·22 ·23 ·24 ·25 ·26 ·27 ·28 ·29 ·30 ·31

Please rate the degree of dysfunction caused by either ACTIVATED or WITHDRAWN behaviors above and below the midline.

Psychosis (√ if Yes)
Hours of Sleep

RATE DEGREE of Dysfunction:

Activated *(IMPULSIVE, AGGRESSIVE)*
SEVERE
HIGH MODERATE
LOW MODERATE
MILD

Days of Month ➡ 1 · 2 · 3 · 4 · 5 · 6 · 7 · 8 · 9 ·10 ·11 ·12 ·13 ·14 ·15 ·16 ·17 ·18 ·19 ·20 ·21 ·22 ·23 ·24 ·25 ·26 ·27 ·28 ·29 ·30 ·31 Baseline

MILD
LOW MODERATE
HIGH MODERATE
SEVERE

Withdrawn *(ANXIOUS, DEPRESSED)*

Number of Switches/Day

Life Events and Predominant Symptoms*
Life Event Impact (-4 to +4)

Days of Month ➡ 1 · 2 · 3 · 4 · 5 · 6 · 7 · 8 · 9 ·10 ·11 ·12 ·13 ·14 ·15 ·16 ·17 ·18 ·19 ·20 ·21 ·22 ·23 ·24 ·25 ·26 ·27 ·28 ·29 ·30 ·31

Prospective Kiddie life chart form for daily tracking

K-LCM™/R: The Child Life Chart Method - Parents RETROSPECTIVE Ratings

Patient Name _____   Date Completed □□/□□/□□

Please Check√ ALL BEHAVIORS AND SYMPTOMS* Observed in Your Child During This THREE- YEAR Period:

ACTIVATED Behaviors Might Include:

YEAR (Below) 1 2 3		YEAR (Below) 1 2 3	
— — — 1 Impulsivity		— — — 13 Stealing	
— — — 2 Irritability		— — — 14 Disregard for authority	
— — — 3 Temper tantrums		— — — 15 Fighting	
— — — 4 Sleeps less than usual		— — — 16 Destruction of property	
— — — 5 Hyperactivity		— — — 17 Excessive risk taking	
— — — 6 Increased aggression		— — — 18 Trouble with the law	
— — — 7 Skips school		— — — 19 Lack of remorse	
— — — 8 Decreased attention span		— — — 20 Frequent lying	
— — — 9 Inappropriate sexual behavior		— — — 21 Racing thoughts	
— — — 10 Unusually happy and enthusiastic		— — — 22 Bizarre behavior	
— — — 11 Excessively talkative		— — — 23 Other: _____	
— — — 12 Unreasonably and excessively self-confident		— — — 24 Other: _____	

WITHDRAWN Behaviors Might Include:

YEAR (Below) 1 2 3		YEAR (Below) 1 2 3	
— — — 25 Periods of sadness		— — — 35 Suicidal gesture	
— — — 26 Low self-esteem/sense of worthlessness		— — — 36 Serious suicide attempt	
— — — 27 More withdrawn than usual		— — — 37 Physical complaints	
— — — 28 Cries more easily than usual		— — — 38 Sleeps more than usual	
— — — 29 Unusually clingy & dependent		— — — 39 Obsessive thoughts	
— — — 30 Less active & energetic than usual		— — — 40 Night terrors	
— — — 31 Excessive guilt		— — — 41 Does not talk or respond	
— — — 32 More anxious (tense/worried) than usual		— — — 42 Paranoid thinking	
— — — 33 Change in appetite		— — — 43 Hearing voices	
— — — 34 Suicidal thinking		— — — 44 Other: _____	
		— — — 45 Other: _____	
		— — — 46 Other: _____	

K-LCM™/R version 2-02

Interventions or Treatments (list below)

For each **MEDICATION**, please enter (by month) the **maximal dose per day taken** by the child. For **OTHER TREATMENT INTERVENTIONS** (e.g., psychotherapy, behavior modification, etc.), please **indicate the # of visits per month.**

Month of Year ——→ 1:2:3:4:5:6:7:8:9:10:11:12 1:2:3:4:5:6:7:8:9:10:11:12 1:2:3:4:5:6:7:8:9:10:11:12 ——→

19___   19___   19___

Please rate the degree of dysfunction caused by either ACTIVATED or WITHDRAWN behaviors above and below the midline.

Dysphoric / Irritable Mood (√) if Yes

Activated (IMPULSIVE, AGGRESSIVE)

SEVERE / MODERATE / MILD   DYSFUNCTION

Month of Year ——→ 1:2:3:4:5:6:7:8:9:10:11:12 1:2:3:4:5:6:7:8:9:10:11:12 1:2:3:4:5:6:7:8:9:10:11:12 Baseline

MILD / MODERATE / SEVERE   DYSFUNCTION

Withdrawn (ANXIOUS, DEPRESSED)

Number of Mood Switches / Month

Cycling Within A Day (√) if Yes

19___   19___   19___

Life Event Impact* (-4 to +4)

Life Events and Predominant Symptoms*

Month of Year ——→ 1:2:3:4:5:6:7:8:9:10:11:12 1:2:3:4:5:6:7:8:9:10:11:12 1:2:3:4:5:6:7:8:9:10:11:12 ——→

Retrospective Kiddie life chart form for monthly tracking

Kiddie Prospective Life Chart

the expected impact of each life event from extremely positive (+4) to neutral (0) to extremely negative (-4). Graph the severity of behaviors and/or symptoms in the activated and withdrawn sections of the life chart.

Retrospective Kiddie Life Chart

The retrospective kiddie life chart is very similar to the prospective life chart on page 13; however, there are some key differences:

1) Ratings are done by month, not daily, as in the prospective form;

2) There are only three levels of episode severity (mild, moderate, and severe) as opposed to four levels in the prospective kiddie life chart;

3) Hours of Sleep and Psychosis boxes have been eliminated;

4) A box for Number of Mood Switches/Month has been added as well as a checkbox for Cycling Within a Day if it occurred in the month you are rating.

Severity of Symptoms and Behaviors:

Assess how much the child's or adolescent's **Activated** or **Withdrawn** behaviors affected his or her ability to function in usual social or educational roles or interactions at home, with peers, or at school. Check the most prominent symptoms and behaviors for each year on the three-year form (see top box of form at left).

Note: For example if the first year on the three-year form you are rating is 1996, this would be year 1; year 3 would be 1998.

Rate the degree of dysfunction caused by these symptoms and behaviors in the Activated and Withdrawn sections of the rating scale for each month of the rated year.

Activated:

Draw a solid line along the dots according to the severity of impairment experienced; use the **top edge** of the **box for activated symptoms**:

Mild level: Very energetic, enhanced functioning or slightly disorganized; happier or more irritable than usual;

Moderate level: Some feedback and own observation that behavior is different or unusual; some problems with goal-oriented activities and social interactions; illness may progress so that much feedback and own observation that behavior is out of control, highly unusual, bizarre, excessive;

Severe level: Family and friends want child or adolescent in the hospital; he or she cannot be managed at home.

Normal/Usual

Draw a line through the dateline in the middle (marked **Month of Year** and **Baseline**).

Withdrawn

Draw a solid line along the dots according to the severity of impairment experienced; use the **bottom edge** of **box for withdrawn symptoms**:

Mild level: Low mood, might seem a little withdrawn but essentially no impairment in all areas of daily activities;

Moderate level: Some extra effort needed in usual roles, noticeable withdrawal, decrease in many activities; illness may progress so that much extra effort needed, marked difficulty in usual activities, missed days from school;

Severe level: Largely unable to function in any capacity.

If hospitalized for Activated or Withdrawn symptoms and behaviors, blacken in boxes. Do not draw a line through the middle of a box.

Dysphoric / Irritable Mood

If your child exhibits both activated symptoms **and** withdrawn symptoms at the same time in a given month, put a check mark in the **Dysphoric / Irritable Mood** box. For example, your child could be highly activated, energetic, and irritable, but also very anxious, fearful, or suicidal at the same time.

Medication:

Enter (by month) the name and dose taken in the **Interventions or Treatments** section. If your child participated in any type of therapy or other behavioral interventions, please record these in the same section as indicated by putting checkmarks in the appropriate month for the year you are rating.

Number of Switches:

If behaviors and symptoms changed from activated to withdrawn or vice versa in the course of a month in a given year, indicate the greatest functional impact of these activated and depressive states in the appropriate rating sections of the life chart by drawing vertical lines to the appropriate impairment level in the rating sections of the K-LCM (i.e., how much did the child's most activated and depressive/withdrawn symptoms in a rated month affect his or her ability to function). Estimate how often the behaviors and symptoms switched in a month and record the approximate number in the **Number of Mood Switches/Month** box.

Cycling Within a Day:

If you noticed your child was dramatically alternating between distinct activated and withdrawn moods within a day in a given month, please place a check mark in the **Cycling Within a Day** box for that month.

Important Events of the Day:

Record important life events (and/or specific behaviors) in the **Life Events and Predominant Symptoms** section. Rate the expected impact of each life event from extremely positive (+4) to neutral (0) to extremely negative (-4). Graph the severity of behaviors and/or symptoms in the activated and withdrawn sections of the life chart. ■

K-LCM™/P: The Child Life Chart Method - *Parent Daily* PROSPECTIVE Ratings

Name _____ Month _____ Year _____

K-LCM™/P version 2-02

Please Check √ ALL BEHAVIORS AND SYMPTOMS* Observed in Your Child THIS MONTH:

ACTIVATED

___ 1 Impulsivity
___ 2 Irritability
___ 3 Temper tantrums
___ 4 Sleeps less than usual
___ 5 Hyperactivity
___ 6 Increased aggression
___ 7 Skips school
___ 8 Decreased attention span
___ 9 Inappropriate sexual behavior
___ 10 Unusually happy and enthusiastic
___ 11 Excessively talkative
___ 12 Unreasonably and excessively self-confident

___ 13 Stealing
___ 14 Disregard for authority
___ 15 Fighting
___ 16 Destruction of property
___ 17 Excessive risk taking
___ 18 Trouble with the law
___ 19 Lack of remorse
___ 20 Frequent lying
___ 21 Racing thoughts
___ 22 Bizarre behavior
___ 23 Other: _____
___ 24 Other: _____

WITHDRAWN

___ 25 Periods of sadness
___ 26 Low self-esteem/ sense of worthlessness
___ 27 More withdrawn than usual
___ 28 Cries more easily than usual
___ 29 Unusually clingy and dependent
___ 30 Less active and energetic than usual
___ 31 Excessive guilt
___ 32 More anxious (tense/worried) than usual
___ 33 Change in appetite
___ 34 Suicidal thinking

___ 35 Suicidal gesture
___ 36 Serious suicide attempt
___ 37 Physical complaints
___ 38 Sleeps more than usual
___ 39 Obsessive thoughts
___ 40 Night terrors
___ 41 Does not talk or respond
___ 42 Paranoid thinking
___ 43 Hearing voices
___ 44 Other: _____
___ 45 Other: _____

Interventions or Treatments (list below)

For each MEDICATION, please enter the **total dose taken** per day.
For OTHER TREATMENT INTERVENTIONS (e.g., psychotherapy, behavior modification, etc.), please **check the days the treatment was received.**

Days of Month → 1 · 2 · 3 · 4 · 5 · 6 · 7 · 8 · 9 · 10 · 11 · 12 · 13 · 14 · 15 · 16 · 17 · 18 · 19 · 20 · 21 · 22 · 23 · 24 · 25 · 26 · 27 · 28 · 29 · 30 · 31

Please rate the degree of dysfunction caused by either ACTIVATED or WITHDRAWN behaviors above and below the midline.

Psychosis (√ if Yes)
Hours of Sleep

RATE DEGREE of Dysfunction:

Activated *(IMPULSIVE, AGGRESSIVE)*

SEVERE
HIGH MODERATE
LOW MODERATE
MILD

DYSFUNCTION

SEVERE
HIGH MOD
LOW MOD
MILD

DYSFUNCTION

Days of Month → 1 · 2 · 3 · 4 · 5 · 6 · 7 · 8 · 9 · 10 · 11 · 12 · 13 · 14 · 15 · 16 · 17 · 18 · 19 · 20 · 21 · 22 · 23 · 24 · 25 · 26 · 27 · 28 · 29 · 30 · 31 · Baseline

Withdrawn *(ANXIOUS, DEPRESSED)*

MILD
LOW MODERATE
HIGH MODERATE
SEVERE

DYSFUNCTION

MILD
LOW MOD
HIGH MOD
SEVERE

DYSFUNCTION

Number of Switches/Day

Life Event Impact* (-4 to +4)

Life Events and Predominant Symptoms*

Days of Month → 1 · 2 · 3 · 4 · 5 · 6 · 7 · 8 · 9 · 10 · 11 · 12 · 13 · 14 · 15 · 16 · 17 · 18 · 19 · 20 · 21 · 22 · 23 · 24 · 25 · 26 · 27 · 28 · 29 · 30 · 31

Prospective Kiddie life chart form for daily tracking

K-LCM™/R: The Child Life Chart Method - Parents RETROSPECTIVE Ratings

Patient Name _____   Date Completed [ ][ ] / [ ][ ] / [ ][ ]

Please Check √ **ALL BEHAVIORS AND SYMPTOMS*** Observed in Your Child During This **THREE- YEAR Period**:

ACTIVATED Behaviors Might Include:

YEAR (Below) 1 2 3		YEAR (Below) 1 2 3	
1 Impulsivity		13 Stealing	
2 Irritability		14 Disregard for authority	
3 Temper tantrums		15 Fighting	
4 Sleeps less than usual		16 Destruction of property	
5 Hyperactivity		17 Excessive risk taking	
6 Increased aggression		18 Trouble with the law	
7 Skips school		19 Lack of remorse	
8 Decreased attention span		20 Frequent lying	
9 Inappropriate sexual behavior		21 Racing thoughts	
10 Unusually happy and enthusiastic		22 Bizarre behavior	
11 Excessively talkative		23 Other: _____	
12 Unreasonably and excessively self-confident		24 Other: _____	

WITHDRAWN Behaviors Might Include:

YEAR (Below) 1 2 3		YEAR (Below) 1 2 3	
25 Periods of sadness		35 Suicidal gesture	
26 Low self-esteem/sense of worthlessness		36 Serious suicide attempt	
27 More withdrawn than usual		37 Physical complaints	
28 Cries more easily than usual		38 Sleeps more than usual	
29 Unusually clingy & dependent		39 Obsessive thoughts	
30 Less active & energetic than usual		40 Night terrors	
31 Excessive guilt		41 Does not talk or respond	
32 More anxious (tense/worried) than usual		42 Paranoid thinking	
33 Change in appetite		43 Hearing voices	
34 Suicidal thinking		44 Other: _____	
		45 Other: _____	
		46 Other: _____	

K-LCM™/R version 2-02

Interventions or Treatments (list below)

For each **MEDICATION**, please enter (by month) the **maximal dose per day taken** by the child. For **OTHER TREATMENT INTERVENTIONS** (e.g., psychotherapy, behavior modification, etc.), please **indicate the # of visits per month**.

Month of Year ——→ 1:2:3:4:5:6:7:8:9:10:11:12. 1:2:3:4:5:6:7:8:9:10:11:12. 1:2:3:4:5:6:7:8:9:10:11:12

19___   19___   19___

Please rate the degree of dysfunction caused by either ACTIVATED or WITHDRAWN behaviors above and below the midline.

Dysphoric / Irritable Mood (√ if Yes)

Activated (IMPULSIVE, AGGRESSIVE)
- SEVERE
- MODERATE
- MILD

DYSFUNCTION

Month of Year ——→ 1:2:3:4:5:6:7:8:9:10:11:12. 1:2:3:4:5:6:7:8:9:10:11:12. 1:2:3:4:5:6:7:8:9:10:11:12: Baseline

- MILD
- MODERATE
- SEVERE

DYSFUNCTION

Withdrawn (ANXIOUS, DEPRESSED)

Number of Mood Switches / Month
Cycling Within A Day (√ if Yes)

19___   19___   19___

Life Event Impact (-4 to +4)

Life Events and Predominant Symptoms*

Month of Year ——→ 1:2:3:4:5:6:7:8:9:10:11:12. 1:2:3:4:5:6:7:8:9:10:11:12. 1:2:3:4:5:6:7:8:9:10:11:12

Retrospective Kiddie life chart form for monthly tracking

3

Bipolarity Index of Suspicion

(The Speer/Post BIS) (Year 2000* Version)

Name of Subject: _____ Age: _____ Rater: _____

Relationship: _____

Date: Month:____/Day:___/Year:____

Check all statements that are applicable to subject:

A. Family history of bipolar illness (BP) in first-degree relative
___ 2 = One member (or one side of family)
___ 4 = Bilineal (both sides) one side BP, one side either unipolar or BP

A Subtotal_____
(Limit 4)

B. Temperament
___ 2 = Hyperthymic (chronically a little hyper)
___ 1 = Dysthymic (chronically a little low)
___ 2 = Cyclothymic (show cycling between both of above)

B Subtotal_____
(Limit 2)

C. Childhood prodrome
___ 1 = Extreme mood lability
___ 1 = Tantrums/violence
___ 1 = Hyperactivity
___ 1.5 = Hypersexuality
___ 1.5 = Delusional thoughts
___ 1 = Marked sleep disturbance
___ 1 = Substance abuse

C Subtotal_____
(Limit 4)

D. Diagnosis
___ 1.5 = Prepubertal dysthymia
___ 1.5 = Prepubertal depression
___ 2 = Prepubertal psychotic depression
___ 0.5 = Rapidly recurrent depressions
___ 2 = Postpartum depression
___ 1 = PMS with menstrually related euphoria

D Subtotal_____
(Limit 2)

E. Rx treatment-related symptoms

    ___ 3 = Antidepressant-induced hypomania

    ___ 2 = Steroid or other Rx   **E Subtotal**_____

                                                                   (Limit 3)

F. Symptoms occurring before, during, or after a depression

    ___ 3 = Decreased need for sleep

    ___ 2 = Increased energy

    ___ 1 = Increased sociability

    ___ 1 = Racing thoughts and lots of ideas

    ___ 1 = Hypersexuality/promiscuity

    ___ 1 = Complaints from friends, family, employers that behavior is different, overbearing, or aggressive

    ___ 1.5 = Periods of euphoria

    ___ 1 = Frivolous or excessive spending

    ___ 1.5 = Inflated self-esteem

    ___ 1 = Multiple projects started   **F Subtotal**_____

                                                                   (Limit 5)

Total # checked _____

Total raw score:_____   **Total scaled score**_____
(sum of all weighted numbers)   Sum of each limited subtotal (limit 20)
                                                 (i.e., not to exceed maximum of any subtotal)

    *This is an unpublished version of a rating scale that lists many items from the literature that have been associated with increased risk for the onset of bipolar disorder. It has not yet been validated, but is offered here for those who wish to do further clinical research with it. Also, if someone scores high on this inventory, it is advisable that they further investigate the possibility that they have early bipolar disorder and should be treated accordingly.

4

Refractory Depression Indexes
A. Bipolar Illness; B. Unipolar Depression

A. Refractory Index for Bipolar Illness (Year 2001 Version)

Column 1

Anticonvulsants	#	Tol.
A. Lithium (max 10)	10	
B. Carbamazepine (max 10)	10	
C. Lamotrigine (Lamictal) (max 10)	10	
D. Valproic Acid (max 10)	10	
Other (Specify)............		
Ca^{++} Dihydropyridine Type (max 5)		
Nimodipine (Nimotop)	5	
Amlodipine (Norvasc)	5	
Isradipine (DynaCirc)	5	
Other (Specify)............		
Nondihydropyridine Type (max 2.5)		
Verapamil (Calan/Isoptin)	3	
Ca^{+} Subtotal Score (max 5)		
F. Atypical Neuroleptic (max 10)		
Olanzapine (Zyprexa)	10	
Risperidone (Risperdal)	10	
Quetiapine (Seroquel)	10	
Other (Specify)............	10	
Atypical Neuro. Subtotal Score (max 10)		
G. Clozapine (max 10)		
Clozapine (Clozaril)	10	
Clozapine Subtotal Score (max 10)		
H. ECT (max 10)	Score:	
Unilateral: # treatments ____	5	
Bilateral # of treatments ____	10	
ECT Subtotal Score (max 10)		
75 Maximum Score		
Overall Column Subtotal Score ____		

Column 2

MAOI	#	Tol.
Isocarboxazid (Marplan)	3	
Phenelzine (Nardil)	3	
Selegilene (Eldepryl)	3	
Tranylcypromine (Parnate)	3	
MAOI Subtotal Score (max 2.5)		
SSRI Fluoxetine (Prozac)	3	
Fluvoxamine (Luvox)	3	
Paroxetine (Paxil)	3	
Sertraline (Zoloft)	3	
Citalopram (Celexa)	3	
Nefazodone (Serzone)	3	
SSRI Subtotal Score (max 2.5)		
D-A Buproprion (Wellbutrin)	3	
Pramipexole (Mirapex)	3	
D-A Subtotal Score (max 2.5)		
SNRI Venlafaxine (Effexor)	3	
SNRI Subtotal Score (max 2.5)		
TCA Amytriptyline (Elavil)	3	
Imipramine (Tofranil)	3	
Desipramine (DMI/Norpramin)	3	
Nortriptyline (Pamelor)	3	
Clomipramine (Anafranil)	3	
Other (Specify).............	3	
TCA Subtotal Score (max 2.5)		
Alt Potentiation Herbal	3	
Folate	3	
Ascorbate	3	
rTMS	3	
Inositol	3	
Omega-3 Fatty Acids	3	
Other (Specify)............	3	
Alt. Subtotal Score (max 2.5)		
15 Maximum Score		
Overall Column Subtotal Score ____		

Column 3

Augmentation (max 10)	#	Tol.
High-Potency Benzodiazepine (max 2.5)		
Alprazolam (Xanax)		2.5
Chlordiazepoxide (Librium)		2.5
Clonazepam (Klonopin)		2.5
Diazepam (Valium)		2.5
Lorazepam (Ativan)		2.5
Temazepam (Restoril)		2.5
Other (Specify)............		2.5
Benzo. Subtotal Score (max 2.5)		
Typical Neuroleptic (max 2.5)		
Chlorpromazine (Thorazine)		2.5
Haloperidol (Haldol)		2.5
Perphenazine (Trilafon)		2.5
Pimozide (Orap)		2.5
Thioridazine (Melaril)		2.5
Thiothixene (Navane)		2.5
Other (Specify)............		2.5
Neuroleptic Subtotal Score (max 2.5)		
Thyroid (max 2.5)		
T_3 (Cytomel)		2.5
T_4 (Synthroid)		2.5
T_3/T_4 (Cytomel/Synthroid)		2.5
High Dose T_4		2.5
Thyroid Subtotal Score (max 2.5)		
Anticonvulsants (max 2.5)		
Gabapentin (Neurontin)		2.5
Topiramate (Topamax)		2.5
Primidone (Mysoline)		2.5
Other (Specify)............		2.5
Anticonvuls. Subtotal Score (max 2.5)		
10 Maximum Score		
Overall Column Subtotal Score ____		

Total Score ____
(all three columns;
Maximum score is 100)

B. Refractory Index for Unipolar Depression (Year 2001 Version)

A. Tricyclic (max 10)

	#	Tol.
(Tertiary Amines) Amytriptyline (Elavil)	10	
Imipramine (Tofranil)	10	
Other (Specify)........	10	
(2° Amines) Desipramine (Norpramin)	10	
Nortriptyline (Pamelor)	10	
Other (Specify)........	10	
Clomipramine (Anafranil)	10	
TCA Subtotal Score:		

B. SSRI (max 10)

	#	
Fluoxetine (Prozac)	10	
Fluvoxamine (Luvox)	10	
Paroxetine (Paxil)	10	
Sertraline (Zoloft)	10	
Citalopram (Celexa)	10	
Nefazodone (Serzone)	10	
Other (Specify)........	10	
SSRI Subtotal Score:		

C. Dopamine-Related (max 10)

	#	
Bupropion (Wellbutrin)	10	
Pramipexole (Mirapex)	10	
Other (Specify)........	10	
D-R Subtotal Score:		

D. SNRI/RIMA/Other (max 10)

	#	
Venlafaxine (Effexor)	10	
Meclobemide	10	
Mirtazepine (Remeron)	10	
Other (Specify)........	10	
SNRI/RIMA Subtotal Score:		

E. MAOI (max 10)

	#	
Clorgyline	10	
Isocarboxazid (Marplan)	10	
Phenelzine (Nardil)	10	
Selegilene (Eldepryl)	10	
Tranylcypromine (Parnate)	10	
Other (Specify)........	10	
MAOI Subtotal Score:		

50 Maximum Score
Overall Subtotal Score ___

F. Potentiation (max 15)

	#	Tol.
Lithium (Eskalith-C)	5	
T₃/T₄ (Cytomel/Synthroid)	5	
Both T₃ and T₄	5	
Anticonvulsant #1........	5	
Anticonvulsant #2........	5	
Dexadrine(Stim/Amphetamine)	5	
Ritalin	5	
Pindolol	5	
Benzos/Barbituates/Anxiolytics		
Alprazolam (Xanax)	5	
Clonazepam (Klonopin)	5	
Lorazepam (Ativan)	5	
Diazepam (Valium)	5	
Temazepam (Restoril)	5	
Buspirone (Buspar)	5	
Other (Specify)........	5	
Atypical Neuroleptics		
Clozapine (Clozaril)	5	
Risperidone (Risperdal)	5	
Olanzapine (Zyprexa)	5	
Sertindole (Serdolect)	5	
Other (Specify)........	5	
Typical Neuroleptics		
Chlorpromazine (Thorazine)	5	
Haloperidol (Haldol)	5	
Perphenazine (Trilafon)	5	
Pimozide (Orap)	5	
Thioridazine (Melaril)	5	
Thiothixene (Navane)	5	
Other (Specify)........	5	
Other (Specify)........	5	
Other (Specify)........	5	

15 Maximum Score
Overall Subtotal score ___

G. Alt. Potentiation

	#	Tol.
St. John's Wort	3	
Other Herbal		
Light	3	
Melatonin	3	
Folate	3	
Ascorbate	3	
Zinc	3	
rTMS	3	
Inositol	3	
Omega-3 Fatty Acids	3	
Sleep Deprivation	3	
Acupuncture	3	
Other (Specify)........	3	
Other........	3	
Other........	3	

5 Maximum Score
Subtotal score ___

H. ECT

	#	Tol.
Unilateral		
1-5 treatments	10	
6-19 treatments	15	
>20 treatments	20	
Bilateral		
1-5 treatments	20	
6-19 treatments	25	
>20 treatments	30	
If treatment modality is not specified, take average of BL and UL treatment		
Average of BL and UL		

30 Maximum Score
Subtotal score ___

● **Add all 4 Column subtotals for:**
TOTAL REFRACTORY SCORE ___
(100 Max)

List number of:
1. Antidepressant Trials ___ (count first column checks)
2. Adjunctive Med Trials ___ (count potentiation and alt.pot.)
3. Total Med Trials ___ (count all 4 columns)
4. Meds to Which Patient. Became Tolerant

607

5

The Mood Disorder
Questionnaire (MDQ)

The MDQ is a useful screening tool (Hirshfeld et al., 2000, 2003). All those with a history of depression should fill out this brief MDQ.

Please answer these questions by circling the appropriate answers

A. Has there ever been a period of time when you were not your usual self and (while not using drugs or alcohol) . . .

1. . . . you felt so good or so hyper that other people thought you were not your normal self, or you were so hyper that you got into trouble? (*circle yes or no for each line please*)   Yes   No

2. . . . you were so irritable that you shouted at people or started fights or arguments?   Yes   No

3. . . . you felt much more self-confident than usual?   Yes   No

4. . . . you got much less sleep than usual and found you didn't really miss it?   Yes   No

5. . . . you were much more talkative or spoke faster than usual?   Yes   No

6. . . . thoughts raced through your head or you couldn't slow your mind down?   Yes   No

7. . . . you were so easily distracted by things around you that you had trouble concentrating or staying on track?   Yes   No

8. . . . you had much more energy than usual?   Yes   No

9. . . . you were much more active or did many more things than usual?   Yes   No

10. . . . you were much more social or outgoing than usual; for example, you telephoned friends in the middle of the night?   Yes   No

11. . . . you were much more interested in sex than usual?   Yes   No

12. . . . you did things that were unusual for you or that other people might have thought were excessive, foolish, or risky?   Yes   No

13. . . . spending money got you or your family into trouble?   Yes   No

B. If you checked YES to more than one of the above, have several of these ever happened during the *same period of time*?   Yes   No

C. How much of a *problem* did any of these cause you—like being unable to work; having family, money, or legal troubles; getting into arguments or fights?

    No Problem   Minor Problem   Moderate Problem   Serious Problem

D. Draw a line connecting any (blood) relative to any problem (this doesn't have to be neat):

       Grandparents   *Parents*   *Aunts/Uncles*   *Brothers/Sisters*   *Children*

    Suicide   Alcohol/drug problems   Mental Hospital   Depression Problems   Manic or bipolar

E. Has a health professional ever told you that you have manic-depressive illness or bipolar disorder?   Yes   No

If you circled 7 or more "YESs" in Part A, and you checked Yes in Part B, and these caused you minor to severe problems in Part C, you should talk to your physician or clinician for a more complete evaluation of the possibility you have a bipolar mood disorder.

Your Name _____   Today's Date _____

Note: This is not a diagnostic instrument but only a screening tool to alert you and your clinician to further explore these symptom areas as the treatment of a bipolar depression is different from that of a unipolar depression.

6

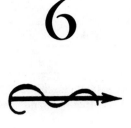

MAOI Diet and Information

Monoamine oxidase inhibitors (MAOIs) are drugs used to treat depression, high blood pressure, and other medical conditions. If you are taking MAOIs, you will follow a special diet.

A side effect of this type of medicine is that a normally harmless substance in food, tyramine (TY-ra-meen), is not broken down by the body by monoamine oxidase. High levels of tyramine release norepinephrine which normally is rapidly removed by monoamine oxidase. High levels of norepinephrine in the blood can lead to very high blood pressure, a severe headache, and possibly bleeding.

To avoid these serious side effects, you should avoid certain foods or eat them only in small amounts. The chart following will help guide you in your food choices.

Important MAOI Diet Points

- Foods that are close to spoiling, are aged (like cheese), or have been stored for a long time have higher levels of tyramine than fresh foods do. Try to prepare and eat fresh foods. Look for the expiration date on food packages. Avoid using dairy products that are close to their expiration date.

- Start the MAOI diet (also called the "low-tyramine" or "tyramine-controlled" diet) when you begin taking MAOI medication.

- Continue the MAOI diet for four weeks (or as directed by your physician) after stopping the MAOI medication.

- If you are on high doses of selegeline (Ensam), this diet should also be followed as the drug loses its selectivity for MAOI-B at high doses and you can still have a tyramine reaction.

Other Critical Information

- If you are on any MAOI, you also must not be on any drug that has potent effects on serotonin, such as the SSRIs or the SNRIs, as the combination can lead to the serotonin syndrome. This could involve fever, tremors, seizures, coma, and even death.

- If you are on a MAOI, you must not take the drug meperidine as this can have a potentially lethal interaction.

MAOI Diet

Food	Allowed	Limit	Avoid
Beverages	milk decaf coffee and tea carbonated drinks	chocolate drinks coffee, tea, and other caffein-ated drinks white wine and clear spirits (limit two 8 oz. servings)	alcoholic drinks, especially beer, ale, wine (Chianti, burgundy, sherry, vermouth, sauterne), and nonalcoholic beer and wine acidophilus milk
Bread	whole-wheat enriched white breads, rolls, crackers, and quick breads	none	cheese breads crackers sourdough and fresh, homemade, yeast-leavened breads
Cereals	cooked and dry cereals	none	none
Cheese and Dairy Products	cottage cheese, farmer or pot cheese, cream cheese, ricotta cheese, and processed cheese	buttermilk (limit to 4 oz.), sour cream, yogurt (national brands only—limit to 4 oz. per day)	all other cheese: aged cheese, Camembert, cheddar, Gouda, Gruyère, mozzarella, Parmesan, provolone, Roquefort, and Stilton
Desserts	cakes and cookies gelatins ice cream and sherbets pastries puddings	chocolate desserts	cheese-filled desserts and cheesecake
Eggs	all	none	quiche with cheese
Fats	all	none	none
Fruits	fresh, frozen, or canned fruits and juices	none	banana peel extract overripe and spoiled fruits
Meats, Fish and Poultry	all fresh or frozen meats, fish, or poultry	aged meats and frankfurters fresh sausage and pepperoni canned sardines canned meats fish roe (caviar) and pâté (limit to 1 oz.) caviar (more than 1 oz.) chicken and beef liver dried, salted, and pickled fish fermented and dry sausages salami dried meats and meat extracts	

Food	Allowed	Limit	Avoid
Potatoes and Substitutes	white and sweet potatoes grits, pasta, and rice	none	none
Soups	all cream and broth soups, except those on the *Avoid* list	none	soups from Italian broad beans and fava beans cheese soup soup made with beer or wine any soup cubes or meat extract packet soups and packaged soups miso soup
Sweets	sugars, hard candies, honey, molasses, and syrups	chocolate candies and chocolate syrups	imported chocolate
Vegetables	all fresh, frozen, canned or dried vegetables and vegetable juices, except those on the *Avoid* list	none	Chinese pea pods fava beans and Italian broad beans sauerkraut fermented soybean products (miso and some tofu products)
Miscellaneous	salt nuts and peanut butter spices, herbs, and flavorings	soy sauce (limit to 1/4 cup) and teriyaki sauce (limit to 1/4 cup) brewer's yeast	Marmite (vegetable extracts) yeast concentrates vitamin supplements with brewer's yeast monosodium glutamate (MSG) all aged products

Summary of Foods Definitely to be Avoided
Beer, red wine
Aged cheeses
Dry sausage, salami
Fava or Italian green beans
Brewer's yeast
Smoked fish
Chicken liver, beef liver
Sauerkraut

7

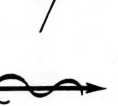

Organizations Offering Information and Support Resources

ORGANIZATIONS

American Academy of Child and Adolescent
   Psychiatry, Facts for Families
Tel: (202) 966-7300
www.aacap.org/

Juvenile Bipolar Research Foundation
Tel: (866) 333-5273
www.bpchildresearch.org/index.html

Child and Adolescent Bipolar Foundation
   (CABF)
Tel: (847) 256-8525
www.cabf.org

Depression Awareness Recognition and Treatment Education Program (D/ART)
Tel: (800) 421-4211 (free brochures)

Depression and Bipolar Support Alliance
   (DBSA); formerly National Depressive and
   Manic-Depressive Association (NDMDA)
Tel: (800) 826-3632; fax: (312) 642-7243
www.dbsalliance.org

National Alliance for Research on Schizophrenia and Depression (NARSAD)
Tel: (800) 829-8289; fax: (516) 487-6930

National Alliance for the Mentally Ill
Tel: (703) 524-7600; (800) 950-NAMI; fax:
   (703) 524-9094
www.nami.org

National Foundation for Depressive Illness
Tel: (800) 239-1265
www.depression.org

National Institute of Mental Health
Tel: (301) 443-4513; fax: (301) 443-4279
Depression brochures: (800) 421-4211; TTY:
   (301) 443-8431; FAX4U: (301) 443-5158
www.nimh.nih.gov

National Mental Health Association
Tel: (703) 684-7722; (800) 969-6642; Fax:
   (703) 684-5968
www.nmha.org

National Suicide Prevention Lifeline
Tel: (800) 273-TALK

INFORMATION

Bipolar Network News (BNN)
Two to four times yearly newsletter on timely
   clinical and research topics and listings of selected abstracts in the literature.
www.bipolarnews.org

The Dana Foundation
www.dana.org

Massachusetts General Hospital Bipolar Clinic
   and Research Program
Tel: (617) 726-6188
www.manicdepressive.org

Systematic Treatment Enhancement Program
for Bipolar Disorder (STEP-BD)
www.stepbd.org

Medscape
Often has articles on bipolar disorder and other
psychopharmacological issues.
www.medscape.com

Texas Department of State Health Services
This Web page contains the TMAP Algorithm
for Bipolar Disorder. Simply put the term
TMAP Algorithm into the small search win-
dow at the upper right-hand corner of the
Web page, which will take you directly to
the TMAP home page.
www.dshs.state.tx.us

References

Aagaard, J., & Vestergaard, P. (1990). Predictors of outcome in prophylactic lithium treatment: A 2-year prospective study. *Journal of Affective Disorders, 18,* 259–266.

Adams, D. H., Perlis, R. H., Houston, J. P., Sutton, V., Farmen, M., & Breier, A. F. (2007). Genetic association study of treatment response with olanzapine/fluoxetine combination or lamotrigine in bipolar I depression. *Presented at 160th Annual Meeting of the American Psychiatric Association, San Diego, CA* NR#777, 55.

Afflelou, S., Auriacombe, M., Cazenave, M., Chartres, J. P., & Tignol, J. (1997). Utilisation de levothyroxine a haute dose dans le traitement des troubles bipolaires a cycles rapides. Revue de la litterature et premieres applications therapeutiques a propos de 6 cas. [Administration of high-dose levothyroxine in treatment of rapid-cycling bipolar disorders. Review of the literature and initial therapeutic application apropos of 6 cases]. *Encephale, 23,* 209–217.

Agricola, R., Mazzarino, M., Urani, R., Gallo, V., & Grossi, E. (1982). Treatment of acute alcohol withdrawal syndrome with carbamazepine: A double-blind comparison with tiapride. *Journal of International Medical Research, 10,* 160–165.

Ahlfors, U. G., Baastrup, P. C., Dencker, S. J., Elgen, K., Lingjaerde, O., Pedersen, V., et al. (1981). Flupenthixol decanoate in recurrent manic-depressive illness. A comparison with lithium. *Acta Psychiatrica Scandinavica, 64,* 226–237.

Akiskal, H. S., Maser, J. D., Zeller, P. J., Endicott, J., Coryell, W., Keller, M., et al. (1995). Switching from "unipolar" to bipolar II. An 11-year prospective study of clinical and temperamental predictors in 559 patients. *Archives of General Psychiatry, 52,* 114–123.

Albright, P. S., & Burnham, W. M. (1983). Effects of phenytoin, carbamazepine, and clonazepam on cortex- and amygdala-kindled seizures in the rat. *Epilepsia, 21,* 681–689.

Alda, M., Passmore, M. J., Garnham, J., Duffy, A., MacDougall, M., Munro, M., et al. (2002). Clinical presentation of bipolar disorders responsive to lithium or lamotrigine. *International Journal of Neuropsychopharmacology, 5,* S58.

Alexander, G. E., Crutcher, M. D., & Delong, M. R. (1990). Basal ganglia-thalamocortical circuits: Parallel substrates for motor, oculomotor, "prefrontal" and "limbic" functions. *Progress in Brain Research, 85,* 119–146.

Altshuler, L. L., Barzokis, G., Grieder, T., Curran, J., & Mintz J. (1998). Amygdala enlargement in bipolar disorder and hippocampal reduction in schizophrenia: an MRI study demonstrating neuroanatomic specificity. *Archives of General Psychiatry 55,* 663–664.

Altshuler, L. L., Cohen, L., Szuba, M. P., Burt, V. K., Gitlin, M., & Mintz, J. (1996). Pharmacologic management of psychiatric illness during pregnancy: Dilemmas and guidelines. *American Journal of Psychiatry, 153,* 592–606.

Altshuler, L. L., Keck, P. E., Jr., McElroy, S. L., Suppes, T., Brown, E. S., Denicoff, K., et al. (1999). Gabapentin in the acute treatment of refractory bipolar disorder. *Bipolar Disorder, 1,* 61–65.

Altshuler, L., Kiriakos, L., Calcagno, J., Goodman, R., Gitlin, M., Frye, M., et al. (2001). The impact of antidepressant discontinuation versus antidepressant continuation on 1-year risk for relapse of bipolar depression: A retrospective chart review. *Journal of Clinical Psychiatry, 62,* 612–616.

Altshuler, L. L., Post, R. M., Black, D. O., et al. (2006). Subsyndromal depressive symptoms are associated with functional impairment in patients with bipolar disorder: Results of a large, multisite study. *Journal of Clinical Psychiatry, 67,* 1551–1660.

Altshuler, L. L., Post, R. M., Leverich, G. S., Mikalauskas, K., Rosoff, A., & Ackerman, L. (1995). Antidepressant-induced mania and cycle acceleration: A controversy revisited. *American Journal of Psychiatry, 152,* 1130–1138.

Altshuler, L. L., Suppes, T., Black, D. O., et al. (2006). Lower switch rate in depressed patients with bipolar II than bipolar I disorder treated adjunctively with second-generation antidepressants. *American Journal of Psychiatry, 163,* 313–315.

Altshuler, L., Suppes, T., Black, D., Nolen, W. A., Keck, P. E., Jr., Frye, M. A., et al. (2003). Impact of antidepressant discontinuation after acute bipolar depression remission on rates of depressive relapse at 1-year follow-up. *American Journal of Psychiatry, 160,* 1252–1262.

Ambrosio, A. F., Soares-da-Silva, P., Carvalho, C. M., & Carvalho, A. P. (2002). Mechanisms of action of carbamazepine and its derivatives, oxcarbazepine, BIA 2–093, and BIA 2–024. *Neurochemistry Research, 27,* 121–130.

American Psychiatric Association (1994). *Diagnostic and statistical manual of mental disorders* (4th ed.). Washington, DC: Author.

Amsterdam, J. (1998). Efficacy and safety of venlafaxine in the treatment of bipolar II major depressive episode. *Journal of Clinical Psychopharmacology, 18,* 414–417.

Amsterdam, J. D., & Garcia-Espana, F. (2000). Venlafaxine monotherapy in women with bipolar II and unipolar major depression. *Journal of Affective Disorders, 59,* 225–229.

Amsterdam, J. D., Garcia-Espana, F., Fawcett, J., Quitkin, F. M., Reimherr, F. W., Rosenbaum, J. F., et al. (1998). Efficacy and safety of fluoxetine in treating bipolar II major depressive episode. *Journal of Clinical Psychopharmacology, 18,* 435–440.

Anand, A., Bukhari, L., Jennings, S. A., Lee, C., Kamat, M., Shekhar, A., et al. (2005). A preliminary study of zonisamide treatment for bipolar depression in 10 patients. *Journal of Clinical Psychiatry 66*(2), 195–198.

Anderson, J. W., Greenway, F. L., Fujioka, K., Gadde, K. M., McKenney, J., & O'Neil, P. M. (2002). Bupropion SR enhances weight loss: A 48-week double-blind, placebo-controlled trial. *Obesity Research, 10,* 633–641.

Andrade, C., & Kurinji, S. (2002). Continuation and maintenance ECT: A review of recent research. *Journal of ECT, 18,* 149–158.

Andrews, J. M., Ninan, P. T., & Nemeroff, C. B. (1997). Venlafaxine: A novel antidepressant that has a dual mechanism of action. *Depression, 4,* 48–56.

Angrist, B., & Schulz, S. C. (1990). The neuroleptic-nonresponsive patient: Characterization and treatment. In D. Spiegel (Ed.), *Progress in psychiatry* (pp. xvii–xxviii). Washington, DC: American Psychiatric Press.

Angst, J., & Marneros, A. (2001). Bipolarity from ancient times to modern times: Conception, birth and rebirth. *Journal of Affective Disorders, 67,* 3–19.

Angst, J., Merikangas, K., Scheidegger, P., & Wicki, W. (1990). Recurrent brief depression: A new subtype of affective disorder. *Journal of Affective Disorders, 19,* 87–98.

Angst, J., Sellaro, R., Stassen, H. H., & Gamma, A. (2005). Diagnostic conversion from depression to bipolar disorders: Results of a long-term prospective study of hospital admissions. *Journal of Affective Disorders, 84,* 149–157.

Antelman, S. M., Eichler, A. J., Black, C. A., & Kocan, D. (1980). Interchangeability of stress and amphetamine in sensitization. *Science, 207,* 329–331.

Appolinario, J. C., Fontenelle, L. F., Papelbaum, M., Bueno, J. R., & Coutinho, W. (2002). Topiramate use in obese patients with binge eating disorder: An open study. *Canadian Journal of Psychiatry, 47,* 271–273.

Arean, P. A., & Alvidrez, J. (2001). Treating depressive disorders: Who responds, who does not respond, and who do we need to study? *Journal of Family Practice, 50,* E2.

Aronson, T. A., Shukla, S., & Hirschowitz, J. (1989). Clonazepam treatment of five lithium-refractory patients with bipolar disorder. *American Journal of Psychiatry, 146,* 77–80.

Asberg, M., Traskman, L., & Thoren, P. (1976). 5HIAA in cerebrospinal fluid. *Archives of General Psychiatry 33,* 1193–1197.

Ashton, A. K., & Wolin, R. E. (1996). Nefazodone-induced carbamazepine toxicity [letter]. *American Journal of Psychiatry, 153,* 733.

Avery, D. H., Isenberg, K. E., Sampson, S. M., Janicak, P. G., Lisanby, S. H., Maixner, D. F., & Loo, C. (2007). TMS in the acute treatment of major depression: Clinical response in an open-label extension trial. *Presented at 160th Annual Meeting of the American Psychiatric Association, San Diego, CA* NR #314, 22.

Avery, D. H., Holtzheimer, P, E, III, Fawaz, W., et al. (2006). A controlled study of repetitive transcranial magnetic stimulation in medication-resistant major depression. *Biological Psychiatry, 59,* 187–194.

Axelson, D., Birmaher, B., Strober, M., et al. (2006). Phenomenology of children and adolescents with bipolar spectrum disorders. *Archives of General Psychiatry, 63,* 1139–1148.

Baastrup, P. C., Hollnagel, P., Sorensen, R., & Schou, M. (1976). Adverse reactions in treatment with lithium carbonate and haloperidol. *Journal of the American Medical Association, 236,* 2645–2646.

Baastrup, P. C., Poulsen, J. C., Schou, M., Thomsen, K.,

& Amdisen, A. (1970). Prophylactic lithium: Double blind discontinuation in manic-depressive and recurrent-depressive disorders. *Lancet, 2*, 326–330.

Baastrup, P. C., & Schou, M. (1967). Lithium as a prophylactic agent: Its effect against recurrent depressions and manic-depressive psychosis. *Archives of General Psychiatry, 16*, 162–172.

Bahk, W.-M., Shin, Y.-C., Woo, J.-M., Yoon, B.-H., Lee, J.-S., Jon, D.-I., et al. (2005). Topiramate and divalproex in combination with risperidone for acute mania: A randomized open-label study. *Progress in Neuropsychopharmacology and Biological Psychiatry, 29*, 115–121.

Balanźa-Martínez, V., Tabarés-Seisdedos, R., Selva-Vera, G., Martińez-Arán, A., Torrent, C., Salazar-Fraile, J., et al. (2005). Persistent cognitive dysfunctions in bipolar I disorder and schizophrenic patients: A 3-year follow-up study. *Psychotherapy and Psychosomatics, 74*, 113–119.

Baldassano, C. F., Ballas, C., Datto, S. M., Kim, D., Littman, L., O'Reardon, J., et al. (2003). Ziprasidone-associated mania: A case series and review of the mechanism. *Bipolar Disorders, 5*, 72–75.

Baldassano, C. F., Nassir, G. S., Chang, A., Lyman, A., & Lipari, M. (2004). Acute treatment of bipolar depression with adjunctive zonisamide: A retrospective chart review. *Bipolar Disorders, 6*, 432–434.

Baldessarini, R. J., Leahy, L., Arcona, S., Gause, D., Zhang, W., & Hennen, J. (2007). Patterns of psychotropic drug prescription for U.S. patients with diagnoses of bipolar disorders. *Psychiatric Services, 58*, 85–91.

Balfour, J. A., & Bryson, H. M. (1994). Valproic acid. A review of its pharmacology and therapeutic potential in indications other than epilepsy. *CNS Drugs, 2*, 144–173.

Ballenger, J. C., & Post, R. M. (1978a). Kindling as a model for alcohol withdrawal syndromes. *British Journal of Psychiatry, 133*, 1–14.

Ballenger, J. C., & Post, R. M. (1978b). Therapeutic effects of carbamazepine in affective illness: Preliminary report. *Communications in Psychopharmacology, 2*, 159–175.

Ballenger, J. C., & Post, R. M. (1984). Carbamazepine in alcohol withdrawal syndromes and schizophrenic psychoses. *Psychopharmacology Bulletin, 20*, 572–584.

Banki, C. M., Bissette, G., Arato, M., & Nemeroff, C. B. (1988). Elevation of immunoreactive CSF TRH in depressed patients. *American Journal of Psychiatry, 145*, 1526–1531.

Banov, M. D., Zarate, C. A., Jr., Tohen, M., Scialabba, D., Wines, J. D., Jr., Kolbrener, M., et al. (1994). Clozapine therapy in refractory affective disorders: Polarity predicts response in long- term follow-up. *Journal of Clinical Psychiatry, 55*, 295–300.

Baptista, T., Rangel, N., Fernandez, V., Carrizo, E., El Fakih, Y., Uzcategui, E., et al. (2007). Metformin as an adjunctive treatment to control body weight and metabolic dysfunction during olanzapine administration: A multicentric, double-blind, placebo-controlled trial. *Schizophrenia Research,* May 7; Epub ahead of print.

Baptista, T., Martínez, J., Lacruz, A., Rangel, N., Beaulieu, S., Serrano, A., et al. (2006). Metformin for prevention of weight gain and insulin resistance with olanzapine: A double-blind placebo-controlled trial. *Canadian Journal of Psychiatry, 51*, 192–196.

Baptista, T., Weiss, S. R., & Post, R. M. (1993). Carbamazepine attenuates cocaine-induced increases in dopamine in the nucleus accumbens: An in vivo dialysis study. *European Journal of Pharmacology, 236*, 39–42.

Baptista, T., Zarate, J., Joober, R., Colasante, C., Beaulieu, S., Paez, X., et al. (2004). Drug induced weight gain, an impediment to successful pharmacotherapy: Focus on antipsychotics. *Current Drug Targets, 5*, 279–299.

Barbee, J. G., Conrad, E. J., & Jamhour, N. J. (2004). Aripiprazole augmentation in treatment-resistant depression. *Annals of Clinical Psychiatry, 16*, 189–194.

Barbee, J. G., IV, Jamhour, N. J., Stewart, J. W., Shelton, R. C., Reimherr, F. W., & Thompson, T. R. (2007). Lamotrigine as an antidepressant augmentation agent in refractory unipolar depression. *Presented at 160th Annual Meeting of the American Psychiatric Association, San Diego, CA* NR#381, 27.

Barker, W. A., & Eccleston, D. (1984). The treatment of chronic depression. An illustrative case. *British Journal of Psychiatry, 144*, 317–319.

Barrickman, L. L., Perry, P. J., Allen, A. J., Kuperman, S., Arndt, S. V., Herrmann, K. J., et al. (1995). Bupropion versus methylphenidate in the treatment of attention-deficit hyperactivity disorder. *Journal of the American Academy of Child and Adolescent Psychiatry, 34*, 649–657.

Bartzokis, G., Beckson, M., Lu, P. H., Edwards, N., Bridge, P., & Mintz, J. (2002). Brain maturation may be arrested in chronic cocaine addicts. *Biological Psychiatry, 51*, 605–611.

Barzman, D. H., DelBello, M. P., Adler, C. M., Stanford, K. E., & Strakowski, S. M. (2006). The efficacy and tolerability of quetiapine versus divalproex for the treatment of impulsivity and reactive aggression in adolescents with co-occurring bipolar disorder and disruptive behavior disorder(s). *Journal of Child and Adolescent Psychopharmacology, 16*, 665–670.

Barzman, D. H., DelBello, M. P., Kowatch, R. A., Gernert, B., Fleck, D. E., Pathak, S., et al. (2004). The effectiveness and tolerability of aripiprazole for pediatric bipolar disorders: A retrospective chart review. *Journal of Child and Adolescent Psychopharmacology, 14,* 593–600.

Bauer, M. S. (1992). Defining seasonal affective disorder(s) [editorial]. *Biological Psychiatry, 31,* 1185–1189.

Bauer, M., Adli, M., Bschor, T., Heinz, A., Rasgon, N., Frye, M., et al. (2003). Clinical applications of levothyroxine in refractory mood disorders. *Clinical Approaches in Bipolar Disorders, 2,* 49–56.

Bauer, M., Baur, H., Berghofer, A., Strohle, A., Hellweg, R., Muller-Oerlinghausen, B., et al. (2002). Effects of supraphysiological thyroxine administration in healthy controls and patients with depressive disorders. *Journal of Affective Disorders, 68,* 285–294.

Bauer, M., Berghofer, A., Bschor, T., Baumgartner, A., Kiesslinger, U., Hellweg, R., et al. (2002). Supraphysiological doses of L-thyroxine in the maintenance treatment of prophylaxis-resistant affective disorders. *Neuropsychopharmacology, 27,* 620–628.

Bauer, M., Fairbanks, L., Berghofer, A., Hierholzer, J., Bschor, T., Baethge, C., et al. (2004). Bone mineral density during maintenance treatment with supraphysiological doses of levothyroxine in affective disorders: A longitudinal study. *Journal of Affective Disorders, 83,* 183–190.

Bauer, M., Hellweg, R., Graf, K. J,, & Baumgartner, A. (1998). Treatment of refractory depression with high-dose thyroxine. *Neuropsychopharmacology, 18,* 444–455.

Bauer, M., London, E. D., Rasgon, N., Berman, S. M., Frye, M. A., Altshuler, L. L., et al. (2005). Supraphysiological doses of levothyroxine alter regional cerebral metabolism and improve mood in bipolar depression. *Molecular Psychiatry, 10,* 456–469.

Bauer, M., Priebe, S., Berghofer, A., Bschor, T., Kiesslinger, U., & Whybrow, P. C. (2001). Subjective response to and tolerability of long-term supraphysiological doses of levothyroxine in refractory mood disorders. *Journal of Affective Disorders, 64,* 35–42.

Bauer, M. S., & Whybrow, P. C. (1986). The effect of changing thyroid function on cyclic affective illness in a human subject. *American Journal of Psychiatry, 143,* 633–636.

Bauer, M. S., & Whybrow, P. C. (1988). Thyroid hormones and the central nervous system in affective illness: Interactions that may have clinical significance. *Integrated Psychiatry, 6,* 75–100.

Bauer, M. S., & Whybrow, P. C. (1990). Rapid cycling bipolar affective disorder. II Treatment of refractory rapid cycling with high-dose levothyroxine: A preliminary study. *Archives of General Psychiatry, 47,* 435–440.

Baumer, F. M., Howe, M., Gallelli, K., Simeonova, D. I., Hallmayer, J., & Chang, K. D. (2006). A pilot study of antidepressant-induced mania in pediatric

bipolar disorder: Characteristics, risk factors, and the serotonin transporter gene. *Biological Psychiatry, 60,* 1005–1012.

Baumgartner, A., Bauer, M., & Hellweg, R. (1994). Treatment of intractable non-rapid cycling bipolar afective disorder with high-dose thyroxine: An open clinical trial. *Neuropsychopharmacology, 10,* 183–189.

Baxter, L. R. (1985). Can lithium carbonate prolong the antidepressant effect of sleep deprivation? *Archives of General Psychiatry, 42,* 635.

Baxter, L. R., Jr., Schwartz, J. M., Phelps, M. E., Mazziotta, J. C., Guze, B. H., Selin, C. E., et al. (1989). Reduction of prefrontal cortex glucose metabolism common to three types of depression. *Archives of General Psychiatry, 46,* 243–250.

Beatty, W. W., Bierley, R. A., & Rush, J. R. (1985). Spatial memory in rats: Electroconvulsive shock selectively disrupts working memory but spares reference memory. *Behavioral and Neural Biology, 44,* 403–414.

Beaudry, P., Fontaine, R., Chouinard, G., & Annable, L. (1985). An open clinical trial of clonazepam in the treatment of patients with recurrent panic attacks. *Progress in Neuropsychopharmacology and Biological Psychiatry, 9,* 589–592.

Bell, C., Vanderlinden, H., Hiersemenzel, R., Otoul, C., Nutt, D., & Wilson, S. (2002). The effects of levetiracetam on objective and subjective sleep parameters in healthy volunteers and patients with partial epilepsy. *Journal of Sleep Research, 11,* 255–263.

Benedetti, F., Barbini, B., Campori, E., Fulgosi, M. C., Pontiggia, A., & Colombo, C. (2001). Sleep phase advance and lithium to sustain the antidepressant effect of total sleep deprivation in bipolar depression: New findings supporting the internal coincidence model? *Journal of Psychiatric Research, 35,* 323–329.

Ben Menachem, E., & Gilland, E. (2003). Efficacy and tolerability of levetiracetam during 1-year follow-up in patients with refractory epilepsy. *Seizure, 12,* 131–135.

Ben-Menachem, E., Maññon-Espaillat, R., Ristanovic, R., Wilder, B. J., Stefan, H., Mirza, W., et al. (1994). Vagus nerve stimulation for treatment of partial seizures. 1. A controlled study of effect on seizures. First International Vagus Nerve Stimulation Study Group. *Epilepsia, 35,* 616–626.

Bennett, G. D., Amore, B. M., Finnell, R. H., Wlodarczyk, B., Kalhorn, T. F., Skiles, G. L., et al. (1996). Teratogenicity of carbamazepine-10,11-epoxide and oxcarbazepine in the SWV mouse. *Journal of Pharmacology and Experimental Therapeutics, 279,* 1237–1242.

Benson, B. E., Willis, M. W., Ketter, T. A., Kimbrell, T. A., George, M. S., Herscovitch, P., & Post, R. M. (2007). Inter regional cerebral metabolic associativity during a continuous performance task, Part II: Differential alterations in bipolar and unipolar disorders. *Psychiatry Research: Neuroimaging*, in press.

Berlant, J. L. (2001). Topiramate in posttraumatic stress disorder: Preliminary clinical observations. *Journal of Clinical Psychiatry, 62*(Suppl. 17), 60–63.

Berlant, J., & Van Kammen, D. P. (2002). Open-label topiramate as primary or adjunctive therapy in chronic civilian posttraumatic stress disorder: A preliminary report. *Journal of Clinical Psychiatry, 63*, 15–20.

Berman, R. M., Marcus, R. M., Swanink, R., McQuade, R. D., and Khan, A. (2007). Efficacy and safety of aripiprazole as adjunctive therapy in MDD; A multicenter, randomized, double-blind, placebo-controlled study. *Presented at 160th Annual Meeting of the American Psychiatric Association, San Diego, CA* NR#310, 22.

Berrettini, W. H., Ferraro, T. N., Goldin, L. R., Weeks, D. E., Detera-Wadleigh, S. D., Nurnberger, J. I., Jr., Gershon, E. S. (1994). Chromosome 18 DNA markers and manic-depressive illness: Evidence for a susceptibility gene. *Proceedings of the National Academy of Sciences USA, 91*, 5918–5921.

Berton,O., McClung, C. A., Dileone, R. J., Krishnan, V., Renthal, W., Russo, S. J., et al. (2006). Essential role of BDNF in the mesolimbic dopamine pathway in social defeat stress. *Science, 311*, 864–868.

Biederman, J., McDonnell, M. A., Wozniak, J., Spencer, T., Aleardi, M., Falzone, R., et al. (2005). Aripiprazole in the treatment of pediatric bipolar disorder: A systematic chart review. *CNS Spectrums, 10*, 141–148.

Biederman, J., Mick, E., Prince, J., Bostic, J. Q., Wilens, T. E., Spencer, T., et al. (1999). Systematic chart review of the pharmacologic treatment of comorbid attention deficit hyperactivity disorder in youth with bipolar disorder. *Journal of Child and Adolescent Psychopharmacology, 9*, 247–256.

Bifulco, A. T., Brown, G. W., & Harris, T. O. (1987). Childhood loss of parent, lack of adequate parental care and adult depression: A replication. *Journal of Affective Disorders, 12*, 115–128.

Birmaher, B. (2004). *New hope for children and teens with bipolar disorder.* New York: Random House.

Birmaher, B., Axelson, D., Strober, M., Gill, M. K., Valeri, S., Chiappetta, L., et al. (2006). Clinical course of children and adolescents with bipolar spectrum disorders. *Archives of General Psychiatry, 63*, 175–183.

Blumberg, H. P., Fredericks, C., Wang, F., Kalmar, J. H., Spencer, L., Papademetris, X., et al. (2005). Preliminary evidence for persistent abnormalities in amygdala volumes in adolescents and young adults with bipolar disorder. *Bipolar Disorders, 7*, 570–576.

Blumberg, H. P., Krystal, J. H., Bansal, R., Martin, A., Dziura, J., Durkin, K., et al. (2006). Age, rapid-cycling, and pharmacotherapy effects on ventral prefrontal cortex in bipolar disorder: a cross-sectional study. *Biological Psychiatry, 59*, 611–618.

Bourgeois, B. F. (1988). Anticonvulsant potency and neurotoxicity of valproate alone and in combination with carbamazepine or phenobarbital. *Clinical Neuropharmacology, 11*, 348–359.

Bowden, C. L. (1995). Predictors of response to divalproex and lithium. *Journal of Clinical Psychiatry, 56*(Suppl. 3), 25–30.

Bowden, C. L., Brugger, A. M., Swann, A. C., Calabrese, J. R., Janicak, P. G., Petty, F., et al. (1994). Efficacy of divalproex vs lithium and placebo in the treatment of mania. *Journal of the American Medical Association, 271*, 918–924.

Bowden, C. L., Calabrese, J. R., McElroy, S. L., Gyulai, L., Wassef, A., Petty, F., et al. (2000). A randomized, placebo-controlled 12-month trial of divalproex and lithium in treatment of outpatients with bipolar I disorder. Divalproex Maintenance Study Group. *Archives of General Psychiatry, 57*, 481–489.

Bowden, C. L., Calabrese, J. R., Sachs, G., Yatham, L. N., Asghar, S. A., Hompland, M., et al. (2003). A placebo-controlled 18-month trial of lamotrigine and lithium maintenance treatment in recently manic or hypomanic patients with bipolar I disorder. *Archives of General Psychiatry, 60*, 392–400.

Bowden, C. L., Lawson, D. M., Cunningham, M., Owen, J. R., & Tracy, K. A. (2002). The role of divalproex in the treatment of bipolar disorder. *Psychiatric Annals, 32*, 742–750.

Bowden, C. L., Myers, J. E., Grossman, F., & Xie, Y. (2004). Risperidone in combination with mood stabilizers: A 10-week continuation phase study in bipolar I disorder. *Journal of Clinical Psychiatry, 65*, 707–714.

Bozikas, V., Petrikis, P., Gamvrula, K., Savvidou, I., & Karavatos, A. (2002). Treatment of alcohol withdrawal with gabapentin. *Progress in Neuropsychopharmacology and Biological Psychiatry, 26*, 197–199.

Bradwejn, J., Shriqui, C., Koszycki, D., & Meterissian, G. (1990). Double-blind comparison of the effects of clonazepam and lorazepam in acute mania. *Journal of Clinical Psychopharmacology, 10*, 403–408.

Brannan, S. K., Mallinckrodt, C. H., Brown, E. B., Wohlreich, M. M., Watkin, J. G., Schatzberg, A. F. (2005). Duloxetine 60 mg once-daily in the treatment of painful physical symptoms in patients with major depressive disorder. *Journal of Psychiatric Research, 39*, 43–53.

Braunig, P., & Kruger, S. (2003). Levetiracetam in the treatment of rapid cycling bipolar disorder. *Journal of Psychopharmacology, 17*, 239–241.

Breier, A., Kelsoe, J. R. J., Kirwin, P. D., Beller, S. A., Wolkowitz, O. M., & Pickar, D. (1988) Early parental loss and development of adult psychopathology. *Archives of General Psychiatry, 45,* 987–993.

Breslau, N., Davis, G. C., Peterson, E. L., & Schultz, L. R. (2000). A second look at comorbidity in victims of trauma: The posttraumatic stress disorder-major depression connection. *Biological Psychiatry, 48,* 902–909.

Brodie, M. J., Forrest, G., & Rapeport, W. G. (1983). Carbamazepine-10, 11-epoxide concentrations in epileptics on carbamazepine alone and in combination with other anticonvulsants. *British Journal of Clinical Pharmacology, 16,* 747–749.

Brodie, M. J., & Yuen, A. W. (1997). Lamotrigine substitution study: Evidence for synergism with sodium valproate? 105 Study Group. *Epilepsy Research, 26,* 423–432.

Brotman, M. A., Fergus, E. L., Post, R. M., & Leverich, G. S. (2000). High exposure to neuroleptics in bipolar patients: A retrospective review. *Journal of Clinical Psychiatry, 61,* 68–72.

Brunet, G., Cerlich, B., Robert, P., Dumas, S., Souetre, E., & Darcourt, G. (1990). Open trial of a calcium antagonist, nimodipine, in acute mania. *Clinical Neuropharmacology, 13,* 224–228.

Bschor, T., Lewitzka, U., Sasse, J., Adli, M., Koberle, U., & Bauer, M. (2003). Lithium augmentation in treatment-resistant depression: Clinical evidence, serotonergic and endocrine mechanisms. *Pharmacopsychiatry, 36*(Suppl. 3), S230–S234.

Bunevicius, R., Kazanavicius, G., Zalinkevicius, R., & Prange, A. J., Jr. (1999). Effects of thyroxine as compared with thyroxine plus triiodothyronine in patients with hypothyroidism. *New England Journal of Medicine, 340,* 424–429.

Burt, T., Lisanby, S. H., & Sackeim, H. A. (2002). Neuropsychiatric applications of transcranial magnetic stimulation: A meta analysis. *International Journal of Neuropsychopharmacology, 5,* 73–103.

Burt, T., Sachs, G. S., & Demopulos, C. (1999). Donepezil in treatment-resistant bipolar disorder. *Biological Psychiatry, 45,* 959–964.

Buse, J. B. (2002). Metabolic effects of antipsychotics: Focusing on hyperglycemia and diabetes. *Journal of Clinical Psychiatry, 63*(Suppl. 4), 37–41.

Cabras, P. L., Hardoy, M. J., Hardoy, M. C., & Carta, M. G. (1999). Clinical experience with gabapentin in patients with bipolar or schizoaffective disorder: Results of an open-label study. *Journal of Clinical Psychiatry, 60,* 245–248.

Cade, J. F. J. (1977). Lithium—past, present and future. In F. N. Johnson & S. Johnson (Eds.), *Lithium in medical practice: Proceedings of the First British Lithium Congress, University of Lancaster, England.* Baltimore: University Park Press.

Calabrese, J. R., Bowden, C. L., Sachs, G. S., Ascher, J. A., Monaghan, E. , & Rudd, G. D. (1999). A double-blind placebo-controlled study of lamotrigine monotherapy in outpatients with bipolar I depression. Lamictal 602 Study Group. *Journal of Clinical Psychiatry, 60,* 79–88.

Calabrese, J. R., Bowden, C. L., Sachs, G., Yatham, L. N., Behnke, K., Mehtonen, O. P., et al. (2003). A placebo-controlled 18-month trial of lamotrigine and lithium maintenance treatment in recently depressed patients with bipolar I disorder. *Journal of Clinical Psychiatry, 64,* 1013–1024.

Calabrese, J. R., Fatemi, S. H., Kujawa, M., & Woyshville, M. J. (1996). Predictors of response to mood stabilizers. *Journal of Clinical Psychopharmacology, 16,* 24S–31S.

Calabrese, J. R., Hirschfeld, R. M., Reed, M., Davies, M. A., Frye, M. A., Keck, P. E., et al. (2003). Impact of bipolar disorder on a U.S. community sample. *Journal of Clinical Psychiatry, 64,* 425–432.

Calabrese, J. R., Keck, P. E., Jr., Macfadden, W., Minkwitz, M., Ketter, T. A., Weisler, R. H., et al. (2005). A randomized, double-blind, placebo-controlled trial of quetiapine in the treatment of bipolar I or II depression. *American Journal of Psychiatry, 162,* 1351–1360.

Calabrese, J. R., Keck, P. E., Jr., McElroy, S. L., & Shelton, M. D. (2001). A pilot study of topiramate as monotherapy in the treatment of acute mania. *Journal of Clinical Psychopharmacology, 21,* 340–342.

Calabrese, J. R., Kimmel, S. E., Woyshville, M. J., Rapport, D. J., Faust, C. J., Thompson, P. A., et al. (1996). Clozapine for treatment-refractory mania. *American Journal of Psychiatry, 153,* 759–764.

Calabrese, J. R., Markivitz, P. J., Kimmel, S. E., & Wagner, S. C. (1992). Spectrum of efficacy of valproate in 78 rapid-cycling bipolar patients. *Journal of Clinical Psychopharmacology, 12,* 53S–56S.

Calabrese, J. R., Rapport, D. J., Shelton, M. D., Kujawa, M., & Kimmel, S. E. (1998). Clinical studies on the use of lamotrigine in bipolar disorder. *Neuropsychobiology, 38,* 185–191.

Calabrese, J. R., Shelton, M. D., Rapport, D. J., Youngstrom, E. A., Jackson, K., Bilali, S., et al. (2005). A 20-month, double-blind, maintenance trial of lithium versus divalproex in rapid-cycling bipolar disorder. *American Journal of Psychiatry, 162,* 2152–2161.

Calabrese, J. R., Soegaard, J., Hompland, M., Mehtonen, O. P., Ruetsch, G., & Paska, W. (2002). Summary and meta-analysis of two large placebo-controlled 18-month maintenance trials of lamotrigine and lithium treatment in bipolar I disorder. *International Journal of Neuropsychopharmacology, 5,* S58.

Calabrese, J. R., Suppes, T., Bowden, C. L., Sachs, G. S., Swann, A. C., McElroy, S. L., et al. (2000).

A double-blind, placebo-controlled, prophylaxis study of lamotrigine in rapid-cycling bipolar disorder. Lamictal 614 Study Group. *Journal of Clinical Psychiatry, 61*, 841–850.

Calabrese, J. R., Woyshville, M. J., Kimmel, S. E., & Rapport, D. J. (1993). Predictors of valproate response in bipolar rapid cycling. *Journal of Clinical Psychopharmacology, 13*, 280–283.

Calabrese, J. R., Woyshville, M. J., & Rapport, R. T. (1994). Clinical efficacy of valproate. In R. T. Joffe & J. R. Calabrese (Eds.), *Anticonvulsants in mood disorders* (pp. 131–146). New York: Marcel Dekker.

Callahan, A. M., Frye, M. A., Marangell, L. B., George, M. S., Ketter, T. A., L'Herrou, T., et al. (1997). Comparative antidepressant effects of intravenous and intrathecal thyrotropin-releasing hormone: Confounding effects of tolerance and implications for therapeutics. *Biological Psychiatry, 41*, 264–272.

Cameron, H. A., & McKay, R. D. (2001). Adult neurogenesis produces a large pool of new granule cells in the dentate gyrus. *Journal of Comparative Neurology, 435*, 406–417.

Carpenter, L. L., Leon, Z., Yasmin, S., & Price, L. H. (2002). Do obese depressed patients respond to topiramate? A retrospective chart review. *Journal of Affective Disorders, 69*, 251–255.

Carrol, B. J. (1978). Neuroendocrine function in psychiatric disorders. In M. A. Lipton, A. DiMascio, & _. Killam (Eds.), *Psychopharmacology: A Generation of Progress.* New York: Raven Press.

Caspi, A., Sugden, K., Moffitt, T. E., Taylor, A., Craig, I. W., Harrington, H., et al. (2003). Influence of life stress on depression: Moderation by a polymorphism in the 5-HTT gene. *Science, 301*, 386–389.

Cavazzoni, P., Tanaka, Y., Roychowdhury, S. M., Breier, A., & Allison, D. B. (2003). Nizatidine for prevention of weight gain with olanzapine: A double-blind placebo-controlled trial. *European Neuropsychopharmacology, 13*, 81–85.

Chadwick, D. W., & Marson, A. G. (2002). Zonisamide add-on for drug-resistant partial epilepsy. *Cochrane Database of Systematic Reviews*, CD001416.

Chang, K., Saxena, K., & Howe, M. (2006). An open-label study of lamotrigine adjunct or monotherapy for the treatment of adolescents with bipolar depression. *Journal of the American Academy of Child and Adolescent Psychiatry, 45*, 298–304.

Charney, D. S., & Woods, S. W. (1989). Benzodiazepine treatment of panic disorder: A comparison of alprazolam and lorazepam. *Journal of Clinical Psychiatry, 50*, 418–423.

Chassan, J. B. (1992). Intensive design: Statistics and the single case. In M. Fava & J. F. Rosenbaum (Eds.), *Research designs and methods in psychiatry* (pp. 173–183). Amsterdam: Elsevier.

Chen, G., Zeng, W. Z., Yuan, P. X., Huang, L. D.,

Jiang, Y. M., Zhao, Z. H., et al. (1999). The mood-stabilizing agents lithium and valproate robustly increase the levels of the neuroprotective protein bcl-2 in the CNS. *Journal of Neurochemistry, 72*, 879–882.

Chen, R. W., & Chuang, D. M. (1999). Long term lithium treatment suppresses p53 and Bax expression but increases Bcl-2 expression. A prominent role in neuroprotection against excitotoxicity. *Journal of Biological Chemistry, 274*, 6039–6042.

Chengappa, R. K. N., Levine, J., Rathore, D., Parepally, H., & Atzert, R. (2001). Long-term effects of topiramate on bipolar mood instability, weight change and glycemic control: A case-series. *European Psychiatry, 16*, 186–190.

Chengappa, K. N., Rathore, D., Levine, J., Atzert, R., Solai, L., Parepally, H., et al. (1999). Topiramate as add-on treatment for patients with bipolar mania. *Bipolar Disorders, 1*, 42–53.

Choi, H, & Morrell, M. J. (2003). Review of lamotrigine and its clinical applications in epilepsy. *Expert Opinion on Pharmacotherapy, 4*, 243–251.

Chouinard, G. (1987). Clonazepam in acute and maintenance treatment of bipolar affective disorder. *Journal of Clinical Psychiatry, 48*, 29–37.

Chuang, D. M, Chen, R. W, Chalecka-Franaszek, E., Ren, M., Hashimoto, R., Senatorov, V., et al. (2002). Neuroprotective effects of lithium in cultured cells and animal models of diseases. *Bipolar Disorders, 4*, 129–136.

Cizza, G., Ravn, P., Chrousos, G. P., & Gold, P. W. (2001). Depression: A major, unrecognized risk factor for osteoporosis? *Trends in Endocrinology and Metabolism, 12*, 198–203.

Cohen, A. N., Hammen, C., Henry, R. M., & Daley, S. E. (2004). Effects of stress and social support on recurrence in bipolar disorder. *Journal of Affective Disorders, 82*, 143–147.

Cohen, B. M, & Baldessarini, R. J. (1985). Tolerance to therapeutic effects of antidepressants. *American Journal of Psychiatry, 142*, 489–490.

Cohrs, S., Tergau, F., Korn, J., Becker, W., & Hajak, G. (2001). Suprathreshold repetitive transcranial magnetic stimulation elevates thyroid-stimulating hormone in healthy male subjects. *Journal of Nervous and Mental Disease, 189*, 393–397.

Coleman, C. C., Cunningham, L. A., Foster, V. J., Batey, S. R., Donahue, R. M., Houser, T. L., et al. (1999). Sexual dysfunction associated with the treatment of depression: A placebo-controlled comparison of bupropion sustained release and sertraline treatment. *Annals of Clinical Psychiatry, 11*, 205–215.

Conway, C. R., Sheline, Y. I., Chibnall, J. T., George, M. S., Bhatt, A. A., Fletcher, J.W., & Mintun, M. A. (2007). Acute, subacute, and chronic brain metabolic change with vagus nerve stimulation in depression. *Presented at 160th Annual Meeting of the American Psychiatric Association, San Diego, CA* NR#334, 23.

Cooke, R. G., Joffe, R. T., & Levitt, A. J. (1992). T3 augmentation of antidepressant treatment in T4-replaced thyroid patients. *Journal of Clinical Psychiatry, 53*, 16–18.

Coplan, J. D., Andrews, M. W., Rosenblum, L. A., Owens, M. J., Friedman, S., Gorman, J. M., et al. (1996). Persistent elevations of cerebrospinal fluid concentrations of corticotropin-releasing factor in adult nonhuman primates exposed to early-life stressors: Implications for the pathophysiology of mood and anxiety disorders. *Proceedings of the National Academy of Science USA, 93*, 1619–1623.

Coppen, A., & Bailey, J. (2000). Enhancement of the antidepressant action of fluoxetine by folic acid: A randomised, placebo controlled trial. *Journal of Affective Disorders, 60*, 121–130.

Coppen, A., Chaudhry, S., & Swade, C. (1986). Folic acid enhances lithium prophylaxis. *Journal of Affective Disorders, 10*, 9–13.

Coppen, A., Prange, A. J., Jr., Whybrow, P. C., & Noguera, R. (1972). Abnormalities of indoleamines in affective disorders. *Archives of General Psychiatry, 26*, 474–478.

Cora-Locatelli, G., Greenberg, B. D., Martin, J., & Murphy, D. L. (1998). Gabapentin augmentation for fluoxetine-treated patients with obsessive-compulsive disorder. *Journal of Clinical Psychiatry, 59*, 480–481.

Coryell, W., Noyes, R., Jr., Clancy, J., Crowe, R., & Chaudhry, D. (1985). Abnormal escape from dexamethasone suppression in agoraphobia with panic attacks. *Psychiatry Research 15*, 301–311.

Coryell, W., Solomon, D., Turvey, C., Keller, M., Leon, A. C., Endicott, J., et al. (2003). The long-term course of rapid-cycling bipolar disorder. *Archives of General Psychiatry, 60*, 914–920.

Cowdry, R. W, & Gardner, D. L. (1988). Pharmacotherapy of borderline personality disorder. Alprazolam, carbamazepine, trifluoperazine, and tranylcypromine. *Archives of General Psychiatry, 45*, 111–119.

Cramer, J. A., De Rue, K., Devinsky, O., Edrich, P., & Trimble, M. R. (2003). A systematic review of the behavioral effects of levetiracetam in adults with epilepsy, cognitive disorders, or an anxiety disorder during clinical trials. *Epilepsy and Behavior, 4*, 124–132.

Cullen, M., Mitchell, P., Brodaty, H., Boyce, P., Parker, G., Hickie, I., et al. (1991). Carbamazepine for treatment-resistant melancholia. *Journal of Clinical Psychiatry, 52*, 472–476.

Cunha, A. B., Frey, B. N., Andreazza, A. C., Goi, J. D., Rosa, A. R., Goncalves, C. A., et al. (2006). Serum brain-derived neurotrophic factor is decreased in bipolar disorder during depressive and manic episodes. *Neuroscience Letters, 398*, 215–219.

Curtin, F, & Schulz, P. (2004). Clonazepam and lorazepam in acute mania: A Bayesian meta-analysis. *Journal of Affective Disorders, 78*, 201–208.

Cutler, N. R., & Post, R. M. (1982). State-related cyclical dyskinesias in manic-depressive illness. *Journal of Clinical Psychopharmacology, 2*, 350–354.

Cutler, N. R., Post, R. M., Rey, A. C., & Bunney, W. E., Jr. (1981). Depression-dependent dyskinesias in two cases of manic depressive illness. *New England Journal of Medicine, 304*, 1088–1089.

Dannon, P. N., Dolberg, O. T., Schreiber, S., & Grunhaus, L. (2002). Three- and six-month outcome following courses of either ECT or rTMS in a population of severely depressed individuals—preliminary report. *Biological Psychiatry, 51*, 687–690.

Dardennes, R., Even, C., Bange, F., & Heim, A. (1995). Comparison of carbamazepine and lithium in the prophylaxis of bipolar disorders. *British Journal of Psychiatry, 166*, 378–381.

Davanzo, P. A., Krah, N., Kleiner, J., & McCracken, J. (1999). Nimodipine treatment of an adolescent with ultradian cycling bipolar affective illness. *Journal of Child and Adolescent Psychopharmacology, 9*, 51–61.

Davidson, J. R., Weisler, R. H., Butterfield, M. I., Casat, C. D., Connor, K. M., Barnett, S., et al. (2003). Mirtazapine vs placebo in posttraumatic stress disorder: A pilot trial. *Biological Psychiatry, 53*, 188–191.

Davies, M. A., Sheffler, D. J., & Roth, B. L. (2004). Aripiprazole: A novel atypical antipsychotic drug with a uniquely robust pharmacology. *CNS Drug Reviews, 10*, 317–336.

Davis, J. M., Wang, Z., & Janicak, P. G. (1993). A quantitative analysis of clinical drug trials for the treatment of affective disorders. *Psychopharmacology Bulletin, 29*, 175–181.

Davis, L. L., Bartolucci, A., & Petty, F. (2005). Divalproex in the treatment of bipolar depression: A placebo-controlled study. *Journal of Affective Disorders, 85*, 259–266.

Davis, L. L., Kabel, D., Patel, D., Choate, A. D., Foslien-Nash, C., Gurguis, G. N., et al. (1996). Valproate as an antidepressant in major depressive disorder. *Psychopharmacology Bulletin, 32*, 647–652.

Davis, M. (1997). Neurobiology of fear responses: The role of the amygdala. *Journal of Neuropsychiatry and Clinical Neuroscience, 9*, 382–402.

Davis, M., Walker, D. L., & Myers, K. M. (2003). Role of the amygdala in fear extinction measured with potentiated startle. *Annals of the New York Academy of Science, 985*, 218–232.

Davis, R., & Risch, S. C. (2002). Ziprasidone induction

of hypomania in depression? *American Journal of Psychiatry, 159,* 673–674.

DeGiorgio, C. M., Schachter, S. C., Handforth, A., Salinsky, M., Thompson, J., Uthman, B., et al. (2000). Prospective long-term study of vagus nerve stimulation for the treatment of refractory seizures. *Epilepsia,* 41, 1195–1200.

DelBello, M. P., Kowatch, R. A., Adler, C. M., Stanford, K. E., Welge, J. A., Barzman, D.H., et al. (2006). A double-blind randomized pilot study comparing quetiapine and divalproex for adolescent mania. *Journal of the American Academy of Child and Adolescent Psychiatry, 45,* 305–313.

DelBello, M. P., Schwiers, M. L., Rosenberg, H. L., & Strakowski, S. M. (2002). A double-blind, randomized, placebo-controlled study of quetiapine as adjunctive treatment for adolescent mania. *Journal of the American Academy of Child and Adolescent Psychiatry, 41,* 1216–1223.

DelBello, M. P., Findling, R. L., Kushner, S., Wang, D., Olson, W. H., Capece, J. A., et al. (2005). A pilot controlled trial of topiramate for mania in children and adolescents with bipolar disorder. *Journal of the American Academy of Child and Adolescent Psychiatry, 44*(6), 539–547.

Denicoff, K. D., Mirsky, A. F., Smith-Jackson, E., Leverich, G. S., Duncan, C. C., Connell, E. G., & Post, R. M. (1999). Relationship between prior course of illness and neuropsychological functioning in patients with bipolar illness. *Journal of Affective Disorders, 56,* 66–73.

Denicoff, K. D., Smith-Jackson, E. E., Bryan, A. L., Ali, S. O., & Post, R. M. (1997). Valproate prophylaxis in a prospective clinical trial of refractory bipolar disorder. *American Journal of Psychiatry, 154,* 1456–1458.

Denicoff, K. D., Smith-Jackson, E. E., Disney, E. R., Ali, S. O., Leverich, G. S., & Post, R. M. (1997). Comparative prophylactic efficacy of lithium, carbamazepine, and the combination in bipolar disorder. *Journal of Clinical Psychiatry, 58,* 470–478.

Denicoff, K. D., Sollinger, A. B., Frye, M. A., Ali, S. O., Smith-Jackson, E. E., Leverich, G. S., et al. (2000). Neuroleptic exposure in bipolar outpatients in a research setting. *Comprehensive Psychiatry, 41,* 248–252.

Di Costanzo, E., & Schifano, F. (1991). Lithium alone or in combination with carbamazepine for the treatment of rapid-cycling bipolar affective disorder. *Acta Psychiatrica Scandinavica, 83,* 456–459.

Di Lorenzo, R., & Genedani, S. (2002). Atypical antipsychotics in the therapy of bipolar disorders: Efficacy and safety. *Expert Review of Neurotherapeutics, 2,* 363–376.

Dilsaver, S. C., Swann, S. C., Chen, Y. W., Shoaib, A., Joe, B., Krajewski, K. J., et al. (1996). Treatment of bipolar depression with carbamazepine: Results of an open study. *Biological Psychiatry, 40,* 935–937.

Dinan, T. G, & Kohen, D. (1989). Tardive dyskinesia in bipolar affective disorder: Relationship to lithium therapy. *British Journal of Psychiatry, 155,* 55–57.

Dreyfus, J. (1981). *A remarkable medicine has been overlooked.* New York: Simon & Schuster.

Dubovsky, S. L. (1993). Calcium antagonists in manic-depressive illness. *Neuropsychobiology, 27,* 184–192.

Dubovsky, S. L. (1995). Calcium channel antagonists as novel agents for manic-depressive disorder. In A. F. Schatzberg & C. B. Nemeroff (Eds.), *Textbook of psychopharmacology* (pp. 377–388). Washington, DC: American Psychiatric Press.

Dubovsky, S. L., Franks, R. D., Lifschitz, M., & Coen, P. (1982). Effectiveness of verapamil in the treatment of a manic patient. *American Journal of Psychiatry, 139,* 502–504.

Dubovsky, S. L., Lee, C., Christiano, J., & Murphy, J. (1991). Elevated platelet intracellular calcium concentration in bipolar depression. *Biological Psychiatry, 29,* 441–450.

Dubovsky, S. L., Murphy, J., Christiano, J., & Lee, C. (1992). The calcium second messenger system in bipolar disorders: Data supporting new research directions. *Journal of Neuropsychiatry and Clinical Neuroscience, 4,* 3–14.

Dudek, S. M., Bear, M. E. (1993). Bidirectional long-term modification of synaptic effectiveness in the adult and immature hippocampus. *Journal of Neuroscience, 13,* 2910–2918.

Duman, R. S. (1998). Novel therapeutic approaches beyond the serotonin receptor. *Biological Psychiatry, 44,* 324–335.

Duman, R. S. (2002). Structural alterations in depression: Cellular mechanisms underlying pathology and treatment of mood disorders. *CNS Spectrums, 7,* 140–142.

Dunn, R. T., Willis, M. W., Benson, B. E., Repella, J. D., Kimbrell, T. A., Ketter, T. A., et al. (2005). Preliminary findings of uncoupling of flow and metabolism in unipolar compared with bipolar affective illness and normal controls. *Psychiatry Research, 140,* 181–198.

Dunner, D. L., & Fieve, R. R. (1974). Clinical factors in lithium carbonate prophylaxis failure. *Archives of General Psychiatry, 30,* 229–233.

Dunner, D. L., Patrick, V., & Fieve, R. R. (1977). Rapid cycling manic depressive patients. *Comprehensive Psychiatry, 18,* 561–566.

Dwight, M. M., Keck, P. E., Jr., Stanton, S. P., Strakowski, S. M., & McElroy, S. L. (1994). Antidepressant activity and mania associated with risperidone treatment of schizoaffective disorder. *Lancet, 344,* 554–555.

Dwork, A. J., Arango, V., Underwood, M., Ilievski, B., Rosoklija, G., Sackeim, H. A., et al. (2004). Absence of histological lesions in primate models of ECT and magnetic seizure therapy. *American Journal of Psychiatry, 161*, 576–578.

Eastwood, S. L., & Harrison, P. J. (2000). Hippocampal synaptic pathology in schizophrenia, bipolar disorder and major depression: A study of complexin mRNAs. *Molecular Psychiatry, 5*, 425–432.

Eberhard, G., Von Knorring, L., Nilsson, H. L., Sundequist, U., Bjorling, G., Linder, H., et al. (1988). A double-blind randomized study of clomipramine versus maprotiline in patients with idiopathic pain syndromes. *Neuropsychobiology, 19*, 25–34.

Ebert, D., Feistel, H., Barocka, A., & Kaschka, W. (1994). Increased limbic blood flow and total sleep deprivation in major depression with melancholia. *Psychiatry Research, 55*, 101–109.

Edwards, R., Stephenson, U., & Flewett, T. (1991). Clonazepam in acute mania: A double blind trial. *Australia New Zealand Journal of Psychiatry, 25*, 238–242.

Egeland, J. A., Blumenthal, R. L., Nee, J., Sharpe, L., & Endicott, J. (1987). Reliability and relationship of various ages of onset criteria for major affective disorder. *Journal of Affective Disorders, 12*, 159–165.

Eidelberg, E., Lesse, H., & Gault, R. P. (1963). An experimental model of temporal lobe epilepsy: Studies of the convulsant properties of cocaine. In G. H. Glaser (Ed.), *EEG and behavior* (pp. 272–283). New York: Basic Books.

Einarson, T. R., Arikiazn, S. R., Casciano, J., & Doyle, J. J. (1999). Comparison of extended-release venlafaxine, selective serotonin reuptake inhibitors, and tricyclic antidepressant in the treatment of depression: A meta-analysis of randomized controlled trials. *Clinical Therapy, 21*, 296–308.

Elger, G., Hoppe, C., Falkai, P., Rush, A. J., & Elger, C. E. (2000). Vagus nerve stimulation is associated with mood improvements in epilepsy patients. *Epilepsy Research, 42*, 203–210.

el Mallakh, R. S., & Karippot, A. (2002). Use of antidepressants to treat depression in bipolar disorder. *Psychiatric Services, 53*, 580–584.

Emrich, H. M. (1990). Studies with oxcarbazepine (Trileptal) in acute mania. *International Clinical Psychopharmacology, 5*, 83–88.

Emrich, H. M., Dose, M., & Von Zerssen, D. (1984). Action of sodium-valproate and of oxcarbazepine in patients with affective disorders. In H. M. Emrich, T. Okuma, & A. A. Muller, (Eds.), *Anticonvulsants in affective disorders* (pp. 45–55). Amsterdam: Excerpta Medica.

Entsuah, A. R., Huang, H., & Thase, M. E. (2001). Response and remission rates in different subpopulations with major depressive disorder administered venlafaxine, selective serotonin reuptake inhibitors, or placebo. *Journal of Clinical Psychiatry, 62*, 869–877.

Eranti, S., Mogg, A., Pluck, G., Landau, S., Purvis, R., Brown, R. G., et al. (2007). A randomized, controlled trial with 6-month follow-up of repetitive transcranial magnetic stimulation and electroconvulsive therapy for severe depression. *American Journal of Psychiatry, 164*, 73–81.

Erfurth, A., Kammerer, C., Grunze, H., Normann, C., & Walden, J. (1998). An open label study of gabapentin in the treatment of acute mania. *Journal of Psychiatric Research, 32*, 261–264.

Evins, A. E., Demopulos, C., Nierenberg, A., Culhane, M. A., Eisner, L., & Sachs, G. (2006). A double-blind, placebo-controlled trial of adjunctive donepezil in treatment-resistant mania. *Bipolar Disorders, 8*, 75–80.

Faedda, G. L., Baldessarini, R. J., Tohen, M., Strakowski, S. M., & Waternaux, C. (1991). Episode sequence in bipolar disorder and response to lithium treatment. *American Journal of Psychiatry, 148*, 1237–1239.

Fares, I., McCulloch, K. M., & Raju, T. N. (1997). Intrauterine cocaine exposure and the risk for sudden infant death syndrome: A meta-analysis. *Journal of Perinatology, 17*, 179–182.

Fattore, C., Cipolla, G., Gatti, G., Limido, G. L., Sturm, Y., Bernasconi, C., et al. (1999). Induction of ethinylestradiol and levonorgestrel metabolism by oxcarbazepine in healthy women. *Epilepsia, 40*, 783–787.

Fava, M., Alpert, J., Nierenberg, A. A., Ghaemi, N., O'Sullivan, R., Tedlow, J., et al. (1996). Fluoxetine treatment of anger attacks: A replication study. *Annals of Clinical Psychiatry, 8*, 7–10.

Fava, M., & Rosenbaum, J. F, (1999). Anger attacks in patients with depression. *Journal of Clinical Psychiatry, 60*, 21–24.

Fava, M., Rosenbaum, J. F., McCarthy, M., Fava, J., Steingard, R., & Bless, E. (1991). Anger attacks in depressed outpatients and their response to fluoxetine. *Psychopharmacology Bulletin, 27*, 275–279.

Fenton, W. S., Dickerson, F., Boronow, J., Hibbeln, J. R., & Knable, M. (2001). A placebo-controlled trial of omega-3 fatty acid (ethyl eicosapentaenoic acid) supplementation for residual symptoms and cognitive impairment in schizophrenia. *American Journal of Psychiatry, 158*, 2071–2074.

Fergus, E. L., Miller, R. B., Luckenbaugh, D. A., Leverich, G. S., Findling, R. L., Speer, A. M., et al. (2003). Is there progression from irritability/dyscontrol to major depressive and manic symptoms? A retrospective community survey of parents of bipolar children. *Journal of Affective Disorders, 77*, 71–78.

Filkowski, M. M., Stan, V. A., Borrelli, D. J., Ostacher,

M. J., El-Mallach, R. S., Baldassano, C. F., & Ghaemi, N. S. (2007). Effect of antidepressant treatment on mood episode cycling in bipolar disorder: A randomized study. *Presented at 160th Annual Meeting of the American Psychiatric Association, San Diego, CA* NR # 121, 9.

Findling, R. L., Kowatch, R. A., & Post, R. M. (2002). *Pediatric bipolar disorder.* London: Martin Dunitz.

Findling, R. L., McNamara, N. K., Stansbrey, R., Gracious, B. L., Whipkey, R. E., Demeter, C. A., et al. (2006). Combination lithium and divalproex sodium in pediatric bipolar symptom restabilization. *Journal of the American Academy of Child and Adolescent Psychiatry, 45,* 142–148.

Findling, R. L., McNamara, N. K., Youngstrom, E. A., Stansbrey, R., Gracious, B. L., Reed, M. D., et al. (2005). Double-blind 18-month trial of lithium versus divalproex maintenance treatment in pediatric bipolar disorder. *Journal of the American Academy of Child and Adolescent Psychiatry, 44,* 409–417.

Findling, R. M., Frazier, T. W., Youngstrom, E. A., McNamara, N. K., Stansbrey, R. J., Gracious, B. L. et al. (2007). Double-blind, placebo-controlled trial of Divalproex monotherapy in the treatment of symptomatic youth at high risk for developing bipolar disorder. *Journal of Clinical Psychiatry, 68,* 783–788.

Fink, M. (2001a). The broad clinical activity of ECT should not be ignored. *Journal of ECT, 17,* 233–235.

Fink, M. (2001b). Convulsive therapy: A review of the first 55 years. *Journal of Affective Disorders, 63,* 1–15.

Fink, M. (2004). ECT after 70 years: What have we learned? *International Journal of Neuropsychopharmacology, 7,* S88.

Fitton, A., & Goa, K. L. (1995). Lamotrigine: An update of its pharmacology and therapeutic use in epilepsy. *Drugs, 50,* 691–713.

Fitzgerald, P. B., Huntsman, S., Gunewardene, R., Kulkarni, J., & Daskalakis, Z. J. (2006). A randomized trial of low-frequency right-prefrontal-cortex transcranial magnetic stimulation as augmentation in treatment-resistant major depression. *International Journal of Neuropsychopharmacology, 9,* 655–666.

Fleischhacker, W. W. (2005). Aripiprazole. *Expert Opinion on Pharmacotherapy, 6,* 2091–2101.

Floris, M., Lejeune, J., & Deberdt, W. (2001). Effect of amantadine on weight gain during olanzapine treatment. *European Neuropsychopharmacology, 11,* 181–182.

Ford, N. (1996). The use of anticonvulsants in posttraumatic stress disorder: Case study and overview. *Journal of Traumatic Stress, 9,* 857–863.

Fountoulakis, K. N., Nimatoudis, I., Iacovides, A., & Kaprinis, G. (2004). Off-label indications for atypical antipsychotics: A systematic review. *Annals of General Hospital Psychiatry, 3,* 4.

Frangou, S., & Lewis, M. (2006). Efficacy of ethyl-eicosapentaenoic acid in bipolar depression: randomised double-blind placebo-controlled study. *British Journal of Psychiatry, 188,* 46–50.

Frangou, S., Raymont, V., & Bettany, D. (2002). The Maudsley bipolar disorder project. A survey of psychotropic prescribing patterns in bipolar I disorder. *Bipolar Disorders, 4,* 378–385.

Frank, E., Kupfer, D. J., Perel, J. M., Cornes, C., Jarrett, D. B., Mallinger, A. G., et al. (1990). Three-year outcomes for maintenance therapies in recurrent depression. *Archives of General Psychiatry, 47,* 1093–1099.

Frankenburg, F. R., Tohen, M., Cohen, B. M., & Lipinski, J. F., Jr. (1988). Long-term response to carbamazepine: A retrospective study. *Journal of Clinical Psychopharmacology, 8,* 130–132.

Frankland, P. W., O'Brien, C., Ohno, M., Kirkwood, A., & Silva, A. J. (2001). Alpha-CaMKII-dependent plasticity in the cortex is required for permanent memory. *Nature, 411,* 309–313.

Freud, S. (1957). Mourning and melancholia In J. Strachey (Ed. & Trans.), *The standard edition of the complete psychological works of Sigmund Freud* (Vol. 14, p. 251). London: Hogarth Press. (Original work published 1917)

Friis, M. L., Kristensen, O., Boas, J., Dalby, M., Deth, S. H., Gram, L., et al. (1993). Therapeutic experiences with 947 epileptic out-patients in oxcarbazepine treatment. *Acta Neurologica Scandinavica, 87,* 224–227.

Fritze, J., Unsorg, B., & Lanczik, M. (1991). Interaction between carbamazepine and fluvoxamine. *Acta Psychiatrica Scandinavica, 84,* 583–584.

Froscher, W., Stoll, K. D., & Hoffmann, F. (1984). Combination therapy with carbamazepine and valproic acid in problem cases at an outpatient epilepsy clinic. *Arzneimittelforschung, 34,* 910–914.

Frye, M. A., Altshuler, L. L., & Bitran, J. A. (1996). Clozapine in rapid cycling bipolar disorder [letter]. *Journal of Clinical Psychopharmacology, 16,* 87–90.

Frye, M. A., Altshuler, L. L., McElroy, S. L., Suppes, T., Keck, P. E., Denicoff, K., et al. (2003). Gender differences in prevalence, risk, and clinical correlates of alcoholism comorbidity in bipolar disorder. *American Journal of Psychiatry, 160,* 883–889.

Frye, M. A., Grunze, H., Suppes, T., McElroy, S. L., Keck, P. E., Jr., Walden, J., et al. (in press). A placebo-controlled evaluation of adjunctive modafinil in the treatment of bipolar depression. *American Journal of Psychiatry.*

Frye, M. A., Ketter, T. A., Altshuler, L. L., Denicoff, K., Dunn, R. T., Kimbrell, T. A., et al. (1998). Clozapine in bipolar disorder: Treatment implications for other atypical antipsychotics. *Journal of Affective Disorders, 48,* 91–104.

Frye, M. A., Ketter, T. A., Kimbrell, T. A., Dunn, R. T., Speer, A. M., Osuch, E. A., et al. (2000). A placebo-controlled study of lamotrigine and gabapentin monotherapy in refractory mood disorders. *Journal of Clinical Psychopharmacology, 20,* 607–614.

Frye, M. A., Ketter, T. A., Leverich, G. S., Huggins, T., Lantz, C., Denicoff, K. D., et al. (2000). The increasing use of polypharmacy for refractory mood disorders: 22 years of study. *Journal of Clinical Psychiatry, 61,* 9–15.

Frye, M. A., Pazzaglia, P. J., George, M. S., Luckenbaugh, D., Vanderham, E., Davis, C. L., et al. (2003). Low CSF somatostatin associated with response to nimodipine in patients with affective illness. *Biological Psychiatry, 53,* 180–183.

Fukumoto, T., Morinobu, S., Okamoto, Y., Kagaya, A., & Yamawaki, S. (2001). Chronic lithium treatment increases the expression of brain-derived neurotrophic factor in the rat brain. *Psychopharmacology (Berlin), 158,* 100–106.

Gamma, F., Buka, S., Goldstein, J. M., Fitzmaurice, G., Seidman, L. J., & Tsuang, M. T. (2007). Early intermodal integration in offspring of parents with schizophrenia. *Presented at 160th Annual Meeting of the American Psychiatric Association, San Diego, CA* NR #486, 35.

Garcia-Borreguero, D., Larrosa, O., de la Llave, Y., Verger, K., Masramon, X., & Hernandez, G. (2002). Treatment of restless legs syndrome with gabapentin: A double-blind, cross-over study. *Neurology, 59,* 1573–1579.

Garcia-Toro, M., Salva, J., Daumal, J., Andres, J., Romera, M., Lafau, O., et al. (2006). High (20-Hz) and low (1-Hz) frequency transcranial magnetic stimulation as adjuvant treatment in medication-resistant depression. *Psychiatry Research, 146,* 53–57.

Gary, K. A., Sevarino, K. A., Yarbrough, G. G., Prange, A. J., Jr., & Winokur, A. (2003). The thyrotropin-releasing hormone (TRH) hypothesis of homeostatic regulation: Implications for TRH-based therapeutics. *Journal of Pharmacology and Experimental Therapeutics, 305,* 410–416.

Gelenberg, A. J., Kane, J. M., Keller, M. B., Lavori, P., Rosenbaum, J. F., Cole, K., et al. (1989). Comparison of standard and low serum levels of lithium maintenance treatment of bipolar disorder. *New England Journal of Medicine, 321,* 1489–1493.

Geller, B., Cooper, T. B., Watts, H. E., Cosby, C. M., & Fox, L. W. (1992). Early findings from a pharmacokinetically designed double-blind and placebo-controlled study of lithium for adolescents comorbid with bipolar and substance dependency disorders. *Progress in Neuropsychopharmacology and Biological Psychiatry, 16,* 281–299.

Geller, B., & DelBello, M. P. (2003). *Bipolar disorder in childhood and early adolescence.* New York: Guilford.

Geller, B., Zimerman, B., Williams, M., DelBello, M. P., Frazier, J., & Beringer, L. (2002). Phenomenology of prepubertal and early adolescent bipolar disorder: Examples of elated mood, grandiose behaviors, decreased need for sleep, racing thoughts and hypersexuality. *Journal of Child and Adolescent Psychopharmacology, 12,* 3–9.

George, M. S., Jones, M., Post, R. M., Mikalauskas, K., & Leverich, G. S. (1992). The longitudinal course of affective illness: Mathematical models involving chaos theory. *World Congress of Biological Psychiatry Abstracts, 31:* 86A–87A.

George, M. S., Nahas, Z., Lisanby, S. H., Schlaepfer, T., Kozel, F. A., & Greenberg, B. D. (2003). Transcranial magnetic stimulation. *Neurosurgical Clinics of North America, 14,* 283–301.

George, M. S., Sackeim, H. A., Marangell, L. B., Husain, M. M., Nahas, Z., Lisanby, S. H., et al. (2000). Vagus nerve stimulation. A potential therapy for resistant depression? *Psychiatric Clinics of North America, 23,* 757–783.

George, M. S., Wassermann, E. M., Kimbrell, T. A., Little, J. T., Williams, W. E., Danielson, A. L., et al. (1997). Mood improvement following daily left prefrontal repetitive transcranial magnetic stimulation in patients with depression: A placebo-controlled crossover trial. *American Journal of Psychiatry, 154,* 1752–1756.

George, M. S., Wassermann, E. M., Williams, W. A., Callahan, A., Ketter, T. A., Basser, P., et al. (1995). Daily repetitive transcranial magnetic stimulation (rTMS) improves mood in depression. *NeuroReport, 6,* 1853–1856.

George, M. S., Wassermann, E. M., Williams, W. A., Steppel, J., Pascual-Leone, A., Basser, P., et al. (1996). Changes in mood and hormone levels after rapid-rate transcranial magnetic stimulation (rTMS) of the prefrontal cortex. *Journal of Neuropsychiatry and Clinical Neuroscience, 8,* 172–180.

Gerlach, J., & Peacock, L. (1995). New antipsychotics: The present status. *International Clinical Psychopharmacology, 10*(Suppl. 3), 39–48.

Gerner, R. H., Post, R. M., & Bunney, W. E., Jr. (1976). A dopaminergic mechanism in mania. *American Journal of Psychiatry, 133,* 1177–1180.

Gershon, E. S., Hamovit, J. H., Guroff, J. J., & Nurnberger, J, I. (1987). Birth-cohort changes in manic and depressive disorders in relatives of bipolar and schizoaffective patients. *Archives of General Psychiatry, 44,* 314–319.

Ghaemi, S. N. (2000). New treatments for bipolar disorder: The role of atypical neuroleptic agents. *Journal of Clinical Psychiatry, 61*(Suppl. 14), S33–S42.

Ghaemi, S. N., Charry, E. L., Katzow, J. A., & Goodwin, F. K. (2000). Does clozapine have antidepressant properties? A retrospective preliminary study. *Bipolar Disorders, 2,* 196–199.

Ghaemi, S. N., Ko, J. Y., & Katzow, J. J. (2002). Oxcarbazepine treatment of refractory bipolar disorder: A retrospective chart review. *Bipolar Disorders, 4,* 70–74.

Ghaemi, S. N., Manwani, S. G., Katzow, J. J., Ko, J. Y., & Goodwin, F. K. (2001). Topiramate treatment of bipolar spectrum disorders: A retrospective chart review. *Annals of Clinical Psychiatry, 13,* 185–189.

Gianfrancesco, F. D., Grogg, A. L., Mahmoud, R. A., Wang, R. H., & Nasrallah, H. A. (2002). Differential effects of risperidone, olanzapine, clozapine, and conventional antipsychotics on type 2 diabetes: Findings from a large health plan database. *Journal of Clinical Psychiatry, 63,* 920–930.

Giannini, A. J., Taraszewski, R., & Loiselle, R. H. (1987). Verapamil and lithium in maintenance therapy of manic patients. *Journal of Clinical Pharmacology, 27,* 980–982.

Gijsman, H. J., Geddes, J. R., Rendell, J. M., Nolen, W. A., & Goodwin, G. M. (2004). Antidepressants for bipolar depression: A systematic review of randomized, controlled trials. *American Journal of Psychiatry, 161,* 1537–1547.

Ginsberg, L. D. (2006). Carbamazepine extended-release capsules in the treatment of bipolar disorder. *Annals of Clinical Psychiatry, 18*(S1), 1040–1237.

Gitlin, M. J., Swendsen, J., Heller, T. L., & Hammen, C. (1995). Relapse and impairment in bipolar disorder. *American Journal of Psychiatry, 152,* 1635–1640.

Gjessing, R. (1938). Disturbances of somatic function in catatonia with a periodic course and their compensation. *Journal of Mental Science, 84,* 608–621.

Glazer, H. I., & Weiss, J. M. (1976). Long-term interference effect: An alternative to "learned helplessness." *Journal of Experimental Psychology (Animal Behavior Processes), 2,* 202–213.

Gloger, S., Grunhaus, L., Birmacher, B., & Troudart, T. (1981). Treatment of spontaneous panic attacks with clomipramine. *American Journal of Psychiatry, 138,* 1215–1217.

Gloor, P., Olivier, A., Quesney, L. F., Andermann, F., & Horowitz, S. (1982). The role of the limbic system in experiential phenomena of temporal lobe epilepsy. *Annals of Neurology, 12,* 129–144.

Goddard, G. V., McIntyre, D. C., & Leech, C. K. (1969). A permanent change in brain function resulting from daily electrical stimulation. *Experimental Neurology, 25,* 295–330.

Goldberg, J. F., & Burdick, K. E. (2002). Levetiracetam for acute mania [letter]. *American Journal of Psychiatry, 159,* 148.

Goldberg, J. F., Burdick, K. E., & Endick, C. J. (2004). Preliminary randomized, double-blind, placebo-controlled trial of pramipexole added to mood stabilizers for treatment-resistant bipolar depression. *American Journal of Psychiatry, 161,* 564–566.

Goldberg, J. F., Harrow, M., & Leon, A. C. (1996). Lithium treatment of bipolar affective disorders under naturalistic followup conditions. *Psychopharmacology Bulletin, 32,* 47–54.

Goldberg, J. F., & Whiteside, J. E. (2002). The association between substance abuse and antidepressant-induced mania in bipolar disorder: A preliminary study. *Journal of Clinical Psychiatry, 63,* 791–795.

Goldstein, J. M., Cristoph, G., Grimm, S., Liu, J. W., Widzowski, D., & Brecher, M. (2007). Unique mechanism of action for the antidepressant properties of the atypical antipsychotic quetiapine. *Presented at 160th Annual Meeting of the American Psychiatric Association, San Diego, CA* NR #336, 24.

Gonzalez, L. P., Veatch, L. M., Ticku, M. K., & Becker, H. C. (2001). Alcohol withdrawal kindling: Mechanisms and implications for treatment. *Alcohol Clinical Experimental Research, 25,* 197S–201S.

Goodnick, P. J. (1995). Nimodipine treatment of rapid cycling bipolar disorder [letter]. *Journal of Clinical Psychiatry, 56,* 330.

Goodwin, F. K., & Jamison, K. R. (1990). *Manic-depressive illness.* New York: Oxford University Press.

Gottschalk, A., Bauer, M. S., & Whybrow, P. C. (1995). Evidence of chaotic mood variation in bipolar disorder. *Archives of General Psychiatry, 52,* 947–959.

Gould, E., & Tanapat, P. (1999). Stress and hippocampal neurogenesis. *Biological Psychiatry, 46,* 1472–1479.

Greene, D. S., & Barbhaiya, R. H. (1997). Clinical pharmacokinetics of nefazodone. *Clinical Pharmacokinetics, 33,* 260–275.

Greene, R. (1998). *The explosive child.* New York: HarperCollins.

Greil, W., Kleindienst, N., Erazo, N., & Muller-Oerlinghausen, B. (1998). Differential response to lithium and carbamazepine in the prophylaxis of bipolar disorder. *Journal of Clinical Psychopharmacology, 18,* 455–460.

Greil, W., Ludwig-Mayerhofer, W., Erazo, N., Engel, R. R., Czernik, A., Giedke, H., et al. (1997). Lithium vs carbamazepine in the maintenance treatment of schizoaffective disorder: A randomised study. *European Archives of Psychiatry and Clinical Neuroscience, 247,* 42–50.

Grimsley, S. R., Jann, M. W., Carter, J. G., D'Mello, A. P., & D'Souza, M. J. (1991). Increased carbamazepine plasma concentrations after fluoxetine coadministration. *Clinical Pharmacology and Therapeutics, 50,* 10–15.

Grof, P., Angst, J., & Haines, T. (1974). The clinical course of depression: Practical issues. In J. Angst

(Ed.), *Classification and prediction of outcome of depression* (Symposia Medica Hoechst, Vol. 8, pp. 141–148). Stuttgart: F.K. Schattauer Verlag.

Grunhaus, L., Dannon, P. N., Schreiber, S., Dolberg, O. H., Amiaz, R., Ziv, R., et al. (2000). Repetitive transcranial magnetic stimulation is as effective as electroconvulsive therapy in the treatment of nondelusional major depressive disorder: An open study. *Biological Psychiatry, 47*, 314–324.

Grunhaus, L., Schreiber, S., Dolberg, O. T., Hirshman, S., & Dannon, P. N. (2002). Response to ECT in major depression: Are there differences between unipolar and bipolar depression? *Bipolar Disorders, 4*(Suppl. 1), 91–93.

Grunhaus, L., Schreiber, S., Dolberg, O. T., Polak, D., & Dannon, P. N. (2003). A randomized controlled comparison of electroconvulsive therapy and repetitive transcranial magnetic stimulation in severe and resistant nonpsychotic major depression. *Biological Psychiatry, 53*, 324–331.

Grunze, H., Kasper, S., Goodwin, G., Bowden, C., Baldwin, D., Licht, R., et al. (2002). WFSBP Task Force on treatment guidelines for bipolar disorders. *World Journal of Biological Psychiatry, 3*, 115–124.

Grunze, H., Langosch, J., Born, C., Schaub, G., & Walden, J. (2003). Levetiracetam in the treatment of acute mania: An open add-on study with an on-off-on design. *Journal of Clinical Psychiatry, 64*, 781–784.

Grunze, H. C., Normann, C., Langosch, J., *Schaefer, M., Amann, B., Sterr, A.*, et al. (2001). Antimanic efficacy of topiramate in 11 patients in an open trial with an on-off-on design. *Journal of Clinical Psychiatry, 62*, 464–468.

Guberman, A. H., Besag, F. M., Brodie, M. J., Dooley, J. M., Duchowny, M. S., Pellock, J. M., et al. (1999). Lamotrigine-associated rash: Risk/benefit considerations in adults and children. *Epilepsia, 40*, 985–991.

Guidotti, A., Auta, J., Davis, J. M., Gerevini, V. D., Dwivedi, Y., Grayson, D. R., et al. (2000). Decrease in reelin and glutamic acid decarboxylase67 (GAD67) expression in schizophrenia and bipolar disorder: A postmortem brain study. *Archives of General Psychiatry, 57*, 1061–1069.

Guille, C., Shriver, A., Demopulos, C., & Sachs, G. (1999). Bupropion vs desipramine in the treatment of bipolar depression. *Bipolar Disorders, 1*(Suppl. 1), 33.

Gupta, A. K., & Jeavons, P. M. (1985). Complex partial seizures: EEG foci and response to carbamazepine and sodium valproate. *Journal of Neurological and Neurosurgical Psychiatry 48*(10), 1010–1014.

Gyulai, L., Bowden, C. L., McElroy, S. L., Calabrese, J. R., Petty, F., Swann, A. C., et al. (2003). Maintenance efficacy of divalproex in the prevention of bipolar depression. *Neuropsychopharmacology, 28*, 1374–1382.

Hallett, M. (1996). Transcranial magnetic stimulation: A useful tool for clinical neurophysiology. *Annals of Neurology, 40*, 344–345.

Hammen, C., & Gitlin, M. (1997). Stress reactivity in bipolar patients and its relation to prior history of disorder. *American Journal of Psychiatry, 154*, 856–857.

Hamner, M. (2002). The effects of atypical antipsychotics on serum prolactin levels. *Annals of Clinical Psychiatry, 14*, 163–173.

Hamner, M. B., Brodrick, P. S., & Labbate, L. A. (2001). Gabapentin in PTSD: A retrospective, clinical series of adjunctive therapy. *Annals of Clinical Psychiatry, 13*, 141–146.

Harrow, M., Goldberg, J. F., Grossman, L. S., & Meltzer, H. Y. (1990). Outcome in manic disorders: A naturalistic follow-up study. *Archives of General Psychiatry, 47*, 665–671.

Harvey, B. H., McEwen, B. S., & Stein, D. J. (2003). Neurobiology of antidepressant withdrawal: Implications for the longitudinal outcome of depression. *Biological Psychiatry, 54*, 1105–1117.

Haykal, R. F., & Akiskal, H. S. (1990). Bupropion as a promising approach to rapid cycling bipolar II patients. *Journal of Clinical Psychiatry, 51*, 450–455.

Henderson, D. C., Copeland, P. M., Daley, T. B., Borba, C. P., Cather, C., Nguyen, D. D., et al. (2005). A double-blind, placebo-controlled trial of sibutramine for olanzapine-associated weight gain. *American Journal of Psychiatry, 162*, 954–962.

Henry, T. R., Bakay, R. A., Votaw, J. R., Pennell, P. B., Epstein, C. M., Faber, T. L., et al. (1998). Brain blood flow alterations induced by therapeutic vagus nerve stimulation in partial epilepsy. I. Acute effects at high and low levels of stimulation. *Epilepsia, 39*, 983–990.

Hertzberg, M. A., Butterfield, M. I., Feldman, M. E., Beckham, J. C., Sutherland, S. M., Connor, K. M., et al. (1999). A preliminary study of lamotrigine for the treatment of posttraumatic stress disorder. *Biological Psychiatry, 45*, 1226–1229.

Hibbeln, J. R., & Salem, N. J. (1995). Dietary polyunsaturated fatty acids and depression: When cholesterol does not satisfy. *American Journal of Clinical Nutrition, 62*, 1–9.

Hillert, A., Maier, W., Wetzel, H., & Benkert, O. (1992). Risperidone in the treatment of disorders with a combined psychotic and depressive syndrome—a functional approach. *Pharmacopsychiatry, 25*, 213–217.

Himmelhoch, J. M., & Garfinkel, M. E. (1986). Sources of lithium resistance in mixed mania. *Psychopharmacology Bulletin, 22*, 613–620.

Himmelhoch, J. M., Thase, M. E., Mallinger, A. G., & Houck, P. (1991). Tranylcypromine versus imipramine in anergic bipolar depression. *American Journal of Psychiatry, 148*, 910–916.

Hirschfeld, R. M., Calabrese, J. R., Weissman, M. M., Reed, M., Davies, M. A., Frye, M. A., et al. (2003). Screening for bipolar disorder in the community. *Journal of Clinical Psychiatry, 64*, 53–59.

Hirschfeld, R. M., Holzer, C., Calabrese, J. R., Weissman, M., Reed, M., Davies, M., et al. (2003). Validity of the mood disorder questionnaire: A general population study. *American Journal of Psychiatry, 160*, 178–180.

Hirschfeld, R. M., Keck, P. E., Jr., Kramer, M., Karcher, K., Canuso, C., Eerdekens, M., et al. (2004). Rapid antimanic effect of risperidone monotherapy: A 3-week multicenter, double-blind, placebo-controlled trial. *American Journal of Psychiatry, 161*, 1057–1065.

Hirschfeld, R. M., Lewis, L., & Vornik, L. A. (2003). Perceptions and impact of bipolar disorder: How far have we really come? Results of the national depressive and manic-depressive association 2000 survey of individuals with bipolar disorder. *Journal of Clinical Psychiatry, 64*, 161–174.

Hirschfeld, R. M., Williams, J. B., Spitzer, R. L., Calabrese, J. R., Flynn, L., Keck, P. E., Jr., et al. (2000). Development and validation of a screening instrument for bipolar spectrum disorder: The Mood Disorder Questionnaire. *American Journal of Psychiatry, 157*, 1873–1875.

Holtzheimer, P. E., III, Russo, J., & Avery, D. H. (2001). A meta-analysis of repetitive transcranial magnetic stimulation in the treatment of depression. *Psychopharmacology Bulletin, 35*, 149–169.

Hoschl, C. (1991). Do calcium antagonists have a place in the treatment of mood disorders? *Drugs, 42*, 721–729.

Hoschl, C., & Kozeny, J. (1989). Verapamil in affective disorders: A controlled, double-blind study. *Biological Psychiatry, 25*, 128–140.

Hough, C., Irwin, R. P., Gao, X.-M., Rogowski, M. A., & Chuang, D.-M. (1993). Carbamazepine inhibition of NMDA-stimulated calcium influx in cerebellar granule cells. *Neuroscience Abstracts, 19*, 1781.

Huey, L. Y., Janowsky, D. S., Mandell, A. J., Judd, L. L., & Pendery, M. (1975). Preliminary studies on the use of thyrotropin releasing hormone in manic states, depression, and the dysphoria of alcohol withdrawal. *Psychopharmacology Bulletin, 11*, 24–27.

Hummel, B., Dittmann, S., Forsthoff, A., Matzner, N., Amann, B., & Grunze, H. (2002). Clozapine as add-on medication in the maintenance treatment of bipolar and schizoaffective disorders: A case series. *Neuropsychobiology, 45*(Suppl.), 37–42.

Hummel, B., Walden, J., Stampfer, R., Dittmann, S., Amann, B., Sterr, A., et al. (2002). Acute antimanic efficacy and safety of oxcarbazepine in an open trial with an on-off-on design. *Bipolar Disorders, 4*, 412–417.

Hunt, N., & Silverstone, T. (1991). Tardive dyskinesia in bipolar affective disorder: A catchment area study. *International Clinical Psychopharmacology, 6*, 45–50.

Huot, R. L., Thrivikraman, K. V., Meaney, M. J., & Plotsky, P. M. (2001). Development of adult ethanol preference and anxiety as a consequence of neonatal maternal separation in Long Evans rats and reversal with antidepressant treatment. *Psychopharmacology (Berlin), 158*, 366–373.

Idzikowski, C., Mills, F. J., & Glennard, R. (1986). 5-Hydroxytryptamine-2 antagonist increases human slow wave sleep. *Brain Research, 378*, 164–168.

Iqbal, M. M., Rahman, A., Husain, Z., Mahmud, S. Z., Ryan, W. G., & Feldman, J. M. (2003). Clozapine: A clinical review of adverse effects and management. *Annals of Clinical Psychiatry, 15*, 33–48.

Isojarvi, J. I. T., Huuskonen, E. J., Pakarinen, A. J., Vuolteenaho, O., & Myllyla, V. V. (2001). The regulation of serum sodium after replacing carbamazepine with oxcarbazepine. *Epilepsia, 42*, 741–745.

Isojarvi, J. I. T., Pakarinen, A. J., Rautio, A., Pelkonen, O., & Myllyla, V. V. (1994). Liver enzyme induction and serum lipid levels after replacement of carbamazepine with oxcarbazepine. *Epilepsia, 35*, 1217–1220.

Isojarvi, J. I., Tauboll, E., Tapanainen, J. S., Pakarinen, A. J., Laatikainen, T. J., Knip, M., et al. (2001). On the association between valproate and polycystic ovary syndrome: A response and an alternative view. *Epilepsia, 42*, 305–310.

Jacobsen, F. M., & Comas-Diaz, L. (1999). Donepezil for psychotropic-induced memory loss. *Journal of Clinical Psychiatry, 60*, 698–704.

Janicak, P. G., Dowd, S. M., Martis, B., Alam, D., Beedle, D., Krasuski, J., et al. (2002). Repetitive transcranial magnetic stimulation versus electroconvulsive therapy for major depression: Preliminary results of a randomized trial. *Biological Psychiatry, 51*, 659–667.

Janicak, P. G., Sharma, R. P., Pandey, G., & Davis, J. M. (1998). Verapamil for the treatment of acute mania: A double-blind, placebo-controlled trial. *American Journal of Psychiatry, 155*, 972–973.

Janowsky, D. S., Leff, M., & Epstein, R. S. (1970). Playing the manic game: interpersonal maneuvers of the acutely manic patient. *Archives of General Psychiatry, 22*, 252–260.

Joffe, H., Cohen, L. S., Suppes, T., McLaughlin, W. L., Lavori, P., Adams, J. M., et al. (2006). Valproate is associated with new-onset oligoamenorrhea with hyperandrogenism in women with bipolar disorder. *Biological Psychiatry, 59*, 1078–1086.

Joffe, R. T. (1998). The use of thyroid supplements to

augment antidepressant medication. *Journal of Clinical Psychiatry, 59*(Suppl. 5), 26–29.

Joffe, R. T., & Singer, W. (1990). A comparison of triiodothyronine and thyroxine in the potentiation of tricyclic antidepressants. *Psychiatry Research, 32*, 241–251.

Joffe, R. T., & Sokolov, T. H. (1994). Thyroid hormones, the brain, and affective disorders. *Critical Review of Neurobiology, 8*, 45–63.

Joffe, R. T., Uhde, T. W., Post, R. M., & Minichiello, M. D. (1987). Motor activity in depressed patients treated with carbamazepine. *Biological Psychiatry, 22*, 941–946.

Johnson, B. A. (2005). Recent advances in the development of treatments for alcohol and cocaine dependence focus on topiramate and other modulators of GABA or glutamate function. *CNS Drugs, 19*, 873–896.

Johnson, B. A., Ait-Daoud, N., Bowden, C. L., DiClemente, C. C., Roache, J. D., Lawson, K., et al. (2003). Oral topiramate for treatment of alcohol dependence: A randomised controlled trial. *Lancet, 361*, 1677–1685.

Johnson, B. A., Rosenthal, N., Capece, J., Wiegand, F., Mao, L., McKay, A., & Ait-Daoud, N. (2007). Topiramate for the treatment of alcohol dependence: Results of a multi-site trial. Presented at 160th Annual Meeting of the American Psychiatric Association, San Diego, CA 2007; NR #546:39.

Kahlbaum, K. (1863). *Die Gruppirung der psychischen Krankheiten und die Einteilung der Seelenstörungen.* Danzig: Verlag von A. Kafemann.

Kahlbaum, K. (1882). Ueber cyklisches Irresein. *Der Irrenfreund: Psychiatrische Monatsschrift für praktische Aerzte, 24*(10), 145–157.

Kalivas, P. W., & Duffy, P. (1989). Similar effects of daily cocaine and stress on mesocorticolimbic dopamine neurotransmission in the rat. *Biological Psychiatry, 25*, 913–928.

Kampman, K. M., Pettinati, H., Lynch, K. G., Dackis, C., Sparkman, T., Weigley, C., et al. (2004). A pilot trial of topiramate for the treatment of cocaine dependence. *Drug and Alcohol Dependence, 75*, 233–240.

Kanba, S., Yagi, G., Kamijima, K., Suzuki, T., Tajima, O., Otaki, J., et al. (1994). The first open study of zonisamide, a novel anticonvulsant, shows efficacy in mania. *Progress in Neuropsychopharmacology and Biological Psychiatry, 18*, 707–715.

Kane, J. M. (1988). The role of neuroleptics in manic-depressive illness. *Journal of Clinical Psychiatry, 49*(Suppl.), S12–S14.

Keck, P. E., Mintz, J., McElroy, S. L., Freeman, M. P., Suppes, T., Frye, M., et al. (2006). Double-blind, randomized, placebo-controlled trials of ethyl-eicosapentanoate in the treatment of bipolar depression and rapid cycling bipolar disorder. *Biological Psychiatry, 60*, 1020–1022.

Keck, P. E., Jr., Calabrese, J. R., Mcquade, R. D., Carson, W. H., Carlson, B. X., Rollin, L. M., et al. (2006). A randomized, double-blind, placebo-controlled 26-week trial of aripiprazole in recently manic patients with bipolar I disorder. *Journal of Clinical Psychiatry, 67*, 626–637.

Keck, P. E., Jr., Marcus, R., Tourkodimitris, S., Ali, M., Liebeskind, A., Saha, A., et al. (2003). A placebo-controlled, double-blind study of the efficacy and safety of aripiprazole in patients with acute bipolar mania. *American Journal of Psychiatry, 160*, 1651–1658.

Keck, P. E., Jr., & McElroy, S. L. (2004). Intramuscular atypical antipsychotics in the management of agitation in bipolar mania. *Clinical Approaches in Bipolar Disorders, 2*, 31–35.

Keck, P. E., Jr., McElroy, S. L., & Friedman, L. M. (1992). Valproate and carbamazepine in the treatment of panic and posttraumatic stress disorders, withdrawal states, and behavioral dyscontrol syndromes. *Journal of Clinical Psychopharmacology, 12*, 36S–41S.

Keck, P. E., Jr., McElroy, S. L., Tugrul, K. C., & Bennett, J. A. (1993). Valproate oral loading in the treatment of acute mania. *Journal of Clinical Psychiatry, 54*, 305–308.

Keck, P. E., Jr., Mintz, J., McElroy, S. L., Freeman, M. P., Suppes, T., Frye, M. A., et al. (2006). Double-blind, randomized, placebo-controlled trials of ethyl-eicosapentanoate in the treatment of bipolar depression and rapid cycling bipolar disorder. *Biological Psychiatry, 60*, 1020–1022.

Keck, P. E., Jr., Perlis, R. H., Otto, M. W., Carpenter, D., Ross, R., & Docherty, J. P. (2004, December). The Expert Consensus Guideline Series: Treatment of Bipolar Disorder 2004. *Postgraduate Medicine*, 1–120.

Keck, P. E. Jr., Taylor, V. E., Tugrul, K. C., McElroy, S. L., & Bennett, J. A. (1993). Valproate treatment of panic disorder and lactate-induced panic attacks. *Biological Psychiatry, 33*, 542–546.

Keck, P. E., Jr., Welge, J. A., McElroy, S. L., Arnold, L. M., & Strakowski, S. M. (2000). Placebo effect in randomized, controlled studies of acute bipolar mania and depression. *Biological Psychiatry, 47*, 748–755.

Keck, P. E., Welge, J. A., Strakowski, S. M., Arnold, L. M., & McElroy, S. L. (2000). Placebo effect in randomized, controlled maintenance studies of patients with bipolar disorder. *Biological Psychiatry, 47*, 756–761.

Keller, M. B., & Boland, R. J. (1998). Implications of failing to achieve successful long-term maintenance treatment of recurrent unipolar major depression. *Biological Psychiatry, 44*, 348–360.

Keller, M. B., & Shapiro, R. W. (1982). "Double depression": Superimposition of acute depressive episodes on chronic depressive disorders. *American Journal of Psychiatry, 139,* 438–442.

Keller, R. W., Jr., Snyder-Keller, A. (2000). Prenatal cocaine exposure. *Annals of the New York Academy of Science, 909,* 217–232.

Kellner, C. H., Knapp, R. G., Petrides, G., Rummans, T. A., Husain, M. M., Rasmussen, K., et al. (2006). Continuation electroconvulsive therapy vs pharmacotherapy for relapse prevention in major depression: A multisite study from the Consortium for Research in Electroconvulsive Therapy (CORE). *Archives of General Psychiatry, 63,* 1337–1344.

Kellner, C. H., Petrides, G., Husain, M., Rummans, T., Fink, M., Knapp, R., et al. (2004). The efficacy of ECT in major depression: Findings from phase I of the C.O.R.E. ECT study. *International Journal of Neuropsychopharmacology, 7,* S87–S88.

Kellner, C. H., Post, R. M., Putnam, F., Cowdry, R., Gardner, D., Kling, M. A., et al. (1987). Intravenous procaine as a probe of limbic system activity in psychiatric patients and normal controls. *Biological Psychiatry, 22,* 1107–1126.

Kendler, K. S., Thornton, L. M., & Gardner, C. O. (2000). Stressful life events and previous episodes in the etiology of major depression in women: An evaluation of the "kindling" hypothesis. *American Journal of Psychiatry, 157,* 1243–1251.

Kendler, K. S., Thornton, L. M., & Gardner, C. O. (2001). Genetic risk, number of previous depressive episodes, and stressful life events in predicting onset of major depression. *American Journal of Psychiatry, 158,* 582–586.

Kessing, L. V., Agerbo, E., & Mortensen, P. B. (2004). Major stressful life events and other risk factors for first admission with mania. *Bipolar Disorders, 6,* 122–129.

Kessing, L. V., & Andersen, P. K. (2004). Does the risk of developing dementia increase with the number of episodes in patients with depressive disorder and in patients with bipolar disorder? *Journal of Neurological and Neurosurgical Psychiatry, 75,* 1662–1666.

Kessing, L. V., Andersen, P. K., Mortensen, P. B., & Bolwig, T. G. (1998). Recurrence in affective disorder. I. Case register study. *British Journal of Psychiatry, 172,* 23–28.

Kessler, R. C., Crum, R. M., Warner, L. A., Nelson, C. B., Schulenberg, J., & Anthony, J. C. (1997). Lifetime co-occurrence of DSM III R alcohol abuse and dependence with other psychiatric disorders in the National Comorbidity Survey. *Archives of General Psychiatry, 54,* 313–321.

Kessler, R. C., Nelson, C. B., McGonagle, K. A., Edlund, M. J., Frank, R. G., & Leaf, P. J. (1996). The epidemiology of co-occurring addictive and mental disorders: Implications for prevention and service utilization. *American Journal of Orthopsychiatry, 66,* 17–31.

Ketter, T. A., Andreason, P. J., George, M. S., Lee, C., Gill, D. S., Parekh, P. I., et al. (1996). Anterior paralimbic mediation of procaine-induced emotional and psychosensory experiences. *Archives of General Psychiatry, 53,* 59–69.

Ketter, T. A., Frye, M. A., Cora-Locatelli, G., Kimbrell, T. A., & Post, R. M. (1999). Metabolism and excretion of mood stabilizers and new anticonvulsants. *Cellular and Molecular Neurobiology, 19,* 511–532.

Ketter, T. A., George, M. S., Kimbrell, T. A., Benson, B. E., & Post, R. M. (1997). Functional brain imaging in mood and anxiety disorders. *Current Review of Mood and Anxiety Disorders, 1,* 95–112.

Ketter, T. A., Jenkins, J. B., Schroeder, D. H., Pazzaglia, P. J., Marangell, L. B., George, M. S., et al. (1995). Carbamazepine but not valproate induces bupropion metabolism. *Journal of Clinical Psychopharmacology, 15,* 327–333.

Ketter, T. A., Kimbrell, T. A., George, M. S., Willis, M. W., Benson, B. E., Danielson, A., et al. (1999). Baseline cerebral hypermetabolism associated with carbamazepine response, and hypometabolism with nimodipine response in mood disorders. *Biological Psychiatry, 46,* 1364–1374.

Ketter, T. A., & Manji, H. K. (2003). Potential mechanisms of action of lamotrigine in the treatment of bipolar disorders. *Journal of Clinical Psychopharmacology, 23,* 484–495.

Ketter, T. E., Pazzaglia, P. J., & Post, R. M. (1992). Synergy of carbamazepine and valproic acid in affective illness: Case report and review of the literature. *Journal of Clinical Psychopharmacology, 12,* 276–281.

Ketter, T. A., & Post, R. M. (1994). Clinical pharmacology and pharmacokinetics of carbamazepine. In R. T. Joffe & J. R. Calabrese (Eds.), *Anticonvulsants in mood disorders* (pp. 147–187). New York: Marcel Dekker.

Ketter, T. A., Post, R. M., Denicoff, K., Pazzaglia, P. J., Marangell, L. B., George, M. S., et al. (1998). Carbamazepine. In P. J. Goodnick (Ed.), *Mania: Clinical and research perspectives* (pp. 263–300). Washington, DC: American Psychiatric Press.

Ketter, T. A., Wang, P. W., & Post, R. M. (2004). Carbamazepine and oxcarbazepine. In A. F. Schatzberg & C. B. Nemeroff (Eds.), *Textbook of psychopharmacology* (pp. 581–606). Washington, DC: American Psychiatric Press.

Kim, T.-S., Kim, D.-J., Yoon, S.-J., & Kim, Y.-K. (2007). Increased plasma brain-derived neurotrophic factor levels following unaided smoking cessation. *Presented at 160th Annual Meeting of the American Psychiatric Association, San Diego, CA* NR # 528, 38.

Kim, Y. H., Lee, J. G., Lee, C. H., & Park, S. W. (2007). Effects of ziprasidone on the immobilization stress-induced BDNF mRNA expression in rat brain. *Presented at 160th Annual Meeting of the American Psychiatric Association, San Diego, CA* NR #354, 25.

Kimbrell, T. A., Ketter, T. A., George, M. S., Little, J. T, Benson, B. E., Willis, M. W., et al. (2002). Regional glucose utilization in patient with a range of severities of unipolar depression. *Biological Psychiatry, 51,* 237–252.

Kimbrell, T. A., Little, J. T., Dunn, R. T., Frye, M. A., Greenberg, B. D., Wassermann, E. M., et al. (1999). Frequency dependence of antidepressant response to left prefrontal repetitive transcranial magnetic stimulation (rTMS) as a function of baseline cerebral glucose metabolism. *Biological Psychiatry, 46,* 1603–1613.

Kishimoto, A., Kamata, K., Sugihara, T., Ishiguro, S., Hazama, H., Mizukawa, R., et al. (1988). Treatment of depression with clonazepam. *Acta Psychiatrica Scandinavica, 77,* 81–86.

Kitayama, N., Vaccarino, V., Kutner, M., Weiss, P., & Bremner, J. D. (2005). Magnetic resonance imaging (MRI) measurement of hippocampal volume in post-traumatic stress disorder: A meta-analysis. *Journal of Affective Disorders, 88,* 79–86.

Kito, M., Maehara, M., & Watanabe, K. (1996). Mechanisms of T-type calcium channel blockade by zonisamide. *Seizure, 5,* 115–119.

Klitgaard, H. (2001). Levetiracetam: The preclinical profile of a new class of antiepileptic drugs? *Epilepsia, 42*(Suppl. 4), 13–18.

Klitgaard, H., Matagne, A., Gobert, J., & Wulfert, E. (1998). Evidence for a unique profile of levetiracetam in rodent models of seizures and epilepsy. *European Journal of Pharmacology, 353,* 191–206.

Knable, M. B., Torrey, E. F., Webster, M. J., & Bartko, J. J. (2001). Multivariate analysis of prefrontal cortical data from the Stanley Foundation Neuropathology Consortium. *Brain Research Bulletin, 55,* 651–659.

Knoll, J., Stegman, K., & Suppes, T. (1998). Clinical experience using gabapentin adjunctively in patients with a history of mania or hypomania. *Journal of Affective Disorders, 49,* 229–233.

Kobayashi, T., Kishimoto, A., & Inagaki, T. (1988). Treatment of periodic depression with carbamazepine. *Acta Psychiatrica Scandinavica, 77,* 364–367.

Koller, E. A., & Doraiswamy, P. M. (2002). Olanzapine-associated diabetes mellitus. *Pharmacotherapy, 22,* 841–852.

Koob, G. F. (2006). The neurobiology of addiction: A neuroadaptational view relevant for diagnosis. *Addiction, 101,* 23–30.

Kosel, M., Frick, C., Lisanby, S. H., Fisch, H. U., &

Schlaepfer, T. E. (2003). Magnetic seizure therapy improves mood in refractory major depression. *Neuropsychopharmacology, 28,* 2045–2048.

Koukopoulos, A., Reginaldi, D., Minnai, G., Serra, G., Pani, L., & Johnson, F. N. (1995). The long term prophylaxis of affective disorders. *Advances in Biochemical Psychopharmacology, 49,* 127–147.

Kowatch, R. A., DelBello, M. P., & Findling, R. L. (2002). Depressive episodes in children and adolescents with bipolar disorders. *Clinical Neuroscience Research, 2,* 158–160.

Kowatch, R. A., Fristad, M., Birmaher, B., Wagner, K. D., Findling, R. L., & Hellander, M. (2005). Treatment guidelines for children and adolescents with bipolar disorder. *Journal of the American Academy of Child and Adolescent Psychiatry, 44,* 213–235.

Kowatch, R. A., Suppes, T., Carmody, T. J., Bucci, J. P., Hume, J. H., Kromelis, M., et al. (2000). Effect size of lithium, divalproex sodium, and carbamazepine in children and adolescents with bipolar disorder. *Journal of the American Academy of Child and Adolescent Psychiatry, 39,* 713–720.

Kozel, F. A., & George, M. S. (2002). Meta-analysis of left prefrontal repetitive transcranial magnetic stimulation (rTMS) to treat depression. *Journal of Psychiatric Practice, 8,* 270–275.

Kozel, F. A., Nahas, Z., deBrux, C., Molloy, M., Lorberbaum, J. P., Bohning, D., et al. (2000). How coil-cortex distance relates to age, motor threshold, and antidepressant response to repetitive transcranial magnetic stimulation. *Journal of Neuropsychiatry and Clinical Neuroscience, 12,* 376–384.

Kraepelin, E. (1921). *Manic-depressive insanity and paranoia* (R. M. Barclay, Trans.). Edinburgh: E.S. Livingstone.

Krahl, S. E., Clark, K. B., Smith, D. C., & Browning, R. A. (1998). Locus coeruleus lesions suppress the seizure-attenuating effects of vagus nerve stimulation. *Epilepsia, 39,* 709–714.

Kramlinger, K. G., & Post, R. M. (1996). Ultra-rapid and ultradian cycling in bipolar affective illness. *British Journal of Psychiatry, 168,* 314–323.

Krupp, E., Heynen, T., Li, X. L., Post, R. M., & Weiss, S. R. (2000). Tolerance to the anticonvulsant effects of lamotrigine on amygdala kindled seizures: Cross-tolerance to carbamazepine but not valproate or diazepam. *Experimental Neurology, 162,* 278–289.

Kubacki, A. (1986). Male and female mania. *Canadian Journal of Psychiatry, 31,* 70–72.

Kubek, M. J., Liang, D., Byrd, K. E., & Domb, A. J. (1998). Prolonged seizure suppression by a single implantable polymeric-TRH microdisk preparation. *Brain Research, 809,* 189–197.

Kuhn, C. M., Butler, S. R., & Schanberg, S. M. (1978). Selective depression of serum growth hormone during maternal deprivation in rat pups. *Science, 201*,1034–1036.

Kukopulos, A., Reginaldi, D., Giradi, P., & Tondo, L. (1975). Course of manic-depressive recurrences under lithium. *Comprehensive Psychiatry, 16*, 517–524.

Kukopulos, A., Reginaldi, D., Laddomada, P., Floris, G., Serra, G., & Tondo, L. (1980). Course of the manic-depressive cycle and changes caused by treatment. *Pharmakopsychiatrie, Neuropsychopharmakology, 13*, 156–167.

Kunzel, H. E., Binder, E. B., Nickel, T., et al. (2003). Pharmacological and nonpharmacological factors influencing hypothalamic-pituitary-adrenocortical axis reactivity in acutely depressed psychiatric in-patients, measured by the Dex-CRH test. *Neuropsychopharmacology, 28*, 2169–2178.

Kupchik, M., Spivak, B., Mester, R., Reznik, I., Gonen, N., Weizman, A., et al. (2000). Combined electroconvulsive-clozapine therapy. *Clinical Neuropharmacology, 23*, 14–16.

Kupfer, D. J., Carpenter, L. L., & Frank, E. (1988). Possible role of antidepressants in precipitating mania and hypomania in recurrent depression. *American Journal of Psychiatry, 145*, 804–808.

Kupfer, D. J., Frank, E., Grochocinski, V. J., Cluss, P. A., Houck, P. R., & Stapf, D. A. (2002). Demographic and clinical characteristics of individuals in a bipolar disorder case registry. *Journal of Clinical Psychiatry, 63*, 120–125.

Kupfer, D. J., Frank, E., Perel, J. M., Cornes, C., Mallinger, A. G., Thase, M. E., et al. (1992). Five-year outcome for maintenance therapies in recurrent depression. *Archives of General Psychiatry, 49*, 769–773.

Kupka, R. W., Luckenbaugh, D. A., Post, R. M., Suppes, T., Altshuler, L. L., Keck, P. E., Jr., et al. (2005).Comparison of rapid-cycling and non-rapid-cycling bipolar disorder based on prospective mood ratings in 539 outpatients. *American Journal of Psychiatry, 162*, 1273–1280.

Kutt, H., Solomon, G., Peterson, H., Dhar, A., & Caronna, J. (1985). Accumulation of carbamazepine epoxide caused by valproate contributing to intoxication syndromes. *Neurology, 35*(Suppl. 1), 286–287.

Kuzniecky, R., Hetherington, H., Ho, S., Pan, J., Martin, R., Gilliam, F., et al. (1998). Topiramate increases cerebral GABA in healthy humans. *Neurology, 51*, 627–629.

Ladd, C. O., Huot, R. L., Thrivikraman, K. V., Nemeroff, C. B., Meaney, M. J., & Plotsky, P. M. (2000). Long-term behavioral and neuroendocrine adaptations to adverse early experience. *Progress in Brain Research, 122*, 81–103.

Lambert, P. A. (1984). Acute and prophylactic therapies of patients with affective disorders using valpromide (dipropylacetamide). In H. M. Emrich, T. Okuma, & A. A. Muller (Eds.), *Anticonvulsants in affective disorders* (pp. 33–44). Amsterdam: Excerpta Medica.

Lamberty, Y., Margineanu, D. G., & Klitgaard, H. (2001). Effect of the new antiepileptic drug levetiracetam in an animal model of mania. *Epilepsy and Behavior, 2*, 454–459.

Landolt, H. (1953). Some clinical electroencephalographical correlations in epileptic psychoses (twilight states). *Electroencephalography and Clinical Neurophysiology, 5*, 121.

Lange, K. J., & McInnis, M. G. (2002). Studies of anticipation in bipolar affective disorder. *CNS Spectrums, 7*, 196–202.

Law, A. J., Weickert, C. S., Hyde, T. M., Kleinman, J. E., & Harrison, P. J. (2004). Reduced spinophilin but not microtubule-associated protein 2 expression in the hippocampal formation in schizophrenia and mood disorders: molecular evidence for a pathology of dendritic spines. *American Journal of Psychiatry, 161*, 1848–1855.

LeDoux, J. E. (1992). Emotion and the amygdala. In J. P. Aggleton (Ed.), *The amygdala: Neurobiological aspects of emotion, memory, and mental dysfunction* (pp. 339–351). New York: Wiley-Liss.

Leppig, M., Bosch, B., Naber, D., & Hippius, H. (1989). Clozapine in the treatment of 121 out-patients. *Psychopharmacology (Berlin), 99*(Suppl.), S77–S79.

Leppik, I. E. (2002). Three new drugs for epilepsy: Levetiracetam, oxcarbazepine, and zonisamide. *Journal of Child Neurology, 17*(Suppl. 1), S53–S57.

Levander, E., Frye, M. A., McElroy, S., Suppes, T., Grunze, H., Nolen, W. A., et al. (in press). Alcoholism and anxiety in bipolar illness: Differential lifetime anxiety comorbidity in bipolar I women with and without alcoholism. *Journal of Affective Disorders.*

Leverich, G. S., Altshuler, L. L., Frye, M. A., Suppes, T., Keck, P. E., Jr., McElroy, S., et al. (2003). Factors associated with suicide attempts in 648 patients with bipolar disorder in the Stanley Foundation Bipolar Network. *Journal of Clinical Psychiatry, 64*, 680–690.

Leverich, G. S., Altshuler, L. L., Frye, M. A., Suppes, T., McElroy, S. L., Keck, P. E., Jr., et al. (2006). Risk of switch in mood polarity to hypomania or mania in patients with bipolar depression during acute and continuation trials of venlafaxine, sertraline, and bupropion as adjuncts to mood stabilizers. *American Journal of Psychiatry, 163*, 232–239.

Leverich, G. S., McElroy, S. L., Altshuler, L. L., Frye, M. A., Grunze, H., Keck, P. E., Jr., et al. (2005). The anticonvulsant zonisamide in bipolar illness: Clinical response and weight loss. *Aspects of Affect, 1*, 53–56.

Leverich, G. S., McElroy, S. L., Suppes, T., Keck, P. E., Jr., Denicoff, K. D., Nolen, W. A., et al. (2002). Early physical and sexual abuse associated with an adverse course of bipolar illness. *Biological Psychiatry, 51*, 288–297.

Leverich, G. S., Perez, S., Luckenbaugh, D. A., & Post, R. M. (2002). Early psychosocial stressors: Relationship to suicidality and course of bipolar illness. *Clinical Neuroscience Research, 2*, 161–170.

Leverich, G. S., & Post, R. M. (1996). Life charting the course of bipolar disorder. *Current Review of Mood and Anxiety Disorders, 1*, 48–61.

Leverich, G. S., & Post, R. M. (1998). Life charting of affective disorders. *CNS Spectrums, 3*, 21–37.

Leverich, G. S., & Post, R. M. (2006). Course of bipolar illness after history of childhood trauma. *Lancet, 367*, 1040–1042.

Leverich, G. S., Post, R. M., Keck, P. E., Jr, Altshuler, L. L, Frye, M. A., Kupka, R. W., et al. (2007). The poor prognosis of childhood-onset bipolar disorder. *Journal of Pediatrics, 150*, 485–490.

Levine, J., Chengappa, K. N., Brar, J. S., Gershon, S., Yablonsky, E., Stapf, D., et al. (2000). Psychotropic drug prescription patterns among patients with bipolar I disorder. *Bipolar Disorders, 2*, 120–130.

Li, H., Chen, A., Xing, G., Wei, M. L., & Rogawski, M. A. (2001). Kainate receptor-mediated heterosynaptic facilitation in the amygdala. *Nature Neuroscience, 4*, 612–620.

Li, H., Weiss, S.R.B., Chuang, D.-M., Post, R. M., & Rogawski, M. A. (1998). Bidirectional synaptic plasticity in the rat basolateral amygdala: characterization of an activity-dependent switch sensitive to the presynaptic metabotropic glutamate receptor antagonist 2S-α-ethylglutamic acid. *Journal of Neuroscience,18*, 1662–1670.

Liewendahl, K., Majuri, H., & Helenius, T. (1978). Thyroid function tests in patients on long-term treatment with various anticonvulsant drugs. *Clinical Endocrinology, 8*, 185–191.

Liewendahl, K., Tikanoja, S., Helenius, T., & Majuri, H. (1985). Free thyroxin and free triiodothyronine as measured by equilibrium dialysis and analog radioimmunoassay in serum of patients taking phenytoin and carbamazepine. *Clinical Chemistry, 31*, 1993–1996.

Lindhout, D., Hoppener, R. J. E. A., & Meinardi, H. (1984). Teratogenicity of antiepileptic drug combinations with special emphasis on epoxidation (of carbamazepine). *Epilepsia, 25*, 77–83.

Linnarsson, S., Bjorklund, A., & Ernfors, P. (1997). Learning deficit in BDNF mutant mice. *European Journal of Neuroscience, 9*, 2581–2587.

Lisanby, S. H., Luber, B., Schlaepfer, T. E., & Sackeim, H. A. (2003). Safety and feasibility of magnetic seizure therapy (MST) in major depression: Randomized within-subject comparison with electroconvulsive therapy. *Neuropsychopharmacology, 28*, 1852–1865.

Lish, J. D., Dime-Meenan, S., Whybrow, P. C., Price, R. A., & Hirschfeld, R. M. A. (1994). The National Depressive and Manic-Depressive Association (DMDA) survey of bipolar members. *Journal of Affective Disorders, 31*, 281–294.

Little, J. T., Ketter, T. A., Kimbrell, T. A., Danielson, A., Benson, B., Willis, M. W., et al. (1996). Venlafaxine or bupropion responders but not nonresponders show baseline prefrontal and paralimbic hypometabolism compared with controls. *Psychopharmacology Bulletin, 32*, 629–635.

Little, J. T., Ketter, T. A., Kimbrell, T. A., Dunn, R. T., Benson, B. E., Willis, M. W., et al. (2005). Bupropion and venlafaxine responders differ in pretreatment regional cerebral metabolism in unipolar depression. *Biological Psychiatry, 57*, 220–228.

Lledo, P. M., Hjelmstad, G. O., Mukherji, S., Soderling, T. R., Malenka, R. C., & Nicoll, R. A. (1995). Calcium/calmodulin-dependent kinase II and long-term potentiation enhance synaptic transmission by the same mechanism. *Proceedings of the National Academy of Science, USA, 92*, 11175–11179.

Loftis, J. M., Huckans, M., Hinrichs, D. J., & Hauser, P. (2007). Elevated levels of plasma interleukin and tumor necrosis factor are associated with increased depressive symptomatology in patients with and without chronic hepatitis C. *Presented at 160th Annual Meeting of the American Psychiatric Association, San Diego, CA* NR#702, 50.

London, E. D., Bonson, K. R., Ernst, M., & Grant, S. (1999). Brain imaging studies of cocaine abuse: Implications for medication development. *Critical Reviews in Neurobiology, 13*, 227–242.

Loosen, P. T. (1988). TRH: Behavioral and endocrine effects in man. *Progress in Neuropsychopharmacology and Biological Psychiatry, 12*(Suppl.), S87–S117.

Loscher, W., & Honack, D. (1993). Profile of ucb L059, a novel anticonvulsant drug, in models of partial and generalized epilepsy in mice and rats. *European Journal of Pharmacology, 232*, 147–158.

Loscher, W., Honack, D., & Rundfeldt, C. (1998). Antiepileptogenic effects of the novel anticonvulsant levetiracetam (ucb L059) in the kindling model of temporal lobe epilepsy. *Journal of Pharmacology and Experimental Therapeutics, 284*, 474–479.

Luckenbaugh, D. A., Findling, R. L., Leverich, G. S., Pizzarello, S. M., & Post, R. M. (2007). *Earliest symptoms discriminating prepubertal onset bipolar illness from ADHD.* Manuscript submitted for publication.

Lynch, B. A., Lambeng, N., Nocka, K., Kensel-Hammes, P., Bajjalieh, S. M., Matagne, A., et al. (2004). The synaptic vesicle protein SV2A is the binding site for the antiepileptic drug levetiracetam. *Proceedings of the National Academy of Sciences, USA, 101*, 9861–9866.

Macdonald, R. L. (2002). Zonisamide: Mechanisms of action. In R. H. Levy, R. H. Mattson, B. S. Meldrum, & E. Perucca (Eds.), *Antiepileptic drugs* (pp. 867–872). Philadelphia: Lippincott Williams & Wilkins.

Macedo, A., Azevedo, M. H., Coelho, I., Duorado, A., Valente, J., Pato, M. T., et al. (1999). Genetic anticipation in Portuguese families with bipolar mood disorder. *CNS Spectrums, 4*, 25–31.

Machado-Vieira, R., Dietrich, M. O., Leke, R., Cereser, V. H., Zanatto, V., Kapczinski, F., et al. (2007). Decreased plasma brain derived neurotrophic factor levels in unmedicated bipolar patients during manic episode. *Biological Psychiatry, 61*, 142–144.

MacLean, P. D. (1973). A triune concept of the brain and behavior: The Clarence M. Hincks Memorial Lecture, T. J. Boag & D. Campell (eds.). University of Toronto Press, Toronto and Buffalo, pp 1–66.

MacQueen, G. M., Campbell, S., McEwen, B. S., et al. (2003). Course of illness, hippocampal function, and hippocampal volume in major depression. *Proceedings of the National Academy of Science USA, 100*, 1387–1392.

Maier, S. F., & Jackson, R. L. (1977). The nature of the initial coping response and the learned helplessness responses. *Animal Learning and Behavior, 5*, 404–414.

Maj, M., Pirozzi, R., & Kemali, D. (1989). Long-term outcome of lithium prophylaxis in patients initially classified as complete responders. *Psychopharmacology (Berlin), 98*, 535–538.

Maj, M., Pirozzi, R., & Magliano, L. (1995). Nonresponse to reinstituted lithium prophylaxis in previously responsive bipolar patients: Prevalence and predictors. *American Journal of Psychiatry, 152*, 1810–1811.

Maj, M., Pirozzi, R., Magliano, L., & Bartoli, L. (1998). Long-term outcome of lithium prophylaxis in bipolar disorder: A 5-year prospective study of 402 patients at a lithium clinic. *American Journal of Psychiatry, 155*, 30–35.

Malberg, J. E., Eisch, A. J., Nestler, E. J., & Duman, R. S. (2000). Chronic antidepressant treatment increases neurogenesis in adult rat hippocampus. *Journal of Neuroscience, 20*, 9104–9110.

Mammen, O. K., Pilkonis, P. A., Chengappa, K. N., & Kupfer, D. J. (2004). Anger attacks in bipolar depression: Predictors and response to citalopram added to mood stabilizers. *Journal of Clinical Psychiatry, 65*, 627–633.

Manji, H. K., Moore, G. J., & Chen, G. (2000). Clinical and preclinical evidence for the neurotrophic effects of mood stabilizers: Implications for the pathophysiology and treatment of manic-depressive illness. *Biological Psychiatry, 48*, 740–754.

Mann, J. J. (1983). Loss of antidepressant effect with long-term monoamine oxidase inhibitor treatment without loss of monoamine oxidase inhibition. *Journal of Clinical Psychopharmacology, 3*, 363–366.

Manna, V. (1991). Disturbi affettivi bipolari e ruolo del calcio intraneuronale. Effetti terapeutici del trattamento con sali di litio e/o calcio antagonista in pazienti con rapida inversione di polarita. [Bipolar affective disorders and role of intraneuronal calcium. Therapeutic effects of treatment with lithium salts and/or calcium antagonist in patients with rapid polar inversion]. *Minerva Med, 82*, 757–763.

Marangell, L. B., George, M. S., Callahan, A. M., Ketter, T. A., Pazzaglia, P. J., L'Herrou, T. A., et al. (1997). Effects of intrathecal thyrotropin-releasing hormone (protirelin) in refractory depressed patients. *Archives of General Psychiatry, 54*, 214–222.

Marcotte, D. (1998). Use of topiramate, a new antiepileptic as a mood stabilizer. *Journal of Affective Disorders, 50*, 245–251.

Marcus, R. N., Owen, R., Swanink, R., McQuade, R. D., & Iwamoto, T. (2007). Two studies to evaluate the safety and efficacy of aripiprazole monotherapy in outpatients with bipolar I disorder with a major depressive episode without psychotic features. *Presented at 160th Annual Meeting of the American Psychiatric Association, San Diego, CA* NR #311, 22.

Markovitz, P. J., Calabrese, J. R., Schulz, S. C., & Meltzer, H. Y. (1991). Fluoxetine in the treatment of borderline and schizotypal personality disorders. *American Journal of Psychiatry, 148*, 1064–1067.

Marneros, A., & Brieger, P. (2002). Prognosis of bipolar disorder: A review. In H. Maj, H. Akiskal, J. J. Lopez-Ibor, & N. Satorius (Eds.), *Bipolar disorder* (Vol. 5, pp. 97–148). WPA Series, Evidence and Experience in Psychiatry. New York: John Wiley & Sons.

Martin, A., Young, C., Leckman, J. F., Mukonoweshuro, C., Rosenheck, R., & Leslie, D. (2004). Age effects on antidepressant-induced manic conversion. *Archives of Pediatric and Adolescent Medicine, 158*, 773–780.

Mason, B., & Ownby, R. L. (2000). Acamprosate for the treatment of alcohol dependence: A review of double-blind, placebo-controlled trials. *CNS Spectrums, 5*, 58–69.

Matsumoto, I., Burke, L., Inoue, Y., & Wilce, P. A. (2001). Two models of ethanol withdrawal kindling. *Nihon Arukoru Yakubutsu Igakkai Zasshi, 36*, 53–64.

Mauri, M. C., Laini, V., Scalvini, M. E., Omboni, A., Ferrari, V. M., Clemente, A., et al. (2001). Gabapentin and the prophylaxis of bipolar disorders in patients intolerant to lithium. *Clinical Drug Investigations, 21*, 169–174.

McCall, W. V., Dunn, A., Rosenquist, P. B., & Hughes,

D. (2002). Markedly suprathreshold right unilateral ECT versus minimally suprathreshold bilateral ECT: Antidepressant and memory effects. *Journal of ECT, 18*, 126–129.

McDermut, W., Pazzaglia, P. J., Huggins, T., Mikalauskas, K., Leverich, G. S., Ketter, T. A., et al. (1995). Use of single case analyses in off-on-off-on trials in affective illness: A demonstration of the efficacy of nimodipine. *Depression, 2*, 259–271.

McElroy, S. L., Altshuler, L. L., Suppes, T., Keck, P. E., Frye, M. A., Denicoff, K. D., et al. (2001). Axis I psychiatric comorbidity and its relationship to historical illness variables in 288 patients with bipolar disorder. *American Journal of Psychiatry, 158*, 420–426.

McElroy, S. L., Arnold, L. M., Shapira, N. A., Keck, P. E., Jr., Rosenthal, N. R., Karim, M. R., et al. (2003). Topiramate in the treatment of binge eating disorder associated with obesity: A randomized, placebo-controlled trial. *American Journal of Psychiatry, 160*, 255–261.

McElroy, S. L., Frye, M. A., Altshuler, L. L., Suppes, T., Hellemann, G., Black, D., et al. (2007). A 24-week, randomized, controlled trial of adjunctive sibutramine versus topiramate in the treatment of weight gain in overweight or obese patients with bipolar disorders. *Bipolar Disorder, 9*, 426–434.

McElroy, S. L., Frye, M., Denicoff, K., Altshuler, L., Nolen, W., Kupka, R., et al. (1998). Olanzapine in treatment-resistant bipolar disorder. *Journal of Affective Disorders, 49*, 119–122.

McElroy, S. L., Frye, M. A., Suppes, T., Dhavale, D., Keck, P. E., Jr., Leverich, G. S., et al. (2002). Correlates of overweight and obesity in 644 patients with bipolar disorder. *Journal of Clinical Psychiatry, 63*, 207–213.

McElroy, S. L., Keck, P. E., Pope, H. G., & Hudson, J. I. (1988). Valproate in the treatment of rapid-cycling bipolar disorder. *Journal of Clinical Psychopharmacology, 8*, 275–279.

McElroy, S. L., Keck, P. E., Jr., Pope, H. G., Jr., & Hudson, J. I. (1989). Valproate in psychiatric disorders: Literature review and clinical guidelines. *Journal of Clinical Psychiatry, 50*, 23–29.

McElroy, S. L., Keck, P. E., Jr., Pope, H. G., Jr., & Hudson, J. I. (1992). Valproate in the treatment of bipolar disorder: Literature review and clinical guidelines. *Journal of Clinical Psychopharmacology, 12*(Suppl. 1), 42S–52S.

McElroy, S. L., Keck, P. E., Pope, H. G., Hudson, J. I., Faedda, G. L., & Swann, A. C. (1992) Clinical and research implications of the diagnosis of dysphoric or mixed mania or hypomania. *American Journal of Psychiatry, 149*, 1633–1644.

McElroy, S. L., Keck, P. E., & Strakowski, S. M. (1996). Mania, psychosis, and antipsychotics. *Journal of Clinical Psychiatry, 57*(Suppl. 3), 14–26.

McElroy, S. L., Pope, H. G., Jr., Keck, P. E., Jr., & Hudson, J. I. (1988). Treatment of psychiatric disorders with valproate: A series of 73 cases. *Psychiatrie and Psychobiologie, 3*, 81–85.

McElroy, S. L., Soutullo, C. A., Keck, P. E., Jr., & Kmetz, G. F. (1997). A pilot trial of adjunctive gabapentin in the treatment of bipolar disorder. *Annals of Clinical Psychiatry, 9*, 99–103.

McElroy, S. L., Suppes, T., Frye, M. A., Altshuler, L. L., Stanford, K., Martens, B., et al. (2007). Open-label aripiprazole in the treatment of acute bipolar depression: A prospective pilot trial. Journal of Affective Disorders, 101, 275–281.

McElroy, S. L., Suppes, T., Keck, P. E., Jr., Black, D., Frye, M. A., Altshuler, L. L., et al. (2005). Open-label adjunctive zonisamide in the treatment of bipolar disorders: A prospective trial. *Journal of Clinical Psychiatry, 66*, 617–624.

McElroy, S. L., Suppes, T., Keck, P. E., Frye, M. A., Denicoff, K. D., Altshuler, L. L., et al. (2000). Open-label adjunctive topiramate in the treatment of bipolar disorders. *Biological Psychiatry, 47*, 1025–1033.

McGavin, J. K., & Goa, K. L. (2002). Aripiprazole. *CNS Drugs, 16*, 779–786.

McIntyre, R. S., Mancini, D. A., McCann, S., Srinivasan, J., Sagman, D., & Kennedy, S. H. (2002). Topiramate versus bupropion SR when added to mood stabilizer therapy for the depressive phase of bipolar disorder: A preliminary single-blind study. *Bipolar Disorders, 4*, 207–213.

McLoughlin, D. M., Eranti, S., Mogg, A., Pluck, G., Purvis, R., Brown, R., et al. (2005). A 6-month, follow-up, pragmatic randomised controlled trial of ECT and rTMS in major depression. *Journal of ECT, 21*, 59.

McMahon, F. J., Hopkins, P. J., Xu, J., Shaw, S., Cardon, L., Simpson, S. G., et al. (1997). Linkage of bipolar affective disorder to chromosome 18 markers in a new pedigree series. *American Journal of Human Genetics, 61*, 1379–1404.

McNamara, B., Ray, J. L., Arthurs, O. J., & Boniface, S. (2001). Transcranial magnetic stimulation for depression and other psychiatric disorders. *Psychological Medicine, 31*, 1141–1146.

Meador, K. J., Baker, G. A., Finnell, R. H., Kalayjian, L. A., Liporase, J. D., Loring, D. W., et al. for the NEAD Study Group. (2006). *In utero* antiepileptic drug exposure. *Neurology, 67*, 407–412.

Meaney, M. J., Aitken, D. H., Van Berkel, C., Bhatnagar, S., & Sapolsky, R. M. (1988). Effects of neonatal handling on age-related impairments associated with the hippocampus. *Science, 239*, 766–768.

Meaney, M. J., Brake, W., & Gratton, A. (2002). Environmental regulation of the development of mesolimbic dopamine systems: A neurobiological mechanism for vulnerability to drug abuse? *Psychoneuroendocrinology, 27,* 127–138.

Mellegers, M. A., Furlan, A. D., & Mailis, A. (2001). Gabapentin for neuropathic pain: Systematic review of controlled and uncontrolled literature. *Clinical Journal of Pain, 17,* 284–295.

Meltzer, H. Y., Alphs, L., Green, A. I., Altamura, A. C., Anand, R., Bertoldi, A., et al. (2003). Clozapine treatment for suicidality in schizophrenia: International Suicide Prevention Trial (InterSePT). *Archives of General Psychiatry, 60,* 82–91.

Meyer, A. (1951). The Life Chart and the obligation of specifying positive data in psychological diagnosis. In E. E. Winters (Ed.), *The collected papers of Adolf Meyer* (Vol. III). Baltimore: Johns Hopkins University Press.

Miklowitz, D. J. (2002). *The bipolar disorder survival guide: What you and your family need to know.* New York: Guilford.

Miklowitz, D. J., Otto, M. W., Frank, E., Reilly-Harrington, N. A., Wisniewski, S. R., Kogan, J. N., et al. (2007). Psychosocial treatments for bipolar depression: A 1-year randomized trial from the systematic treatment enhancement program. *Archives of General Psychiatry, 64,* 419–426.

Miller, D. D. (2000). Review and management of clozapine side effects. *Journal of Clinical Psychiatry, 61*(Suppl. 8), 14–17.

Mimaki, T., Suzuki, Y., Tagawa, T., Karasawa, T., & Yabuuchi, H. (1990). Interaction of zonisamide with benzodiazepine and GABA receptors in rat brain. *Medical Journal of Osaka University, 39,* 13–17.

Mishory, A., Winokur, M., & Bersudsky, Y. (2003). Prophylactic effect of phenytoin in bipolar disorder: A controlled study. *Bipolar Disorders, 5,* 464–467.

Mishory, A., Yaroslavsky, Y., Bersudsky, Y., & Belmaker, R. H. (2000). Phenytoin as an antimanic anticonvulsant: A controlled study. *American Journal of Psychiatry, 157,* 463–465.

Moller, H.-J., & Grunze, H. (2000). Have some guidelines for the treatment of acute bipolar depression gone too far in the restriction of antidepressants? *European Archives of Psychiatry and Clinical Neuroscience, 250,* 57–68.

Motamedi, M., Nguyen, D. K., Zaatreh, M., Singh, S. P., Westerveld, M., Thompson, J. L., et al. (2003). Levetiracetam efficacy in refractory partial-onset seizures, especially after failed epilepsy surgery. *Epilepsia, 44,* 211–214.

Mukherjee, S., Rosen, A. M., Caracci, G., & Shukla, S. (1986). Persistent tardive dyskinesia in bipolar patients. *Archives of General Psychiatry, 43,* 342–346.

Mullen, J., Jibson, M. D., & Sweitzer, D. (2001). A comparison of the relative safety, efficacy, and tolerability of quetiapine and risperidone in outpatients with schizophrenia and other psychotic disorders:

The quetiapine experience with safety and tolerability (QUEST) study. *Clinical Therapy, 23,* 1839–1854.

Muller, D. J., de Luca, V., Sicard, T., King, N., Strauss, J., & Kennedy, J. L. (2006). Brain-derived neurotrophic factor (BDNF) gene and rapid-cycling bipolar disorder: family-based association study. *British Journal of Psychiatry, 189,* 317–323.

Murphy, D. J., Gannon, M. A., & McGennis, A. (1989). Carbamazepine in bipolar affective disorder [letter]. *Lancet, 2,* 1151–1152.

Myrick, H., & Anton, R. F. (2000). Clinical management of alcohol withdrawal. *CNS Spectrums, 5,* 22–32.

Naber, D., Leppig, M., Grohmann, R., & Hippius, H. (1989). Efficacy and adverse effects of clozapine in the treatment of schizophrenia and tardive dyskinesia—a retrospective study of 387 patients. *Psychopharmacology (Berlin), 99*(Suppl.), S73–S76.

Nahas, Z., Kozel, F. A., Li, X., Anderson, B., & George, M. S. (2003). Left prefrontal transcranial magnetic stimulation (TMS) treatment of depression in bipolar affective disorder: A pilot study of acute safety and efficacy. *Bipolar Disorders, 5,* 40–47.

Nahas, Z., Marangell, L. B., Husain, M. M., Rush, A. J., Sackeim, H. A., Lisanby, S. H., et al. (2005). Two-year outcome of vagus nerve stimulation (VNS) for treatment of major depressive episodes. *Journal of Clinical Psychiatry, 66,* 1097–1104.

Nahas, Z., Teneback, C. C., Kozel, A., Speer, A. M., DeBrux, C., Molloy, M., et al. (2001). Brain effects of TMS delivered over prefrontal cortex in depressed adults: role of stimulation frequency and coil-cortex distance. *Journal of Neuropsychiatry and Clinical Neuroscience, 13,* 459–470.

Nakajima, T., Post, R. M., Pert, A., Ketter, T. A., & Weiss, S. R. (1989). Perspectives on the mechanism of action of electroconvulsive therapy: Anticonvulsant, peptidergic, c-fos proto-oncogene effects. *Convulsive Therapy, 5,* 274–295.

Nelson, J. C., Mazure, C. M., Bowers, M. B., Jr., & Jatlow, P. I. (1991). A preliminary, open study of the combination of fluoxetine and desipramine for rapid treatment of major depression. *Archives of General Psychiatry, 48,* 303–307.

Nemeroff, C. B., Evans, D. L., Gyulai, L., Sachs, G. S., Bowden, C. L., Gergel, I. P., et al. (2001). Double-blind, placebo-controlled comparison of imipramine and paroxetine in the treatment of bipolar depression. *American Journal of Psychiatry, 158,* 906–912.

Nemeroff, C. B., Kinkead, B., & Goldstein, J. (2002). Quetiapine: Preclinical studies, pharmacokinetics, drug interactions, and dosing. *Journal of Clinical Psychiatry, 63*(Suppl. 13), 5–11.

Nemets, H., Nemets, B., Apter, A., Bracha, Z., & Belmaker, R. H. (2006). Omega-3 treatment of childhood depression: A controlled, double-blind pilot study. *American Journal of Psychiatry, 163*, 1098–1100.

Nemets, B., Stahl, Z., & Belmaker, R. H. (2002). Addition of omega-3 fatty acid to maintenance medication treatment for recurrent unipolar depressive disorder. *American Journal of Psychiatry, 159*, 477–479.

Neppe, V. M. (1983). Carbamazepine as adjunctive treatment in nonepileptic chronic inpatients with EEG temporal lobe abnormalities. *Journal of Clinical Psychiatry, 44*, 236–331.

Neumann, J., Seidel, K., & Wunderlich, H.-P. (1984). Comparative studies of the effect of carbamazepine and trimipramine in depression. In H. M. Emrich, T. Okuma, & A. A. Muller (Eds.), *Anticonvulsants in affective disorders* (pp. 160–166). Amsterdam: Excerpta Medica.

Neves-Pereira, M., Mundo, E., Muglia, P., King, N., Macciardi, F., & Kennedy, J. L. (2002). The brain-derived neurotrophic factor gene confers susceptibility to bipolar disorder: evidence from a family-based association study. *American Journal of Human Genetics, 71*, 651–655.

Nibuya, M., Morinobu, S., & Duman, R. S. (1995). Regulation of BDNF and trkB mRNA in rat brain by chronic electroconvulsive seizure and antidepressant drug treatments. *Journal of Neuroscience, 15*, 7539–7547.

Nickel, M. K., Muehlbacher, M., Nickel, C., Kettler, C., Gil, F. P., Bachler, E., et al. (2006). Aripiprazole in the treatment of patients with borderline personality disorder: A double-blind, placebo-controlled study. *American Journal of Psychiatry, 163*, 833–838.

Nielsen, O. A., Johannessen, A. C., & Bardrum, B. (1988). Oxcarbazepine-induced hyponatremia, a cross-sectional study. *Epilepsy Research, 2*, 269–271.

Ninan, P. T. (2000). Use of venlafaxine in other psychiatric disorders. *Depression and Anxiety, 12*(Suppl. 1), 90–94.

Nobler, M. S., Sackeim, H. A., Prohovnik, I., Moeller, J. R., Mukherjee, S., Schnur, D. B., et al. (1994). Regional cerebral blood flow in mood disorders, III. Treatment and clinical response. *Archives of General Psychiatry, 51*, 884–897.

Nolen, W. A., Luckenbaugh, D. A., Altshuler, L. L., Suppes, T., McElroy, S. L., Frye, M. A., et al. (2004). Correlates of 1-year prospective outcome in bipolar disorder: Results from the Stanley Foundation Bipolar Network. *American Journal of Psychiatry, 161*, 1447–1454.

Nomikos, G. G., Damsma, G., Wenkstern, D., & Fibiger, H. C. (1989). Acute effects of bupropion on extracellular dopamine concentrations in rat striatum and nucleus accumbens studied by in vivo microdialysis. *Neuropsychopharmacology, 2*, 273–279.

Nomikos, G. G., Damsma, G., Wenkstern, D., & Fibiger, H. C. (1992). Effects of chronic bupropion on interstitial concentrations of dopamine in rat nucleus accumbens and striatum. *Neuropsychopharmacology, 7*, 7–14.

Nutt, J. G. (1995). Pharmacodynamics of levodopa in Parkinson's disease. *Clinical and Experimental Pharmacology and Physiology, 22*, 837–840.

Nylander, P. O., Engstrom, C., Chotai, J., Wahlstrom, J., & Adolfsson, R. (1994). Anticipation in Swedish families with bipolar affective disorder. *Journal of Medical Genetics, 31*, 686–689.

Obrocea, G. V., Dunn, R. M., Frye, M. A., Ketter, T. A., Luckenbaugh, D. A., Leverich, G. S., et al. (2002). Clinical predictors of response to lamotrigine and gabapentin monotherapy in refractory affective disorders. *Biological Psychiatry, 51*, 253–260.

O'Connell, R. A., Mayo, J. A., Flatow, L., Cuthbertson, B., & O'Brien, B. E. (1991). Outcome of bipolar disorder on long-term treatment with lithium. *British Journal of Psychiatry, 159*, 123–129.

Okada, M., Hirano, T., Kawata, Y., Murakami, T., Wada, K., Mizuno, K., et al. (1999). Biphasic effects of zonisamide on serotonergic system in rat hippocampus. *Epilepsy Research, 34*, 187–197.

Okada, M., Kawata, Y., Mizuno, K., Wada, K., Kondo, T., & Kaneko, S. (1998). Interaction between Ca2+, K+, carbamazepine and zonisamide on hippocampal extracellular glutamate monitored with a microdialysis electrode. *British Journal of Pharmacology, 124*, 1277–1285.

Okada, M., Kaneko, S., Hirano, T., Mizuno, K., Kondo, T., Otani, K., et al. (1995). Effects of zonisamide on dopaminergic system. *Epilepsy Research, 22*, 193–205.

Okuma, T. (1993). Effects of carbamazepine and lithium on affective disorders. *Neuropsychobiology, 27*, 138–145.

Okuma, T., Inanaga, K., Otsuki, S., & Sarai, K. (1979). Comparison of the antimanic efficacy of carbamazepine and chlorpromazine: A double-blind controlled study. *Psychopharmacology, 66*, 211–217.

Okuma, T., Kishimoto, A., Inoue, K., Matsumoto, H., & Ogura, A. (1973). Anti-manic and prophylactic effects of carbamazepine (Tegretol) on manic depressive psychosis. A preliminary report. *Folia Psychiatrica et Neurologica Japonica, 27*, 283–297.

Olver, J. S., Cryan, J. F., Burrows, G. D., & Norman, T. R. (2000). Pindolol augmentation of antidepressants: A review and rationale. *Australia and New Zealand Journal of Psychiatry, 34*, 71–79.

Ostroff, R. B., & Nelson, J. C. (1999). Risperidone augmentation of selective serotonin reuptake inhibitors in major depression. *Journal of Clinical Psychiatry, 60*, 256–259.

Osuch, E. A., Brotman, M. A., Podell, D., Geraci, M., Touzeau, P. L., Leverich, G. S., et al. (2001). Prospective and retrospective life-charting in posttraumatic stress disorder (the PTSD-LCM): A pilot study. *Journal of Trauma and Stress, 14*, 229–239.

Osuch, E. A., McCann, U. D., Benson, B. E., Podell, D. M., Morgan, C. M., Willis, M. W., et al. (2001). Regional cerebral blood flow correlated with flashback intensity in patients with posttraumatic stress disorder. *Biological Psychiatry, 50*, 246–253.

Owen, R. R., Jr., Beake, B. J., Marby, D., Dessain, E. C., & Cole, J. O. (1989). Response to clozapine in chronic psychotic patients. *Psychopharmacology Bulletin, 25*, 253–256.

Pae, C. U., Kim, J. J., Lee, K. U., Lee, C. U., Bahk, W. M., Lee, S. J., et al. (2003). Effect of nizatidine on olanzapine-associated weight gain in schizophrenic patients in Korea: A pilot study. *Human Psychopharmacology, 18*, 453–456.

Pande, A. C., Crockatt, J. G., Janney, C. A., Werth, J. L., & Tsaroucha, G. (2000). Gabapentin in bipolar disorder: A placebo-controlled trial of adjunctive therapy. Gabapentin Bipolar Disorder Study Group. *Bipolar Disorders, 2*, 249–255.

Pande, A. C., Davidson, J. R., Jefferson, J. W., Janney, C. A., Katzelnick, D. J., Weisler, R. H., et al. (1999). Treatment of social phobia with gabapentin: A placebo-controlled study. *Journal of Clinical Psychopharmacology, 19*, 341–348.

Pande, A. C., Pollack, M. H., Crockatt, J., Greiner, M., Chouinard, G., Lydiard, R. B., et al. (2000). Placebo-controlled study of gabapentin treatment of panic disorder. *Journal of Clinical Psychopharmacology, 20*, 467–471.

Papakostas, G. I., Petersen, T. J., Kinrys, G., Burns, A. M., Worthington, J. J., Alpert, J. E., et al. (2005). Aripiprazole augmentation of selective serotonin reuptake inhibitors for treatment-resistant major depressive disorder. *Journal of Clinical Psychiatry, 66*, 1326–1330.

Papez, J. W. (1937). A proposed mechanism of emotion. *Archives of Neurological Psychiatry, 38*, 725–744.

Papolos, D. F., & Papolos, J. (1999). *The bipolar child.* New York: Broadway Books.

Parekh, P. I., Ketter, T. A., Altshuler, L., Frye, M. A., Callahan, A., Marangell, L., et al. (1998). Relationships between thyroid hormone and antidepressant responses to total sleep deprivation in mood disorder patients. *Biological Psychiatry, 43*, 392–394.

Park, S.W., Lee, S. K., Kim, J. M., Yoon, J. S., & Kim, Y. H. (2006). Effects of quetiapine on the brain-derived neurotrophic factor expression in the hippocampus and neocortex of rats. *Neuroscience Letters, 402*, 25–29.

Pascual-Leone, A., Grafman, J., Cohen, L. G., Roth, B. J., & Hallett, M. (1997). Transcranial magnetic stimulation: A new tool for the study of higher cognitive functions in humans. In N. Grafman & F. Boller (Eds.), *Handbook of neuropsychology* (pp. 267–290). New York, Elsevier.

Pascual-Leone, A., Rubio, B., Pallardo, F., & Catala, M. D. (1996). Rapid-rate transcranial magnetic stimulation of left dorsolateral prefrontal cortex in drug-resistant depression. *Lancet, 348*, 233–237.

Pauk, J., Kuhn, C. M., Field, T. M., & Schanberg, S. M. (1986). Positive effects of tactile versus kinesthetic or vestibular stimulation on neuroendocrine and ODC activity in maternally-deprived rat pups. *Life Sciences, 39*, 2081–2087.

Pavuluri, M. N., O'Connor, M. M., & Sweeney, J. A. (2007). Neurocognitive outcome of lamotrigine in pediatric bipolar disorder. *Presented at 160th Annual Meeting of the American Psychiatric Association, San Diego, CA* NR # 732, 52.

Pazzaglia, P. J., George, M. S., Post, R. M., Rubinow, D. R., & Davis, C. L. (1995). Nimodipine increases CSF somatostatin in affectively ill patients. *Neuropsychopharmacology, 13*, 75–83.

Pazzaglia, P. J., & Post, R. M. (1992). Contingent tolerance and reresponse to carbamazepine: A case study in a patient with trigeminal neuralgia and bipolar disorder. *Journal of Neuropsychiatry and Clinical Neuroscience, 4*, 76–81.

Pazzaglia, P. J., Post, R. M., Ketter, T. A., Callahan, A. M., Marangell, L. B., Frye, M. A., et al. (1998). Nimodipine monotherapy and carbamazepine augmentation in patients with refractory recurrent affective illness. *Journal of Clinical Psychopharmacology, 18*, 404–413.

Pazzaglia, P. J., Post, R. M., Ketter, T. A., George, M. S., & Marangell, L. B. (1993). Preliminary controlled trial of nimodipine in ultra-rapid cycling affective dysregulation. *Psychiatry Research, 49*, 257–272.

Pearson, H. J. (1990). Interaction of fluoxetine with carbamazepine. *Journal of Clinical Psychiatry, 51*, 126.

Pecknold, J. C., & Fleury, D. (1986). Alprazolam-induced manic episode in two patients with panic disorder. *American Journal of Psychiatry, 143*, 652–653.

Peet, M., & Horrobin, D. F. (2002). A dose-ranging study of the effects of ethyl-eicosapentaenoate in patients with ongoing depression despite apparently adequate treatment with standard drugs. *Archives of General Psychiatry, 59*, 913–919.

Peet, M., Murphy, B., Shay, J., & Horrobin, D. (1998). Depletion of omega-3 fatty acid levels in red blood cell membranes of depressive patients. *Biological Psychiatry, 43*, 315–319.

Penfield, W. (1955). The role of the temporal cortex in

certain physical phenomena. *Journal of Mental Science, 101*, 451–465.

Perlis, R. H., Smoller, J. W., Fava, M., Rosenbaum, J. F., Nierenberg, A. A., & Sachs, G. S. (2004). The prevalence and clinical correlates of anger attacks during depressive episodes in bipolar disorder. *Journal of Affective Disorders, 71*, 291–295.

Pert, A. (1998). Neurobiological substrates underlying conditioned effects of cocaine. *Advances in Pharmacology, 42*, 991–995.

Perucca, E. (1997). A pharmacological and clinical review on topiramate, a new antiepileptic drug. *Pharmacology Research, 35*, 241–256.

Peselow, E. D., Fieve, R. R., Difiglia, C., & Sanfilipo, M. P. (1994). Lithium prophylaxis of bipolar illness. The value of combination treatment. *British Journal of Psychiatry, 164*, 208–214.

Pfeiffer, H., Scherer, J., & Albus, M. (2004). [High dose L-thyroxine in therapy refractory depression. Case analysis and catamnesis as quality control]. *Nervenarzt, 75*, 242–248.

Pflug, B., & Tolle, R. (1971). Disturbance of the 24-hour rhythm in endogenous depression and the treatment of endogenous depression by sleep deprivation. *International Pharmacopsychiatry, 6*, 187–196.

Philpot, V. B. (1993). Thyrotropin-releasing hormone in a patient with bipolar disorder. *Journal of Neuropsychiatry, 5*, 349–350.

Pickar, D. (1995). Prospects for pharmacotherapy of schizophrenia. *Lancet, 345*, 557–562.

Pinel, J. P. (1980). Alcohol withdrawal seizures: Implications of kindling. *Pharmacology, Biochemistry, and Behavior, 13*(Suppl. 1), 225–231.

Plotsky, P. M., & Meaney, M. J. (1993), Early, postnatal experience alters hypothalamic corticotropin-releasing factor (CRF) mRNA, median eminence CRF content and stress-induced release in adult rats. *Molecular Brain Research, 18*, 195–200.

Pollack, M. H. (1993). Innovative uses of benzodiazepines in psychiatry. *Canadian Journal of Psychiatry, 38*(Suppl. 4), S122–S126.

Pope, H. G., Jr., McElroy, S. L., Keck, P. E., Jr., & Hudson, J. I. (1991). Valproate in the treatment of acute mania. A placebo-controlled study. *Archives of General Psychiatry, 48*, 62–68.

Post, R. M. (1975). Cocaine psychoses: A continuum model. *American Journal of Psychiatry, 132*, 225–231.

Post, R. M. (1977). Progressive changes in behavior and seizures following chronic cocaine administration: Relationship to kindling and psychosis. In E. H. Ellinwood & M. M. Kilbey (Eds.), *Cocaine and other stimulants* (pp. 353–372). New York: Plenum Press.

Post, R. M. (1987). Mechanisms of action of carbamazepine and related anticonvulsants in affective illness. In H. Meltzer & W. E. Bunney, Jr. (Eds.), *Psycho-pharmacology: A generation of progress* (pp. 567–576). New York, Raven Press.

Post, R. M. (1988). Time course of clinical effects of carbamazepine: Implications for mechanisms of action. *Journal of Clinical Psychiatry, 49*(Suppl.), 35–48.

Post, R. M. (1990). Alternatives to lithium for bipolar affective illness. In A. Tass, S. M. Goldfinger, & C. A. Kaufmann (Eds.), *Review in psychiatry* (Vol. 9, pp. 170–202). Washington, DC: American Psychiatric Assocation Press.

Post, R. M. (1992). Transduction of psychosocial stress into the neurobiology of recurrent affective disorder. *American Journal of Psychiatry, 149*, 999–1010.

Post, R. M. (1996). Impact of psychosocial stress on gene expression: Implications for PTSD and recurrent affective disorder. In T. W. Miller (Ed.), *Theory and assessment of stressful life events* (pp. 37–91). New York: International University Press.

Post, R. M. (1999). Valproate use in psychiatry: A focus on bipolar illness. In W. Loscher (Ed.), *Valproate* (pp. 167–201). Basel, Switzerland: Birkhauser Verlag.

Post, R. M. (2002). Depression in bipolar illness: The stepchild. *Clinical Neuroscience Research, 2*, 122–126.

Post, R. M. (2004a). Differing psychotropic profiles of the anticonvulsants in bipolar and other psychiatric disorders. *Clinical Neuroscience Research, 4*, 9–30.

Post, R. M. (2004b). Practical approaches to polypharmacy in the long-term management of bipolar disorder. *Drug Benefit Trends, 16*, 329–342.

Post, R. M. (2004c). The status of the sensitization/kindling hypothesis of bipolar disorder. *Current Psychosis and Therapeutics Reports, 2*, 135–141.

Post, R. M. (2007). Role of BDNF in bipolar and unipolar disorder: Clinical and theoretical implications. Journal of Psychiatric Research.

Post, R. M. (2007). Kindling and sensitization as models for affective episode recurrence, cyclicity, and tolerance phenomena. *Neuroscience and Biobehavioral Reviews, 31*, 858–873.

Post, R. M., Altshuler, L. L., Frye, M. A., Suppes, T., Rush, A. J., Keck, P. E., Jr., et al. (2001). Rate of switch in bipolar patients prospectively treated with second-generation antidepressants as augmentation to mood stabilizers. *Bipolar Disorders, 3*, 159–265.

Post, R. M., Altshuler, L. L., Frye, M. A., Suppes, T., McElroy, S. L., Keck, P. E., Jr., et al. (2005). Preliminary observations on the effectiveness of levetiracetam in the open adjunctive treatment of refractory bipolar disorder. *Journal of Clinical Psychiatry, 66*, 370–374.

Post, R. M., Altshuler, L. L., Frye, M. A., Suppes, T., McElroy, S., Keck, P. E., Jr., et al. (2006). New findings from the Bipolar Collaborative Network:

clinical implications for therapeutics. *Current Psychiatric Reports, 8,* 489–497.

Post, R. M., Altshuler, L. L., Leverich, G. S., Frye, M. A., Nolen, W. A., Kupka, R. W., et al. (2006). Mood switch in bipolar depression: Comparison of adjunctive venlafaxine, bupropion and sertraline. *British Journal of Psychiatry, 189,* 124–131.

Post, R. M., Berrettini, W. H., Uhde, T. W., & Kellner, C. H. (1984). Selective response to the anticonvulsant carbamazepine in manic-depressive illness: A case study. *Journal of Clinical Psychopharmacology, 4,* 178–185.

Post, R. M., Chalecka-Franaszek, E., & Hough, C. (2002). Mechanisms of action of anticonvulsants and new mood stabilizers. In J. C. Soares & S. Gershon (Eds.), *Handbook of medical psychiatry* (pp. 767–791). New York: Marcel Dekker.

Post, R. M., Chang, K. D., Findling, R. L., Geller, B., Kowatch, R. A., Kutcher, S. P., et al. (2004). Prepubertal bipolar I disorder and bipolar disorder NOS are separable from ADHD. *Journal of Clinical Psychiatry, 65,* 898–902.

Post, R. M., Denicoff, K. D., Frye, M. A., & Leverich, G. S. (1997). Re-evaluating carbamazepine prophylaxis in bipolar disorder. *British Journal of Psychiatry, 170,* 202–204.

Post, R. M., Denicoff, K., Frye, M., Leverich, G. S., Cora-Locatelli, G., & Kimbrell, T. A. (1999). Long-term outcome of anticonvulsants in affective disorders. In J. F. Goldberg & M. Harrow (Eds.), *Bipolar disorders: Clinical course and outcome* (pp. 85–114). Washington, DC: American Psychiatric Press.

Post, R. M., Denicoff, K. D., & Leverich, G. S. (2000). Special issues in trial design and use of placebo in bipolar illness. *Biological Psychiatry, 47,* 727–732.

Post, R. M., Denicoff, K. D., Leverich, G. S., Altshuler, L. L., Frye, M. A., Suppes, T. M., et al. (2002). Presentations of depression in bipolar illness. *Clinical Neuroscience Research, 2,* 142–157.

Post, R. M., Denicoff, K. D., Leverich, G. S., Altshuler, L. L., Frye, M. A., Suppes, T. M., et al. (2003). Morbidity in 258 bipolar outpatients followed for 1 year with daily prospective ratings on the NIMH Life Chart Method. *Journal of Clinical Psychiatry, 64,* 680–690.

Post, R. M., & Frye, M. A. (2005). Carbamazepine. In B. J. Sadock & V. A. Sadock (Eds.), *Kaplan and Sadock's comprehensive textbook of psychiatry* (pp. 2732–2746). New York: Lippincott Williams & Wilkins.

Post, R. M., Frye, M. A., Denicoff, K. D., Kimbrell, T. A., Cora-Locatelli, G., & Leverich, G. S. (1997). Anticonvulsants in the long-term prophylaxis of depression. In A. Honig & H. M. Van Praag (Eds.), *Depression: Neurobiological, psychopathological and therapeutic advances* (pp. 483–498). Sussex, England: John Wiley & Sons.

Post, R. M., Frye, M. A., Denicoff, K. D., Leverich, G. S., Kimbrell, T. A., & Dunn, R. T. (1998). Beyond lithium in the treatment of bipolar illness. *Neuropsychopharmacology, 19,* 206–219.

Post, R. M., Frye, M. A., Leverich, G. S., & Denicoff, K. D. (1998). The role of complex combination therapy in the treatment of refractory bipolar illness. *CNS Spectrums, 3,* 66–86.

Post, R. M., Kennedy, C., Shinohara, M., Squillace, K., Miyaoka, M., Suda, S., et al. (1984). Metabolic and behavioral consequences of lidocaine-kindled seizures. *Brain Research, 324,* 295–303.

Post, R. M., Ketter, T. A., Denicoff, K., Leverich, G. S., & Mikalauskas, K. (1993). Assessment of anticonvulsant drugs in patients with bipolar affective illness. In I. Hindmarch & P. D. Stonier (Eds.), *Human psychopharmacology: Methods and measures* (pp. 211–245). Chichester, England: John Wiley & Sons.

Post, R. M., Ketter, T. A., Joffe, R. T., & Kramlinger, K. L. (1991). Lack of beneficial effects of l-baclofen in affective disorder. *International Clinical Psychopharmacology, 6,* 197–207.

Post, R. M., Ketter, T. A., Uhde, T., & Ballenger, J. C. (2007). Thirty years of clinical experience with carbamazepine in the treatment of bipolar illness: Principles and practice. *CNS Drugs, 21*(1), 47–71.

Post, R. M., Kopanda, R. T., & Lee, A. (1975). Progressive behavioral changes during chronic lidocaine administration: Relationship to kindling. *Life Sciences, 17,* 943–950.

Post, R. M., & Leverich, G. S. (2006). The role of psychosocial stress in the onset and progression of bipolar disorder and its comorbidities: The need for earlier and alternative modes of therapeutic intervention. *Developmental Psychopathology, 18,* 1181–1211.

Post, R. M., Leverich, G. S., Altshuler, L., & Mikalauskas, K. (1992). Lithium-discontinuation-induced refractoriness: Preliminary observations. *American Journal of Psychiatry, 149,* 1727–1729.

Post, R. M., Leverich, G. S., Nolen, W. A., Kupka, R. W., Altshuler, L. L., Frye, M. A., et al. (2003). A reevaluation of the role of antidepressants in the treatment of bipolar depression: Data from the Stanley Bipolar Treatment Network. *Bipolar Disorders, 5,* 396–406.

Post, R. M., Leverich, G. S., Pazzaglia, P. J., Mikalauskas, K., & Denicoff, K. (1993). Lithium tolerance and discontinuation as pathways to refractoriness. In N. J. Birch & C. Hughes (Eds.), *Lithium in medicine and biology* (pp. 71–84). Carnforth: Marius Press.

Post, R. M., Leverich, G. S., Rosoff, A. S., & Altshuler, L. L. (1990). Carbamazepine prophylaxis in refractory affective disorders: A focus on long-term follow-up. *Journal of Clinical Psychopharmacology, 10,* 318–327.

Post, R. M., L'Herrou, T., Luckenbaugh, D. A., Frye, M. A., Leverich, G. S., & Mikalauskas, K. (1998). Statistical approaches to trial durations in episodic affective illness. *Psychiatry Research, 78*, 71–87.

Post, R. M., & Luckenbaugh, D. A. (2003). Unique design issues in clinical trials of patients with bipolar affective disorder. *Journal of Psychiatric Research, 37*, 61–73.

Post, R. M., Luckenbaugh, D. A., Leverich, G. S., Altshuler, L. L., Frye, M. A., Suppes, T., et al. (2007). Differential rate of childhood-onset bipolar illness in the U.S. versus Europe. *British Journal of Psychiatry*, in press.

Post, R. M., Pazzaglia, P. J., Ketter, T. A., Denicoff, K., Weiss, S. R. B., Hough, C., et al. (2000). Carbamazepine and nimodipine in refractory affective illness: Efficacy and mechanisms. In U. Halbreich & S. Montgomery (Eds.), *Pharmacotherapy for mood, anxiety, and cognitive disorders* (pp. 77–110). Washington, DC: American Psychiatric Press.

Post, R. M., & Post, S. L. W. (2004). Molecular and cellular developmental vulnerabilities to the onset of affective disorders in children and adolescents: Some implications for therapeutics. In: H. Steiner, eds. *Handbook of Mental Health Interventions in Children and Adolescents*. San Francisco: Jossey-Bass, 140–192.

Post, R. M., Putnam, F., Contel, N. R., & Goldman, B. (1984). Electroconvulsive seizures inhibit amygdala kindling: Implications for mechanisms of action in affective illness. *Epilepsia, 25*, 234–239.

Post, R. M., Roy-Byrne, P. P., & Uhde, T. W. (1988). Graphic representation of the life course of illness in patients with affective disorder. *American Journal of Psychiatry, 145*, 844–848.

Post, R. M., Rubinow, D. R., & Ballenger, J. C. (1984). Conditioning, sensitization, and kindling: Implications for the course of affective illness. In R. M. Post & J. C. Ballenger (Eds.), *Neurobiology of mood disorders* (pp. 432–466). Baltimore: Williams and Wilkins.

Post, R. M., Rubinow, D. R., Roy-Byrne, P. P., Linnoila, M., Rosoff, A., & Cowdry, R. W. (1989). Dysphoric mania: Clinical and biological correlates. *Archives of General Psychiatry, 46*, 353–358.

Post, R. M., Rubinow, D. R., Uhde, T. W., Ballenger, J. C., & Linnoila, M. (1986). Dopaminergic effects of carbamazepine. Relationship to clinical response in affective illness. *Archives of General Psychiatry, 43*, 392–396.

Post, R. M., & Speer, A. M. (2007). Repetitive transcranial magnetic stimulation and related somatic therapies: Prospects for the future. In: George, M. S., Belmaker, R. H., ed. *Transcranial magnetic stimulation in clinical psychiatry*. Washington, DC: American Psychiatric Publishing, Inc., 225–255.

Post, R. M., & Speer, A. M. (2002). A brief history of anticonvulsant use in affective disorders. In M. R. Trimble & B. Schmitz (Eds.), *Seizures, affective disorders and anticonvulsant drugs*, p. 53–81. Surrey, UK: Clarius Press.

Post, R. M., Speer, A. M., Hough, C. J., & Xing, G. (2003). Neurobiology of bipolar illness: implications for future study and therapeutics. *Annals of Clinical Psychiatry, 15*, 85–94.

Post, R. M., Speer, A. M., & Leverich, G. S. (2003). Bipolar illness: Which critical treatment issues need studying? *Clinical Approaches in Bipolar Disorders, 2*, 24–30.

Post, R. M., Speer, A. M., & Leverich, G. S. (2006). Complex combination therapy: The evolution toward rational polypharmacy in lithium-resistant bipolar illness. In H. S. Akiskal & M. Tohen (Eds.), *Bipolar psychopharmacotherapy: Caring for the patient* (pp. 135–167). London: Wiley & Sons.

Post, R. M., Speer, A. M., Obrocea, G. V., & Leverich, G. S. (2002). Acute and prophylactic effects of anticonvulsants in bipolar depression. *Clinical Neuroscience Research, 2*, 228–251.

Post, R. M., Uhde, T. W., Ballenger, J. C., Chatterji, D. C., Greene, R. F., & Bunney, W. E., Jr. (1983). Carbamazepine and its -10,11-epoxide metabolite in plasma and CSF. Relationship to antidepressant response. *Archives of General Psychiatry, 40*, 673–676.

Post, R. M., Uhde, T. W., Roy-Byrne, P. P., & Joffe, R. T. (1986). Antidepressant effects of carbamazepine. *American Journal of Psychiatry, 143*, 29–34.

Post, R. M., Uhde, T. W., Roy-Byrne, P. P., & Joffe, R. T. (1987). Correlates of antimanic response to carbamazepine. *Psychiatry Research, 21*, 71–83.

Post, R. M., & Weiss, S. R. (1992). Ziskind-Somerfeld Research Award 1992. Endogenous biochemical abnormalities in affective illness: Therapeutic versus pathogenic. *Biological Psychiatry, 32*, 469–484.

Post, R. M., & Weiss, S. R. B. (1996). A speculative model of affective illness cyclicity based on patterns of drug tolerance observed in amygdala-kindled seizures. *Molecular Neurobiology, 13*, 33–60.

Post, R. M., & Weiss, S. R. B. (1997). Kindling and stress sensitization. In R. T. Joffe & L. T. Young (Eds.), *Bipolar disorder: Biological models and their clinical application* (pp. 93–126). New York: Marcel Dekker.

Post, R. M., & Weiss, S. R. B. (2004). Convergences in course of illness and treatments of the epilepsies and recurrent affective disorders. *Clinical Electroencephalography, 35*, 14–24.

Post, R. M., Weiss, S. R., & Chuang, D. M. (1992). Mechanisms of action of anticonvulsants in affective disorders: Comparisons with lithium. *Journal of Clinical Psychopharmacology, 12*(Suppl.), 23S–35S.

Post, R. M., Weiss, S. R. B., Clark, M., Chuang, D. M.,

Hough, C., & Li, H. (2000). Lithium, carbamazepine, and valproate in affective illness: Biochemical and neurobiological mechanisms. In H. Manji, C. L. Bowden, & R. H. Belmaker (Eds.), *Bipolar medications: Mechanisms of action* (pp. 219–248). Washington, DC: American Psychiatric Press.

Post, R. M., Weiss, R. B., & Leverich, G. S. (1994). Recurrent affective disorder: Roots in developmental neurobiology and illness progression based on changes in gene expression. *Development and Psychopathology, 6,* 781–813.

Post, R. M., Weiss, S. R. B., Leverich, G. S., George, M. S., Frye, M. A., & Ketter, T. A. (1996). Developmental psychobiology in cyclic affective illness: Implications for early therapeutic intervention. *Development and Psychopathology, 8,* 273–305.

Post, R. M., Weiss, S. R.B., & Pert, A. (1992). Sensitization and kindling effects of chronic cocaine administration. In J. M. Lakoski, M. P. Galloway, & F. J. White (Eds.), *Cocaine: Pharmacology, physiology, and clinical strategies* (pp. 115–161). Caldwell, NJ: Telford Press.

Post, R. M., Weiss, S. R. B., Pert, A., & Uhde, T. W. (1987). Chronic cocaine administration: Sensitization and kindling effects. In A. Raskin & S. Fisher (Eds.), *Cocaine: Clinical and biobehavioral aspects* (pp. 109–173). New York: Oxford University Press.

Poyurovsky, M., Isaacs, I., Fuchs, C., Schneidman, M., Faragian, S., Weizman, R., et al. (2003). Attenuation of olanzapine-induced weight gain with reboxetine in patients with schizophrenia: A double-blind, placebo-controlled study. *American Journal of Psychiatry, 160,* 297–302.

Practice guideline for the treatment of patients with bipolar disorder (revision). (2002). *American Journal of Psychiatry, 159,* 1–50.

Prange, A. J., Jr., Lara, P. P., Wilson, I. C., Alltop, L. B., & Breese, G. R. (1972). Effects of thyrotropin-releasing hormone in depression. *Lancet, 2,* 999–1002.

Preskorn, S. D., Baker, B., Omo, K., Kolluri, S., Menniti, F., & Landen, J. (2007). A placebo-controlled trial of the NR2B specific NMDA antagonist CP-101, 606 plus paroxetine for treatment resistant depression. *Presented at 160th Annual Meeting of the American Psychiatric Association, San Diego, CA* NR #362, 25.

Pridmore, S., Bruno, R., Turnier-Shea, Y., Reid, P., & Rybak, M. (2000). Comparison of unlimited numbers of rapid transcranial magnetic stimulation (rTMS) and ECT treatment sessions in major depressive episode. *International Journal of Neuropsychopharmacology, 3,* 129–134.

Prien, R. F., Caffey, E. M., & Klett, C. J. (1972). Comparison of lithium carbonate and chlorpromazine in the treatment of mania. *Archives of General Psychiatry, 26,* 146–153.

Prien, R. F., & Gelenberg, A. J. (1989). Alternatives to lithium for preventive treatment of bipolar disorder. *American Journal of Psychiatry, 146,* 840–848.

Prien, R. F., Himmelhoch, J. M., & Kupfer, D. J. (1988). Treatment of mixed mania. *Journal of Affective Disorders, 15,* 9–15.

Prien, R. F., Klett, C. J., & Caffey, E. M. J. (1973). Lithium carbonate and imipramine in prevention of affective episodes: A comparison in recurrent affective illness. *Archives of General Psychiatry, 29,* 420–425.

Prudic, J., Haskett, R. F., Mulsant, B., Malone, K. M., Pettinati, H. M., Stephens, S., et al. (1996). Resistance to antidepressant medications and short-term clinical response to ECT. *American Journal of Psychiatry, 153,* 985–992.

Prudic, J., Olfson, M., Marcus, S. C., Fuller, R. B., & Sackeim, H. A. (2004). Effectiveness of electroconvulsive therapy in community settings. *Biological Psychiatry, 55,* 301–312.

Rajkowska, G. (2000). Postmortem studies in mood disorders indicate altered numbers of neurons and glial cells. *Biological Psychiatry, 48,* 766–777.

Rami-Gonzalez, L., Bernardo, M., Boget, T., Salamero, M., Gil-Verona, J. A., & Junque, C. (2001). Subtypes of memory dysfunction associated with ECT: Characteristics and neurobiological bases. *Journal of ECT, 17,* 129–135.

Ranga, K., Krishnan, R., Swartz, M. S., Larson, M. J., & Santoliquido, G. (1984). Funeral mania in recurrent bipolar affective disorders: Reports of three cases. *Journal of Clinical Psychiatry, 45,* 310–311.

Rasgon, N. L., Altshuler, L. L., Fairbanks, L., Elman, S., Bitran, J., Labarca, R., et al. (2005). Reproductive function and risk for PCOS in women treated for bipolar disorder. *Bipolar Disorders, 7,* 246–259.

Raskin, J., Goldstein, D. J., Mallinckrodt, C. H., & Ferguson, M. B. (2003). Duloxetine in the long-term treatment of major depressive disorder. *Journal of Clinical Psychiatry, 64,* 1237–1244.

Raskind, M. A., Peskind, E. R., Hoff, D. J., Hart, K. L., Holmes, H. A., Warren, D., et al. (2007). A parallel group placebo controlled study of prazosin for trauma nightmares and sleep disturbance in combat veterans with post-traumatic stress disorder. *Biological Psychiatry, 61,* 928–934.

Raskind, M. A., Peskind, E. R., Kanter, E. D., Petrie, E. C., Radant, A., Thompson, C. E., et al. (2003). Reduction of nightmares and other PTSD symptoms in combat veterans by prazosin: A placebo-controlled study. *American Journal of Psychiatry, 160,* 371–373.

Rattya, J., Turkka, J., Pakarinen, A. J., Knip, M., Kotila, M. A., Lukkarinen, O., et al. (2001). Reproductive effects of valproate, carbamazepine, and oxcarbazepine in men with epilepsy. *Neurology, 56,* 31–36.

Rauch, S. L., Van der Kolk, B. A., Fisler, R. E., Alpert, N. M., Orr, S. P., Savage, C. R., et al. (1996). A symptom provocation study of posttraumatic stress disorder using positron emission tomography and script-driven imagery. *Archives of General Psychiatry, 53,* 380–387.

Regenold, W., Thapar, R. K., Marano, C., Gavirneni, S., & Kondapavuluru, P. V. (2002). Increased prevalence of type 2 diabetes mellitus among psychiatric inpatients with bipolar I affective and schizoaffective disorder independent of psychotropic drug use. *Journal of Affective Disorders, 70,* 19–26.

Regier, D. A., Farmer, M. E., Rae, D. S., Locke, B. Z., Keith, S. J., Judd, L. L., et al. (1990). Comorbidity of mental disorders with alcohol and other drug abuse: Results from the Epidemiologic Catchment Area (ECA) study. *Journal of the American Medical Association, 264,* 2511–2518.

Rehm, O. (1919). *Das Manisch-Melancholische Irresein: Eine Monographische Studie.* Berlin: Verlag von Julius Springer.

Reiter, S. R., Pollack, M. H., Rosenbaum, J. F., & Cohen, L. S. (1990). Clonazepam for the treatment of social phobia. *Journal of Clinical Psychiatry, 51,* 470–472.

Richelson, E. (1996). Preclinical phgarmacology of neuroleptics: Focus on new generation compounds. *Journal of Clinical Psychiatry, 57*(Suppl. 11), 4–11.

Richmond, R., & Zwar, N. (2003). Review of bupropion for smoking cessation. *Drug and Alcohol Review, 22,* 203–220.

Rickarby, G. A. (1977). Four cases of mania associated with bereavement. *Journal of Nervous and Mental Disease, 165,* 255–262.

Riemann, D., Wiegand, M., Lauer, C. J., & Berger, M. (1994). Naps after total sleep deprivation in depressed patients: Are they depressiogenic? *Psychiatry Research, 49,* 109–120.

Rigo, J. M., Hans, G., Nguyen, L., Rocher, V., Belachew, S., Malgrange, B., et al. (2002). The anti-epileptic drug levetiracetam reverses the inhibition by negative allosteric modulators of neuronal GABA- and glycine-gated currents. *British Journal of Pharmacology, 136,* 659–672.

Rouillon, F., Lejoyeux, M., & Filteau, M. J. (1992). Unwanted effects of long-term treatment. In S. A. Montgomery & F. Rouillon (Eds.), *Long-term treatment of depression* (pp. 81–111). Chichester: John Wiley & Sons.

Roy-Byrne, P. P., Joffe, R. T., Uhde, T. W., & Post, R. M. (1984). Carbamazepine and thyroid function in affectively ill patients: Clinical and theoretical implications. *Archives of General Psychiatry, 41,* 1150–1153.

Roy-Byrne, P. P., Uhde, T. W., & Post, R. M. (1984). Carbamazepine for aggression, schizophrenia, and nonaffective syndromes. *International Drug Therapy Newsletter, 19,* 9–12.

Roy-Byrne, P. P., Uhde, T. W., & Post, R. M. (1986). Effects of one night's sleep deprivation on mood and behavior in panic disorder: Patients with panic disorder compared with depressed patients and normal controls. *Archives of General Psychiatry, 43,* 895–899.

Rubinow, D. R., Post, R. M., Gold, P. W., Ballenger, J. C., & Reichlin, S. (1985). Effects of carbamazepine on cerebrospinal fluid somatostatin. *Psychopharmacology (Berlin), 85,* 210–213.

Rudas, S., Schmitz, M., Pichler, P., & Baumgartner, A. (1999). Treatment of refractory chronic depression and dysthymia with high-dose thyroxine. *Biological Psychiatry, 45,* 229–233.

Rudolph, R. L. (2002). Achieving remission from depression with venlafaxine and venlafaxine extended release: A literature review of comparative studies with selective serotonin reuptake inhibitors. *Acta Psychiatr Scand,* (Suppl.), 24–30.

Rush, A. J., George, M., Sackeim, H., Marangell, L., Husain, M., Giller, C., et al. (2000). Vagus nerve stimulation (VNS) for treatment-resistant depressions: A multicenter study. *Biological Psychiatry, 47,* 276–286.

Rush, A. J., Marangell, L. B., Sackeim, H. A., George, M. S., Brannan, S. K., Davis, S. M., et al. (2005). Vagus nerve stimulation for treatment-resistant depression: A randomized, controlled acute phase trial. *Biological Psychiatry, 58,* 347–354.

Rush, A. J., Sackeim, H. A., Marangell, L. B., George, M. S., Brannan, S. K., Davis, S. M., et al. (2005). Effects of 12 months of vagus nerve stimulation in treatment-resistant depression: A naturalistic study. *Biological Psychiatry, 58,* 355–363.

Ryan, M. C., Collins, P., & Thakore, J. H. (2003). Impaired fasting glucose tolerance in first-episode, drug-naive patients with schizophrenia. *American Journal of Psychiatry, 160,* 284–289.

Rybakowski, J. K., Borkowska, A., Czerski, P. M., Skibinska, M., & Hauser, J. (2003). Polymorphism of the brain-derived neurotrophic factor gene and performance on a cognitive prefrontal test in bipolar patients. *Bipolar Disorders, 5,* 468–472.

Sachar, E. J., Hellman, L., Roffwarg, H. P., Halpern, F. S., Fukushima, D. K., & Gallagher, T. F. (1973). Disrupted 24-hour patterns of cortisol secretion in psychotic depression. *Archives of General Psychiatry, 28,* 19–24.

Sachs, G. S. (1990). Use of clonazepam for bipolar affective disorder. *Journal of Clinical Psychiatry, 51*(Suppl.), 31–34.

Sachs, G. S., Lafer, B., Stoll, A. L., Banov, M., Thibault, A. B., Tohen, M., et al. (1994). A double-blind trial of bupropion versus desipramine for bipolar depression. *Journal of Clinical Psychiatry, 55,* 391–393.

Sachs, G. S., Nierenberg, A. A., Calabrese, J. R., Marangell, L. B., Wisniewski, S. R., Gyulai, L., et al. (2007). Effectiveness of adjunctive antidepressant treatment for bipolar depression. *New England Journal of Medicine, 356,* 1711–1722.

Sachs, G. S., Rosenbaum, J. F., & Jones, L. (1990). Adjunctive clonazepam for maintenance treatment of bipolar affective disorder. *Journal of Clinical Psychopharmacology, 10,* 42–47.

Sachs, G., Sanchez, R., Marcus, R., Stock, E., McQuade, R., Carson, W., et al. (2006). Aripiprazole in the treatment of acute manic or mixed episodes in patients with bipolar I disorder: A 3-week placebo-controlled study. *Journal of Psychopharmacology, 20,* 536–546.

Sachs, G. S., Weilburg, J. B., & Rosenbaum, J. F. (1990). Clonazepam vs neuroleptics as adjuncts to lithium maintenance. *Psychopharmacology Bulletin, 26,* 137–143.

Sackeim, H. A., Devanand, D. P., Lisanby, S. H., Nobler, M. S., Prudic, J., Heyer, E. J., et al. (2001). Treatment of the modal patient: does one size fit nearly all? *Journal of ECT, 17,* 219–222.

Sackeim, H. A., Decina, P., Portnoy, S., Neeley, P., & Malitz, S. (1987). Studies of dosage, seizure threshold, and seizure duration in ECT. *Biological Psychiatry, 22,* 249–268.

Sackeim, H. A., Haskett, R. F., Mulsant, B. H., Thase, M. E., Mann, J. J., Pettinati, H. M., et al. (2001). Continuation pharmacotherapy in the prevention of relapse following electroconvulsive therapy: A randomized controlled trial. *Journal of the American Medical Association, 285,* 1299–1307.

Sackeim, H. A., Keilp, J. G., Rush, A. J., George, M. S., Marangell, L. B., Dormer, J. S., et al. (2001). The effects of vagus nerve stimulation on cognitive performance in patients with treatment-resistant depression. *Neuropsychiatry, Neuropsychology, and Behavioral Neurology, 14,* 53–62.

Sackeim, H. A., Prudic, J., Devanand, D. P., Decina, P., Kerr, B., & Malitz, S. (1990). The impact of medication resistance and continuation pharmacotherapy on relapse following response to electroconvulsive therapy in major depression. *Journal of Clinical Psychopharmacology, 10,* 96–104.

Sackeim, H. A., Prudic, J., Devanand, D. P., Kiersky, J. E., Fitzsimons, L., Moody, B. J., et al. (1993). Effects of stimulus intensity and electrode placement on the efficacy and cognitive effects of electroconvulsive therapy. *New England Journal of Medicine, 328,* 839–846.

Sackeim, H. A., Prudic, J., Devanand, D. P., Nobler, M. S., Lisanby, S. H., Peyser, S., et al. (2000). A prospective, randomized, double-blind comparison of bilateral and right unilateral electroconvulsive

therapy at different stimulus intensities. *Archives of General Psychiatry, 57,* 425–434.

Sackeim, H. A., Prudic, J., Fuller, R., Keilp, J., Lavori, P. W., & Olfson, M. (2007). The cognitive effects of electroconvulsive therapy in community settings. *Neuropsychopharmacology, 32,* 244–254.

Salloum, I. M., Cornelius, J. R., Daley, D. C., Kirisci, L., Himmelhoch, J. M., & Thase, M. E. (2005). Efficacy of valproate maintenance in patients with bipolar disorder and alcoholism: A double-blind placebo-controlled study. *Archives of General Psychiatry, 62,* 37–45.

Samia, R. L., Joca, L. L., Skalisz, V. B., Maria Aparecida, B. F., & Vital, R. A. (2000). The antidepressive-like effect of oxcarbazepine: Possible role of dopaminergic neurotransmission. *European Neuropsychopharmacology, 10,* 223–228.

Santarelli, L., Saxe, M., Gross, C., Surget, A., Battaglia, F., Dulawa, S., et al. (2003). Requirement of hippocampal neurogenesis for the behavioral effects of antidepressants. *Science, 301,* 805–809.

Saravanan, P., Simmons, D. J., Greenwood, R., Peters, T. J., & Dayan, C. M. (2005). Partial substitution of thyroxine (T4) with triiodothyronine in patients on T4 replacement therapy: Results of a large community-based randomized controlled trial. *Journal of Clinical Endocrinology and Metabolism, 90,* 805–812.

Saravay, S. M., Marie, J., Steinberg, M. D., & Rabiner, C. J. (1987). "Doom anxiety" and delirium in lidocaine toxicity. *American Journal of Psychiatry, 144,* 159–163.

Sayar, K., Aksu, G., Ak, I., & Tosun, M. (2003). Venlafaxine treatment of fibromyalgia. *Annals of Pharmacotherapy, 37,* 1561–1565.

Schachter, S. C. (2000). The next wave of anticonvulsants: Focus on levetiracetam, oxcarbazepine and zonisamide. *CNS Drugs, 14,* 229–249.

Schaff, M. R., Fawcett, J., & Zajecka, J. M. (1993). Divalproex sodium in the treatment of refractory affective disorders. *Journal of Clinical Psychiatry, 54,* 380–384.

Schaffer, C. B., Mungas, D., & Rockwell, E. (1985). Successful treatment of psychotic depression with carbamazepine. *Journal of Clinical Psychopharmacology, 5,* 233–235.

Schatzberg, A. F., & Nemeroff, C. B. (Eds.). (2004). *Textbook of psychopharmacology.* Washington DC: American Psychiatric Association Press.

Schatzberg, A. F., & Zaninelli, R. (2007). Agomelatine, a novel antidepressant, is effective in MDD across gender and severity of depression. *Presented at 160th Annual Meeting of the American Psychiatric Association, San Diego, CA* NR #382, 27.

Schlanger, S., Shinitzky, M., & Yam, D. (2002). Diet enriched with omega-3 fatty acids alleviates convulsion symptoms in epilepsy patients. *Epilepsia, 43,* 103–104.

Schmahmann, J. D., & Sherman, J. C. (1998). The cerebellar cognitive affective syndrome. *Brain, 121,* 561–579.

Schmidt, P. J., Nieman, L. K., Danaceau, M. A., Adams, L. F., & Rubinow, D. R. (1998). Differential behavioral effects of gonadal steroids in women with and in those without premenstrual syndrome. *New England Journal of Medicine, 338,* 209–216.

Schou, M. (1973). *Prophylactic lithium maintenance treatment in recurrent endogenous affective disorders: Its role in psychiatric research and treatment* (S. Gershon & B. Shopsin, Eds.). New York: Plenum.

Schou, M. (2001). Lithium treatment at 52. *Journal of Affective Disorders, 67,* 21–32.

Schulze-Rauschenbach, S. C., Harms, U., Schlaepfer, T. E., Maier, W., Falkai, P., & Wagner, M. (2005). Distinctive neurocognitive effects of repetitive transcranial magnetic stimulation and electroconvulsive therapy in major depression. *British Journal of Psychiatry, 186,* 410–416.

Schweizer, E., Pohl, R., Balon, R., Fox, I., Rickels, K., & Yeragani, V. K. (1990). Lorazepam vs alprazolam in the treatment of panic disorder. *Pharmacopsychiatry, 23,* 90–93.

Schweizer, E., Rickels, K., Case, W. G., & Greenblatt, D. J. (1991). Carbamazepine treatment in patients discontinuing long-term benzodiazepine therapy. Effects on withdrawal severity and outcome. *Archives of General Psychiatry, 48,* 448–452.

Sedler, M. J. (1983). Falret's discovery: The origins of the concept of bipolar affective illness. *American Journal of Psychiatry, 140,* 1127–1133.

Seligman, M. E., & Beagley, G. (1975). Learned helplessness in the rat. *Journal of Comparative and Physiological Psychology, 88,* 534–541.

Seligman, M. E., & Maier, S. F. (1967). Failure to escape traumatic shock. *Journal of Experimental Psychology, 74,* 1–9.

Semple, C. A., Morris, S. W., Porteous, D. J., & Evans, K. L. (2000). In silico identification of transcripts and SNPs from a region of 4p linked with bipolar affective disorder. *Bioinformatics, 16,* 735–738.

Semple, W. E., Goyer, P., McCormick, R., Morris, E., Compton, B., Muswick, G., et al. (1993). Preliminary report: Brain blood flow using PET in patients with posttraumatic stress disorder and substance-abuse histories. *Biological Psychiatry, 34,* 115–118.

Sernyak, M. J., Leslie, D. L., Alarcon, R. D., Losonczy, M. F., & Rosenheck, R. (2002). Association of diabetes mellitus with use of atypical neuroleptics in the treatment of schizophrenia. *American Journal of Psychiatry, 159,* 561–566.

Sernyak, M. J., & Woods, S. W. (1993). Chronic neuroleptic use in manic-depressive illness. *Psychopharmacology Bulletin, 29,* 375–381.

Sharma, V., Persad, E., Mazmanian, D., & Karunaratne, K. (1993). Treatment of rapid cycling bipolar disorder with combination therapy of valproate and lithium. *Canadian Journal of Psychiatry, 38,* 137–139.

Sheitman, B. B., & Lieberman, J. A. (1998). The natural history and pathophysiology of treatment resistant schizophrenia. *Journal of Psychiatric Research, 32,* 143–150.

Sheline, Y. I., Gado, M. H., & Kraemer, H. C. (2003). Untreated depression and hippocampal volume loss. *American Journal of Psychiatry, 160,* 1516–1518.

Sheline, Y. I., Sanghavi, M., Mintun, M. A., & Gado, M. H. (1999). Depression duration but not age predicts hippocampal volume loss in medically healthy women with recurrent major depression. *Journal of Neuroscience, 19,* 5034–5043.

Shelton, R. C., Tollefson, G. D., Tohen, M., Stahl, S., Gannon, K. S., Jacobs, T. G., et al. (2001). A novel augmentation strategy for treating resistant major depression. *American Journal of sychiatry, 158,* 131–134.

Shin, L. M., Kosslyn, S. M., McNally, R. J., Alpert, N. M., Thompson, W. L., Rauch, S. L., et al. (1997). Visual imagery and perception in posttraumatic stress disorder: A positron emission tomographic investigation. *Archives of General Psychiatry, 54,* 233–241.

Sienaert, P., Vansteelandt, K., Demyttenaere, K., & Peuskens, J. (2007). Comparison of bifrontal and unilateral ultra-brief pulse electroconvulsive therapy for depression. *Presented at 160th Annual Meeting of the American Psychiatric Association, San Diego, CA* NR#821, 58.

Silberman, E. K., Post, R. M., Nurnberger, J., Theodore, W., & Boulenger, J. P. (1985). Transient sensory, cognitive and affective phenomena in affective illness: A comparison with complex partial epilepsy. *British Journal of Psychiatry, 146,* 81–89.

Simon, J. S., & Nemeroff, C. B. (2005). Aripiprazole augmentation of antidepressants for the treatment of partially responding and nonresponding patients with major depressive disorder. *Journal of Clinical Psychiatry, 66*(10): 1216–1220.

Simpson, G. M., & Lindenmayer, J. P. (1997). Extrapyramidal symptoms in patients treated with risperidone. *Journal of Clinical Psychopharmacology, 17,* 194–201.

Smith, M. A., Kim, S. Y., van Oers, H. J., & Levine, S. (1997). Maternal deprivation and stress induce immediate early genes in the infant rat brain. *Endocrinology, 138,* 4622–4628.

Smith, M. A., Makino, S., Altemus, M., Michelson, D., Hong, S. K., Kvetnansky, R., et al. (1995). Stress and antidepressants differentially regulate neurotrophin 3 mRNA expression in the locus coeruleus. *Proceedings of the National Academy of Sciences, USA, 92,* 8788–8792.

Smith, M. A., Makino, S., Kvetnansky, R., & Post, R. M. (1995a). Effects of stress on neurotrophic factor expression in the rat brain. *Annals of the New York Academy of Science, 771,* 234–239.

Smith, M. A., Makino, S., Kvetnansky, R., & Post, R. M. (1995b). Stress and glucocorticoids affect the expression of brain-derived neurotrophic factor and neurotrophin-3 mRNAs in the hippocampus. *Journal of Neuroscience, 15,* 1768–1777.

Sonne, S. C., & Brady, K. T. (1999). Substance abuse and bipolar comorbidity. *Psychiatric Clinics of North America, 22,* 609–627.

Sorg, B. A., & Kalivas, P. W. (1991). Effects of cocaine and footshock stress on extracellular dopamine levels in the ventral striatum. *Brain Research, 559,* 29–36.

Soria, C. A., & Remedi, C. (2002). Levetiracetam as mood stabilizer in the treatment of pharmacogenic hypomania in bipolar disorder II in elderly patients. *International Journal of Neuropsychopharmacology, 5,* S57.

Sovner, R. (1988). A clinically significant interaction between carbamazepine and valproic acid [letter]. *Journal of Clinical Psychopharmacology, 8,* 448–449.

Speer, A. M., Benson, B. E., Kimbrell, T. A., Wassermann, E. M., Willis, M. W., Herscovitch, P., et al. (in press). Opposite effects of high and low frequency rTMS on mood in depressed patients: Relationship to baseline cerebral activity on PET. *Journal of Affective Disorders*

Speer, A. M., Kimbrell, T. A., Wassermann, E. M., Repella, D., Willis, M. W., Herscovitch, P., et al. (2000). Opposite effects of high and low frequency rTMS on regional brain activity in depressed patients. *Biological Psychiatry, 48,* 1133–1141.

Speer, A. M., Wassermann, E. M., Benson, B. E., Herscovitch, P., & Post, R. M. (2006). *Antidepressant efficacy of high and low frequency rTMS at 110% of motor threshold vs sham stimulation over left prefrontal cortex.* Manuscript submitted for publication.

Spoov, J., & Lahdelma, L. (1998). Should thyroid augmentation precede lithium augmentation—a pilot study. *Journal of Affective Disorders, 49,* 235–239.

Sporn, J., Smith, M., Jean-Mary, J., Greenberg, B., Cora-Locatelli, G., & Murphy, D. (2001). A double-blind, placebo-controlled trial of gabapentin (GBP) augmentation of fluoxetine for treatment of obsessive-compulsive disorder (OCD) [Abstract]. *NCDEU Abstracts.*

Squillace, K., Post, R. M., Savard, R., & Erwin-Gorman, M. (1984). Life charting of the longitudinal course of recurrent affective illness. In R. M. Post &

J. C. Ballenger (Eds.), *Neurobiology of mood disorders.* Baltimore: Williams & Wilkins.

Stahl, S. M., Entsuah, R., & Rudolph, R. L. (2002). Comparative efficacy between venlafaxine and SSRIs: A pooled analysis of patients with depression. *Biological Psychiatry, 52,* 1166–1174.

Stancer, H. C., & Persad, E. (1982). Treatment of intractable rapid-cycling manic-depressive disorder with levothyroxine. *Archives of General Psychiatry, 39,* 311–312.

Stanton, T. L., Winokur, A., & Beckman, L. (1980). Reversal of natural CNS depression by TRH action in the hippocampus. *Brain Research, 181,* 470–475.

Stoddard, F. J., Post, R. M., & Bunney, W. E., Jr. (1977). Slow and rapid psychobiological alterations in a manic-depressive patient: Clinical phenomenology. *British Journal of Psychiatry, 130,* 72–78.

Stoll, A. L., Mayer, P. V., Kolbrener, M., Goldstein, E., Suplit, B., Lucier, J., et al. (1994). Antidepressant-associated mania: A controlled comparison with spontaneous mania. *American Journal of Psychiatry, 151,* 1642–1645.

Stoll, A. L., Severus, W. E., Freeman, M. P., Rueter, S., Zboyan, H. A., Diamond, E., et al. (1999). Omega 3 fatty acids in bipolar disorder: A preliminary double-blind, placebo-controlled trial. *Archives of General Psychiatry, 56,* 407–412.

Strafella, A. P., Paus, T., Barrett, J., & Dagher, A. (2001). Repetitive transcranial magnetic stimulation of the human prefrontal cortex induces dopamine release in the caudate nucleus. *Journal of Neuroscience, 21,* RC157.

Strandjord, R. E., Aanderud, S., Myking, O. L., & Johannessen, S. I. (1981). Influence of carbamazepine on serum thyroxine and triiodothyronine in patients with epilepsy. *Acta Neurologica Scandinavica, 63,* 111–121.

Stuppaeck, C., Barnas, C., Miller, C., Schwitzer, J., & Fleischhacker, W. W. (1990). Carbamazepine in the prophylaxis of mood disorders. *Journal of Clinical Psychopharmacology, 10,* 39–42.

Stuppaeck, C. H., Pycha, R., Miller, C., Whitworth, A. B., Oberbauer, H., & Fleischhacker, W. W. (1992). Carbamazepine versus oxazepam in the treatment of alcohol withdrawal: A double-blind study. *Alcohol and Alcoholism, 27,* 153–158.

Suh, J. J., Pettinati, H. M., Kampman, K. M., & O'Brien, C. P. (2006). The status of disulfiram: A half of a century later. *Journal of Clinical Psychopharmacology, 26,* 290–302.

Suppes, T. (2002). Review of the use of topiramate for treatment of bipolar disorders. *Journal of Clinical Psychopharmacology, 22,* 599–609.

Suppes, T., Baldessarini, R. J., Faedda, G. L., & Tohen, M. (1991). Risk of recurrence following discontinuation of lithium treatment of bipolar disorder. *Archives of General Psychiatry, 48*, 1082–1088.

Suppes, T., Erkan, O. M., & Carmody, T. (2004). Response to clozapine of rapid cycling versus noncycling patients with a history of mania. *Bipolar Disorders, 6*, 329–332.

Suppes, T., Leverich, G. S., Keck, P. E., Jr., Nolen, W. A., Denicoff, K. D. S., Altshuler, L. L., et al. (2001). The Stanley Foundation Bipolar Treatment Outcome Network: II. Demographics and illness characteristics of the first 261 patients. *Journal of Affective Disorders, 67*, 45–59.

Suppes, T., McElroy, S. L., Gilbert, J., Dessain, E. C., & Cole, J. O. (1992). Clozapine in the treatment of dysphoric mania. *Biological Psychiatry, 32*, 270–280.

Suppes, T., Mintz, J., McElroy, S. L., Altshuler, L. L., Kupka, R. W., Frye, M. A., et al. (2005). Mixed hypomania in 908 patients with bipolar disorder evaluated prospectively in the Stanley Foundation Bipolar Treatment Network: A sex-specific phenomenon. *Archives of General Psychiatry, 62*, 1089–1096.

Suppes, T., Phillips, K. A., & Judd, C. R. (1994). Clozapine treatment of nonpsychotic rapid cycling bipolar disorder: A report of three cases. *Biological Psychiatry, 36*, 338–340.

Suppes, T., Webb, A., Paul, B., Carmody, T., Kraemer, H., & Rush, A. J. (1999). Clinical outcome in a randomized 1-year trial of clozapine versus treatment as usual for patients with treatment-resistant illness and a history of mania. *American Journal of Psychiatry, 156*, 1164–1169.

Swann, A. C. (1995). Mixed or dysphoric manic states: Psychopathology and treatment. *Journal of Clinical Psychiatry, 56*(Suppl. 3), 6–10.

Swann, A. C., Bowden, C. L., Calabrese, J. R., Dilsaver, S. C., & Morris, D. D. (1999). Differential effect of number of previous episodes of affective disorder on response to lithium or divalproex in acute mania. *American Journal of Psychiatry, 156*, 1264–1266.

Szasz, T. (1974). *The Myth of Mental Illness.* New York: Harper Collins Publishers.

Szuba, M. P., Amsterdam, J. D., Fernando, A. T., III, Gary, K. A., Whybrow, P. C., & Winokur, A. (2005). Rapid antidepressant response after nocturnal TRH administration in patients with bipolar type I and bipolar type II major depression. *Journal of Clinical Psychopharmacology, 25*, 325–330.

Szuba, M. P., Baxter, L. R., Altshuler, L. L., Allen, E. M., Guze, B. H., Schwartz, J. M., et al. (1994). Lithium sustains the acute antidepressant effects of sleep deprivation: Preliminary findings from a controlled study. *Psychiatric Responsivity, 51*, 283–295.

Szuba, M. P., O'Reardon, J. P., Rai, A. S., Snyder-Kastenberg, J., Amsterdam, J. D., Gettes, D. R., et al. (2001). Acute mood and thyroid stimulating hor-

mone effects of transcranial magnetic stimulation in major depression. *Biological Psychiatry, 50*, 22–27.

Szymanski, S., Lieberman, J. A., Alvir, J. M., Mayerhoff, D., Loebel, A., Geisler, S., et al. (1995). Gender differences in onset of illness, treatment response, course, and biologic indexes in first-episode schizophrenic patients. *American Journal of Psychiatry, 152*, 698–703.

Tamminga, C. A. (2003). Similarities and differences among antipsychotics. *Journal of Clinical Psychiatry, 64*(Suppl. 17), 7–10.

Tesar, G. E., & Rosenbaum, J. F. (1986). Successful use of clonazepam in patients with treatment-resistant panic disorder. *Journal of Nervous and Mental Disease, 174*, 477–482.

Thase, M. E. (2001). The clinical, psychosocial, and pharmacoeconomic ramifications of remission. *American Journal of Managed Care, 7*, S377–S385.

Thase, M. E., Macfadden, W., Weisler, R. H., Chang, W., Paulsson, B., Khan, A., et al. (2006). Efficacy of quetiapine monotherapy in bipolar I and II depression: a double-blind, placebo-controlled study (the BOLDER II study). *Journal of Clinical Psychopharmacology, 26*, 600–609.

Thompson, P. J., Baxendale, S. A., Duncan, J. S., & Sander, J. W. (2000). Effects of topiramate on cognitive function. *Journal of Neurology, Neurosurgery, and Psychiatry, 69*, 636–641.

Tohen, M., Baker, R. W., Altshuler, L. L., Zarate, C. A., Suppes, T., Ketter, T. A., et al. (2002). Olanzapine versus divalproex in the treatment of acute mania. *American Journal of Psychiatry, 159*, 1011–1017.

Tohen, M., Chengappa, K. N., Suppes, T., Baker, R. W., Zarate, C. A., Bowden, C. L., et al. (2004). Relapse prevention in bipolar I disorder: 18-month comparison of olanzapine plus mood stabiliser v. mood stabiliser alone. *British Journal of Psychiatry, 184*, 337–345.

Tohen, M., Chengappa, K. N., Suppes, T., Zarate, C. A., Jr., Calabrese, J. R., Bowden, C. L., et al. (2002). Efficacy of olanzapine in combination with valproate or lithium in the treatment of mania in patients partially nonresponsive to valproate or lithium monotherapy. *Archives of General Psychiatry, 59*, 62–69.

Tohen, M., Goldberg, J. F., Gonzalez-Pinto Arrillaga, A. M., Azorin, J. M., Vieta, E., Hardy-Bayle, M. C., et al. (2003). A 12-week, double-blind comparison of olanzapine vs haloperidol in the treatment of acute mania. *Archives of General Psychiatry, 60*, 1218–1226.

Tohen, M., Ketter, T. A., Zarate, C. A., Suppes, T., Frye, M., Altshuler, L., et al. (2003). Olanzapine versus divalproex sodium for the treatment of acute mania and maintenance of remission: A 47-week study. *American Journal of Psychiatry, 160*, 1263–1271.

Tohen, M., Marneros, A., Bowden, C., Baker, R. W., Williamson, D., Evans, A. R., et al. (2004). Olanzapine versus lithium in relapse prevention in bipolar disorder: A randomized double-blind controlled 12-month clinical trial. *World Journal of Biological Psychiatry, 5*, 51.

Tohen, M., Sanger, T. M., McElroy, S. L., Tollefson, G. D., Chengappa, K. N., Daniel, D. G., et al. (1999). Olanzapine versus placebo in the treatment of acute mania. Olanzapine HGEH Study Group. *American Journal of Psychiatry, 156*, 702–709.

Tohen, M., Vieta, E., Calabrese, J., Ketter, T. A., Sachs, G., Bowden, C., et al. (2003). Efficacy of olanzapine and olanzapine-fluoxetine combination in the treatment of bipolar I depression. *Archives of General Psychiatry, 60*, 1079–1088.

Tohen, M., & Zarate, C. A. (1998). Antipsychotic agents and bipolar disorder. *Journal of Clinical Psychiatry, 59*(Suppl. 1), 38–48.

Tondo, L., Baldessarini, R. J., Floris, G., & Rudas, N. (1997). Effectiveness of restarting lithium treatment after its discontinuation in bipolar I and bipolar II disorders. *American Journal of Psychiatry, 154*, 548–550.

Tondo, L., Hennen, J., & Baldessarini, R. J. (2001). Lower suicide risk with long-term lithium treatment in major affective illness: A meta-analysis. *Acta Psychiatrica Scandinavica, 104*, 163–172.

Tondo, L., Hennen, J., & Baldessarini, R. J. (2003). Rapid-cycling bipolar disorder: Effects of long-term treatments. *Acta Psychiatrica Scandinavica, 108*, 4–14.

Tortella, F. C., & Long, J. B. (1985). Endogenous anticonvulsant substance in rat cerebrospinal fluid after a generalized seizure. *Science, 228*, 1106–1108.

Tremont, G., & Stern, R. A. (2000). Minimizing the cognitive effects of lithium therapy and electroconvulsive therapy using thyroid hormone. *International Journal of Neuropsychopharmacology, 3*, 175–186.

Trimble, M. (2000). Anticonvulsants and behaviour? The profile of new drugs with respect to psychosis and depression. *International Journal of Neuropsychopharmacology, 3*, S261.

Tsankova, N. M., Berton, O., Reuthal, W., Kumar, A., Neve, R. L., & Nestler, E. J. (2006). Sustained hippocampal chromatin regulation in a mouse model of depression and antidepressant action. *National Neuroscience, 9*, 519–525.

Ulrichsen, J., Woldbye, D. P., Madsen, T. M., Clemmesen, L., Haugbol, S., Olsen, C. H., et al. (1998). Electrical amygdala kindling in alcohol-withdrawal kindled rats. *Alcohol and Alcoholism, 33*, 244–254.

Uzcategui, E. (2007). Metformin plus sibutramine in the treatment of weight gain and metabolic dysfunction during olanzapine administration: A double-blind, placebo controlled pilot study. *Presented at 160th Annual Meeting of the American Psychiatric Association, San Diego, CA* NR # 389, 27.

van der Loos, M., & Nolen, W. (2007). Lamotrigine as add-on to lithium in bipolar depression. *Presented at 160th Annual Meeting of the American Psychiatric Association, San Diego, CA* NR # 286, 20.

van der Loos, M. L., Kolling, P., Knoppert-van der Klein, E. A., & Nolen, W. A. (2007). Lamotrigine as add-on to lithium in bipolar depression. *Presented at 160th Annual Meeting, American Psychiatric Assn, San Diego, CA.* NR#286, 20.

van der Loos, M. L., Kolling, P., Knoppert-van der Klein, E. A., & Nolen, W. A. (2007). Lamotrigine in the treatment of bipolar disorder, a review. *Tijdschr Psychiatr, 49*, 95–103.

Vanderburg, D., Rappard, F., Warrington, L., Herman, B., & Yang, R. (2007). Ziprasidone in hospitalized patients with schizophrenia: Evidence supporting rapid dose titration. *Presented at 160th Annual Meeting of the American Psychiatric Association, San Diego, CA* NR #465, 33.

Van Gaal, L. F., Rissanen, A. M., Scheen, A. J., Ziegler, O., & Rossner, S. (2005). Effects of the cannabinoid-1 receptor blocker rimonabant on weight reduction and cardiovascular risk factors in overweight patients: 1-year experience from the RIO-Europe study. *Lancet, 365*, 1389–1397.

Veatch, L. M., & Gonzalez, L. P. (1999). Nifedipine alleviates alterations in hippocampal kindling following repeated ethanol withdrawal. *Alcoholism, Clinical and Experimental Research, 24*, 484–491.

Vestergaard, P. (1992). Treatment and prevention of mania: A Scandinavian perspective. *Neuropsychopharmacology, 7*, 249–259.

Vieta, E., Bourin, M., Sanchez, R., Marcus, R., Stock, E., McQuade, R., et al. (2005). Effectiveness of aripiprazole v. haloperidol in acute bipolar mania: Double-blind, randomised, comparative 12-week trial. *British Journal of Psychiatry, 187*, 235–242.

Vieta, E., Brugue, E., Goikolea, J. M., Sanchez-Moreno, J., Reinares, M., Comes, M., et al. (2004). Acute and continuation risperidone monotherapy in mania. *Human Psychopharmacology, 19*, 41–45.

Vieta, E., Goikolea, J. M., Corbella, B., Benabarre, A., Reinares, M., Martinez, G., et al. (2001). Group for the Study of Risperidone in Affective Disorders (GSRAD). Risperidone safety and efficacy in the treatment of bipolar and schizoaffective disorders: Results from a 6-month, multicenter, open study. *Journal of Clinical Psychiatry, 62*, 818–825.

Vieta, E., Goikolea, J. M., Martínez-Arán, A., Comes, M., Verger, K., Masramon, X., et al. (2006). A double-blind, randomized, placebo-controlled, prophylaxis study of adjunctive gabapentin for bipolar disorder. *Journal of Clinical Psychiatry, 67*, 473–477.

Vieta, E., Manuel Goikolea, J., Martinez-Aran, A., Comes, M., Verger, K., Masramon, X., et al. (2006). A double-blind, randomized, placebo-controlled, prophylaxis study of adjunctive gabapentin for bipolar disorder. *Journal of Clinical Psychiatry, 67,* 473–477.

Vieta, E., Martinez-Aran, A., Goikolea, J. M., Torrent, C., Colom, F., Benabarre, A., et al. (2002). A randomized trial comparing paroxetine and venlafaxine in the treatment of bipolar depressed patients taking mood stabilizers. *Journal of Clinical Psychiatry, 63,* 508–512.

Vieta, E., Sanchez-Moreno, J., Goikolea, J. M., Colom, F., Martinez-Aran, A., Benabarre, A., et al. (2004). Effects on weight and outcome of long-term olanzapine-topiramate combination treatment in bipolar disorder. *Journal of Clinical Psychopharmacology, 24,* 374–378.

Viguera, A. C., Cohen, L. S., Baldessarini, R. J., & Nonacs, R. (2002). Managing bipolar disorder during pregnancy: Weighing the risks and benefits. *Canadian Journal of Psychiatry, 47,* 426–436.

Volpicelli, J. R., Alterman, A. I., Hayashida, M., & O'Brien, C. P. (1992). Naltrexone in the treatment of alcohol dependence. *Archives of General Psychiatry, 49*(11):876–880.

Voris, J., Smith, N. L., Rao, S. M., Thorne, D. L., & Flowers, Q. J. (2003). Gabapentin for the treatment of ethanol withdrawal. *Substance Abuse, 24,* 129–132.

Vythilingam, M., Heim, C., Newport, J., Miller, A. H., Anderson, E., Bronen, R., et al. (2002). Childhood trauma associated with smaller hippocampal volume in women with major depression. *American Journal of Psychiatry, 159,* 2072–2080.

Waddington, J. L., & Youssef, H. A. (1988). Tardive dyskinesia in bipolar affective disorder: Aging, cognitive dysfunction, course of illness, and exposure to neuroleptics and lithium. *American Journal of Psychiatry, 145,* 613–616.

Wagner, K. D., Kowatch, R. A., Emslie, G. J., Findling, R. L., Wilens, T. E., McCague, K., et al. (2006). A double-blind, randomized, placebo-controlled trial of oxcarbazepine in the treatment of bipolar disorder in children and adolescents. *American Journal of Psychiatry, 163,* 1179–1186.

Wagner, K. D., Kowatch, R. A., & Findling, R. L. (2005, October 18–23). *Oxcarbazepine in youth with bipolar disorder.* Presented at the Joint Annual Meeting of the American Academy of Child and Adolescent Psychiatry and Canadian Academy of Child and Adolescent Psychiatry, Toronto, Ontario, Canada.

Walton, S. A., Berk, M., & Brook, S. (1996). Superiority of lithium over verapamil in mania: A randomized, controlled, single-blind trial. *Journal of Clinical Psychiatry, 57,* 543–546.

Wan, R. Q., Noguera, E. C., & Weiss, S. R. (1998). Anticonvulsant effects of intra-hippocampal injection of TRH in amygdala kindled rats. *Neuroreport, 9,* 677–682.

Wang, S. J., Huang, C. C., Hsu, K. S., Tsai, J. J., & Gean, P. W. (1996). Inhibition of N-type calcium currents by lamotrigine in rat amygdalar neurones. *Neuroreport, 7,* 3037–3040.

Wehr, T. A. (1989). Sleep loss: A preventable cause of mania and other excited states. *Journal of Clinical Psychiatry, 50*(Suppl.), 8–16.

Wehr, T. A. (1991). Sleep-loss as a possible mediator of diverse causes of mania. *British Journal of Psychiatry, 159,* 576–578.

Wehr, T. A. (1993). Can antidepressants induce rapid cycling? *Archives of General Psychiatry, 50,* 495–496.

Wehr, T. A., & Goodwin, F. K. (1987). Can antidepressants cause mania and worsen the course of affective illness? *American Journal of Psychiatry, 144,* 1403–1411.

Wehr, T. A., Sack, D. A., Rosenthal, N. E., & Cowdry, R. W. (1988). Rapid cycling affective disorder: Contributing factors and treatment responses in 51 patients. *American Journal of Psychiatry, 145,* 179–184.

Weisler, R. H., Risner, M. E., Ascher, J. A., & Houser, T. L. (1994). Use of lamotrigine in the treatment of bipolar disorder. *APA New Research Program and Abstracts,* Abstract NR611: 216.

Weiss, S. R., Clark, M., Rosen, J. B., Smith, M. A., & Post, R. M. (1995). Contingent tolerance to the anticonvulsant effects of carbamazepine: Relationship to loss of endogenous adaptive mechanisms. *Brain Responsivity Review, 20,* 305–325.

Weiss, S. R. B., Post, R. M., Marangos, P. J., & Patel, J. (1986). Peripheral-type benzodiazepines: Behavioral effects and interactions with the anticonvulsant effects of carbamazepine. In J. A. Wada (Ed.), *Kindling III* (pp. 375–389). New York: Raven Press.

Weiss, S. R., Post, R. M., Sohn, E., Berger, A., & Lewis, R. (1993). Cross-tolerance between carbamazepine and valproate on amygdala-kindled seizures. *Epilepsy Research, 16,* 37–44.

Wesner, R. B., & Noyes, R, Jr. (1988). Tolerance to the therapeutic effect of phenelzine in patients with panic disorder. *Journal of Clinical Psychiatry, 49,* 450–451.

West, C. P., & Hillier, H. (1994). Ovarian suppression with gonadotrophin-releasing hormone agonist goserelin (Zoladex) in management of the premenstrual tension syndrome. *Human Reproduction, 9,* 1058–1063.

White, H. S. (1999). Comparative anticonvulsant and mechanistic profile of the established and newer antiepileptic drugs. *Epilepsia, 40*(Suppl. 5), S2–S10.

Whybrow, P. C. (1994). The therapeutic use of triiodothyronine and high dose thyroxine in psychiatric disorder. *Acta Medica Austriaca, 21,* 47–52.

Wickramaratne, P. J., Weissman, M. M., Leaf, P. J., & Holford, T. R. (1989). Age, period and cohort effects on the risk of major depression: Results from five United States communities. *Journal of Clinical Epidemiology, 42,* 333–343.

Wilens, T. E., Biederman, J., Kwon, A., Ditterline, J., Forkner, P., Moore, H., et al. (2004). Risk of substance use disorders in adolescents with bipolar disorder. *Journal of the American Academy of Child and Adolescent Psychiatry, 43,* 1380–1386.

Winsberg, M. E., Degolia, S. G., Strong, C. M., & Ketter, T. A. (2001). Divalproex therapy in medication-naive and mood-stabilizer-naive bipolar II depression. *Journal of Affective Disorders, 67,* 207–212.

Wisner, K. L., Peindl, K. S., Perel, J. M., Hanusa, B. H., Piontek, C. M., & Baab, S. (2002). Verapamil treatment for women with bipolar disorder. *Biological Psychiatry, 51,* 745–752.

Worthington, J. J., 3rd, Kinrys, G., Wygant, L. E., & Pollack, M. H. (2005). Aripiprazole as an augmentor of selective serotonin reuptake inhibitors in depression and anxiety disorder patients. *International Clinical Psychopharmacology, 20,* 9–11.

Wu, J. C., Gillin, J. C., Buchsbaum, M. S., Hershey, T., Johnson, J. C., & Bunney, W. E., Jr. (1992). Effect of sleep deprivation on brain metabolism of depressed patients. *American Journal of Psychiatry, 149,* 538–543.

Wyatt, R. J. (1997). Research in schizophrenia and the discontinuation of antipsychotic medications. *Schizophrenia Bulletin, 23,* 3–9.

Xing, G. Q., Russell, S., Hough, C., O'Grady, J., Zhang, L., Yang, S., et al. (2002). Decreased prefrontal CaMK-IIá mRNA in bipolar illness. *NeuroReport, 13,* 501–505.

Xu, H., Qing, H., Lu, W., Keegan, D., Richardson, J. S., Chlan-Fourney, J., et al. (2002). Quetiapine attenuates the immobilization stress-induced decrease of brain-derived neurotrophic factor expression in rat hippocampus. *Neuroscience Letter, 321,* 65–68.

Yan, Q. S., Zheng, S. Z., & Yan, S. E. (2004). Prenatal cocaine exposure decreases brain-derived neurotrophic factor proteins in the rat brain. *Brain Research, 1009,* 228–233.

Yamamoto, T., Pipo, J. R., Akaboshi, S., & Narai, S. (2001). Forced normalization induced by ethosuximide therapy in a patient with intractable myoclonic epilepsy. *Brain Development, 23,* 62–64.

Yassa, R., Ghadirian, A. M., & Schwartz, G. (1983). Prevalence of tardive dyskinesia in affective disorder patients. *Journal of Clinical Psychiatry, 44,* 410–412.

Yatham, L. N., Binder, C., Kusumakar, V., & Riccardelli, R. (2004). Risperidone plus lithium versus risperidone plus valproate in acute and continuation treatment of mania. *International Clinical Psychopharmacology, 19,* 103–109.

Yehuda, R. (2000). Biology of posttraumatic stress disorder. *Journal of Clinical Psychiatry, 61*(Suppl. 7), 14–21.

Young, L. T., Joffe, R. T., Robb, J. C., MacQueen, G. M., Marriott, M., & Patelis-Siotis, I. (2000). Double-blind comparison of addition of a second mood stabilizer versus an antidepressant to an initial mood stabilizer for treatment of patients with bipolar depression. *American Journal of Psychiatry, 157,* 124–126.

Young, L. T., Robb, J. C., Patelis-Siotis, I., MacDonald, C., & Joffe, R. T. (1997). Acute treatment of bipolar depression with gabapentin. *Biological Psychiatry, 42,* 851–853.

Young, R. C., Biggs, J. T., & Ziegler, V. E. (1978). A rating scale for mania: Reliability, validity and sensitivity. *British Journal of Psychiatry, 133,* 429–435.

Zakrzewska, J. M., & Patsalos, P. N. (1989). Oxcarbazepine: A new drug in the management of intractable trigeminal neuralgia. *Journal of Neurology, Neurosurgery, and Psychiatry, 52,* 472–476.

Zarate, C. A., Jr., Payne, J. L., Singh, J., Quiroz, J. A., Luckenbaugh, D. A., Denicoff, K. D., et al. (2004). Pramipexole for bipolar II depression: A placebo-controlled proof of concept study. *Biological Psychiatry, 56,* 54–60.

Zarate, C. A., Jr., Singh, J. B., Carlson, P. J., Brutsche, N. E., Ameli, R., Luckenbaugh, D. A., et al. (2006). A randomized trial of an N-methyl-D-aspartate antagonist in treatment-resistant major depression. *Archives of General Psychiatry, 63,* 856–864.

Zarate, C. A., Tohen, M., & Baldessarini, R. J. (1995). Clozapine in severe mood disorders. *Journal of Clinical Psychiatry, 56,* 411–417.

Zarate, C. A., Tohen, M., Banov, M. D., Weiss, M. K., & Cole, J. O. (1995). Is clozapine a mood stabilizer? *Journal of Clinical Psychiatry, 56,* 108–112.

Zhang, L. X., Levine, S., Dent, G., Zhan, Y., Xing, G., Okimoto, D., et al. (2002). Maternal deprivation increases cell death in the infant rat brain. *Brain Research. Developmental Brain Research, 133,* 1–11.

Zhang, L. X., Xing, G. Q., Levine, S., Post, R. M., & Smith, M. A. (1998). Effects of maternal deprivation on neurotrophic factors and apoptosis-related genes in rat pups [Abstract]. *Society for Neuroscience Abstracts, 24*(176.8), 451.

Zhang, Z. J., Kang, W. H., Tan, Q. R., Li, Q., Gao, C. G., Zhang, F. G., et al. (2007). Adjunctive herbal medicine with carbamazepine for bipolar disorders: A double-blind, randomized, placebo-controlled study. *Journal of Psychiatric Research, 41,* 360–369.

Zhang, Z.-J., Xing, G. Q., Russell, S., Obeng, K., & Post, R. M. (2003). Unidirectional cross-tolerance from levetiracetam to carbamazepine in amygdala-kindled seizures. *Epilepsia, 44*, 1487–1493.

Zis, A. P., Cowdry, R. W., Wehr, T. A., Muscettola, G., & Goodwin, F. K. (1979). Tricyclic-induced mania and MHPG excretion. *Psychiatry Research, 1*, 93–99.

Zohar, J., Insel, T. R., Zohar-Kadouch, R. C., Hill, J. L., & Murphy, D. L. (1988). Serotonergic responsivity in obsessive-compulsive disorder. Effects of chronic clomipramine treatment. *Archives of General Psychiatry, 45*, 167–172.

Index

Figures and tables are indicated with "f" and "t," respectively, following the page reference.